W0007714

THE SCOPE OF
EPIDEMIOLOGICAL
PSYCHIATRY

THE SCOPE OF EPIDEMIOLOGICAL PSYCHIATRY

*Essays in Honour of
Michael Shepherd*

Edited by
PAUL WILLIAMS
GREG WILKINSON
KENNETH RAWNSLEY

ROUTLEDGE
London and New York

First published 1989
by Routledge
11 New Fetter Lane, London EC4P 4EE
29 West 35th Street, New York, NY 10001

Printed and bound in Great Britain by Mackays of Chatham PLC, Kent
Filmset by Mayhew Typesetting, Bristol, BS1 6JZ

British Library Cataloguing in Publication Data

The Scope of epidemiological psychiatry :
   essays in honour of Michael Shepherd.
   1. Man. Mental disorders. Epidemiology
   I. Williams, P. (Paul), *1947–* .
   II. Wilkinson, Greg, *1951–* . III. Rawnsley,
   Kenneth IV. Shepherd, Michael, *1923–*
   362.2′0422

   ISBN 0–415–01814–5

Library of Congress Cataloging in Publication Data

The Scope of epidemiological psychiatry :
   essays in honour of Michael Shepherd /
   edited by Paul Williams, Greg Wilkinson, Kenneth Rawnsley.
        p.   cm.
     Includes index.
      1. Psychiatric epidemiology.
   I. Shepherd, Michael, 1923–   .
   II. Williams, Paul, D.P.M.
   III. Wilkinson, Greg, 1951–   .
   IV. Rawnsley, Kenneth.
   RC455.2.E64S36 1989   362.2′042–dc19   89–18495

   ISBN 0–415–01814–5

Contents

SECTION TWO: EPIDEMIOLOGICAL STUDIES OF MENTAL DISORDER

CHARTING HISTORICAL TRENDS

COMPLETING THE CLINICAL PICTURE OF DISEASE AND THE DELINEATION OF NEW SYNDROMES

IDENTIFICATION OF CAUSAL FACTORS AND THE COMPUTATION OF INDIVIDUAL MORBID RISKS

SECTION THREE: THE EVALUATION OF PSYCHIATRIC INTERVENTION

SPECIFIC TREATMENT APPROACHES

SERVICE ORGANIZATION

SECTION FOUR: THE INTERNATIONAL PERSPECTIVE

SECTION FIVE: THE SCIENTIFIC APPROACH TO EPIDEMIOLOGICAL AND SOCIAL PSYCHIATRY: THE CONTRIBUTION OF MICHAEL SHEPHERD

Tables and figures

Contributors

Monica Briscoe, Lecturer, General Practice Research Unit, Institute of Psychiatry, London

William Bynum, Assistant Director, Wellcome Institute for the History of Medicine, London

Tai-Ann Cheng, Associate Professor of Psychiatry, National Taiwan University Hospital, Taipei

Anthony Clare, Professor of Psychological Medicine, St Bartholomew's Hospital Medical College, London

Brian Cooper, Professor of Epidemiological Psychiatry, Zentralinstitut für Zeelischegesundheit, Mannheim

Roslyn Corney, Senior Lecturer, General Practice Research Unit, Institute of Psychiatry, London

Graham Dunn, Senior Lecturer, Biometrics Unit, Institute of Psychiatry, London

Robin Eastwood, Professor of Psychiatry, Departments of Psychiatry, Preventive Medicine & Biostatistics, University of Toronto, Clark Institute of Psychiatry, Toronto

Leon Eisenberg, Presley Professor of Social Medicine & Professor of Psychiatry, Harvard Medical School, Boston

Ian Falloon, Consultant Physician (Mental Health), Buckingham Mental Health Service, Buckingham

Jonathan Gabe, Lecturer in Sociology, General Practice Research Unit, Institute of Psychiatry, London

Eric Glover, Senior Programmer/Analyst, Biometrics Unit, Institute of Psychiatry, London

David Goldberg, Professor of Psychiatry, The University Hospital of South Manchester, Manchester

David Hand, Professor of Statistics, The Open University, Milton Keynes

Assen Jablensky, Director, WHO Collaborating Centre for Mental Health, Medical Academy, Sofia

Rachel Jenkins, Principal Medical Officer, Mental Health Division, Department of Health & Social Security, London

Michael King, Senior Lecturer, General Practice Research Unit, Institute of Psychiatry, London

Gerald Klerman, Professor of Psychiatry, Department of Psychiatry, Cornell University Medical College, Westchester Division, White Plains, New York

Morton Kramer, Professor Emeritus, School of Hygiene & Public Health, Department of Mental Hygiene, The Johns Hopkins University, Baltimore

Malcolm Lader, Professor of Psychopharmacology, Institute of Psychiatry, London

Annette Lawson, Institute of Human Development, University of California, Berkeley, Berkeley

Glyn Lewis, Research Worker, General Practice Research Unit, Institute of Psychiatry, London

Michael MacDonald, Professor of History, Department of History, University of Michigan, Ann Arbor

Anthony Mann, Professor of Psychiatry, Royal Free Hospital School of Medicine, London

Jair Mari, Associate Professor, Department of Social Medicine, Santa Casa de Sao Paulo, Sao Paulo

David Morrell, Professor of General Practice, Division of General Practice, United Medical & Dental Schools of Guy's & St. Thomas's Hospitals, London

Joanna Murray, Research Worker, General Practice Research Unit, Institute of Psychiatry, London

Anthony Pelosi, Research Worker, General Practice Research Unit, Institute of Psychiatry, London

Kenneth Rawnsley, Past President, Royal College of Psychiatrists, Emeritus Professor of Psychological Medicine, University of Wales College of Medicine, Cardiff

Darrel Regier, Director, Division of Clinical Research, National Institute for Mental Health, Alcohol, Drug Abuse, and Mental Health Administration, Rockville

Geoffrey Rose, Professor of Epidemiology, London School of Hygiene and Tropical Medicine, London

Gerald Russell, Professor of Psychiatry, Institute of Psychiatry, London

Norman Sartorius, Director, Division of Mental Health, World Health Organization, Switzerland

Biswajit Sen, Girindrasekhar Clinic, Calcutta

Deborah Sharp, Lecturer, Division of General Practice, United Medical & Dental Schools of Guy's & St. Thomas's Hospitals, London

David Skuse, Wellcome Trust Senior Lecturer, Department of Child Psychiatry, Institute of Child Health, London

Nigel Smeeton, Lecturer, General Practice Research Unit, Institute of Psychiatry, London

Jean Starobinski, Professor of the History of Ideas, Faculté des Lettres, University of Geneva, Geneva

Geraldine Strathdee, Research Worker, General Practice Research Unit, Institute of Psychiatry, London

Erik Strömgren, Professor of Psychiatry, Institute of Psychiatric Demography, Psychiatric Hospital, Risskov

Michele Tansella, Professor of Psychological Medicine, Cattedra di Psicologia Medica, Istituto di Psichiatria, Policlinico Borgo Roma, Verona

David Watt, Honorary Consultant Psychiatrist, Department of Medical Genetics, The Churchill Hospital, Oxford

Myrna Weissman, Professor of Epidemiology in Psychiatry, College of Physicians and Surgeons of Columbia University, New York

Greg Wilkinson, Senior Lecturer, General Practice Research Unit, Institute of Psychiatry, London

Paul Williams, Honorary Senior Lecturer, General Practice Research Unit, Institute of Psychiatry, London

John Wing, Professor of Social Psychiatry, M.R.C. Social Psychiatry Unit, Institute of Psychiatry, London

Foreword 1

The production of a Festschrift to signal the retirement of Professor Michael Shepherd is a felicitous way of honouring a renowned teacher. Close colleagues and students have come forward to describe their personal researches, selecting topics which reflect Michael Shepherd's influence on their work and thinking. Most of the contributors have been associated closely with him in the Institute of Psychiatry; they are drawn from a conspicuously wide range of scientific disciplines, medical and non-medical, which bear on the far-reaching applications of epidemiological methods to mental health problems. Other contributors have also collaborated fruitfully with Michael Shepherd and share his predilection for epidemiological studies. For a few the association has been more transient; their contributions are all the more significant as they reflect distinctive and independent viewpoints and ideas which nevertheless show striking consistencies with Michael Shepherd's scientific approach to psychiatry.

This book reminds me of another Festschrift, written some twenty years ago by grateful students and colleagues of Sir Aubrey Lewis on his retirement, in recognition of the unique way he had shaped British psychiatry.[1] The editors were Michael Shepherd and David L. Davies, both ardent admirers of Aubrey Lewis. We shall indeed appreciate better Michael Shepherd's view of psychiatry and psychiatrists if we recall the very high affection and regard in which he held Aubrey Lewis. It was quite natural that he should model himself on his mentor, even though they differed so much in their temperaments and backgrounds. Michael Shepherd has honoured Lewis's memory in several addresses and publications,[2] notably in his 1976 Adolf Meyer Lecture[3] and the paper he read, also in 1976, at the Aubrey Lewis Memorial Meeting of the Royal College of Psychiatrists.[4] There we have recorded Michael Shepherd's analysis of the personal and intellectual qualities of Aubrey Lewis, which made him the principal architect of British psychiatry at a time when it was first developing into a scientifically credible discipline. A comparison of the attributes of these two teachers is inescapable. Both were gifted with qualities of erudition and creative scepticism, often displayed with brilliance. Professionally they shared an eclectic approach tied to a multidimensional view of the causation of mental illness. In consequence, it was hardly surprising that the discipline of social psychiatry received a new impetus which was to set the scene for vigorous growth and expansion. As teachers they both exploited the Socratic method of conducting an argument as an effective device for imparting information and, beyond this, setting the limits of knowledge. Their scepticism – always rigorous but more a stimulant than a destructive force – led them to question the claims of uncritical enthusiasts, whether in the field of psychotherapy or in treatment with drugs. For them questioning was not a clogging weakness, and they seldom failed 'to pick up and examine the little hedgehogs of doubt that sit by the therapist's path'.[5]

Michael Shepherd obtained his medical training at Oxford University Medical School and the Radcliffe Infirmary. In 1952, after house appointments and national service in the RAF, he joined the staff of the Maudsley Hospital. He has remained there ever since, apart from a one-year attachment to the School of Public Health at Johns Hopkins University, Baltimore, from where he completed a wide-ranging survey of American psychiatry. From reading the Festschrift to Aubrey Lewis it may indeed be argued that during the 1950s and 1960s the Maudsley was unrivalled in providing the best stimulation and environment for a psychiatrist eager to advance his subject, and there was little point in going elsewhere. In 1967 Michael Shepherd was appointed Professor of Epidemiological Psychiatry, the subject which he had done so much to establish at the Institute and which would alter, expand, and extend at the hands of increasing numbers of research students so that his imprint is now clearly visible in several departments of psychiatry in Britain and abroad. He holds a very broad view of the subject matter of epidemiology. In addition to the older recognized spheres of concern – the search for causal factors and the completion of the spectrum of disease – it embraces the establishment of outcome and the evaluation of the efficacy of treatment, including applications of the controlled clinical trial.[6,7] The last are usually viewed as the preserves of the clinical psychiatrists. But for Michael Shepherd such lines of division are artificial: he has argued convincingly that the store of knowledge on which clinical practice relies can be enlarged and given precision by contributions from the whole field of epidemiology. The signs of this breadth of outlook were evident in his earlier researches,[8] including his personal contributions to the clarification of morbid jealousy and clinical trials of neuroleptics. They were followed by a seminal international study of observer variations in psychiatric diagnosis. His awareness of the pitfalls of hospital-based studies led him to question cogently the value of psychiatric classifications based on hospital cases. In recent years he discovered the value of psychiatric research in the more representative population of patients who consult their general practitioners. This approach culminated in his establishing the General Practice Research Unit within the Department of Psychiatry in the Institute. This Festschrift happily reflects Michael Shepherd's breadth of outlook through its wide-ranging contributions. It also supports his dictum that 'In no branch of Medicine is epidemiology needed more than in psychiatry'.[6]

The appearance of this Festschrift also provides an apt illustration of Michael Shepherd's personal influence on the numerous contributors who, irrespective of their current professional seniority, began their research careers as trainees under his supervision. His standing as a teacher is indelibly established. He excels in the set-piece lecture, when he presents carefully honed ideas in an entertaining style: hence the frequency with which he is invited to deliver named lectures and keynote addresses. To colleagues within the Institute of Psychiatry and the Maudsley Hospital, his reputation as an outstanding teacher is based on a number of assessments. Foremost is his ability to attract within his fold young men and women eager to benefit from the intellectual stimulation obtained from contact with a man of ideas who will set them on a secure path of research. Generations of registrars at the Maudsley, attached to his clinical unit, have learned from him the complexities inherent in the assessment of psychiatric patients, the avoidance of glib diagnostic labels, and the moulding effects of personality and social background in determining not only the content but also, at times, the form of psychiatric illness.

Any appreciation of Michael Shepherd's achievements as an educator would be incomplete without acknowledging his success as foundation editor of *Psychological Medicine*, a journal internationally recognized for its high scientific standards and the quality of its articles. In more recent years this journal has further increased its impact through the linked publication of a series of monographs and the ambitious *Handbook of Psychiatry* in five volumes.

The epidemiological method tends to emphasize the study of groups of patients rather than the individual. I have called attention to Michael Shepherd's impressive gifts in assessing the individual patient and his qualities as a clinician. Lest anyone should believe these are overshadowed by his scientific excellence, I wish to quote from an autobiography of a gifted author who recounted her experiences as a patient at the Maudsley. She used a pseudonym, not hard to decipher in the light of her liking for French poetry. She describes her first meeting with her psychiatrist:

Dr Berger, a tall dark pale man, with a chillingly superior glance and quellingly English voice, made another appointment to see me. Feelings of past unpleasantness and fear had been aroused in me by this visit to a psychiatrist: attracting his attention and observing his serious face had reduced my store of confidence. I knew, however, that if anyone could discover the 'truth' it would be he, alone or with his colleagues.[9]

On behalf of all his colleagues at the Institute and the Maudsley, I wish Michael a prosperous retirement and many years of creative activity. I am confident that he will continue to enrich psychiatry.

Gerald Russell

NOTES

1. Shepherd, M. and Davies, D.L. (eds) (1968) *Studies in Psychiatry*, London: Oxford University Press.
2. Shepherd, M. (1975) 'In Memoriam: Aubrey Lewis (1900–1975)', *American Journal of Psychiatry* 132 (8): 872.
3. Shepherd, M. (1977) 'A representative psychiatrist: the career and contributions of Sir Aubrey Lewis', *American Journal of Psychiatry* 134 (1): 7–13.
4. Shepherd, M. (1977) 'Aubrey Lewis: the makings of a psychiatrist', *British Journal of Psychiatry* 131: 238–42.
5. Lewis, A.J. (1958) 'Between guesswork and certainty in psychiatry', *Lancet* i: 171–5 and 227–30.
6. Shepherd, M. (1978) 'Epidemiology and clinical psychiatry', *British Journal of Psychiatry* 133: 289–98.
7. Shepherd, M. (1984) 'Editorial: the contribution of epidemiology to clinical psychiatry', *American Journal of Psychiatry* 141 (12): 1574–5.
8. Shepherd, M. (1969) 'Research in the field of psychiatry', *British Medical Journal* 4: 161–3.
9. Frame, J. (1985) *The Envoy from Mirror City: Autobiography 3*, London: The Women's Press, p. 99.

Foreword 2

For many a foreigner, Michael Shepherd is the perfect example of an Englishman. On the other hand, some of my English friends disagree and even see him as faintly foreign in his manner and speech. He is at home in many lands: when he first came to Yugoslavia he introduced me to artists I had never met before, although they were in and from the town in which I grew up and lived. Not only are his students spread all over the globe, but the remarkable width of his interests has brought him to places and people whom others of our profession rarely meet.

But even in places which he has not visited, his work has left indelible traces. They are particularly visible in three of his areas of interest, all essential to the development of psychiatry and of health care in general. These are: the area of mental disorder in general practice; the improvement of psychiatric diagnosis and classification; and the publication of matters of interest to psychiatry. In the first of these his work has helped to transform the education of general practitioners and to give priority to mental health programmes in many parts of the world; in the second it has helped to make psychiatry a more respectable discipline; and in the third (in particular with the appearance – now seventeen years ago – of *Psychological Medicine*, which he edits with so much brio and rigorous scientific attention), it has set a new standard in writing about psychiatric issues.

There are many things which could be admired in Professor Shepherd – his erudition, scientific acumen, and sense of humour, for example. Yet, if I was to search for the one which had most impact on his students, I would select his keen critical sense. It is not a tool which he has to apply with effort: its use comes easily. He has an ear for disharmony in science, clinical work, and health policy. The many foreign students who came to work under his supervision were not only trained in psychiatry – they were also offered an opportunity to learn how to think critically, with sound scepsis and reasoned caution. Years later, when most other knowledge gained in the course has become obsolete or forgotten, the Shepherdian stamp of critical and salutary scepticism is still present in all his old students, immediately recognizable and infinitely useful.

Contemporaries, students, and present-day younger collaborators have been invited to contribute to this volume. Most of them are British, a few are American, and a few are from other countries. There is no doubt that the papers assembled are as good as anyone in this field of endeavour could hope for. Other books may follow: however important this Festschrift may be, it is only one event in the stream of publications which have been, in one way or another, stimulated by Professor Shepherd and which will be appearing in different languages and different lands for many years to come.

Norman Sartorius

General introduction

Professor Michael Shepherd retired from the chair of Epidemiological Psychiatry at the Institute of Psychiatry (University of London) in September 1988. The impact of his work has led to a wide recognition of his enormous contribution to, and influence on, psychiatry. We thought it appropriate, therefore, to mark the occasion of his retirement by a work of academic scholarship.

While Michael Shepherd's work has spanned many areas of psychiatry, it is perhaps in the field of epidemiological and social psychiatry that his contribution has been greatest. The study of mental illness requires a wide variety of approaches, and the epidemiological approach is one of the most important. While it is concerned with definition, classification, aetiology, natural history, as well as the treatment and outcome of disease, the essential attribute of epidemiology is that it addresses the problem of disease in the context of the community as a whole. Thus, at a time when the trend in psychiatry is away from hospital treatment and towards care in the community, the epidemiological investigation of mental illness is increasingly important. We have, therefore, attempted to bring together theoretical considerations, scientific studies, and service evaluations.

The book is divided into five sections. The first is concerned with the scientific principles which underpin, and are a necessary 'tool-kit' for, investigations in epidemiological and social psychiatry, while the second is divided into three subsections, each of which is concerned with a particular area of enquiry within the general field. These areas of enquiry are taken from the 'Uses of Epidemiology' described by Jeremy Morris, and serve to emphasize the link between epidemiological psychiatry and medical epidemiology, while the content of each of the sections exemplifies the close relationship between scientific enquiry and clinical psychiatry.

The third section is concerned with the evaluation of psychiatric intervention, and is divided into subsections which focus respectively on the organization of services and the evaluation of specific treatments.

Although the contributors to the first three sections are drawn from many countries, the fourth section is specifically concerned with epidemiological and social psychiatric perspectives from an international point of view, while the fifth and final section is an overview which assesses the contribution of Michael Shepherd to the subjects under discussion.

The authors can be regarded as falling into three groups. First, there is a group of eminent investigators who, while perhaps not having worked directly with Michael Shepherd at the Institute of Psychiatry, have been closely associated with him in other ways. Second, there is a group who have worked under his supervision in the past and who have now themselves attained positions of seniority, while the third group consists of younger workers who are currently members of, or are closely associated with, the General Practice Research Unit at the Institute of Psychiatry.

In structuring this book and commissioning the authors, we kept very much in mind the idea that this Festschrift should be a substantial addition to the literature in its own right, rather than a collection of reminiscences or personal statements. We believe we have achieved this: we hope that Michael Shepherd would agree, and that he would regard the contributions as fine examples of the scientific approach to psychiatry that he has striven to develop, to advocate, and to teach.

Paul Williams
Greg Wilkinson
Kenneth Rawnsley

Section One

The Scientific Principles of Epidemiological and Social Enquiry in Psychiatry

Introduction

We have categorized the scientific principles which underpin epidemiological and social psychiatry into three groups. The first subsection deals with historical origins. While case definition is of considerable current concern to psychiatric epidemiologists, Jean Starobinski describes how the definition of 'madness' was a source of debate well over 2,000 years ago. He also demonstrates the emphasis given by Hippocrates to 'arithmetic' in medicine. In the subsequent chapter, William Bynum describes the Victorian origins of psychiatric epidemiology.

The second subsection consists of three papers on the social sciences. As early as 1879, Henry Maudsley acknowledged that it was 'proper to emphasise the fact that insanity is really a social phenomenon, and to insist that it cannot be investigated satisfactorily and apprehended rightly except it be studied from a social point of view' (Maudsley 1879: vi).

One of the most influential figures in establishing the social scientific basis of psychiatry was Sir Aubrey Lewis (Shepherd 1980). Lewis's first research project was an anthropological study of the aborigines of South Australia: it is not inappropriate, therefore, that Annette Lawson discusses sociology and socio-anthropology in the first chapter in this subsection.

In contrast to the collectivist nature of these disciplines, psychology is essentially individualistic. It is perhaps for this reason that its contribution to social and epidemiological psychiatry has been relatively neglected, an omission which is remedied by Monica Briscoe in the subsequent chapter.

The increasing awareness that resources are not limitless has given rise to heightened interest in the economic evaluation of mental health care. Thus, Greg Wilkinson and Anthony Pelosi provide an overview of the principles and techniques of economic appraisal.

Sir Francis Galton observed that 'until the phenomena of any branch of knowledge have been submitted to measurement and number, it cannot assume the status and dignity of science'. Quantitative methods form the basis of virtually all investigations in epidemiological psychiatry: these are the topic of the third subsection. Geoffrey Rose discusses the need to adopt a population-based strategy, while Morton Kramer draws on administrative mental health statistics to illustrate the biostatistical approach. The value of fully utilizing such data in psychiatry was emphasized by Sir Aubrey Lewis over forty years ago, when he observed that 'so far as psychiatry is conceived as a branch of social medicine and public health, it must rely for its advancement upon methods which require accurate statistics such as it is the business of official intelligence to supply' (Lewis 1945: 492).

As Shepherd has noted, administrative statistics have been utilized in psychiatry since the nineteenth century. He commented further that 'the use of modern survey methods to study the nature and distribution of extramural psychiatric morbidity with more sensitive instruments represents the logical extension of this work' (Shepherd 1983: 20).

Thus, a host of techniques have been developed for identifying and estimating the extent of untreated psychiatric morbidity. These, broadly referred to as 'screening', are dealt with by David Goldberg.

Investigations using such techniques almost invariably involve computer analysis. Latterly, computers have also been used to collect such data – for example, there now exist several systems whereby respondents are assessed by means of direct interaction with a computer. These and other relevant aspects of information technology are dealt with by David Hand and Eric Glover in the last chapter of this section.

REFERENCES

Lewis, A. (1945) 'Psychiatric investigation in Britain', *American Journal of Psychiatry* 101: 486–93.
Maudsley, H. (1879) *The Pathology of Mind*, London: Macmillan.
Shepherd, M. (1980) 'From social medicine to social psychiatry: the achievement of Sir Aubrey Lewis', *Psychological Medicine*, 10: 211–18.
Shepherd, M. (1983) *The Psychosocial Matrix of Psychiatry: Collected Papers*, London: Tavistock.

Historical Origins

1

Who Is Mad? The Exchange Between Hippocrates and Democritus

Jean Starobinski*

As is known, the pseudo-hippocratic letters relating to Hippocrates' interview at Abdera with Democritus exercised considerable influence in the sixteenth and seventeenth centuries. Burton, in particular, makes the interview the central account in his 'satyricall preface' at the beginning of the *Anatomy of Melancholy*. The text, in spite of being a sort of historical novel – the work of a 'forger' said the philologists – rather than an authentic document, has had a deserved success. It is vouched for in a fable by La Fontaine, *Démocrite et les Abdéritains* (Democritus and the Abderites, viii, 26), and by a satirical novel by Wieland (*Die Abderiter*, 1774).

Who is mad? Who knows how to recognize madness? What authority permits a decision? That is what is at issue in the letters.[1] The first letter is addressed to Hippocrates by the Council and people of Abdera. It is an appeal for help and the admission of general distress. An important man is ill, and his illness imperils the entire city, which had placed in him its hope of 'eternal glory'. The city fears that it will be abandoned, so much does its own existence depend on that of the superior man in whom they had hitherto recognized a superior wisdom. Now Democritus is sick, says the letter 'because of the excess of wisdom that possesses him' (p. 320).

The alleged cause is not discreditable. In the eyes of the Abderites, predisposed to moderation, all excess, even of a virtue, is pernicious. This conviction, in the circumstances, gives rise to an imputation of illness, of delirium (*paracopè*), of paralysis of discernment (*apoplexia dianoias*). The Abderites believe that they already know the cause of the malady. They have pronounced judgement ('he is ill') before describing the symptoms. But they do not forget to go on to the description, in which figure, correctly placed, some of the ideas which doxographic tradition ascribes to Democritus. The 'clinical picture' indistinctly reveals the behaviour, the words, and the convictions of the alleged patient. 'He is oblivious of everything, even of himself, he stays awake by night as by day, laughing at everything, however

* Translated from the French by E.S. Hague

important or trivial.' He thinks that 'the whole of life is nothing', he says that 'the air is full of shadowy likenesses' (*eidolon*):

> He listens to the sound of the birds, and, rising frequently at night, when alone he seems to be singing softly; at other times he says that he is travelling through infinite space and that there are innumerable Democrituses that resemble him. And his colour is as much changed as his mode of thought.

The disturbing signs, beginning with oblivion, can essentially be defined as the ignoring of normally accepted limits. Public opinion is alarmed at seeing them ignored: the boundaries between night and day, serious and comic, happy and unhappy events, earth and the subterranean world, human speech and bird song, singular and plural.

In the face of all these alarming signs, the only recourse for the Abderites is the physician, that is, the man who possesses the power to cure. They count on him to save 'the body of wisdom', and to become in this way the new founder (*Ktistes*) of the whole city. To make up Hippocrates' mind, they promise a substantial reward.

In Hippocrates' letter in reply, he promises to come but refuses payment. Democritus is a work of nature; in the circumstances, the physician considers himself summoned by nature. And he also calls in question the opinion reached by the Abderites. The physician wishes to retain complete freedom to arbitrate on the situation, to recognize the presence or absence of a morbid state: it may be that the Abderites are mistaken (*apatei*) in considering Democritus to be ill.

In another letter, addressed privately to Philopoemen, his host and friend in Abdera, Hippocrates says how difficult it is to distinguish the signs of 'excessive wisdom' from those of maladies produced by the black bile. He inclines to the first hypothesis, which does not prevent him from providing himself with hellebore, that is, the medicament regarded as efficacious in driving out melancholy. Those who seclude themselves, those who are silent, those who flee human society may be now contemplative, now raving sick men.

Addressing another correspondent (Dionysios of Halicarnassus), whom he asks to come to look after his house and his wife in his absence, Hippocrates once again expresses his doubts and criticizes popular opinion; when men talk of excess they always speak from the standpoint of what they lack; 'Thus the coward will see excess in courage, the miser will see excess in open-handedness' (letter 13, p. 335). Hippocrates puts clearly in doubt the norm which individuals cite as an authority when they make an accusation of deviation or aberration. He himself will formulate his opinion and his *prognosis* only after he has seen and listened to Democritus. The principle of the personal and direct examination is formulated clearly here.

In a letter to another recipient named Damagetes (letter 14), Hippocrates nevertheless expresses uneasiness about a symptom described by the Abderites: an undifferentiated laugh at every event in life. This means a lack of the sense of proportion that men must always retain. In advance, Hippocrates admonishes Democritus and imputes to him, as do the Abderites, a melancholic 'immoderacy':

> You laugh when someone is ill, you are delighted when someone dies . . .
> What an unpleasant man you are, O Democritus, and how far from
> wisdom, if you think that such things are not evils. Most certainly you are
> tormented by the black bile (*melancholais*).

Hippocrates could have been the sole arbiter. The author of the letters does not restrict himself to that. He gives Hippocrates assistance and Asclepios appears in a dream, escorted appropriately by enormous serpents and accompanied by the allegorical figures of Truth and Opinion.[2] The god declares that, as far as Democritus is concerned, his help will be of no use, for Democritus is utterly sound in mind. The dream is perfectly clear, but, when Hippocrates wakes, he still feels in need of an explanation. The author of the letters does not flinch from any effect: he reveals in his physician hero a perfect oneirocritic. Hippocrates declares to his correspondent: 'I do not reject dreams, above all those that keep an order. Medicine and divination are close cousins, for Apollo is the common father of the two arts' (letter 15, p. 343).

The introduction of the term divination (*mantikè*) is disturbing. For the terms *mantis* (diviner) and *mantikè* have been associated since antiquity with *mania* (madness) and *mainesthai* (to be a prey to fury, passion). Thus, the art of divination, considered as closely related to medicine, and which permits the declaration that Democritus is not mad, itself maintains a special semantic relationship with frenzy.

A letter on the best way to gather hellebore gives an idea of Hippocrates' technical knowledge (letter 16). We learn even more about the same subject in a later letter (letter 21). The author means to give us the highest idea of the pharmacological competence of the great physician, in the field that particularly relates to mental disturbances. But the question of diagnosis and of the indications for such treatment is still not touched upon. What can decide this is the interview with the patient.

This interview is described at length in the letter that is the culmination of the collection. This letter to Damagetes (letter 17) is the one most often quoted, imitated, translated, by writers from Sebastian Frank to Robert Burton. It deserves a painstaking commentary, for it relates a kind of drama, with many details of the staging, each of which is highly significant.

While, far off, the Abderites lament or try to make the alleged sick man laugh, the physician and the philosopher engage in conversation: this will

17

take the form of a philosophical disputation, by means of question and answer. Reading the letter we learn from the start the conclusions which Hippocrates has reached: 'It is as we thought, Damagetes: Democritus was not raving, but he scorned everything, and he taught us, and, through us, all men' (p. 349).

Hippocrates will give a perfect demonstration of his method: he brushes aside the bystanders. He wants to see and hear the man he is examining, 'to be near his words and his body' (p. 353). We see that the physical examination and the interview with the patient are closely linked. From a distance Hippocrates had already observed the individual's general appearance, the place of his activities, the things that interest him. The signs before they engage in conversation had still been ambiguous: they could lend themselves to an unfavourable interpretation. Democritus, seated under a very low plane-tree, is a man 'in a coarse tunic, alone, his body neglected, on a stone seat, his colour very yellow, emaciated, with a long beard'. So, later, did the famous painting and engraving by Salvator Rosa depict him. But this unusual man receives Hippocrates with perfect courtesy, asks his name, invites him to sit near him. He asks him whether he has come to see him about a public or private matter (*idion oud è epidemion*).

Hippocrates introduces himself as an ambassador, and, with an astute question, satisfies himself that his patient has no disturbance of memory or orientation: he knows who Philopoemen is and in what part of the town he lives. When interrogated about the book open in front of him and which he is engaged in writing, Democritus answers that it is a book on madness. The animals that he dissects in search of 'the nature and seat of bile' (p. 355) will enable him to gain a better understanding of the 'cause of madness'.

Democritus is trying to resolve a 'physiological' problem: bile 'exists in all naturally, but varies in degree in each one: if it is in excess, illnesses will occur, and it is a substance now good, now bad'. Most certainly, it is a question of rudimentary quantitative reasoning in the framework of a humoral postulate without real proof. No more is needed, however, for Hippocrates to admire the wisdom and profound tranquillity of the person with whom he is talking – tranquillity, he confesses immediately, that he does not himself enjoy. That is the turning point of the conversation, from which he will acknowledge the superiority of the philosopher, free of all ties, over the physician, still a captive to the cares of practical living: his thought is still engrossed in 'fields, house, children, debts, maladies, the dead, servants, marriages, and everything else.'

The philosopher's superiority, as can be clearly seen, is that of the *vita contemplativa* (*bioas theoretikos*) over the active life. From this, Democritus has no difficulty in exposing the innumerable vanities of human ambition, the folly of the quest for power, riches, pleasures. Hippocrates tries to plead the cause of practical life: 'to act is imposed by necessity.' Democritus replies that men are ridiculous through their lack of foresight, through their inability to face the consequences of their actions. His laughter, at all that happens to men, is therefore perfectly appropriate. But in thus exculpating himself from the accusation of madness, he throws the accusation back to everyone else: 'the whole world is ill without knowing it', says Hippocrates, coming to the logical conclusion. And in such a case, what can we hope for? Where is one to send 'a delegation' to find the remedy?

Such a complete generalization of illness (from which the contemplative philosopher alone excepts himself) leaves no room for any health in the world. There is 'an infinity of worlds' declares Democritus, a poor consolation. From this text, which dates from the beginning of the Christian era, one can infer how Christ, God incarnate, but whose kingdom is not of this world, would answer to this radical condemnation of the world's madness. It is to him that prayer could 'send a delegation'. The man in search of salvation should repudiate the alleged wisdom of the world, which is madness, and opt for 'the madness of the Cross'.

Democritus has found tranquillity in retreat and in the investigation of physical causes. His complaint against men becomes all the more implacable. The vehemence of the accusation leads to the avowed desire to harm mankind. The tranquil philosopher becomes a misanthrope: he would find pleasure in aggravating the evil in order to inflict the deserved punishment:

> As for me, I do not think that I even laugh enough, and I should like to be able to find something that would afflict them, something that was neither medicine to cure them nor a Peon to prepare remedies for them. (p. 373).

The justifications found for Democritus' vengeful argument are analogous to those formulated very much later by the Marquis de Sade: 'Don't you see that the world (*Kosmos*) is full of hostility to man (*misanthropos*) and has marshalled against him infinite evils' (p. 375).

How is it possible to orientate oneself in the world when all boundaries between good and evil are thus obliterated? The moral rule will be that of indifference to all that may happen to us and of knowing how to draw in ourselves 'the limits of calm and agitation' (p. 367).

Did Democritus, in the general purpose of his diatribe against the madness of the world, keep entirely calm? Hippocrates does not express the doubts that we might have. He is persuaded that he has found in Democritus a man who surpasses him: 'He smiled at my speaking thus and he appeared to me, Damagetes, as a divine being, and I forgot that he was a man.'

Instead of applying the treatment, Hippocrates received it: it was the physician who at the end of the interview went away provided with a beneficial remedy. He humbly declares to the man he was questioning: 'I have received from you the remedy that will increase my own understanding' (p. 379). Are we to believe that the author of the pseudo-hippocratic letters intended to demonstrate the superiority of philosophy, 'medicine of the intellect' over the art of medicine, the medicine of the 'body'?

The fact is that the author of the letters is bent on attributing to Democritus a twofold competence: he makes him a master of wisdom, and he attributes to him a medical work on madness (composed, it must be added, of long extracts from well-known hippocratical writings), a short treatise 'on the nature of man', as well as a letter lavishing advice on Hippocrates as if the latter needed a course in improvement.

The physician must judge maladies not only by sight but from the facts themselves, he must examine the rhythms of the malady in general, whether it is in its initial stage, its middle stage, or its wane, and, having observed the differences, the season, age, as well as the body as a whole, must then apply the treatment. (p. 383).

The anonymous author has obviously tried to show that the philosopher 'physiologist', starting from his knowledge of the world and the whole of nature can be a complete physician, as qualified as the specialist who has descended from Asclepios; but, in addition, philosophy possesses the knowledge of the rules of behaviour, that is, wisdom, which puts at a disadvantage those who possess only the medical art. In the preamble to his short letter on 'the nature of man' (letter 23), Democritus demonstrates the link between the two disciplines:

All men ought to know the art of medicine, O Hippocrates, and especially those who have acquired learning and are versed in its doctrines, for it is both beautiful and advantageous to life. I think that knowledge of philosophy is sister to medicine and lives under the same roof; indeed, philosophy frees the soul from passions and medicine rids the body of maladies. (p. 395)

One can see it, the miniature novel in the form of letters, which contains some very remarkable things formulated rather daringly, has managed to turn upside down the initial situation. The populace of Abdera, who demanded treatment for Democritus' madness, appears as the real patient in need of hellebore; it is the collective opinion that is unhealthy. The physician, who at first delivered his advice with perfect assurance, accepts the role of pupil. The philosopher, whose behaviour at first seemed abnormal, is revealed as the custodian of truth. The deceptive appearances have been dissipated.

Even in antiquity, the Abderites did not enjoy a reputation for intelligence. They have nevertheless found a defender, in the person of the French philosopher Pierre Bayle. In the article 'Abdera' in his famous *Dictionary*, he writes, apropos of the suspicion of madness held against Democritus: 'People would do the same today about a philosopher who made fun of everything.' (*Dictionary*: note K).

As usually happens in a pleasant fable, the pseudo-hippocratic novel makes use of the principle of all or nothing. If Democritus is mad, the council and citizens of Abdera are justified in being alarmed by his behaviour. If, on the other hand, Democritus is not mad, the whole community, in allowing itself to be deceived by appearances, must accept the accusation of madness. Such sweeping reversals of a situation have characterized present-day 'radical' thought whenever it has let itself be carried away by the temptation to mythify. 'Radical' thought, of course, no longer shares the elitist interpretation that long characterized the lesson drawn from the story of Hippocrates and Democritus. La Fontaine, in telling it, declares that he 'always hated general opinion'. Such a story shows that 'the people are an untrustworthy judge' (Book VIII, 26). In its rhetoric, 'radical' thought usually indicts 'society' while approving of the *vox populi*.

The present reader's attention may reasonably dwell on a detail in the last of Hippocrates' letters (letter 22). It is written to his son Thessalus, and contains recommendations on the basic knowledge necessary for medicine: geometry and arithmetic. Geometry 'will be useful in the location of bones, their displacement, and the whole arrangement of the limbs.' As for the 'order of arithmetic', it will be applicable enough to the periods, to the regular changes of fevers, to patients' crises, and to preventive measures (p. 393). Here, no doubt, it is a matter of a rudimentary arithmetic applied to forecasting the course of illnesses.

Hippocrates' counsel is sufficiently general to include half of the medieval *quadrivium* as well as the astrological calculations practised by the iatro-mathematicians of the Renaissance. The whole range of the possible application of mathematics to medicine (for us who know what happened in history) appears in embryo in the initial exhortation.

Occupy yourself, my son, with the study of geometry and arithmetic, for it will not only make your life glorious and most useful in human affairs, but it will also make your mind more penetrating and more perceptive to profit from all that is useful in medicine.

The physicians who, towards the end of the eighteenth century, at the time of the 'return to Hippocrates', devoted themselves to the statistics of illnesses in correlation with the winds, rain, temperature, have certainly illustrated in yet another way this paternal injunction.

Hippocrates, whose example has so often been invoked in favour of 'clinical' observation, can certainly not be regarded as the inspiration for quantification in physiology. His interest, as has so often been repeated, is focused on qualitative phenomena that can be directly evaluated by sensory contact. But the text (certainly apocryphal) which we just read opens the path to everything from eighteenth-century calculation of probabilities to contemporary epidemiology. It points to the need to bring medicine, in its own domain, to the 'degree of certainty' – to use Cabanis's expression – that it can obtain through the legitimate use of epidemiology. To the words in which the imaginary Hippocrates of the novel exhorts his son, one is tempted to add these: 'Medicine and philosophy most certainly live under the same roof, and if the philosopher can give the physician a lesson in serenity, he will have performed a worthy deed, but if the physician deliberately uses the science of numbers he will be able to talk on equal terms with those who use this same science of numbers to decipher the laws of the cosmos. He will even be able, among the Abderites, to discern those who are less mad than others. And when the philosopher declares that "man is illness entire", he will be able to answer him by saying that such a generalization removes every chance of calmness which the philosopher, in his capacity as a man, wishes to attain. The humoral doctrine, and the very one that Democritus professes, sees illness as disproportion. That is why my dear Thessalus, I have bound you to have recourse to arithmetic. It will enable you to recognize relationships, proportions, and not to scorn any of the Abderites.'

NOTES

1. They are numbered 10 to 23 in the series 'Lettres, décrets et harangues' in E. Littré (ed.) (1861) Oeuvres Complètes: volume IX, Paris, 321–99.
2. The apparition of Asclepios in a dream generally manifests itself to patients who have come to consult him by incubation in his temple. I am unaware of any other example of Asclepios appearing to a physician, cf. Edelstein, L. and Edelstein, E. (1945) Asclepius: A Collection and Interpretation of the Testimonies, volume 2, Baltimore: Johns Hopkins University Press.
N.B. A good analysis, together with bibliographical references, can be found in Pigeaud, J. (1981) La maladie de l'âme (The Malady of the Soul), Paris: Les Belles-Lettres, 452–77.

2

Victorian Origins of Epidemiological Psychiatry

William Bynum

In the nineteenth century, had there been chairs in psychiatry, the Professor of Epidemiological Psychiatry would have been called something like 'Professor of the Statistics of Insanity'. The *Oxford English Dictionary* is only moderately helpful in explaining why someone should now occupy a chair in Epidemiological Psychiatry. 'Epidemiological' ('of or pertaining to epidemiology') is given a first English usage of 1881; 'epidemiology' ('that branch of medical science which treats of epidemics') is first dated 1873, in the title of J.P. Parkin's book *Epidemiology, or the Remoter Causes of Epidemic Diseases*. 'Epidemic', both as noun and adjective, goes back much further, of course, and in its plural form, was the title of Hippocratic treatises. The editors of the *Oxford English Dictionary* failed to notice that there was established, in 1850, the London Epidemiological Society, which published transactions and did much to stimulate interest in the subject. Epidemiology itself, however, did not routinely deal with mental disorder. The first paper in the Society's *Transactions* of any psychiatric relevance did not appear until the 1901–2 session, when (Sir) Frederick Mott published his study on 'Dysentery in Asylums'. Unsurprisingly, the first rather than the second noun of the title was the operative word.

'Psychiatry' was even slower than 'epidemics' and its derivatives in establishing itself in the English language. Although the OED cites an 1846 usage, and both 'psychiatric' and 'psychiatrics' date from the 1847 English translation of Ernst von Feuchtersleben's *Lehrbuch der ärztlichen Seelenkunde*, as late as 1892, Daniel Hack Tuke's monumental *Dictionary of Psychological Medicine* gives only 'Psychiatrie (Ger.), Psychological Medicine'. The sparse entry in Hack Tuke's *Dictionary* reminds us that, whatever the Victorians did, they did not call it epidemiological psychiatry.

Tuke's *Dictionary* does, however, contain clues to the antecedents of the modern discipline. Three articles in particular are relevant to the history of epidemiological psychiatry: 'Epidemic insanity', 'Statistics of insanity', and 'Suicide'. Between them, they raise what strike me as the major preoccupations of those a century ago who sought to come to grips with the complex relationships between mental disorder, society, and populations.

Of epidemic insanity I shall say little, merely referring those interested to some passages in Shepherd's work (e.g. Shepherd 1978: 289), to the writings of the late George Rosen (Rosen 1968), and to the monograph of Robert Nye (Nye 1975). The article in the *Dictionary* on 'Epidemic insanity' leaned heavily on Hecker's great *Epidemics of the Middle Ages* in discussing what Gustave Le Bon would call the crowd psychology associated with such phenomena as the Flagellants, Dancing Mania, Tarantism, and the Convulsionnaires. That Hecker himself included his chapters on medieval episodes of 'psychic contagion' within a work primarily devoted to more conventional epidemic disorders reinforces the primary point of this essay, namely, that the historical roots of epidemiological psychiatry cannot be divorced from the scientific, medical, and social concerns of the last century.

I shall use the entries on 'Statistics of insanity' and on 'Suicide' to examine briefly the uses to which psychiatric statistics were put by those who collected them and the extent to which epidemiological concerns have enlivened some recent historical writings. The statistically-minded editor of the *Dictionary*, Daniel Hack Tuke, wrote both of the entries.

THE STATISTICS OF INSANITY

For the most part, what we may anachronistically call Victorian epidemiological psychiatry confined itself to the asylum. The only notable exception was suicide, only a fraction of which occurred within a psychiatric institution or was committed by patients recently released from one. Suicide apart, however, statistical concern was primarily directed towards patients already formally identified as suffering from mental disorder. The use of epidemiological techniques to elucidate disorders such as pellagra and kuru belongs to the present century (Roe 1973; Gajdusek 1975).

The scientific fascination with the security of numbers goes back to the Scientific Revolution of the sixteenth and seventeenth centuries. In the physical sciences, mathematics reigned supreme, with Newton's reputation extending far beyond the range of individuals able to fathom the nuances of his thought. Demographic and social studies by men such as John Graunt (1620–74) and Sir William Petty (1623–87) possessed a distinct quantitative flavour (Laslett, 1971), and in medicine, the 'iatromathematicians' visualized the human body as a machine understandable through physics and mathematics (Shryock 1948). Iatromathematics had fallen from grace by the middle of the eighteenth century, although the beginnings of multiple case reporting, from about that time, initiated another tradition of numbers in medicine most famously represented by the *method numérique* of Pierre Louis (1787–1872) (Tröhler 1978).

Despite these and similar developments within science and medicine, it is no exaggeration to speak of a 'statistical movement' in early Victorian Britain which went far beyond the realizations of earlier individuals. The decennial censuses, first conducted in 1801, became more accurate by the third or fourth headcount, and the civil registration of births, marriages and deaths, from 1837, brought some coherence to mortality patterns (Nissel 1987). Government departments, such as the General Register Office and the Board of Trade, possessed their quota of numerate civil servants, and government commissions and enquiries, such as that which looked into the operation of the Old Poor Law (1832), began to want more systematic information (MacDonagh 1977). Edwin Chadwick (1800–90) on the Poor Law Commission and William Farr (1807–83) at the GRO are merely two outstanding examples of the passion for numbers which characterizes the period. They were active both within and outside government circles, especially in the statistical societies which sprang up in London, Manchester, Glasgow, and elsewhere (Cullen 1975). Chadwick was particularly under the influence of utilitarianism, a reforming force which Hervey detects in the Metropolitan Commissioners of Lunacy, the body established in 1828 to oversee the asylums and madhouses of the metropolis. Both inspection and statistics came within the Commission's ken, supplemented in the provinces by local magistrates (Hervey 1987). The impetus towards centralization and standardization was consolidated by the 1845 Acts, which extended the Lunacy Commissioners' purview to the provinces, gave them greater powers, and required counties to build, from the rates, asylums for the care, cure, and custody of pauper lunatics.

The compulsion to provide specialized care for pauper lunatics led (at least initially) to the rapid expansion of the asylum system, since a number of counties had declined to act on earlier, permissive, legislation, and, at the time of the 1845 Act, certified pauper lunatics were almost as commonly housed in work- or poor-houses as in asylums (Scull 1979). The sheer number of asylums was bound to increase, but the increase in the average size of each asylum (from under 300 patients in 1850 to over 800 in 1890), or the fact that some counties, such as Middlesex, found it necessary to build more than one asylum, point to the principal epidemiological issues worrying Victorian alienists and statisticians: was insanity increasing, and, if so, why? That there were more individuals certified as insane was beyond dispute, but there were several reasons why this might have happened. Better diagnostic techniques, a greater public awareness of the indications of insanity, and a more efficient machinery to place pauper lunatics within the asylums (where they came under the Commissioners' view) could all have contributed to a larger number of identified lunatics. Better sanitary and environmental conditions and nursing care within the asylums could prolong the average lifespan of the insane, so that at any given time, there would be more of them.

The importance of these factors was agreed by the commentators at the time, and has been accepted more recently by Hare, Scull, and others who

25

have reopened the question (Hare 1983; Scull 1979; Scull 1984; Torrey 1980). The rate of insanity (number of insane divided by total population) was clearly rising during the second half of the nineteenth century; but the incidence of new cases was another issue. Hack Tuke was aware of this basic distinction, although his own terms were *existing* and *occurring* insanity, respectively. Indeed, I think he would have understood perfectly the Scull-Hare debate, and certainly appreciated the flaws in the statistics of insanity available to him. He discounted as totally unreliable any figures before 1859, because readmissions and transfers too often got lumped together with new cases, as each asylum reported its annual statistics. Early in the century, cure rates often suffered from a similar problem, since if the same patient were admitted and discharged 'cured' several times in a single year, he could count as multiple cures. (A helpful analysis of this issue may be found in the article on 'Curability of the insane' by Pliny Earle in Hack Tuke's *Dictionary*.)

In essence, Tuke insisted, the only squarely relevant figure for deciding whether the alleged increase in insanity was real or not was the rate of new cases, a figure continuously available only from 1878. No long-term trend was consequently available to Tuke in 1892, but the modest rise of new cases from 3.29 to 3.46 per 10,000 living (average for 1881–5 and 1886–90, respectively) was not, in his opinion, especially significant. My own assessment of the 'alleged increase in insanity' debate suggests that psychiatrists like Tuke, who denied a major increase in its real incidence, had much the better of the argument, although, as Hare has noted, there were those who felt that a great wave of insanity was spreading across Britain during Victoria's reign (Hare 1983). Hare himself is one of the 'realists', of course, suggesting that the disorder we now call schizophrenia was uncommon before the nineteenth century, and common by the time Bleuler actually gave it its modern name. (Incidentally, *dementia praecox* does not rate a mention in Tuke's *Dictionary*, although *hebephrenia* is given a brief definition.)

Whether the national statistics collected by the Lunacy Commissioners and others will bear the weight of Hare's interpretation is a matter of debate, but, as Tuke pointed out, the raw figures from mid-century until its last decade, while they do show a continuing increase in the number of lunatics, point to a diminishing rate of increase after about 1880. This strikes me as significant, given the fact that this ran counter to the dominant alarmist paradigm of the time, the concept of progressive hereditary degeneration as first comprehensively formulated by Morel (Morel 1857; Dowbiggin 1985).

Tuke recognized two further parameters which bore on the 'increase' question, although he was not sanguine that either one could be used very productively in the 1890s to answer it. The first concerned the relationships between the British experience and those of other countries. Scattered through the *Dictionary* were articles on the provision of psychiatric services for most European countries, the United States, Canada, Australia, etc. The difficulties in using different national statistics in any comparative analysis were insurmountable, since, as Tuke pointed out, different criteria were used in collecting them. American statistics, for example, contained many cases of acute alcoholism which in Britain would not have been admitted to any asylum and would, therefore, be absent from official figures. Accordingly, Tuke refused to speculate on the varying rates of insanity in different countries, even if reliable and comparable figures might have borne on the nagging subtext of the 'increase' question, viz., did insanity and civilization go hand in hand? His summary comment on the issue reflects his own healthy scepticism:

> It may be stated, without danger of contradiction, that the proportion of idiots and lunatics to the population in uncivilized nations is less than in those who are civilized. At the same time there are many reasons why the actual number accumulated in the latter should be vastly greater than in the former without a corresponding difference in the liability to mental disorders. If we consider only this liability we should recommend savages to remain uncivilized, but on the other hand we should decidedly recommend the class corresponding to savages (city-arabs, &c.) in a civilized community to enter the ranks of the educated and well-fed classes.
>
> (Tuke 1892: 1206)

Tuke was also aware that, beyond the visible cases of certified insanity, there existed what he called a 'considerable mass of borderland cases', and that these 'nervous disorders' were also alleged to be on the increase. While not denying that the incidence of nervous disorders might be rising, Tuke recognized that that aspect of the debate was informed only by 'impressions' and 'general observations', and, hence, no definite conclusions could be drawn. He would have appreciated both the problems and the importance of more recent comparative and cross-cultural epidemiological studies (e.g. Hoch and Zubin 1961; Hare and Wing 1970), and of research looking at the incidence of psychiatric morbidity within general practice (e.g. Shepherd *et al.* 1966) and the community (e.g. Srole *et al.* 1962; Plunkett and Gordon 1960).

Tuke's article on the 'statistics of insanity' was not simply about the alleged increase in insanity, however. It also dealt with a whole series of parameters – considered in the mass – about the influence of such factors as age, sex, marital status, and treatment, on the course and outcome of mental disease. Its causation, too, came under his statistical purview, as did the relative frequency of different forms of mental disorder. Causes were broken down into the typical Victorian categories of *moral* and *physical*, and almost 90 per cent of the forms could be accounted for by the broad diagnostic labels of mania, melancholia, or dementia. For virtually all of his statistics Tuke relied on the figures collected by the Lunacy Commissioners, but, when local medical superintendents had attempted to go further than was required by the statutory machinery, Tuke was ready to report more refined statistical findings. Thus, Dr Boyd of the Somerset County Asylum had broken down diagnostic categories (adding monomania, general paralysis, moral insanity, epilepsy, and delirium tremens to the grouping); and Dr Major of the West Riding Asylum had examined the role of alcoholic excess in the life histories of patients admitted to his care. Other studies which Tuke could refer to included the pioneering work of William Farr (1841) on the mortality of insanity; the classic monograph of John Thurnam (1845) on the statistics of insanity; the researches of Sir Arthur Mitchell (1877) on the Scottish scene; and the sensitive and numerate survey of Noel Humphreys (1890) on the 'increase' debate.

In the end, Tuke was aware that his statistics did not permit him to answer many questions, and that they represented the cumulative experience of many asylums and many medical superintendents. They were collected by many hands, albeit along guidelines laid down by the Lunacy Commissioners, and related primarily to patients just before, during, and just after psychiatric hospitalization. Even though the 1871 census had attempted to measure the extent of 'insanity and idiocy' in the general population, Tuke's statistics were essentially those of the asylum and its psychiatry. In only one significant area did he and his colleagues turn their numerical gaze on a phenomenon occurring largely outside the asylum. This was the question of suicide.

SUICIDE

Suicide occupies a special place within the history of the social sciences, principally because of Durkheim's classic monograph, which was first published five years after Tuke's *Dictionary* (Durkheim 1952). Tuke could consequently make no use of it, but he did have access to the man who was also Durkheim's most frequently cited authority, Enrico Morselli, the Italian psychiatrist whose own study of suicide had been translated into English in 1881 (Morselli 1881; Guarnieri 1988). In fact, except for the historical sections detailing attitudes towards, and legislation relating to, suicide from antiquity to the nineteenth century, most of Tuke's entry was derived from Morselli's monograph. He was also able to refer his readers to some English work, notably in the monographs of Forbes Winslow (1840), the mid-century psychiatric entrepreneur (Smith 1981; Shepherd 1986), and of W.W. Westcott (1885), the deputy coroner for Central Middlesex, as well as the article of William Ogle (1886), one of Farr's successors at the General Register Office.

Reflecting the broad concerns of Tuke's principal authorities, his article was permeated with a social, comparative, and statistical orientation. His first table summarized the incidence of suicide in nineteen countries or areas, and included the fact that suicide was more than twenty-nine times more common in Saxony than Portugal. These crude figures were subsequently analysed, for many of the geographical areas, in terms of sex and age ratios, and variations in suicide in terms of seasonality, time of day, religion, political life, race, trade cycles, marital state, occupation, urbanization, population density, social condition, and alcohol consumption. The mode by which men and women chose to take their own lives was also subjected to numerical analysis.

Throughout Europe and North America – indeed, wherever statistics were being compiled – there was evidence that suicide was on the increase. The only exceptions reported by Tuke were Holland, where it had been stationary between 1870 and 1880, and Russia, Finland, and Norway, where its frequency had diminished during the 1870s. Morselli's own conclusion, quoted by Tuke, was that 'madness and suicide are met with the more frequently in proportion as civilization progresses' (Morselli 1881: 117; as quoted by Tuke 1892: 1224). Tuke was prepared to accept that significant geographical, occupational, ethnological, sexual, and religious variations existed in the incidence of suicide, but at the same time he fought shy of some of Morselli's sweeping conclusions for the simple fact that the figures themselves were subject to too many sources of error: under-reporting, doubtful circumstances, subterfuge, as well as the inadequate bureaucratic machinery for collecting statistics in many countries. 'All that we are justified in concluding is the apparent greater liability [to suicide] of the more cultured races of mankind', Tuke commented.

Victorian and Edwardian suicide has recently been brilliantly examined by Olive Anderson (1987), who has amply substantiated Tuke's suspicions about the quality of the statistics, even as they relate to Tuke's own country, let alone to other parts of Europe. Nevertheless, Anderson has been able to make creative historical use of the statistical legacy bequeathed to us by our Victorian forebears and has gone beyond what was available to Tuke in analysing some particularly full sets of surviving coroners' returns (one in Southwark, one in Sussex) from coroners especially concerned with the incidence and the individual circumstances of suicide. Incidentally, Anderson's shrewd examination of national patterns and regional variations of Victorian and Edwardian suicide shows the inadequacy of Durkheim's notion of anomie in explaining suicide as a social phenomenon, at least for England and Wales. Rates were higher in the wealthy, established, and rural southeast than they were in the turbulent areas of England's industrial north.

Anderson's study also demonstrates how historians can with good effect use earlier epidemiological data as well as subject historical collections of materials to their own analyses. MacDonald's investigations of suicide in the seventeenth and eighteenth centuries (described in more detail by him later in this book) confirm the second point (MacDonald 1977; MacDonald 1986; MacDonald 1988), and his dissection of the case notes of Richard Napier

(1559–1634) in essence presents a psychiatric epidemiology of an early-seventeenth-century general practice (MacDonald 1981). Neither Anderson nor MacDonald view suicide as a subject within the exclusive ken of psychiatry. Nor did Tuke: his article was broad in its terms of reference, suggesting that perhaps no more than 20 per cent of suicide cases could be attributed to insanity. Kushner (1986) has recently suggested that American psychiatrists failed to see the relevance of social studies such as Durkheim's, turning instead to psychoanalysis in their attempt to understand the psychodynamics of the desire to destroy oneself. The history of most of British psychiatry in the present century remains to be written, and the study of suicide is no exception. Nevertheless, Tuke's article suggests that, at the close of the last century, psychiatrists were cognizant of the importance of both social and psychopathological factors in the phenomenon.

CONCLUSION

This brief essay has done no more than point to some of the themes and literature relating to epidemiological psychiatry before the subject was actually called that. For the Victorians, epidemiology was concerned almost exclusively with infectious diseases. In the present century, the methods of the discipline have been refined and the objects of its analysis revealingly extended to many other kinds of disorders, such as neoplasms and diseases of the cardio-vascular system. Within British psychiatry, much of the impetus has come from the Institute of Psychiatry and the Maudsley Hospital, where Shepherd, Wing, Hare, and many others have continued traditions which were well established during the Aubrey Lewis era (Shepherd 1977; Shepherd and Davies 1968). But the fundamental importance of the subject was appreciated by Thurnam, Hack Tuke, and others a century and more ago. Despite shifts in vocabulary, Victorian psychiatrists may be said to have pioneered the epidemiological investigation of non-infectious disorders.

REFERENCES

Anderson, O. (1987) *Suicide in Victorian and Edwardian Britain*, Oxford: Clarendon Press.
Cullen, M.J. (1975) *The Statistical Movement in Early Victorian Britain*, Hassocks: Harvester Press.
Dowbiggin, I. (1985) 'Degeneration and hereditarianism in French mental medicine 1840–90', in W.F. Bynum, R. Porter and M. Shepherd (eds) *The Anatomy of Madness*, London: Tavistock, vol. I, 188–232.
Durkheim, E. (1952) *Suicide: A Study in Sociology*, translated by J.A. Spaulding and G. Simpson, London: Routledge & Kegan Paul.
Gajdusek, D.C. (ed.) (1975) *Correspondence on the Discovery and Original Investigations on Kuru: Smadel-Gajdusek Correspondence, 1955–1958*, Bethesda,

Maryland: National Institutes of Health.

Guarnieri, P. (1988) 'Between soma and psyche: Morselli and psychiatry in late-nineteenth-century Italy', in W.F. Bynum, R. Porter and M. Shepherd (eds) *The Anatomy of Madness*, London: Tavistock, vol. III, 102–24.

Hare, E.H. (1983) 'Was insanity on the increase?', *British Journal of Psychiatry* 142: 439–55.

Hare, E.H. and Wing, J.K. (eds) (1970) *Psychiatric Epidemiology*, London: Oxford University Press.

Hecker, J.F.K. (1859) *The Epidemics of the Middle Ages* (trans. B.G. Babington), London: Trübner.

Hervey, N. (1987) 'The Lunacy Commission 1845–60, with special reference to the implementation of policy in Kent and Surrey', two vols, PhD thesis, University of Bristol.

Hoch, P.H. and Zubin, J. (eds) (1961) *Comparative Epidemiology of the Mental Disorders*, New York: Grune and Stratton.

Humphreys, N. (1890) 'Statistics of Insanity in England, with special reference to its alleged increasing prevalence', *Journal of the Royal Statistical Society* 53: 201–45.

Kushner, H. (1986) 'American psychiatry and the cause of suicide, 1844–1917', *Bulletin of the History of Medicine* 60: 36–57.

Laslett, P. (1971) *The World We Have Lost*, London: Methuen.

MacDonagh, O. (1977) *Early Victorian Government 1830–1870*, London: Weidenfeld & Nicolson.

MacDonald, M. (1977) 'The inner side of wisdom: suicide in early modern England', *Psychological Medicine* 7: 562–82.

MacDonald, M. (1981) *Mystical Bedlam: Madness, Anxiety and Healing in Seventeenth-Century England*, Cambridge and New York: Cambridge University Press.

MacDonald, M. (1986) 'The secularization of suicide in England 1660–1800', *Past and Present* 111: 50–100.

MacDonald, M. (1988) 'Introduction' to facsimile reprint of John Sym (1637) *Lifes Preservative Against Self-killing*, London: Routledge.

Mitchell, A. (1877) 'Contributions to the statistics of insanity', *Journal of Mental Science* 22: 507–15.

Morel, B.A. (1857) *Traité des dégénérescences physiques, intellectuelles, et morales de l'espèce humaine*, Paris: Baillière.

Morselli, E. (1881) *Suicide: An Essay on Comparative Moral Statistics*, London: Kegan Paul.

Nissel, M. (1987) *People Count: A History of the General Register Office*, London: Her Majesty's Stationery Office.

Nye, R.A. (1975) *The Origins of Crowd Psychology: Gustave Le Bon and the Crisis of Mass Democracy in the Third Republic*, London and Beverly Hills: Sage.

Ogle, W.H. (1886) 'Suicides in England and Wales in relation to age, sex, season and occupation', *Journal of the [Royal] Statistical Society* 49: 101–35.

Plunkett, J. and Gordon, J.E. (1960) *Epidemiology and Mental Illness*, New York: Basic Books.

Roe, D. (1973) *A Plague of Corn: The Social History of Pellagra*, Ithaca: Cornell University Press.

Rosen, G. (1968) *Madness in Society: Chapters in the Historical Sociology of Mental Illness*, London: Routledge & Kegan Paul.

Scull, A. (1979) *Museums of Madness: The Social Organization of Insanity in Nineteenth-Century England*, London: Allen Lane.

Scull, A. (1984) 'Was insanity increasing? A response to Edward Hare', *British Journal of Psychiatry* 144: 432–6.

Shepherd, M. (1957) *A Study of the Major Psychoses in an English County* (Maudsley Monograph No. 3), London: Chapman and Hall.

Shepherd, M. (1977) *The Career and Contributions of Sir Aubrey Lewis*, London: Bethlem Royal and Maudsley Hospitals.

Shepherd, M. (1978) 'Epidemiology and clinical psychiatry', *British Journal of Psychiatry* 133: 289–98. (Reprinted in Shepherd (1983).)

Shepherd, M. (1983) *The Psychosocial Matrix of Psychiatry: Collected Papers*, London: Tavistock.

Shepherd, M. (1986) 'Psychological medicine *redivivus*: concept and communication', *Journal of the Royal Society of Medicine* 79: 639–45.

Shepherd, M. and Davies, D.L. (eds) (1968) *Studies in Psychiatry*, London: Oxford University Press.

Shepherd, M., Cooper, B., Brown, A.C., and Kalton, G.W. (1966) *Psychiatric Illness in General Practice*, London: Oxford University Press.

Shryock, R. (1948) *The Development of Modern Medicine: An Interpretation of the Social and Scientific Factors Involved*, London: Victor Gollancz.

Smith, R. (1981) *Trial by Medicine: Insanity and Responsibility in Victorian Trials*, Edinburgh: Edinburgh University Press.

Srole, L., Langner, T.S., Michael, S.T., Opler, M.K., and Rennie, T.A.C. (1962) *Mental Health in the Metropolis: The Midtown Manhattan Study*, New York: McGraw-Hill.

Thurnam, J. (1845) *Observations and Essays on the Statistics of Insanity*, London: Simpkin, Marshall & Co.

Torrey, E.F. (1980) *Schizophrenia and Civilization*, New York: Jason Aronson.

Tröhler, U. (1978) 'Quantification in British medicine and surgery 1750–1830, with special reference to its introduction into therapeutics', PhD thesis, University of London.

Tuke, D.H. (ed.) (1892) *A Dictionary of Psychological Medicine*, two vols, London: J. & A. Churchill.

Wescott, W.W. (1885) *Suicide: Its History, Literature, Jurisprudence, Causation and Prevention*, London: H.K. Lewis.

Winslow, F. (1840) *The Anatomy of Suicide*, London: Henry Renshaw.

The Social Sciences

3

A Sociological and Socio-anthropological Perspective

Annette Lawson

'. . . epidemiology represents a corpus of methods rather than a theory of science'   Felton Earls[1]

In 1958 I began work on my doctoral dissertation in the field known then as social psychiatry.[2] It was a time of great optimism. Mental illness, we believed ('we' – both social scientists and psychiatrists), could be unravelled. We could discover what it was about the social world (we spoke of social 'factors') that made people ill, that brought them into the mental hospital, that influenced the course of their illness, that enabled them to recover.[3] We also believed that much mental illness went undiscovered – it was out there in the community. Shepherd (1966: 173) wrote: 'The proportion of cases referred to psychiatrists is not more than one tenth of the total identified.'[4] We needed to discover the rates, persuading those with the means to provide the skilled and expert help that would make the sick better.

This may be an exaggeration. Certainly there were conflicts within psychiatry, especially about the aetiology of mental illness and, hence, about the best and most appropriate forms of treatment. Psychiatry was also battling with other medical disciplines for recognition and a higher place in the hierarchy. And I am assuming a homogeneity to sociology that has never been achieved. That is, several strands, including social research, armchair theorizing, and social anthropology, have divided the camp in a society that, until late in this century, failed to offer institutional means for establishing the discipline, partly because so many alternative routes to government and influence were available.[5] None the less, sociology was at its height of respectability; there was a rapid growth in the discipline and Britain, it was said by Prime Minister Harold Macmillan, had 'never had it so good'. Money was made available to do research.

Hence, in the 1950s and 1960s, as much in the United States as in the United Kingdom, the classic sociological/epidemiological studies of mental illness in populations by Faris and Dunham (1967), Alexander Leighton (1959), D.C. Leighton *et al.* (1963), Hollingshead and Redlich (1958), and the Midtown Manhattan Studies (1962) by Srole and colleagues included both social scientists and psychiatrists as principal investigators. Although there has been a continuing struggle between the relativity of the cultural anthropologist and the universality of the medical epidemiologist, in Britain both leading psychiatrists like Aubrey Lewis and Morris Carstairs and anthropologists like C.G. Seligman and W.H. Rivers thought major new advances in understanding mental illness would be achieved by collaboration between social science and psychiatry.[6] It was a time of partnership with shared ideas about the nature of mental illness – a 'medical' model of a disease entity to be defined and diagnosed by expert psychiatrists and investigated by expert social scientists who understood about population studies and the importance of scientific methods of investigation, especially of quantitative methods. It is fair to say that neither Lewis nor Carstairs could have predicted the enormous theoretical shift that would occur to throw social science into rethinking its premises and hence its methodologies.

In this chapter, I sketch the developments in both epidemiology and sociology (the former concentrating on methods, the latter on theory) that have led to a certain dissolution of the partnership, exacerbated, perhaps, by the increasing importance of a medical background for the epidemiologist and the lack of psychiatrists working with or as anthropologists or sociologists.[7]

These developments lead me to make paradoxical and related claims: first, that epidemiological psychiatry is both well founded in sociological and social anthropological scientific features *and* that it fails adequately to answer problems by not employing the best of sociological and social anthropological theories and methods; second, that epidemiology largely contributes to advancing knowledge in a progressive way *and* that by failing to pay attention to the meaning and context of social action[8] it may function retrogressively.

A PARTNERSHIP BETWEEN EPIDEMIOLOGY AND SOCIAL SCIENCE

In the beginning, that is, in 1951 in Britain but more than fifty years earlier in France, Durkheim's *Suicide* was published.[9] One of the most famous of sociological texts, it is also a forerunner of epidemiological psychiatry. Well-known as it is to readers of this collection, it is important to recall what Durkheim did. Following in the footsteps of the great nineteenth-century 'moral statisticians' such as Quetelet in Belgium, Durkheim took published rates of suicide and showed that individuals undertaking the most deeply psychological and philosophically important action of ending their own lives did so in non-random ways. Protestants more often than Catholics,[10] married men less often than the unmarried,[11] intellectuals and the well-educated more than the less-well-educated, the divorced – that is, those without families – more often than would have been expected by mere chance. Durkheim, of course, did not stop there.[12] He set out to explain the variation in the rates that he had mapped. Suicide, he argued, was, in the sense he had shown, not merely an individual act, to be understood in terms only of each unique person's history and current position, or of their particular psychopathology, but also deeply social. It was an act undertaken in particular social conditions that had the effect of undermining the individual's sense of purpose and of meaning. The conditions were typified by 'anomie',[13] a state of normlessness, a state where clear moral goals, where social cohesion and social connectedness were lacking. In other words, a single theoretical construct – anomie – explained the relative lack of clear moral goals, and of relatedness to others that would be found in greater measure among Catholics than Protestants, the married than the unmarried.

Using this technique, Durkheim demonstrated the task of the sociologist; it is, as Merton later put it, 'to explain the rates'. It is not the purpose of the sociologist to explain the action of any given and particular individual. Indeed, Durkheim recognized that it was this that should be done by psychologists. Thus, he mapped also the terrain of these two disciplines.

Of course, the rates must first be discovered. Durkheim employed published figures, or those collected by governmental agencies. But the social survey and the discrete study of specially selected populations became the hallmark of sociological work, for it was recognized early that data collected for one purpose (administration, for example) were by no means complete or satisfactory for quite other goals. None the less, official data or specially chosen samples both rested on the assumption of the concrete reality of the social fact. There was a real rate out there in the real world to be discovered if only the correct tools and methods for investigation were employed. Having determined what this accurate rate was, the sociologist should explain it. Of course, it was not only the methods of the survey that might be at fault and thus produce untrue rates, but the analysis could also be erroneous. Durkheim has been criticized on both counts. In addition, the explanation might usefully indicate social measures for combating or lowering the rate, since the problem to be investigated was, usually, already identified as a social problem – something undesirable that was pathological for the body politic. Thus, Durkheim thought that new groupings, such as the syndicate, would develop to enable the modern person to be integrated when disintegration threatened, thus lowering the suicide rate. In other words, the whole endeavour was not only scientific but also deeply political. This, too, has been the focus of more recent attention.[14]

Following in Durkheim's footsteps, both epidemiologists and social scientists, at least of that group conducting empirical work, identified suffering, knew that it should be scientifically investigated and believed that knowledge would in and of itself lead to the better society, for the more information, the greater the tolerance that would be exercised. The good that was truth was both a means and an end. W.H. Sprott (1962)[15] thought the central message of British sociology up to that time had been that, through the best evidence one could accumulate about the social world, increased rationality and widened sympathy would be achieved.

The partnership between epidemiologist and sociologist was also healthy for another reason: there was a certain division of labour based on an acceptance of the different expertise each discipline brought to the enquiry. Thus, social scientists were not competent to define mental illness – that was for the expert psychiatrist. Just as the criminologist accepted the expert definition of lawyers as to what constituted crime, and of the executive arm of the state as to which criminal problems would benefit from sociological investigation, so social scientists as socio-technicians[16] worked in the service of psychiatry. The psychiatrist, on the other hand, accepted that the social scientist had particular methodological expertise – a knowledge of how to *do* the necessary science. Indeed, psychiatry accepted that, as its disease categories were so tenuous and not generally marked by physical signs, the sociologist's concepts of impairment or disability marked by social dysfunction could be the key to unravelling the rates of mental illness.[17] It was in this sense that sociology was a 'positive' science: it was an objective, value-free endeavour that could study social problems and produce knowledge enabling governments to make what *evidently* would be the right decisions. To use a distinction employed by Morris Janowitz (1970: 243–59)[18] and developed by Philip Abrams (1985: 182–3),[19] this was social science as 'engineering' that would, it was intended, lead to 'enlightenment'.

EPIDEMIOLOGY: EMBEDDED IN MEDICINE, FOCUSING ON MEASUREMENT

As long as these attitudes were shared, the goals and, hence, the methods of social science and epidemiology were also shared. But, as epidemiology has become increasingly embedded in medicine, the stress has been to develop harder and more rigorously bounded *medical* categories of disease that seek for universality and hence ignore the specificity and particularity of social context and historical moment.

This is how Eaton describes these assumptions:

Epidemiology is a branch of medicine, and, thus, the assumptions of the medical model of disease are implicit. The most important assumption is that the disease under study actually exists – or, to put it another way . . . it is useful to engage in study involving the given disease category. In psychiatry this assumption is assuredly more tenuous than in other areas of medicine, because psychiatric diseases tend to be defined by failure to locate a physical cause, and validation of a given category of disease is therefore more subtle and complex.   Eaton (1986)[20]

In fact, it is by no means only the psychiatric categories that are so intractable. The NMR scanner throws the idea of multiple sclerosis as a disease constituted by its symptoms into disarray when it makes visible not one but many and old lesions existing at the time of the first symptoms. The new technique is taken to demonstrate an underlying pathology but symptoms and signs appear ever more disassociated. The HIV antibodies are found in people who have no symptoms and may never develop any symptoms of AIDS. Concepts such as carrier, potential patient, non-malignant or pre-cancerous growth, and sub-clinical illness are not, it seems to me, more robust than, say, schizoid personality, and some have social consequences as or more alarming.

None the less, epidemiological psychiatry does maintain a concept, especially with schizophrenia, of a single and universal entity, and that there *is* a physical cause to be located at some future date through clinical and experimental work in biochemistry or physiology. Indeed, Wing says that an 'essential element in any disease theory is the hypothesis that the cluster of traits is "symptomatic" of some underlying biological disturbance' (Wing 1978: 22). The less there is a social component, the better.[21] It is, thus, of critical importance that most effort is expended on constructing measures that most accurately reflect this specific disease entity. Given its model of the hard sciences, epidemiology, like sociology in its earlier manifestations, has concentrated on quantitative techniques, not on the kinds of interpretative, descriptive, narrative, or historical analyses that are more typical of anthropology and of qualitative sociology.

Hence, and because of somewhat gross differences in the rates of various clinically judged mental illnesses around the world in earlier studies that were explained by variations in diagnostic practice and inadequate case-finding,[22] psychiatric epidemiologists have developed such important diagnostic community-based tools as CATEGO, SADS, SADD, and the PSE including Wing's ID modification, as well as measures that can be applied by relatively unskilled people such as the GHQ.

The finest examples of studies using and developing such sophisticated instruments are, perhaps, the collaborative WHO[23] and the US–UK diagnostic projects, attempting to establish rates of mental illness in different societies.[24] The use of these standardized instruments, of case-registers,[25] of techniques of case-finding through local healers, alternative sources of care, and community leaders, as well as of statistical techniques for analysing data that deal more adequately with the problems of when illness events occur and how the course of illness can best be mapped, has resulted in diminished overall differences between study centres in the rates of the various diagnostic groups. There remain, however, wider variations in the affective or mood change and neurotic categories than in the psychotic,[26] suggesting more strongly than before that distress is manifested as somatic complaints as often as it is in emotional disturbance around the world, but that there may be a 'core' illness called schizophrenia by western psychiatrists.[27] Early reports from the WHO collaborative study indicate, however, that its course varies substantially in urban and industrialized societies where it seems to take longer, the recovery rate is worse and disability greater than in rural and developing societies.[28]

The fact that it is now the affective disorders and the course of mental illness generally that vary most across cultures is best understood within a theory that explains mood disturbance and illness recognition, treatment, and outcome as the consequence of social events and social context, for it is these that vary most across cultures, not biology. When psychiatry insists on the discovery of biochemical or other individual and organic phenomena as *causing* illness, it misses the possibility of much more plausible, parsimonious, and, to my mind, scientific reasoning. To insist, in a word, on one possible type of cause is to scientize rather than to do good science.

Given the goals of epidemiology set out by Morris (1957)[29] and described in detail later by Shepherd (1982),[30] it makes sense that the questions asked are directed not only towards the fundamental issues of the nature of the disease, clues as to its aetiology, and the boundaries of the normal and the pathological[31] but also to more practical questions of treatment, provision of services, and the evaluation of various therapeutic interventions.

DIVERGENT QUESTIONS, GOALS, THEORIES, AND METHODS

Epidemiologists want to know 'how many? where? when? what happens? why? what is needed there to prevent and treat the illness?' Social scientists, however, not being medically trained, have a different agenda. They want to know 'how does this become recognized and classified as an illness? what does the person in whom the illness is said to reside and who believes himself or herself sick feel and think? what do those who consider that person sick feel and think? what actions are taken by each? what meaning do such actions have? how do the illness and its pattern of social interaction and treatment vary with other features of the social structure and cultural beliefs of that society, class or gender group? what is the structure and nature of the relationship between providers and receivers of therapeutic care?' Thus the differences between the epidemiological and the sociological or social anthropological approach and the methodologies most recently employed lie in the purposes for which each undertakes research and the uses to which it is hoped the work will be put. These goals are both affected by and affect a general theory (usually not spelt out or attended to by the epidemiologist) of the nature of illness; indeed, of human nature. Because this underlying general theory, and the purposes and outcome of epidemiological and sociological research, varies, the actual techniques employed in any given study have also, since Durkheim's *Suicide*, become increasingly divergent.

While epidemiologists have continued to map the distribution of mental illness with a special interest in schizophrenia, indicating that it is, for example, more common among young people, among lower socio-economic groups, among men rather than women, and in the central hotel and boarding house districts near the great railway terminals of cities,[32] sociologists have gone inside the mental institution unravelling its own madness,[33] have attached much importance to the societal reaction in the development of a 'career' that is stigmatized,[34] have shown how women's madness is stereo-typically along lines permitted females and men's madness along stereotypic-ally male lines,[35] that diagnostic and treatment patterns for black and other ethnic minority groups vary from those of the 'normal' (and more powerful) white groups with similar symptoms and the same diagnosis,[36] and have con-centrated on the defining process itself,[37] and on paths to medical care.[38]

At the same time, there have been critiques of science that showed its activity as necessarily political. The very questions that are asked and left un-examined indicate this; thus, the over-representation of women among the depressed population is well reported in the literature, but the fact that unmarried men are over-represented, and the possible origins of this in the male psyche or environment, are not widely discussed in epidemiological research. Duster, in another context, uses the example of IQ studies to demonstrate that while correlational studies have been used to show the superiority of whites over blacks, the available evidence showing that Jews do better in schools than Gentiles has not been used to show the intellectual superiority of the Jews over Gentiles (Duster 1984).[39] Furthermore, since race is not a genetically homogeneous category, and since intelligence is not an objective phenomenon, such correlational studies depend for their validation on socio-political considerations. Littlewood (1986)[40] argues that not only should psychiatry apply social anthropology, but apply it to itself. If this were done, it would be seen that 'much of the endeavour of academic psychology and psychiatry is the reification and amplification of what is basically European folk psychology'.

Why did these two disciplines diverge in this way? Two answers are needed. First, the work of ancestors other than Durkheim became increasingly impor-tant and was developed during the 1960s and 1970s. Second, the upheaval in political and economic life that included the rapid growth of sociology in British universities was particularly favourable to the pursuit of these directions.

SOCIOLOGY: THE PURSUIT OF MEANING AND THE GROWTH OF QUALITATIVE METHODS

I have already pointed to the underlying model of disease and of human nature that underpins epidemiological work. It was this model that came under increasing attack as the work of ancestors other than Durkheim became increas-ingly important. Alfred Schutz[41] drew on Weber – particularly on his

41

concepts of *verstehen* (or empathetic understanding) and of the social actor's subjectivity, as well as on the work of Husserl, to produce a sociological phenomenology.[42] In this approach, it is the meaning of social action that is central and must be examined.[43] At the same time, the influence of George Herbert Mead became widely diffused. The 'I' of Mead's social actor is fundamentally constructed as the 'me' acts and reflects in relation always to the social world. It was, thus, not possible to accept uncritically the observer's truth; there had to be a detailed mapping of social *inter*action in order to build a meaningful picture of social *action*. Such an approach was particularly fruitful in deviancy studies where the concept of 'societal re-action' became central to understanding and explaining criminalization[44] or, indeed, the process of becoming and being a mental patient.[45]

The concepts that were developed by this school included 'career' and 'stigma'. These arose in conditions of secondary deviance. First, someone becomes disturbed or commits some law infraction. This is primary deviance. Various processes occur that might include that person coming before a psychiatrist or a judge. These people, occupying significant and powerful roles in the social structure, label the patient/offender. Now the possibility of secondary deviance occurs. The person may, in conditions where the behaviour that is labelled is stigmatized, take on the status of patient or criminal as their master-status. The label is sticky; it is not thrown off. New ways of behaving that confirm rather than deny the label are engaged in. The person enters a patient or criminal career. Such concepts led to a severely critical approach to the acceptance of expert definitions of the problem. It was the law-*makers* as much as the law-*breakers* who had to be studied, the labelling process as much as the characteristics of those labelled.

Work on mental illness in the late 1960s was also heavily influenced by the 'anti-psychiatry' of many psychiatrists such as Thomas Szasz in America and Ronald Laing in the UK. Their approaches were by no means unitary but Laing (among others) stressed the meaningfulness and centrality of the patient's own experience. At the same time in Britain, too, the new deviancy theorists[46] and critical criminologists,[47] putting a neo-Marxist view forward, were creating an entirely new climate in which to think about and investigate mental illness and the lives of mentally ill people.

Of course, none of these perspectives was without critics[48] and none is a complete explanation for the phenomenon of mental illness, but they have much to offer and they led to very different research agendas that stressed ethnographic and participant observer techniques, derived more from social anthropology than from survey research and the analysis of large-scale data sets. In Britain, there was a decisive move away from statistics and numeracy (also criticized on theoretical grounds)[49] in favour of qualitative work, perhaps, as I explore below, the result of the influx of not particularly numerate students, and faculty who were very much leaders of the new schools of thought.[50] In addition, there was a further, even more radical attack on traditional methods of sociological enquiry.

Originally an offspring of the phenomenology and interactionist schools, ethnomethodology[51] made the construction of the rate itself into the *topic* of research. A rate was no longer a resource, a step necessary as a spring-board for analysis and explanation. Indeed, when, in 1967, Douglas[52] returned to *Suicide*, intending not to undermine but to re-examine Durkheim's thesis, he ended by focusing on the social process of negotiation whereby the dead person becomes a suicide statistic – a process ignored by Durkheim. It was the detailed examination of this process (not of the relationship of the dead person to their families and social worlds) that laid bare the structure and culture, the norms of the society. In his examination he unravelled the 'everyday' and 'common-sense' decisions of family and friends, of clerks, coroners, and registrars. It was the rules according to which their judgements were made that illuminated social life.[53]

Such an approach directly contradicts that of trans- or cross-cultural psychiatry that now holds, for example, that schizophrenia, although it might be called by other names and have somewhat different cultural content and different outcomes, is found in roughly similar rates everywhere and that this fact will not be altered by the tools employed in its discovery.[54] Rather, the tools must be perfected *in order to* discover it. Yet it is clear that the tools employed do, quite fundamentally, alter what is discovered. At its most obvious, if a diagnostic interview schedule did not ask about drinking habits, there would be no alcoholism rate. DIS, the Diagnostic Interview Schedule,[55] used in the large-scale American Epidemiologic Catchment Area studies, is linked to DSM-III, and this manual changes each time it is issued by the American Psychiatric Association. Had the newly proposed diagnoses making women who remained in abusive relationships and men who committed rape but who fantasized about it beforehand[56] into mentally sick people been adopted in DSM III-R, the overall rates of mental illness for women and men would have increased overall. Perhaps there would be more sick than well people in each of the Epidemiologic Catchment Areas currently using DIS. As it is, Huffine has suggested that the equalization in the ratio of mental illness as between women and men appearing in these studies results from the fact that DIS, unlike other tools such as the Cornell Medical Index, emphasizes patterns of drug and alcohol use as mental illnesses and hence increases the male rate, thus reducing the female:male ratio.[57]

With ethnomethodology, sociology had seemingly come full circle, for we were no longer debunking or establishing common sense but investigating it. Sociology itself became just another way of accounting for life, no more and no less interesting. There were simply many ways of constructing meaning.

Given that literary scholars were busy analysing texts divorced from the social or psychological world and meanings within which they had been constructed, it is perhaps scarcely surprising that sociology, too, should have been required to examine different kinds of 'facts' and to face what it had

43

hitherto taken for granted. Both activities were perhaps the product of an era at the end of optimism, in economic crisis and forced back on itself, an era which began to demonstrate impatience with the social and increasing dependence on and faith in the technological and the scientific.

This was all right if what you wanted from your work was to construct meaning, or, rather, to analyse how, in everyday life, it was done. But most sociologists still had other goals in mind, other questions they wished to pose. For these, among whom I number myself, ethnomethodology has been influential – it has meant that, even after a rate has been empirically questioned, it can never be uncritically accepted – but it has not led us to despair of posing the grander questions that Durkheim or Weber wished to pose. Wanting to pose such questions brings us back to the goals also of the epidemiologist, because, as I have pointed out, the very decision to pose certain and not other questions is political.

POLITICAL AND SOCIAL CHANGE

So, too, must the politics of the times enter as having both enabled and constrained the divergence of epidemiology and sociology, for their agendas arose within markedly different institutional settings. Epidemiology, to be taken at all seriously and to obtain resources and maintain precarious funding, had, like medicine itself (and especially those branches to which epidemiology was most closely allied – community and preventive medicine and, in our case, psychiatry) to turn away from its humanistic past and follow a model of 'hard science'. Technology (ushered in by the Wilson government in 1964) was the way of the future, whether translated as sophisticated computerized statistical packages, more standardized forms of measurement, or in hardware proper. That social science was also perceived as part of the technological revolution and given space and resources in the new technological universities founded at that time ignored the fact that the mass of students attracted to this field came from the humanities, had their eyes on the helping professions, journalism, or administration, were not particularly numerate, and were not budding scientists. Furthermore, top-ranking sociologists were part of the critique of society, including the critique of medicine and psychiatry explored here, that was also anti-'positivist' – a term that became merely abusive. This critique was allied to other broad, important socio-political changes elsewhere.

The Vietnamese conflict fundamentally altered the American political scene and it was accompanied and followed by sexual permissiveness and the cry for civil rights, particularly for black people but also for women, homosexuals, and people of various ethnic minorities. All these liberation movements stressed the importance of the history and experience of the people themselves. Women could not be spoken for; they had a voice of their own. This was no less true for black people who had been silenced for so long. Homosexuality was a political choice and a particular, valid way of living in the world; it was not a mental illness or a condition that needed expert diagnosis and treatment. Hence its eventual disappearance from the American DSM in 1973 as a psychiatric diagnosis. These movements did not have the same powerful impact in Britain that they had in the United States, but London was the 'swinging city' and married women began to re-enter the market places of the world in increasing numbers.[58]

In addition, as the social climate changed, for example towards homosexuals, so there was, in fact, less distress among them of the kind that might lead to the psychiatric consulting room, because there was reduced stigma and greater opportunity for self-expression if not much greater opportunity in the social structure. (AIDS, of course, may swing opinion against gay men again.) Feminist scholars began to develop new theories about the psychology and development of women[59] that lend support to the newer feminist therapies that, instead of simply noticing women seemed to blame themselves for domestic strife and reported to professionals more often than men about relational problems,[60] offered both an explanation and strategies of treatment to address rather than suppress the problem.[61] Most recently, the idea that lay people – that is, *non-experts* in any particular social or medical problem – and those who actually suffer from such problems have to speak for themselves, are entitled to speak for themselves, and can affect their own destinies has resulted in powerful self-help groups, some still closely bound to the medical experts through advisory panels, others deliberately refusing such association because it gives less freedom for self-determination.[62]

In other words, there is no going back, though, in times of economic strain, regression is likely. Since the development of epidemiology has continued alongside that of sociology within these changing times, does it matter that the disciplines have followed rather different paths in their exploration of mental illness? What consequences in the sum of human happiness flow from that? There are, I think, both scientific and therapeutic consequences. Taking account of these consequences permits us to recognize the best areas in which the partnership might be revived.

REVIVING THE PARTNERSHIP

Littlewood has pointed out that the approaches that allocate to the culture a surrounding or content role – that is, that permit an acknowledgement, for example, that a certain diagnosis might be difficult to make when dealing with a person from a different ethnic background, or that a person's delusions may be culture specific – but not a generative one, have considerable difficulties in accounting not only for culture-bound syndromes such as *latah*,[63] but also for the appearance and disappearance of psychopathologies: 'such as agoraphobia, Briquet's syndrome, anorexia nervosa, exhibitionism, self-poisoning or, perhaps, the chronic pain syndromes.'[64] Or, we might add, homosexuality. Who is to say how much misery was created by the recognition of homosexuality as a psychiatric disease? If these are scientific difficulties, the therapies that follow are likely, at the least, to be inappropriate and, at worst, to be iatrogenic. Fernando[65] challenges the very concept of depression among black people in Britain but also, given the high rates identified, moves to express this dilemma with respect to treatment. He suggests that racism acts as a 'poison'. Therefore:

> In dealing with a depressed person one should try to identify the blows to self esteem in recent events that arise from racism. An awareness of what happens is important because the patient has to develop strategies to safeguard self-esteem; finding alternative sources of self-pride may mean identifying with (for example) black movements, seeking ethnic therapists, or finding models (to identify with) that do not represent the dominant racial groups . . . Avoiding the issue by advising patients to 'accept' and lower expectations without understanding the situation is not helpful. Treatment within a model of depression caused by learned helplessness is to encourage strategies for self-assertion and control over events – not a 'coming to terms' or changing cognitive sets. (Fernando 1986: 130–1)

Fernando, together with others interested in the concept of 'stress', employs epidemiological knowledge and strategies but grounds them in culture and in the specific meaning experiences have for the patient. This, it seems, is one area where the partnership between psychiatry and sociology and social anthropology proper (not merely as servicers of psychiatry) can flourish.

What the social conditions are that make for either particularly high or low rates of an illness *within* one culture or its more rapid or slower recovery rates remains an urgent topic of both epidemiological and sociological investigation. The sophistication of the concepts employed here has developed from straightforward 'stress', usually translated as 'life events' or 'social class' or 'marital status', to a multifactorial examination of particular stressors for particular gender and class and ethnic groups in given situations of 'vulnerability' that have powerful effects on self-esteem (Brown and Harris 1978)[66] and of complex interrelationships with psychological meaning, such as mastery and control over events and of one's own life (Thoits 1987).[67]

Of course, simple measurement of life events and outcomes does not *explain* the rates so obtained, any more than simply collecting data about diagnostic categories explains any differences found. It is this explanatory level that brings us back to our ancestors – both Durkheim and Weber. For Brown and Harris, for example, it is not simply that women, in the face of a severe life difficulty, are more vulnerable to depression if they lack a confiding relationship, a job outside the home, and have three children or more under 14 living at home; rather, it is the meaning of this that has to be understood. What is it about being a woman, about the relationship between women and men, about the place of paid employment, about roles (this is explored by Thoits) that is important? And, further, what are the psychological mechanisms (that might, of course, have organic concomitants) that are invoked in such situations? In a word, data-driven research – research that is done because there is a technique of measurement or analysis waiting to be employed – may add nothing to understanding.

Second, although the epidemiologist, working with a disease model, will expect to explain the incidence of any particular illness discovered by ignoring differences in meaning and reducing the possibilities to the smallest factor unravelled in *micro-analysis* of the genetics, biology, physiology, or chemistry undertaken in detailed laboratory studies of the blood groups, diets, viral exposure, hormone imbalance, brain chemistry, and so forth of the populations found to be most at risk compared with those least at risk, there is another direction to pursue.

The investigator can accept the definition as given of the disturbance but move to a broad *macro-analysis* that places the rate in the particular context in which it has been located and where it was generated, and is directed to taking account of particular meanings. Socio-anthropologist Nancy Scheper-Hughes's study of schizophrenia in rural Ireland furnishes an excellent example of the kind of work I have in mind (Scheper-Hughes 1979).[66]

Scheper-Hughes analyses the published figures that repeatedly show the highest rates of schizophrenia among Irish people, not only in Ireland but also in the United States after emigration. She stresses, too, another epidemiological finding: that the huge excess of schizophrenics in Ireland is among *single* people and men. This is not an illness of women or married people. Nor does it appear as early as it does elsewhere – rather it occurs first in young, bachelor men in their thirties. Nor do those who become sick marry and have children; they are outcasts from the pairing and child-bearing system. So a genetic disposition seems unlikely to provide an adequate explanation. Scheper-Hughes wants to understand and explain this differential, without denying a biological basis to the illness, but in terms of the cultural and structural worlds within which the Irish person is nurtured and in which they must survive. Using Thematic Apperception Tests and lengthy interviews, together with her own skills in participant observation, as she lived with her husband and two small children among the people of 'Ballybran', she identifies the heightened risk in terms of a whole complex of cultural and economic conditions. Patterns of farming, of emigration, of Catholicism and repressed sexuality, the specific position of individuals based on their gender and birth-order combine to drive the youngest sons mad and to exclude them from marriage and a satisfying maturity. She turns also to labelling theory for help in understanding why certain kinds of mental aberration are not identified as requiring hospital admission – the 'Saints' of her title – where others are.

Perhaps there is no answer in rural Ireland other than the massive hospitalization and drug therapies currently pursued, for the economic life of

47

those areas is, she thinks, doomed; they are dying. On the other hand, perhaps profound socio-political change would reduce the rates of schizophrenia faster than any other treatment currently available.

In sum, the epidemiologist who can incorporate the best of sociological theorizing about the nature of the relationship between a particular set of structural and cultural conditions and the individual becoming disturbed, breaching social norms, being identified as mentally ill and requiring treatment, and the sociologist or social anthropologist who maintains always a critical and sceptical eye to any observation but who can join in the rigorous and, usually, numerically skilled work of the epidemiologist, have as much to offer one another in 1988 as they did in in 1958.

Acknowledgement: I am grateful to Colin Samson and Scott Pimley for help in the preparation of this chapter and to John Clausen for his comments on an earlier draft.

NOTES

1. Earls, F. (1987) 'Epidemiology of psychiatric disorders in children and adolescents', in G. Klerman, M. Weissman, P. Appelbaum, and L. Roth (eds) *Social, Epidemiologic and Legal Psychiatry*, vol. 5 of *Psychiatry*, New York: Basic Books, 133.

2. Lawson, A. (1966) *The Recognition of Mental Illness in London* (Maudsley Monograph No. 15), London: Oxford University Press. See pp. 1–2 for a definition of social psychiatry.

3. John Clausen summarizes social psychiatry now as embracing 'all those aspects of diagnosis, the aetiology, course and treatment of mental illness that are influenced by socio-cultural context in which each person develops', in 'Social psychiatry revisited', address to the Conference on Social Psychiatry, Tunghai University, Taiwan, 6 June 1987.

4. Shepherd, M., Cooper, B., Brown, A.C., and Kalton, G.W. (1966) *Psychiatric Illness in General Practice*, London: Oxford University Press.

5. See Martin Blumer's edited collection in honour of Philip Abrams (1985) *Essays on the History of Sociological Research*, Cambridge: Cambridge University Press, especially Halsey, A.H. 'Provincials and professionals: the British post-war sociologists', 151–64.

6. Using psychoanalysis, similar hopes were shared by members of the 'Culture and Personality' school represented particularly by Clyde Kluckhohn (1949), Margaret Mead (1928), Ruth Benedict (1934) and Abraham Kardiner, Ralph Linton, and C. DuBois (1945).

7. See Littlewood, R. (1986) 'Russian dolls and Chinese boxes: an anthropological approach to the implicit models of comparative psychiatry', in J. Cox (ed.) *Transcultural Psychiatry*, Bromley: Croom Helm. He points to increasing specialization, particularly in Britain: 'The syllabus for the examination for Membership to the Royal College of Psychiatrists in Britain includes social anthropology but no essay question has ever been set' (p. 38). In the United States, by contrast, chairs are held jointly in psychiatry and anthropology and Arthur Kleinman edits *Culture, Medicine and Psychiatry* from Harvard.

8. I use the term 'social action' in the Weberian sense: behaviour is the knees bent, the arms flexed, and the palms of the hands joined, the head bent and the eyes shut,

lips moving. Social action is praying. The praying might be considered a symptom of illness if the person does it in the middle of a busy street or continuously. It has a whole range of possible meanings depending on the particular individuals involved, their unique circumstances, desires, and beliefs.

9. First published in 1897 following an article that appeared in 1888 on suicide and the birth rate, which was falling as the suicide rate was rising, and a course of lectures in 1889–90.

10. In fact, Durkheim did not have the data to permit him to identify the person who had committed suicide with their actual religious affiliation; the measure was only one of the preponderance of one religion over another within a geographical area. Clearly, it is possible, if improbable, that all suicides were actually of Catholics in a predominantly Protestant area and vice versa. For a recent critique of Durkheim using similar contemporary data to those available to Durkheim, see Day, L.H. (1987) 'Durkheim on religion and suicide – a demographic critique', *Sociology* 21: 449–61.

11. Married women did not show this difference and the rates were not greatly different for men.

12. Durkheim did not actually begin there either. He had fairly well developed ideas about his theory before he used the empirical data. In other words, this was both deductive and inductive work.

13. He also described 'egoistic', 'altruistic', and 'fatalistic' forms of suicide but it is anomic suicide and anomie that has entered everyday sociology and captured the imagination as surely as has Marx's concept of 'alienation'. Steven Lukes, in his classic work on Durkheim (first published by Allen Lane in 1973), points out that 'anomie differs from egoism and altruism in that it depends not on how individuals are attached to society but on how it regulates them' (Lukes, Penguin edition, 1977: 207). (Fatalism occurs in over-regulation where the individual becomes powerless.) Thus, anomie is most clearly sociological; it is the result of social forces, of the 'social fact', as concrete as any material stick or stone, external to the individual and constraining (or enabling) action.

14. See Townsend, P. (1985) 'Surveys of poverty to promote democracy', and Baric, L.F. (1985) 'Reading the palm of the invisible hand: indicators, progress and prediction', both in M. Bulmer (ed.) *Essays on the History of Sociological Research*, Cambridge: Cambridge University Press.

15. Sprott, W.H. (1962) *Sociology at the Seven Dials*, London: Athlone Press.

16. Abrams, P. (1985) 'The uses of British sociology', in M. Bulmer (ed.), op. cit.

17. Srole *et al.* used impairment measures in the Midtown studies. See Srole, L., Langner, T.S., Michael, S.T., Opler, M.K., and Rennie, T.A.C. (1962) *Mental Health in the Metropolis: The Midtown Manhattan Study*, New York: McGraw-Hill.

18. Janowitz, M. (1970) *Political Conflict*, Chicago: Quadrangle.

19. Abrams, P. (1985) 'The uses of British sociology', in M. Bulmer (ed.), op. cit.

20. Eaton, W. (1986) *The Sociology of Mental Disorders*, New York: Praeger, p. 42.

21. Wing, J.K. (1978) *Reasoning About Madness*, London: Oxford University Press.

22. Richard Neugebauer, Bruce Dohrenwend, and Barbara Snell Dohrenwend, reviewing the prevalence of disorders in the American adult population, state that 'different concepts and methods have led to very different estimates of amounts of disorder in these studies'. From 'Formulation of hypotheses about the true prevalence of functional psychiatric disorders among adults in the United States', in B. Dohrenwend, B.S. Dohrenwend, M.S. Gould, B. Link, R. Neugebauer, and R. Wunsch-Hitzig (eds) (1980) *Mental Illness in the United States: Epidemiological Estimates*, New York: Praeger, pp. 45–94.

23. World Health Organization (1973) *International Pilot Study of Schizophrenia*, Geneva: WHO; also the current WHO *Collaborative Study*.

24. For the US–UK Diagnostic Project, see Cooper, J.E., Kendell, R., Gurland, B.J., Sharpe, L., Copeland, J.R.M., and Simon, R. (1972) *Psychiatric Diagnosis in New York and London* (Maudsley Monograph No. 20), London: Oxford University Press; WHO (1979) *Schizophrenia: International Follow-Up Study*, Chichester: Wiley.

25. Julian Leff has pointed out that the difference in mania found between Aarhus, Denmark, and Camberwell, London, in the IPSS (16 per cent: 5 per cent) disappeared when case registers were established in both centres, suggesting the first difference 'was an artefact attributable to differences in referral and admission practices'. Leff, J. (1986) 'The epidemiology of mental illness across cultures', in J. Cox (ed.), op. cit., 23–36.

26. Leff, in the work quoted above, summarizes these difficulties in cross-cultural work, pointing out that many societies have no words to express western concepts such as anxiety or depression and that even when local scales are devised, translation to produce universal categories remains fraught with difficulty.

27. Thus studies within urban areas using standardized measures have produced rates of schizophrenia that are comparable with other similar areas. See Hodiamont, P., Peer, N., and Syben, N. (1987) 'Epidemiological aspects of psychiatric disorder in a Dutch health area', *Psychological Medicine* 17: 495–505.

28. Sartorius, N., Jablensky, A., Korten, A., Ernberg, G., Anker, M., Cooper, J.E., and Day, R. (1986) *Psychological Medicine* 16 (4): 909–28.

29. Morris, J.N. (1957) *Uses of Epidemiology*, Edinburgh: Churchill Livingstone.

30. Shepherd, M. (1982) 'The application of the epidemiological method in psychiatry', in T.A. Baasher, *et al.* (eds) *Epidemiology and Mental Health Services: Principle and Applications for Developing Countries* (*Acta Psychiatrica Scandinavia* Supplement 296, vol. 65).

31. Shepherd, M., Oppenheim, A.N., and Mitchell, S. (1971) *Childhood Behaviour and Mental Health*, London: University of London Press. Listing the prevalence of so-called symptoms of childhood disturbance such as bed-wetting in boys made it possible to see that what was common at four was relatively uncommon at fourteen. Such findings have clear implications for the construction of a medical problem and for treatment. 'With these data,' Shepherd noted later, 'it has proved possible to construct a picture of behavioural *norms*' (Baasher, op. cit., p. 11).

32. Eaton, W. (1986) *The Sociology of Mental Disorders*, New York: Praeger, and Cockerham, W. .(1981) *The Sociology of Mental Disorder*, Englewood Cliffs, NJ: Prentice Hall, summarize these major and consistent findings.

33. Goffman, E. (1961) *Asylums: Essays on the Social Situation of Mental Patients and Other Inmates*, New York: Doubleday; Rosenhan, D. (1973) 'On being sane in insane places', *Science* 179: 250–8.

34. Lemert, E. (1967) *Human Deviance, Social Problems and Social Control*, Englewood Cliffs, NJ: Prentice Hall; Goffman, E. (1968) *Stigma: Notes on the Management of Spoiled Identity*, Harmondsworth: Penguin.

35. Chesler, P. (1973) *Women and Madness*, New York: Avon Books; Showalter, E. (1986) *The Female Malady: Women, Madness and English Culture, 1830–1980*, New York: Pantheon; Penfold, S. and Walker, G. (1984) *Women and the Psychiatric Paradox*, Milton Keynes: Open University Press; Joan Busfield argues that the typical excess of affective disorder in women and of schizophrenia in men may be the result of 'differential involvement of the psychiatric profession with women' (Busfield, J. 'Gender, mental illness and psychiatry', in M. Evans and C. Ungerson (eds) (1983) *Sexual Divisions: Patterns and Processes*, London: Tavistock, 106–35).

36. See Littlewood, R. and Lipsedge, M. (1982) *Aliens and Alienists: Ethnic Minorities and Psychiatry*, Harmondsworth: Penguin; Fernando, S. (1986) 'Depression in ethnic minorities', in J. Cox (ed.), op. cit., pp. 107–38; Schwab, J., Bell, R., Warheit, E., and Schwab, R. (1979) *Social Order and Mental Health: The Florida Health Study*, New York: Brunner/Mazel; Littlewood, R. and Cross, S. (1980) 'Ethnic

minorities and psychiatric services', *Sociology of Health and Illness* 2 (2): 194–201.

37. Smith, D.K. (1978) 'K is mentally ill', *Sociology* 12 (1).

38. Lawson, A. (op cit., 1966); Gurin, G., Veroff, J., and Feld, S.C. (1960) *Americans View Their Mental Health*, New York: Basic Books; Douvan, E. and Kulka, R. (1981) *Mental Health in America*, New York: Basic Books.

39. Duster, T. (1984) 'Biological knowledge', in T. Duster and K. Garret (eds) *Cultural Perspectives on Biological Knowledge*, Norwood, NJ: Ablex.

40. Littlewood, R. (1986) 'Russian dolls and Chinese boxes', in J. Cox (ed.), op. cit., 43.

41. Schutz, A. (1945) 'On multiple realities', *Philosophy and Phenomenological Research* 5: 533–76.

42. See Giddens, A. (1976) *New Rules of Sociological Method*, London: Hutchinson, pp. 23–33, for an account and critique of phenomenology.

43. See Brown, G. and Harris, T. (1978) *The Social Origins of Depression*, London: Tavistock, chapter five on 'meaning', for a discussion of this approach.

44. Leading scholars are: Schur, E. (1969) 'Reactions to deviance: a critical assessment', *American Journal of Sociology* 49: 499–507; Becker, H. (ed.) (1963) *Outsiders: Studies in the Sociology of Deviance*, Glencoe, Ill.: Free Press; Erikson, K. (1962) 'Notes on the sociology of deviance', in Becker (op. cit., 1963), and (1966) *Wayward Puritans*, New York: Wiley; Kitsuse, J. (1962) 'Societal reaction to deviant behaviour', in Becker (op. cit. 1963); and Lemert, E. (1951) *Social Pathology*, New York: McGraw-Hill. The last-named was the originator of the idea of primary and secondary deviance but his ideas were not really taken up until after they were further developed in 1967 in *Human Deviance, Social Problems and Social Control*, Englewood Cliffs, NJ: Prentice-Hall.

45. Scheff, T. (1966) *Being Mentally Ill*, Chicago: Aldine.

46. Cohen, S. (1971) *Images of Deviance*, Harmondsworth: Penguin (for the National Deviancy Conference).

47. Taylor, I., Walton, P., and Young, J. (1973) *The New Criminology*, London: Routledge & Kegan Paul; Taylor, I., Walton, P., and Young, J. (1975) *Critical Criminology*, London: Routledge & Kegan Paul.

48. Especially Walter Gove who conducted careful studies of various aspects of the labelling process, demonstrating its inadequacy to account, for example, for the difference in female and male rates of mental illness: Gove, W. (ed.) (1974) *The Labelling of Deviance: Evaluating a Perspective*, London and Beverly Hills: Sage; Gove, W. (ed.) (1982) *Deviance and Mental Illness*, London and Beverly Hills: Sage.

49. Hindess, B. (1973) *The Use of Official Statistics in Sociology*, London: Macmillan. And see also Box, S. (1971) *Deviance, Reality and Society*, New York: Holt, Rinehart and Winston, chapter five.

50. The paradox that British sociology is considered among the best in the world at the same time as its numeracy and sophistication in quantitative research are less advanced is set out in the ESRC report, *Horizons and Opportunities in the Social Science* (1987), chaired by Griffith Edwards.

51. Garfinkel, H. (1968) *Studies in Ethnomethodology*, Englewood Cliffs, NJ: Prentice-Hall; Cicourel, A. (1964) *Method and Measurement in Sociology*, Glencoe, Ill.: Free Press; Cicourel, A. (1968) *The Social Organization of Juvenile Justice*, New York: Wiley; Turner, R. (ed.) (1974) *Ethno-methodology*, Harmondsworth: Penguin.

52. Douglas, J. (1967) *The Social Meanings of Suicide*, Princeton: Princeton University Press. See also Atkinson, J.M. (1978) *Discovering Suicide: Studies in the Social Organisation of Sudden Death*, London: Macmillan.

53. Coulter, J. (1973) *Approaches to Insanity*, Chichester: Wiley, employs the ethnomethodological perspective in relation to other categories of mental illness.

54. Murphy, J.M. (1986) 'Cross-cultural psychiatry', in G. Klerman, M. Weissman,

P. Appelbaum, and L. Roth (eds) *Social, Epidemiological and Legal Psychiatry*, vol. 5 of *Psychiatry*, New York: Basic Books, chapter two.

55. Robins, L., Helzer, J., Croughan, J., and Ratcliff, K. (1981) 'National Institute of Mental Health Diagnostic Interview Schedule', *Archives of General Psychiatry* 38: 381–9.

56. 'Self-defeating disorder aka masochism' and 'paraphilic coercive disorder aka rapism'. The former remains in Appendix A. The latter has not been incorporated although sadism (excluding sexual sadism) is also in Appendix A. Various other paraphilic disorders that can include the commission of rape remain.

57. Huffine, C. (1987), personal communication.

58. Hakim, C. 'Social monitors: population censuses as social surveys', in M. Bulmer (ed.) op. cit., 43–44, notes that women were as involved in the labour force in mid-nineteenth-century England as they are now.

59. Miller, J.B. (1976) *Towards a New Psychology of Women*, Boston: Beacon (Harmondsworth: Penguin, 1978); Chodorow, N. (1978) *The Reproduction of Mothering: Psychoanalysis and the Sociology of Gender*, Berkeley: University of California Press; Gilligan, C. (1982) *In a Different Voice*, Harvard: Harvard University Press.

60. Lehtiner, V. and Konkama, M. (1987) 'Mental disorders in a sample representative of the whole adult Finnish population', in B. Cooper (ed) *Psychiatric Epidemiology: Progress and Prospects*, Bromley: Croom Helm.

61. Penfold, S. and Walker, G. (1984) *Women and the Psychiatric Paradox*, Milton Keynes: Open University Press.

62. The MS Society is an example of the former kind of self-help patient group, ARMS (Action for Research in Multiple Sclerosis) an example of the latter. In practice, members of both groups (and some join both) who have MS have become considerable experts in their illness, and both groups provide advice and support and raise funds for research. ARMS decides independently of medical advice which projects to pursue.

63. Although Kenny, cited by Littlewood, has suggested '*latah* in its cross-cultural distribution is no more of a paradox than is the fact that all people have hands, but only some cultures have exploited the fact in requiring them to be shaken in formal greeting'. Littlewood, R. (1985), in *Psychiatric Medicine* 17 (1), reviewing Simons, R.C. and Hughes, C.C. (eds) (1985) *The Culture Bound Syndromes: Folk Illnesses of Psychiatric and Anthropological Interest*, Dordrecht, Boston: Reidel.

64. Littlewood, R. (1986) 'Russian dolls and Chinese boxes', in J. Cox (ed.), op. cit., p. 50.

65. Fernando, S. (1986) 'Depression in Ethnic Minorities', in J. Cox (ed.), op. cit., 107–38.

66. Brown, G. and Harris, T., op. cit.

67. Thoits, P. (1987) 'Gender and marital status differences in control and distress: common stress versus unique stress explanations', *Journal of Health and Social Behavior*, 28: 17–22, argues that life events are not, in and of themselves, damaging to people of certain status groups (women, the unmarried, lower social class, etc.). Rather, the relationship with psychological disturbance is mediated by such factors as whether or not the events in question are controllable and whether or not the person has mastery over situations. For example, both depression and anxiety are positively correlated to a sense of mastery. Among married males there is a negative relationship with anxiety and depression but a positive relationship with mastery. Thus, it is particular roles that individuals hold that account for much of the stress (p. 18).

68. Scheper-Hughes, N. (1979) *Saints, Scholars and Schizophrenics: Mental Illness in Rural Ireland*, Berkeley: University of California Press.

4

The Contribution of Psychology

Monica Briscoe

'Many of the facts, and even some of the principles, that psychologists have discovered when they may have thought they were discovering something else are useful.' (Skinner 1987: 782)

Definitions of a science are often misleading. In no case is this more true than that of psychology, for much confusion exists as to what should be its proper subject matter. The roots of this are largely historical. During the heyday of behaviourism, it was fashionable to define psychology narrowly as the science of behaviour. For a long time scientific psychologists ignored questions that were of central importance to the understanding of mind, while their activities were almost restricted to the study of learning in the rat. More recently, subjective factors have been readmitted so that psychology is now commonly regarded as the science of behaviour and experience (Pritchard 1986). However, within the discipline there are inevitably many different areas using different levels of explanation. This variety has prompted Beloff (1973) to propose that there is no single science of psychology but rather a number of sciences, each asking different questions, using different methods, and making different assumptions. Certainly, discipline boundaries are somewhat arbitrary and artificial, especially in the human sciences, and the essential core of psychology is particularly difficult to identify. However, Radford (1987: 283) has specified its particular focus of interest as being 'the individual as an emergent product of physiology and society'.

Not only is the essence of psychology difficult to define, but its relationship with the world to which it might be expected to relate is also particularly problematic. This is partly because the topics of theoretical interest tend to be very specific, seeking to explain only a tiny portion of behaviour as it occurs in a carefully defined and restricted situation. Thus it has been said, with some truth, that academic psychology 'consists in knowing more and more about less and less' (Watson 1963: 487). As a result, psychologists are not taken very seriously as experts, especially because the everyday experience of relating to other people necessitates everyone being his or her own psychologist. A scientific approach stresses certainty and lawfulness but most people do not view human behaviour as either comprehensible or predictable. It might be expected that a world full of essentially human problems and a science devoted to the analysis of (human) behaviour would be addressing each other constantly and productively. Yet, in practice, students of the subject tend to find that psychology is interesting but not particularly useful (Radford 1985). Because its subject matter lies within common experience, it is not only dismissed as nothing more than common sense but also compared unfavourably with other sciences. Ironically, a further degree of prejudice actually arises from the confusion of psychology with psychiatry, so that the former is tainted with the stigma of mental illness in the lay mind.

Psychiatrists are no more immune to such misconceptions than any other section of the population. And yet psychiatry is as much a branch of psychology as of medicine. A basic premise in psychology is that an appreciation of the wide variation in 'normality' is fundamental to the understanding of abnormal functioning. Major branches are concerned with the assessment of individual differences in personality and intelligence. This philosophy also underlies the procedures for post-graduate training in applied psychology. For example, as a prerequisite of their specialization, those wishing to become educational psychologists are required to undertake several years' teaching of normal children on top of their basic studies in general psychology. Medical education, on the other hand, concentrates on the diagnosis and treatment of pathological conditions; the study of normal functioning is abandoned at a relatively early stage. Nevertheless, some of the most successful examples of applied psychology are to be found in the clinical sphere. Psychologists have developed a wide range of behaviour and cognitive therapies, originally derived from learning theory but more recently incorporating a cognitive perspective also (Eysenck 1975). Other examples include the application of intelligence testing to the diagnostic process in neuropsychiatry. Thus, despite its comparative youth, psychology has established itself as a basic science of psychiatry, in a relationship paralleling that between physiology and somatic disease (Lewis 1967).

Farrell (1985: 14) has observed that it is its psychological subject matter which makes psychiatry important and distinctive in medicine, even though, 'as a psychological enquiry, psychiatry is still in a very primitive stage'. In view of this, it is hardly surprising that a number of ideological positions have evolved, including the biological, the dynamic, the behavioural, and the social, each of which places a different emphasis on the respective contributions of man, culture, and nature to the phenomenon of mental illness (Clare 1976). Interest in social psychiatry stems from the belief that mental illness is a product of civilization, a viewpoint which has been traced back to Democritus in the fifth century BC (Schwab and Schwab 1978). It seeks to discover the social causes of disorder in the hope that this will lead to the rational development of social methods of prevention, and that increased understanding of social influences on course and outcome will suggest appropriate techniques of treatment and rehabilitation. The topics of interest include all aspects of the social causes, concomitants and consequences of psychiatric disorder, together with social techniques for dealing with them. Social psychiatrists are also concerned with planning and evaluating social and medical services as well as the assessment of the psychiatric implications of public policy in such areas as employment, education, and housing.

There are three major causal hypotheses which have received a great deal of attention in this field. The first is that the loss of one's mother in childhood predisposes the individual to depressive illness in later life (Tennant, Bebbington and Hurry 1980), an approach with its roots in the psychoanalytic tradition (Bowlby 1958). The second is that recent exposure to adverse experiences or events leads to an increased incidence of psychiatric disorder. This model postulates that a vulnerable individual will develop an episode of disease only if it is triggered by a life-event stressor. However, findings from a number of studies indicate that less than ten per cent of the variance in the occurrence of episodes is linked to such adverse experiences (Rabkin and Struening 1976). Since there seem to be many individuals who do not develop disorders after such exposure, it seems that there must also be some quite powerful modifying influences. Third, there has been considerable interest in investigating the importance of social networks as just such a moderating variable for absorbing the impact of stress. Thus, it has been suggested that a deficiency in social relationships might be a causal factor in the onset of neurosis, although the evidence for this is limited (Henderson, Byrne and Duncan-Jones 1981).

These three views as to aetiology are in no way mutually exclusive (Brown and Harris 1978). It is, however, clear from them that social psychiatrists rely on no single underlying theory. Indeed, they draw on diverse disciplines, including biology, psychology, and sociology. The relation to sociology is particularly close because there is a common concern with the various social phenomena reflected in the relationship of society to mental illness and its sufferers. Hence, there are instances of considerable overlap in both topic and method, as, for example, in Durkheim's (1897) classic study of suicide. This involved the empirical exploration of the social correlates of suicide as well as theorizing about the influence of collective processes on the individual's tendency towards self-destruction. The distinction between sociology and social psychology is by no means clear-cut, but central to the former is the view that explanations at the societal level of analysis are satisfactory and not reducible to psychological or biological concepts. Important contributions to the ideas used in social psychiatry have also come from sociological approaches to deviance, stratification, collective behaviour, and institutions, as well as studies of the family, small groups, and social networks.

The main tool of the social psychiatrist is, however, the epidemiological method, which is essentially the study of human populations based on rates of illness. Epidemiology differs from clinical medicine in that its focus is not primarily on the characteristics of patients but on 'the patterns of disease occurrence in human populations and of the factors that influence these patterns' (Lilienfeld and Lilienfeld 1980: 3). The clinical approach cannot answer epidemiological questions since the information available is restricted to patients under medical care. Hence, clinical findings cannot be contrasted with those in other members of the same population who are free from the condition under consideration. Barker and Rose (1984) have pointed out that in order to conduct standardized examinations of large numbers of (mostly healthy) people, epidemiologists have to accept lower standards of diagnostic accuracy than clinicians. Conversely, 'problems of case definition and quality control of measurements must be considered more rigorously in population than in clinical studies' (Barker and Rose 1984: 30). The underlying philosophy of epidemiology is actually closely akin to that of the *nomothetic* approach within psychology. This seeks to build up an objective and quantitative picture of the parameters of a population. The aim of nomothetic research is the establishment of universal laws, generally through the use of the quantitative (mostly multivariate) and experimental methods of psychology. Such a strategy stands in contrast to the *idiographic* approach, in which the focus of concern is on the description of unique events and specific individuals, a position closely analogous to that of the clinician. Within psychology, researchers favouring the idiographic position tend to prefer a subjective approach and stress the need for intuitive understanding of each individual. It is, however, important to appreciate that the size of the population studied is not necessarily a criterion to be used in differentiating the nomothetic from the idiographic. This applies even when the population under consideration is restricted to a single individual. Thus, Freud (1900) was endeavouring to discover the general principles underlying dreaming on the basis of data derived primarily from himself. Moreover, among experimental psychologists, we find the example of Ebbinghaus (1885), who used just one subject in his search for general laws of memory. Although no absolute distinctions can be drawn, this may be contrasted with the essentially idiographic work of Luria (1969), who spent over thirty years studying a single case involving an unusual capacity for remembering.

What then does psychology have to offer epidemiological psychiatry? The primary contribution is methodological. A large body of knowledge has been developed both in the field and under laboratory conditions about observational methods, including interviewing techniques, questionnaire design, and attitude measurement (Davies 1972). Sadly, the psychological literature in these areas remains largely unknown to psychiatrists, resulting, at best, in unnecessary duplication of effort (e.g. at the pilot stage of a questionnaire) or, at worst, in the use of clumsy and badly constructed instruments. A specific example of the lack of communication between psychologists and psychiatrists interested in epidemiology concerns the failure of the latter to make use of standard psychometric tests for case identification. Thus, for example, it would seem that some of the tests of cognitive function developed by clinical psychologists might have considerable potential for exploring the epidemiology of dementia. In practice, however, these validated tests are often ignored and assessments attempted through the use of psychiatrists' own instruments.

The clinical interview is the major psychiatric tool for arriving at a diagnosis. Diagnosis is an application of both psychology and psychiatry. However, the categorization of mental disorder and the phenomenological investigations on which diagnoses are based arise largely from psychiatry, whereas the development of systematic interviews and the determination of their reliability and validity stem primarily from psychology (Oppenheim 1966). In itself the interview is a form of natural conversation and its special characteristics have only recently been appreciated. Psychology's successes in providing psychometric methods for assessing intelligence and personality by the use of systematic tests and inventories served to challenge the somewhat haphazard way in which interviews had been carried out by psychiatrists. The development of psychometric methods has also served to encourage the construction of self-rating inventories to be completed by patients as well as checklists for interviewers. Self-report instruments, such as the General Health Questionnaire (Goldberg 1972), have the advantage of eliminating interview bias and interpretation. The emphasis is on the individual's response rather than on the response of the interviewer to the patient's behaviour. Inevitably, however, such measures are useful principally for surveys of psychiatric morbidity in the general population, rather than being suitable for the classification of inpatients.

A major area of research in social psychology deals with the way people interpret the causality of events, and such research has great importance for psychiatry (Nisbett and Valins 1971). Attribution theory is concerned with meaning in social action and the motives and traits attributed to oneself and others under various conditions (Heider 1958). An attribution approach examines the way people appraise their inner states and behaviour and explain changes in feelings and experience (Harvey and Weary 1985). It is also concerned with the effects of such definitions on subsequent feelings and behaviour. The way symptoms and behaviour are conceptualized may have an important influence on the course of disorder, help-seeking, and rehabilitation. Thus, changes in assumptions about the capacity of the mentally ill to remain in the community are as much a product of changing attributions as of new knowledge. Historically, many attributions made to the helplessness, irresponsibility, and dangerousness of the mentally ill actually served to exacerbate such reactions by isolating and stigmatizing patients. Conversely, it is now clear that normalization of symptoms and an emphasis on positive aspects of behaviour and experience may do a lot to maintain and enhance social functioning. Thus, for example, it is increasingly recognized that the improvement of the mental health services depends on the strengthening of the family doctor in his therapeutic role rather than on a large proliferation and expansion of specialist psychiatric services (Shepherd 1987).

It is also clear that the difficulties faced by any individual may be determined as much by social structure as by personal traits. Increasingly, the problems characteristically experienced by members of particular groups are being examined in terms of the ways in which social attributions and environmental organization limit the opportunities for such individuals to adjust to their circumstances. Such a trend can be made out in the literature concerning sex differences in psychiatric disorder. Numerous studies report a higher prevalence of psychological distress in women (Weissman and Klerman 1977). This is particularly true of the neuroses and manic depressive psychoses (i.e., disorders which involve personal discomfort). By contrast, the sex difference is either reversed or non-existent when personality disorders and schizophrenia are under consideration (Dohrenwend and Dohrenwend 1976). It has been argued that these differences reflect the general strains in the social role of women in contemporary society, which include the stresses and frustrated expectations of the housewife role and the discrepancies between education and preparation of women for adult roles and the realities of their daily lives. Thus, it has been suggested that marriage is much more protective for men than for women, and there are also indications that single women fare better than single men (Briscoe 1982). Certainly, attitudes to women are still more negative than those towards men, while inequality between the sexes is often attributed to women's primary role of housewife rather than worker, which itself has disastrous consequences for their self-image. Women's disadvantaged status has been perceived as contributing to a low level of psychological well-being both directly, in that women find their situation inherently depressing, and indirectly through the socially conditioned mechanism of *learned helplessness* (Seligman 1975) whereby young girls are socialized to value the stereotype of femininity and develop a cognitive set against assertiveness and independence.

Apart from general approaches, methodological issues, and measurement techniques, psychology also has substantive contributions to make to epidemiological and social psychiatry. Among the most fundamental come from the study of psycholinguistics. It is known that people all share identical types of processing capacities and, on the whole, have similar personal and social needs. Thus, for example, groups of speakers need to refer to objects and actions in their environment, and hence certain kinds of linguistic units reflect the basic human need to communicate experience. Specific languages may differ considerably in their precise form, but *all* languages share the common requirement to refer to objects. This reflection of common human desires, aspirations, and anxieties among all languages has been termed *linguistic universality.* Naturally, particular cultures differ in their needs according to environmental factors, so that the kinds of things for which people have words may differ from one linguistic community to another. The existence of such linguistic differences, which directly reflect cultural differences, has led to the concept of *linguistic relativity.* Thus, for example, distinguishing various forms of rice is relatively unimportant in western technological cultures but much more important where rice is a staple diet. The Hanunoo of the Philippine Islands have names for ninety-two varieties of rice, but all ninety-two varieties are, for the English speaker, simply *rice* (Brown 1965). In this context, it has been observed that the English language is extremely rich in words to describe mood states. Thus, 'in addition to "depressed" one can be despondent, despairing, disconsolate, dispirited, disillusioned, gloomy, melancholy, miserable, morbid, morose, unhappy, sad, and so on' (Rack 1982: 106). In many non-European languages, however, the emotional vocabulary is far more restricted. In Yoruba, for example, one word suffices for both 'angry' and 'sad', two emotions which most Europeans would consider to be quite distinct. In Ghana, just three words cover all shades of unpleasant emotion, their meaning perhaps being conveyed by the somewhat ambiguous English term, 'upset'. In contrast to its rich vocabulary of introspective words, English is very vague with regard to family relationships. Terms such as 'cousin' and 'brother-in-law' cover a variety of different relationships and role obligations, which would merit different words in most family-oriented cultures. Hence, the concept of linguistic relativity shows that, rather than some languages being primitive, each culture develops a rich vocabulary around the issues which seem particularly important to these people at that time.

The essential question in this field is, therefore, whether the experience of emotional distress is the same even if the vocabulary is different? If language serves to chart an experience introspectively, then it is at least possible that the internal experiences concerned are modified by the words available. As Rack has put it, 'if the only available word is "upset", is the experience equally non specific? Does the Pakistani not know whether he is anxious or miserable? . . . Two depressed patients (English and Pakistani) may be having similar emotional experiences, but we cannot be sure they are identical' (Rack 1982: 107–8). Rather than words merely reflecting patterns of thought and interest within a given society (as common sense might suggest), in its extreme form the notion of linguistic relativity implies that patterns of thought are actually shaped by the words a society has agreed to use. Thus, language serves not only to report experience but also to define it (Whorf 1956). As a result of this there will obviously be difficulties in translation. Rack (1982) has observed that it might actually be quite pointless to ask an Urdu speaker (for instance) whether his feelings are mainly those of 'anxiety' or of 'sadness', although a great deal of psychiatric diagnosis depends heavily on just such a question. Similar problems arise even among different sections within English society; inarticulate groups are less able to translate their knowledge into thoughts so that much emotional and introspective knowledge remains unnamed for them (Bernstein 1971). The notion of linguistic relativity suggests that thought and language are not independent processes, with the latter being the overt manifestation of the former. Rather, it appears that our thinking about the world is only possible through the ways in which we reflect it in language. Such findings are of major importance in many applied fields, including education and general medicine, but perhaps nowhere more than in psychiatry because of the central role of language in its diagnostic process.

Mechanic (1985) has argued that psychiatry is primarily an applied social science and therefore its concerns cannot be differentiated from those of the social and behavioural sciences more generally. Psychology is both a social and a behavioural science and hence basic to both epidemiology and social medicine. There is still much truth, however, in Ebbinghaus' (1908) famous dictum that psychology has a long past but only a short history. Its long past lies in the philosophical tradition, its short history is that of the experimental method. Inevitably, therefore, its contribution to social and epidemiological psychiatry is found less in the direct application of psychological findings than in the lending and exchanging of methods for joint investigation.

REFERENCES

Barker, D.J.P. and Rose, G. (1984) *Epidemiology in Medical Practice*, third edition, Edinburgh: Churchill Livingstone.
Beloff, J. (1973) *Psychological Sciences: A Review of Modern Psychology*, London: Crosby Lockwood Staples.
Bernstein, B.B. (1971) *Class, Codes and Control*, St Albans: Paladin.
Bowlby, J. (1958) 'The nature of the child's tie to his mother', *International Journal of Psychoanalysis* 39: 1–34.
Briscoe, M.E. (1982) *Sex Differences in Psychological Well-Being*, (Psychological Medicine Monograph Supplement 1).
Brown, G.W. and Harris, T. (1978) *Social Origins of Depression: A Study of Psychiatric Disorder in Women*, London: Tavistock.
Brown, R. (1965) *Social Psychology*, New York and London: Collier-Macmillan.
Clare, A.W. (1976) *Psychiatry in Dissent: Controversial Issues in Thought and Practice*, London: Tavistock.
Davies, R.M. (1972) *Fundamentals of Attitude Measurement*, New York: Wiley.
Dohrenwend, B.P. and Dohrenwend, B.S. (1976) 'Sex differences and psychiatric disorders', *American Journal of Sociology* 81: 1447–54.
Durkheim, E. (1897) *Le suicide: étude de sociologie*, Paris: Alcan, translated by J.A. Spaulding and G. Simpson (1951) *Suicide*, Glencoe, Ill.: Free Press.
Ebbinghaus, H. (1885) *Uber das Gedachtnis: Untersuchungen zur experimentallen Psychologie*, Leipzig: Duncker & Humblot, translated by H.A. Ruger and C.E. Bussenius (1964) *Memory: A Contribution to Experimental Psychology*, New York: Dover.

Ebbinghaus, H. (1908) *Abriss der Psychologie*, Leipzig: Veit & Co., translated by M. Miller (1908) *Psychology: An Elementary Textbook*, Boston: Heath.
Eysenck, H.J. (1975) 'Psychological theories and behaviour therapy', *Psychological Medicine* 5: 219-21.
Farrell, B.A. (1985) 'Philosophy and psychiatry: some reflections on the nature of psychiatry', in M. Shepherd (ed.) *Handbook of Psychiatry Volume 5: The Scientific Foundations of Psychiatry*, Cambridge: Cambridge University Press, pp. 3-15.
Freud, S. (1900) *The Interpretation of Dreams*, translated by J. Strachey (1953), London: Hogarth.
Goldberg, D. (1972) *The Detection of Psychiatric Illness by Questionnaire* (Maudsley Monograph No. 21), London: Oxford University Press.
Harvey, J.H. and Weary, G. (1985) *Attribution, Basic Issues and Applications*, London: Academic Press.
Heider, F. (1958) *The Psychology of Interpersonal Relations*, New York: Wiley.
Henderson, S., Byrne, D.G., and Duncan-Jones, P. (1981) *Neurosis and the Social Environment*, Sydney: Academic Press.
Lewis, A. (1967) 'Empirical or rational? The nature and basis of psychiatry', *Lancet* ii: 1-9.
Lilienfeld, A.M. and Lilienfeld, D.E. (1980) *Foundations of Epidemiology*, second edition, Oxford: Oxford University Press.
Luria, A.R. (1969) *The Mind of a Mnemonist*, translated from the Russian by L. Solitariff, London: Jonathan Cape.
Mechanic, D. (1985) 'Social science in relation to psychiatry', in M. Shepherd (ed.) *Handbook of Psychiatry Volume 5: The Scientific Foundations of Psychiatry*, Cambridge: Cambridge University Press, pp. 69-79.
Nisbett, R.E. and Valins, S. (1971) 'Perceiving the causes of one's own behavior', in E.E. Jones, D.E. Kanouse, H.H. Kelley, R.E. Nisbett, S. Valins, and B. Weiner (eds) *Attribution: Perceiving the Causes of Behavior*, Morristown, NJ: General Learning Press, pp. 63-78.
Oppenheim, A.N. (1966) *Questionnaire-Design and Attitude Measurement*, London: Heinemann.
Pritchard, M.J. (1986) *Medicine and the Behavioural Sciences*, London: Edward Arnold.
Rabkin, J.G. and Struening, E.L. (1976) 'Life events, stress and illness', *Science* 194: 1013-20.
Rack, P. (1982) *Race, Culture and Mental Disorder*, London: Tavistock.
Radford, J. (1985) 'Is the customer right? Views and expectations of psychology', *Psychology Teaching*, special edition, 15-27.
Radford, J. (1987) 'An education in psychology', *Bulletin of the British Psychological Society* 40: 282-9.
Schwab, J.J. and Schwab, M.E. (1978) *Sociocultural Roots of Mental Illness: An Epidemiologic Survey*, New York: Plenum.
Seligman, M.E.P. (1975) *Helplessness: On Depression, Development and Death*, San Francisco: W.H. Freeman & Co.
Shepherd, M. (1987) 'Mental illness and primary care', *American Journal of Public Health* 77 (1): 12-13.
Skinner, B.F. (1987) 'Whatever happened to psychology as the science of behavior?' *American Psychologist* 42 (8): 780-6.
Tennant, C., Bebbington, P., and Hurry, J. (1980) 'Parental death in childhood and risk of adult depressive disorders: a review', *Psychological Medicine* 10: 289-99.
Watson, R.I. (1963) *The Great Psychologists*, Philadelphia: Lippincott.

Weissman, M.M. and Klerman, G.L. (1977) 'Sex differences and the epidemiology of depression', *Archives of General Psychiatry* 34: 98–111.
Whorf, B.L. (1956) *Language, Thought and Reality: Selected Writings of Benjamin Lee Whorf*, edited by J.B. Carroll, New York: MIT Press.

5

Economic Appraisal

Greg Wilkinson and Anthony Pelosi

Economic appraisal consists of methods for formulating problems of choice, and for identifying and organizing the data required to aid decision-making. In health care it is concerned with the explicit specification and examination of different options with a view to assisting choice; with the systematic analysis of the costs and consequences of the different ways of achieving competing objectives; and with judgements about how to allocate scarce resources among competing ends.

Although well known, the principles and techniques of economic appraisal have been insufficiently employed in the field of mental health (May 1970; Regional Office for Europe, World Health Organization 1976; Frank 1981; National Institute of Mental Health 1981), and there are a variety of reasons for this. Economic considerations may conflict with the traditional medical approach: some doctors object to being involved in economic appraisal, believing that their overriding concern is clinical care, though it is being increasingly recognized within the profession that it is irresponsible to be unconcerned about the cost of clinical activities (Jennett 1984). In addition, the scope of economic evaluation in mental health programmes is limited by a lack of accepted medical and epidemiological measures of process and outcome, as well as of the economic impact of identification and treatment (Wilkinson and Pelosi 1987). As a result, the most effective and efficient ways of delivering mental health care are not clear.

CONCEPTUAL FRAMEWORK FOR ECONOMIC APPRAISAL

General framework

Land, labour, and capital resources are consumed by health care in order to produce improvements in health. Health care may be conceptualized as a commodity, albeit with some unusual and interesting characteristics, and its consequences may be categorized and measured as: *health effects* – in natural units; *benefits* – associated economic benefits; and *utilities* – satisfaction with health effects.

Table 5.1 Health care as a commodity

* Resources devoted to it are substantial and appear to be growing
* Governments are the principal source of financial support for the industry
* Private and voluntary organizations are major providers of the commodity
* The effectiveness of the commodity is uncertain
* New producers of the commodity are entering the industry in large numbers
* Each claims to provide a different effective version of the generic commodity
* Supply of the commodity has shifted from large institutional bases to small dispersed settings
* The commodity is so important to certain individuals that access cannot be legally denied because of inability to pay
* Most consumers purchase the commodity at zero price
* Government agencies are under pressure to restrict the access of consumers and to facilitate competition among suppliers, aiming to contain expenditure
* Government and non-profit suppliers have been slow to adopt thorough economic appraisal

Adapted from National Institute of Mental Health (1981)

Scarcity and choice

Economics concerns the relationship between diverse ends and scarce means which have alternative uses. This starting point implies that choices have to be made between various courses of action, and that decisions about the types and the extent of health care provided should be guided by explicit economic consideration of the options available. Discussion then centres on the social and political principles governing choice, especially the issues: 'whose choice?' (individual, institutional, recipient group, governmental); the related problem of the differing valuation of utilities; and on considerations of equity and distributive justice.

It follows from the above that cost is mostly usefully understood in terms of '*opportunity cost*'. This is the benefit that would be derived from a unit of resource in its best alternative use: it is axiomatic that choice results in an opportunity cost equal to the value of the alternative forgone.

Effectiveness and economic efficiency

To obtain the most effective use from the scarce resources expended on health, it is necessary to express effects in the form of costs and conse-quences *to the population* of a particular type of activity, and the improvements that could be obtained if more resources were to be made available (Cochrane 1972). From this perspective, the rational assessment of effectiveness in mental health care is best based on epidemiological methods. The role of health economics is to complement medical and epidemiological evaluation and to provide an estimate of efficiency. Economic efficiency requires the minimization of costs and the maximization of beneficial

Table 5.2 Measuring the costs and consequences of health care

Costs	Consequences
Costs – for organization and operation of service	(1) *Effects*
– professional time	– changes in physical, psychological, and social functioning
– supplies, equipment, power	
– capital costs	
Costs – borne by patients and families	(2) *Benefits* – for organization and operation of service
– expenses	– for original condition
– put into treatment	– for unrelated condition
– time off work*	*Benefits* – for patients and families
– psychic costs*	– savings in expenditure or leisure time
Other costs	– savings in lost work time*
– changes in resource use outside health sector	
	(3) *Utility*
	– changes in the quality of life of patients and families

Adapted from Drummond *et al.* (1987)
* Indirect costs or benefits

consequences, with the implication that choices in health care should be made so as to derive the maximum possible benefit from the resources at disposal. It follows that inefficiency denotes waste of scarce resources.

Measuring costs and consequences of health care

In health care it is often possible to measure direct and indirect costs and consequences in monetary units, but many difficulties arising in the valuation of less tangible items remain to be resolved.

The margin

It is necessary to introduce the concept of the margin, which is the increment added to costs or consequences by a unit increase in provision. For example, the marginal cost of one additional person using an under-used CT scanner is lower than the average cost since the resources have already been committed to the facility: average cost is higher than marginal cost because the overheads have been spread over a relatively small number of users (Glass and Goldberg 1977).

The significance of this is that investment of resources should be increased when marginal benefit exceeds marginal cost. The most efficient level of provision is attained when marginal cost is equal to marginal benefit.

Table 5.3 A model for cost accounting

Income and expenses of patient and family	Costs to the rest of the community
Patients' earnings after tax	Hospital costs
Family's earnings after tax	Other health service costs
Social security receipts	Local authority costs
Charges for local authority services	Social security payments
Travel costs	Less taxation received
Total	Total

Adapted from Glass and Goldberg (1977)
Costs are indicated as −ve and benefits as +ve

A model accounting system

A model accounting system for each patient studied, which can be extended for each year of the investigation and for each form of treatment under consideration has been developed by Glass and Goldberg (1977) (see Table 5.3).

Costs

The range of costs measured in a given study depends on the viewpoint of the analysis. For example, an item may be a cost to the patient but not to the providing agency; costs common to specified programmes need not be considered; and some categories of costs may be excluded because they will not substantially affect decision-making.

In economic appraisal, costs refer to resources consumed and are not restricted to expenditure. For example, they include resource use not easily reflected in market price, such as use of leisure time and voluntary activity. The appropriate concept is that of opportunity cost, though this may be difficult to estimate. Similarly, marginal or incremental costs are more relevant than average costs (see above).

Although the costing of most resource use is straightforward, more difficult problems are raised by the derivation of values for non-market items, capital outlays, average/marginal cost distinctions, overhead costs, the estimation of indirect costs, and, importantly, allowance for the differential timing of costs (discounting). These topics are covered by Williams and Anderson (1975) and Drummond *et al.* (1987).

Effects

The measurement of health care effects is principally a matter of medical and epidemiological concern. In the framework of economic appraisal, an effect should, whenever possible, apply to a final health output (e.g. life years

66

gained) or, less satisfactorily, to a closely related intermediate output (e.g. cases detected or patients treated).

In mental health care this usually requires valid and reliable measures of the patient's psychological, social, and physical functioning, and the burden of care on the patient's family. Since the ideal assessment is unattainable, it is important that explicit consideration should be given to the theoretical assumptions underlying the research instruments and other measures employed.

Benefits

The economic benefits of health care may be measured according to market valuations, clients' willingness-to-pay estimates, policy-makers' views, and professional opinion. The principles underlying the differing methods are described by Sugden and Williams (1979).

Market valuations exist or can be derived or estimated for most resource items. Nevertheless, a number of difficulties remain: for example, it may prove difficult to allow for the effects of health care on subsequent earnings and income (Glass and Goldberg 1977). If one form of treatment permits the patient to return to work earlier, the patient is better off by the difference between his after-tax income and his previous social security receipts and the community is better off in relation to the extent of his taxation and the reduced social security bill. In practice, to make an accurate assessment, it may be necessary to record earnings and social receipts annually for patients and their families. For these purposes social security benefits may be regarded as a cost to the 'rest of the community', since they are a transfer payment between the community as a whole and a particular patient and family.

A further question arises: how far should the valuation of intangible items be pursued (Drummond et al. 1987)? This depends on the amount of resources available to seek the relevant information, the extent to which that information is likely to alter the results of the study, and the likelihood that more informed decision-making will result. The extent to which quantification of intangible benefits is superior to qualitative assessment is not clearly established.

Even more difficult to value is the change in health status (including satisfaction in relationships, leisure, and occupation) of individuals receiving health care. Much attention has centred on the lack of an agreed measure of health benefits, particularly when different patient groups are compared, and the development of health status measurement as an empirical and explicit contribution to the resolution of some of these disagreements (Hurst 1983; Rosser 1983).

Utility

The perfect global measure of health would reflect the quality of life expectancy as well as its quantity, and would result in the derivation of a cardinal index based on a comparison of the relative valuations attached to different health states (Williams 1983).

Such utility values for health states may be obtained by judgement, from the literature, or by empirical measures (Weinstein and Fineberg 1980). Utilities sought depend on the approach of the study – the majority of utility analyses concern public policy decisions and so require a societal perspective. At the same time, it has to be stressed that the reliability and validity of measures of utility are uncertain: their main current justification is that they require explicit and objective specification (Drummond *et al.* 1987).

Techniques of economic appraisal

Five related techniques of economic appraisal are shown in table 5.4. These methods illustrate how the nature of health care consequences affects their measurement, valuation, and comparison to costs. Although economic appraisal of mental health services is discussed primarily in relation to cost-effectiveness and cost-benefit analysis, the evaluation of mental health programmes is rarely amenable to either of these techniques in their idealized form. There is seldom a single objective, and the different objectives cannot easily be combined or measured directly in monetary terms. Table 5.5 details a number of recent examples of economic appraisal in mental health.

Combining monetary and non-monetary costs and consequences

Full economic appraisal in mental health care would involve estimation of the

Table 5.4 Techniques of economic appraisal

---

* *Cost-analysis* – refers only to costs.
* *Cost-minimization analysis* refers to the identification of the least cost alternative of equally effective programmes with identical consequences.
* *Cost-effectiveness analysis* refers to the identification of comparative costs per unit effect of interest, where dissimilar programme costs are related to a single common effect, which differs in extent between alternative programmes. Cost-effectiveness compares the cost of achieving a goal by alternative means.
* *Cost-benefit analysis* refers to the identification of monetary costs and consequences of alternative programmes with disparate consequences, in order to express results in relation to a common (monetary) denominator: the ratio of monetary costs/benefits or the net benefit (or loss). To simplify, if benefits exceed costs, a cost-benefit analysis implies that the programme should be carried out.
* *Cost-utility analysis* refers to the identification of the utility or value of a specified level of health status, allowing for 'quality of life' adjustments to diverse treatment consequences and providing a common denominator (e.g. *QALYs*) for comparison of unlike consequences in different programmes.

Table 5.5 Recent examples of economic appraisal in mental health

Authors	Effectiveness and efficiency comparison
	Institutional care
Endicott *et al.* (1976)	Brief hospital care* with or without day care versus standard hospital care for newly admitted patients
	Community care
Weisbrod *et al.* (1980)	Community based* versus mental hospital treatment for chronically disabled patients
Fenton *et al.* (1982)	Home based* versus hospital psychiatric treatment for patients designated to receive hospital care
Hoult *et al.* (1983)	Comprehensive community treatment* versus hospital care for patients presenting for admission to hospital
(i) Schizophrenia	*Diagnosis related*
Jones *et al.* (1980)[1]	Two different services treating patients with schizophrenia: one, a psychiatric unit attached to a teaching district hospital*; the other, an area mental hospital with modern rehabilitation facilities
Falloon *et al.* (1985)	Behavioural family therapy* versus individual supportive psychotherapy as adjunct treatments in the aftercare management of schizophrenia in patients who continue to live in stressful family environments after treatment of the florid episode of schizophrenia
(ii) Neuroses	
Mangen *et al.* (1983)	Treatment by community psychiatric nurses* versus routine outpatient psychiatrist follow-up for patients with chronic neuroses
Ginsberg *et al.* (1984)	Behavioural therapy from a nurse therapist* versus routine general practitioner care for patients with neuroses (mainly phobics and obsessive-compulsives) in primary care
Dick *et al.* (1985)	Day hospital* versus hospital care for patients admitted as emergencies with neuroses, personality disorder or adjustment reaction

* Superior alternative in economic appraisal
[1] Not a randomised trial

costs of all services provided to achieve a specific aim and estimating the monetary value of all direct benefits (such as reduced use of hospital beds) and indirect benefits (such as reduced family burden). All these values should be corrected for inflation and interest discounted on funds saved or spent on future costs and benefits (Cardin *et al.* 1985). This objective has proved infeasible even in the most thorough analyses (Weisbrod *et al.* 1980).

As a practical solution, Glass and Goldberg (1977) characterize a method for interpreting the results of a study of alternative mental health services in which a conventional (monetary) economic appraisal is carried out, but non-monetary costs and consequences are measured separately. Following their scheme, two outcomes are possible. First, one service may be preferable – with monetary and non-monetary effects pointing in the same direction, or with no significant difference in one of the effects. In this case, one service dominates the other and should be preferred. Second, one service may be less expensive, but may provide a lower quality of service. An explicit judgement is then required about whether the extra quality that may be gained from the alternative service is worth the extra price – with worth being considered in relation to whether there are more valuable services which could be provided with the extra funds. These considerations may generate ideas for new services which combine the advantages of the previously specified services and are more cost-effective.

LIMITATIONS OF ECONOMIC APPRAISAL

The techniques of economic appraisal assume but do not establish the effectiveness of health services. Their value is clearly dependent upon the methodological criteria adopted in a particular investigation. Thus, economic appraisal can produce misleading findings if the range of costs and consequences relevant to a given study is not viewed comprehensively, if those not easily measured in monetary terms are omitted, and if there is no explicit presentation of variables for which quantitative measures are unavailable.

Moreover, the assumption is made in economic appraisal that resources freed or saved by preferred services are not wasted but are used in alternative beneficial ways. If these resources are squandered on ineffective programmes, overall health costs will increase without any improvement in the health status of the recipient group.

There are two further considerations. Although economic appraisal may help choice between services, it is less helpful in deciding whether to have a service at all. Also, the techniques of economic appraisal consume resources and should themselves be similarly appraised. They are likely to be of most benefit when programme objectives require clarification, options are significantly different, or large resource commitments are under consideration (Drummond *et al.* 1987).

Equity

The identity of recipient groups may be an important factor in assessing the social desirability of health policy, and the equitable distribution of costs and benefits across particular recipient groups thus becomes one of the competing dimensions upon which policy decisions are made. It is apparent that there may be a conflict between the pursuit of equity and of efficiency.

Clearly the pursuit of equity requires political definition as a goal of health care. Broad objectives of equitable health care provision may include equality of expenditure per capita; equality of input per capita; equality of input for equal need; equality of access for equal need; equality of use for equal need; equality of marginal met need; and equality of health (Culyer 1976). Equal treatment of equals (e.g. two groups of patients from the same area and with the same condition) may promote efficiency; unequal treatment of unequals (a group of patients with chronic schizophrenia versus a group with chronic renal failure) may mean that equity is exchanged for efficiency.

In addition, it is important to recognize that other areas of economics are relevant to mental health. For example, Segall and Vienonen (1987) have drawn attention to the development of an epidemiology of inequalities: the study of inequalities in income, wealth, and access to resources.

Ethics

Medical ethics is usually thought of in terms of individual virtue and duty, while economics embraces a broader concept of social ethics (Tancredi 1974). Economic appraisal may, therefore, appear to conflict with clinical judgement when medical values are challenged as not being conducive to the goal of maximizing health with the resources available. But as Mooney has argued in a related context:

> It is not a question of ethics *or* economics. Without a wider use of economics in health care inefficiencies will abound and decisions will be made less explicitly and hence less rationally than is desirable: we will go on spending large sums to save life in one way when similar lives but in greater numbers could be saved in another way. The price of inefficiency, inexplicitness and irrationality in health care is paid in death and sickness. Is *that* ethical?
> (Mooney 1980: 179)

Acknowledgement: Dr Wilkinson is supported by the Department of Health and Social Security. Dr Pelosi is a Wellcome Research Fellow.

REFERENCES

Cochrane, A.L. (1972) *Effectiveness and Efficiency: Random Reflections on Health Services*, London: The Nuffield Provincial Hospitals Trust.

Cardin, V.A., McGill, C.W., and Falloon, I.R.H. (1985) 'An economic analysis: costs, benefits, and effectiveness', in I.R.H. Falloon (ed.) *Family Management of Schizophrenia: A Study of Clinical, Social, Family, and Economic Benefits*, Baltimore: Johns Hopkins University Press.

Culyer, A.J. (1976) *Need and the National Health Service*, London: Martin Robertson.

Dick, P., Cameron, L., Cohen, D., Barlow, M., and Ince, A. (1985) 'Day and full-time treatment: a controlled comparison', *British Journal of Psychiatry* 147: 246–9.

71

Drummond, M.F. (1981) *Studies in Economic Appraisal in Health Care*, Oxford: Oxford University Press.

Drummond, M.F., Ludbrook, A., Lowson, K., and Steele, A. (1986) *Studies in Economic Appraisal in Health Care*, Oxford: Oxford University Press.

Drummond, M.F., Stoddart, G.L., and Torrance, G.W. (1987) *Methods for the Economic Evaluation of Health Care Programmes*, Oxford: Oxford University Press.

Endicott, J., Herz, M.I., and Gibbon, M. (1976) 'Brief versus standard hospitalisation: the differential costs', *American Journal of Psychiatry* 133: 518–21.

Falloon, I.R.H. (ed.) (1985) *Family Management of Schizophrenia: A Study of Clinical, Social, Family, and Economic Benefits*, Baltimore: Johns Hopkins University Press.

Fenton, F.R., Tessier, L., Contandriopoulos, A., Nguyen, H., and Struening, E.L. (1982) 'A comparative trial of home and hospital psychiatric treatment: financial costs', *Canadian Journal of Psychiatry* 27: 177–87.

Frank, F. (1981) 'Cost-benefit analysis in mental health services: a review of the literature', *Administration in Mental Health* 8: 161–76.

Ginsberg, G., Marks, I., and Waters, H. (1984) 'Cost-benefit analysis of a controlled trial of nurse therapy for neuroses in primary care', *Psychological Medicine* 14: 683–90.'

Glass, N.J. and Goldberg, D. (1977) 'Cost-benefit analysis and the evaluation of psychiatric services', *Psychological Medicine* 7: 701–7.

Hoult, J., Reynolds, I., Charbonneau-Powis, M., Weekes, P., and Briggs, J. (1983) 'Psychiatric hospital versus community treatment: the results of a randomised trial', *Australian and New Zealand Journal of Medicine* 17: 160–7.

Hurst, J. (1983) 'A government economist's attitude to the new measures', in G.T. Smith (ed.) *Measuring the Social Benefits of Medicine*, London: Office of Health Economics.

Jennett, B. (1984) 'Economic appraisal', *British Medical Journal* 288: 1781–2.

Jones, R., Goldberg, D., and Hughes, B. (1980) 'A comparison of two different services treating schizophrenia: a cost-benefit approach', *Psychological Medicine* 10: 493–505.

Mangen, S.P., Paykel, E.S., Griffith, J.H., Burcell, A., and Mancini, P. (1983) 'Cost-effectiveness of community psychiatric nurse or out-patient psychiatric care of neurotic patients', *Psychological Medicine* 13: 407–16.

May, P.R.A. (1970) 'Cost-efficiency of mental health delivery systems: 1. A review of the literature on hospital care', *American Journal of Public Health* 60: 2060–7.

Mooney, G.H. (1980) 'Cost-benefit analysis and medical ethics', *Journal of Medical Ethics* 6: 177–9.

National Institute of Mental Health, Series EN No. 1 (1981) *Economics and Mental Health* (DHHS Publication No. (ADM) 81–1114), Washington, DC: Superintendent of Documents, US Government Printing Office.

Regional Office for Europe, World Health Organization (1976) *Cost/Benefit Analysis in Mental Health Services: Report of a Working Group*, Copenhagen: Regional Office for Europe, World Health Organization.

Rosser, R. (1983) 'A history of the development of health indicators', in G.T. Smith (ed.) *Measuring the Social Benefits of Medicine*, London: Office of Health Economics.

Segall, M. and Vienonen, M. (rapporteurs) (1987) 'Haikko Declaration on actions for primary health care', *Health Policy and Planning* 2: 258–65.

Sugden, R. and Williams, A.H. (1979) *The Principles of Practical Cost-Benefit Analysis*, Oxford: Oxford University Press.

Tancredi, L.E. (ed.) (1974) *Ethics in Health Care*, Washington: National Academy of Sciences.

Weinstein, M.C. and Fineberg, H.V (1980) *Clinical Decision Analysis*, Philadelphia: W.B. Saunders Company.

Weisbrod, B.A. (1982) 'A guide to benefit-cost analysis, as seen through a controlled experiment in treating the mentally ill', *Journal of Health Politics, Policy & Law* 7: 808–45.

Weisbrod, B.A., Test, M.A., and Stein, L.I. (1980) 'Alternative to mental hospital treatment: II. Economic benefit-cost analysis', *Archives of General Psychiatry* 37: 400–5.

Wilkinson, G. and Pelosi, A.J. (1987) 'The economics of mental health services', *British Medical Journal* 294: 139–40.

Williams, A. and Anderson, R. (1975) *Efficiency in the Social Services*, Oxford: Basil Blackwell.

Quantitative Methods

6

The Mental Health of Populations

Geoffrey Rose

Epidemiology is the basic science of public health. Its origin in the mid-nineteenth century came about through the merging of three streams of thought: the concern of clinicians, who could not cure common diseases and therefore looked to their prevention; the new-found application of statistics to medical research, which offered some scientific rigour to the study of rather poor data; and the concern of social reformers and environmentalists, which provided the possibility of preventive action. The subject continues to need the collaboration of these three groups – clinicians, statisticians, and public health activists.

Epidemiology required the development of new research methods, appropriate to the study of groups or populations rather than individual patients; more importantly, it required a capacity to stand back and consider a population as the unit of study. Clinicians find this hard, because for them the natural unit of concern is the individual. It has proved particularly hard for psychiatrists, because their thinking is inevitably and properly more individualistic than that of the other clinical specialities. Psychiatry has, nevertheless, shown more interest in epidemiology than most other branches of medicine; but it has approached it largely from the standpoint of its particular concern for sick individuals.

Many urgent epidemiological questions confront a clinical psychiatrist. For example, in regard to depression, 'How many unrecognized and untreated cases are there in the community? How can they be identified? What sort of individuals get depression, and why? What is the condition's natural history, and can it be altered?' To answer such questions requires epidemiological methods such as surveys, the development and evaluation of screening instruments, case-control and cohort studies, clinical follow-up studies, and intervention trials. Thanks to such methods, now widely used by clinical researchers, the prevalence and natural history of psychiatric disorders are understood far better than 20 years ago; and one can hope that this extension of understanding has improved their recognition and clinical care. It has not, however, contributed much to their prevention: though it may have benefited sick individuals, it has done little for the mental health of populations. The purpose of this essay is to consider this wider field.

AIMS AND METHODS

The most commonly used methods of epidemiological enquiry are the cross-sectional (prevalence) survey and the case-control study. Each of these is concerned primarily with disease in individuals: the survey describes the frequency and distribution of cases, and the case-control study seeks to identify their distinguishing characteristics as clues to causation. Neither approach yields any direct evidence on the underlying factors which determine the incidence rate; study of these first causes calls for comparisons between whole populations with differing rates.

Such comparisons may be across countries (international), across sectors of populations (such as social classes or regions), or across time. Fortunately for epidemiology, most diseases seem to have incidence rates which vary widely across place or time, reflecting the socio-economic heterogeneity which is generally the underlying reason for the environmental exposures or patterns of behaviour which are the proximal causes of illness. This heterogeneity of incidence rates is the necessary condition for discovering the underlying causes; for a cause which is uniformly distributed does not influence the distribution of disease, and hence it is unrecognizable (even though if it were recognized it might be controlled).

Unfortunately, in cross-population studies the problem of confounding is much greater than in studies at the level of individuals: matching is difficult, and the true explanation of a correlation may be unsuspected. One can hope that the findings of cross-population and individual studies will reinforce one another, but this will happen only if there is a similar inequality of exposure to the cause both between and within populations. This is often not the case, and so there is a broad tendency for personal susceptibility factors to dominate the occurrence of individual cases but to explain little of the population differences in incidence, the latter being more under the control of socio-cultural and environmental influences.

CASES AND DISTRIBUTIONS

Clinical diagnosis splits the world into two: with regard to each disease there are those who have it and those who do not. This dichotomy serves well enough in clinical practice, both because treatment decisions are dichotomous and because selective referral brings to the doctor only the more severe examples of a condition. Thus, the distribution of a rating scale for depression in a hospital ward is likely to have two modes, corresponding to patients

MENTAL HEALTH OF POPULATIONS

admitted for severe depression and the others (whose problems are different).

In population studies the situation is not like this, and rating scales for mental illness show continuous, unimodal distributions. 'It follows that to ask what fraction of a population is psychiatrically disturbed is a meaningless question' (Goldberg 1972: 3). This is, nevertheless, exactly what most surveys have attempted to do, because the investigators were determined to force on to the population those descriptive labels with which they were clinically familiar. 'The term "case" can be used in any way that the purposes of a clinician (*sic*) require' (Wing *et al.* 1978: 203), with the aim of identifying 'what proportion of a population would be thought to have a clinically significant psychiatric disturbance if they were interviewed by a psychiatrist' (Goldberg 1972: 3).

In this way the population reality has been constrained to fit the clinical preconception. In fact, it will not fit it, simply because disease in the population is nearly always a quantitative and not a qualitative phenomenon, the question being not 'Has he got it?' but 'How much of it has he got?' An individual's status should thus be described by numbers not labels, for 'in the community the epidemiologist is faced with large numbers of respondents who present with fewer, minor, and non-specific symptoms' (Williams *et al.* 1980: 101).

To anyone familiar with the field of blood pressure research, the story sounds familiar. Hypertension was once considered to be a distinct entity, and Pickering's suggestion that it was only the high tail of a distribution was at first very unpopular. 'Essential hypertension', he wrote 'is a type of disease not hitherto recognised in medicine in which the defect is quantitative not qualitative. It is difficult for doctors to understand because it is a departure from the ordinary process of binary thought to which they are brought up. Medicine in its present state can count up to two but not beyond' (Pickering 1968: 4). Since the Pickering revolution, however, the blood pressure of populations has increasingly been described in terms of its distributions (means and standard deviations) rather than by prevalence rates.

There are two reasons to plead for a similar development in epidemiological psychiatry. The first is statistical: when the Present State Examination, for example, is used in a survey it is a gross waste of information to report only the numbers of persons above and below a certain cutting point, for this fails to use the available grading of individuals within each of these broad categories. Case definition may be necessary for operational decisions (as in screening), but it is too inefficient to earn priority in research: a distribution should always be analysed first by statistics which describe its central tendency and its dispersion.

A second and far more important reason for describing mental illness quantitatively is conceptual rather than technical. So long as attention is confined to the conspicuous cases, the underlying causes of incidence and the means of controlling them will continue to evade attention. Partly this may

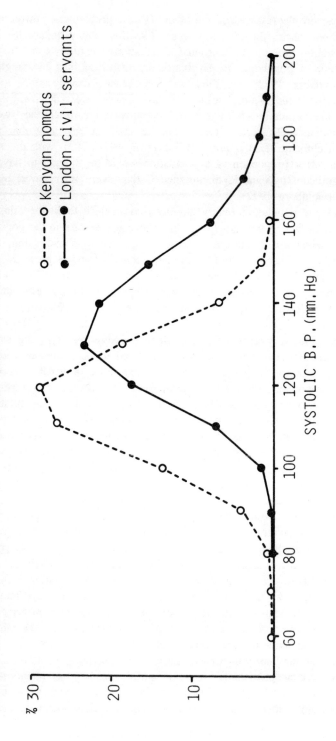

Figure 6.1 Distributions of systolic blood pressure in middle-aged men: (a) Kenyan nomads, (b) London civil servants.

be a willed defensive reaction: concentrating on sick and treatable patients diverts attention from the baffling problems of widespread minor neurosis and depression (which may be society's problem rather than the psychiatrist's).

A favourable shift in the whole distribution of risk may, nevertheless, be the only way to help those many individuals with a problem too small to qualify them for treatment as 'cases'. Even a small shift of this kind may produce an unexpectedly large reduction in the population burden, even though it offers little to each participating individual (the *prevention paradox*, Rose 1981). It also offers a powerful means to reduce the prevalence of 'cases'; in a normal distribution, half of those in the top decile will move to below that level if the population mean falls by as little as one-third of a standard deviation.

SPECIFIC EXAMPLES

The blood pressure analogy

Figure 6.1 shows the distribution of systolic blood pressure among Kenyan nomads and London civil servants. Nearly all research into the causes of hypertension has concentrated on the effort to explain why it is that within one population some individuals have much higher blood pressure than others. This question could be asked as well in Kenya as in London, since inter-individual variation is wide in both places; and the answers might well be similar. But even if the determinants of individual blood pressure could be fully understood, we should be no nearer explaining why hypertension is common in London but virtually absent in the Kenyan nomads; for the answer to this question must be sought in characteristics of the population as a whole, as a result of which the whole distribution is shifted up or down. The coefficient of variation is often a rather robust statistic, implying that the prevalence of high values ('cases') is determined by the value of the population mean.

The question, 'What determines the overall level of disease in a population?' is thus quite different from the question, 'What determines individual cases?' It is studied by different methods, it may yield a different answer, and the implications for prevention are quite different (Rose 1985).

Suicide and depression

In the nineteenth century medical interest in public health was stronger than nowadays. A century ago Durkheim (1951) found that suicide rates were stable and distinctive characteristics of populations. He, therefore, saw suicide as a collective phenomenon, in which personal factors were less important. More recent research has concentrated on the personal factors, with less interest than one would wish in the population experience. As with blood pressure, it is population factors which determine incidence rates.

81

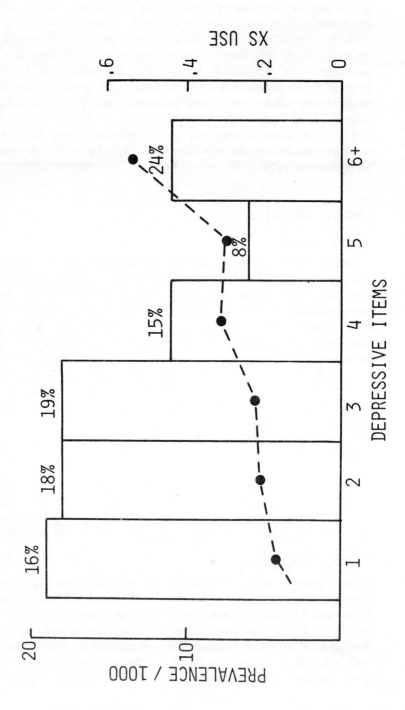

Figure 6.2 Prevalence of various numbers of positive depressive items (bars), frequency of excess use of social supports, above rate for zero depressive items' (interrupted line), and proportions of excess use of social supports attributable to different levels of depression (figures above bars). Derived from data of Brenner (1985)

Brenner (1985) applied a depression inventory in an American population and related the score (number of positive items) to the probability of using social supports. From his data it is possible to derive the results shown in figure 6.2. Of the total excess use of social supports associated with having more than zero depressive items, only a quarter arises among those individuals likely to be recognized as 'cases of depression' (6+ items). Two-thirds of the excess population burden of disability arises in individuals who have only between one and four positive items; they would not be recognized as cases of depression.

This is yet another example of a common phenomenon whereby a large number of people exposed to a small risk may generate a greater population burden than a small number exposed to a conspicuous risk (Rose 1981). The high-risk minority certainly need help; but to confine attention to this high-risk group may be to miss most of the problem.

The example of depression and its relation to use of social supports emphasizes the importance of widespread though slight individual disability. A possible 'collective disability' needs also to be considered. For any population there is *a mean depression score*, which not only determines the prevalence of clinical cases of depression and the total burden of depression-related individual disability, but which must also be some measure of 'population morale'; for presumably a more depressed community will collectively function less well than a community where spirits are higher. For all these reasons we need to know more about the determinants of this mean depression score, and its relation to collective societal functioning.

Alcohol

The alcohol intake of most populations follows a positively-skewed unimodal distribution. The mean intake varies, and these variations determine the prevalence of heavy drinking. To concentrate aetiological research and control efforts on the heavy drinkers is to fail to confront the real issue, for no country has yet achieved the truncated distribution of alcohol intake which such an approach impliedly seeks. Kreitman (1986) has reviewed the benefits of such an (unachievable) truncation, whereby no one would exceed the accepted 'safe limits' of intake; and he concludes that these benefits would be matched by an across-the-board reduction of 30 per cent of current alcohol intake – which is an achievable target, if society willed it.

For obvious reasons, society prefers to concentrate its attention on the minority of heavy drinkers, thereby exonerating the 'moderate drinkers'. This is doubly mistaken. First, the tail belongs to the distribution, however much the distribution may prefer to disown it! The alcohol intake and drinking attitudes of Mr and Mrs Average determine just how many problem drinkers there will be in that population. Secondly, as was seen for depression and social malfunction (figure 6.2), so it may well also be that the large number of moderate drinkers collectively generate more health and social problems than the small but conspicuous group of problem drinkers. If only the world really were divided into those with problems, and the rest of us – but the evidence does not support that view.

In regard to alcohol and road traffic accidents, society castigates and punishes the small minority of drivers with high blood alcohol levels, thereby exonerating the far larger number who drink and drive, but with levels inside the legal limit. The assumption – quite unproven – is that within this limit there is no important relation between blood alcohol and proneness to accidents. Data are needed on the distribution of blood alcohol levels in drivers who have accidents and in a representative sample of other drivers, and it would then be possible to calculate a dose-risk curve, linking exposure with outcome. Such data are not available, illustrating the currently blinkered approach which sees the alcohol problem only as the problem of heavy drinkers. In the absence of information on that crucial dose-response curve, one cannot know the limitations of current control policy. There is a similar need for research into the relation of moderate drinking to other behavioural problems.

It has become clear that heavy drinking destroys neurones and that alcoholics often have shrunken brains. But what is the shape of the dose-response curve linking alcohol intake and neuronal loss? Do moderate drinkers suffer moderate brain damage? Does every drink kill a few more brain cells? And if so, does it matter? If the effect were identifiable in individuals, one feels that it would be important; but if, say, a 10 per cent increase in average alcohol intake of a population led to a 1 per cent decline in average cognitive capacity, that effect – which might be statistically present in the population – would be inapparent in individuals. In discussing the mean depression score of a population, it was thought that this might well be important for collective functioning. Does the same apply to a small shift in the population distribution of cognitive functioning?

Aggression and violence

Like depression scores and alcohol intakes, the distribution of aggression is probably unimodally distributed; and if different societies were compared, it would probably be found that this distribution shifted up and down as a whole, for within one society there is a limited toleration of behavioural variations. For aggression, as for blood pressure, the coefficient of variation is probably a rather robust statistic.

This line of reasoning has major implications for research. It implies that we need to study not only the characteristics of 'psychopathic individuals', who are just the tail end of the distribution; more importantly, we need to study the determinants of the average tolerance of aggression in a society, for this determines the occurrence of 'psychopathy' and extreme violence. Football hooliganism (and wars) may diminish only when the whole population distribution of aggression can be changed.

84

CONCLUSION

The epidemiology of the mental health of populations could lay the basis, in a way that it has not so far done, for understanding and hence perhaps controlling the mass determinants of population means, prevalence rates, and incidence rates. What determines the population's mean level of depression, alcohol intake, or tolerance of violence? What is the relation between these average levels of exposure and the associated ill health or social malfunction? What is the psychiatric counterpart of the identification and control of water pollution, which so impressively reduced the incidence of cholera?

At this point psychiatric epidemiology and psychiatric preventive action merge into social research and social policy. The two cannot exist apart.

REFERENCES

Brenner, B. (1985) 'Continuity between the presence and absence of the depressive syndrome', paper presented at the 113th Annual Meeting of the American Public Health Association, Washington DC, November 1985.

Durkheim, E. (1951) *Suicide: A Study in Sociology*, translated by J.A. Spaulding and G. Simpson, Glencoe, Ill.: Free Press.

Goldberg, D. (1972) *The Detection of Psychiatric Illness by Questionnaire*, London: Oxford University Press.

Kreitman, N. (1986) 'Alcohol consumption and the preventive paradox', *British Journal of Addiction* 81: 353–63.

Pickering, G.W. (1968) *High Blood Pressure*, Edinburgh: Churchill Livingstone.

Rose, G. (1981) 'Strategy of prevention: lessons from cardiovascular disease', *British Medical Journal* 282: 1847–51.

Rose, G. (1985) 'Sick individuals and sick populations', *International Journal of Epidemiology* 14: 32–8.

Williams, P., Tarnopolsky, A., and Hand, D. (1980) 'Case definition and case identification in psychiatric epidemiology: review and assessment', *Psychological Medicine* 10: 101–14.

Wing, J.K., Mann, S.A., Leff, J.P., and Nixon, J.M. (1978) 'The concept of a "case" in psychiatric population surveys', *Psychological Medicine* 8: 203–17.

7

The Biostatistical Approach

Morton Kramer

The report of the Milbank Memorial Fund Commission on *Higher Education in Public Health* describes the many applications of biostatistics to investigations of problems in the health field:

> Biostatistics use statistical methodology to investigate problems in public health and medical care. In addition to collecting, analyzing, and retrieving data, designing experiments, and developing appropriate comparisons among population groups, biostatistics applies the techniques of inference and probability to the examination of biologic data. While interacting most continuously and closely with epidemiology, biostatistic interests extend into the congruent areas of vital statistics and demography, computer programming, computer systems and analysis, and program planning and evaluation. Through the continuing collaboration of epidemiologists and biostatisticians, the science and skill of designing experiments, analytic surveys, and data analysis have progressed to an advanced level. The actual work of these two types of specialists mesh so closely at times that it may be difficult for the outsider to distinguish between them. Through a fruitful working relationship, each in fact has come to learn a great deal about the other's methods and activities. Both as an arm of epidemiology and as a separate science, biostatistics serves as the major method of quantifying and analyzing health information specifically for application within public health.　　　　(Milbank Memorial Fund Commission 1976: 62)

This statement makes it quite clear that biostatistics plays an essential role both in quantifying and evaluating community-wide health problems and in the design and implementation of basic, clinical, laboratory, and field research. This chapter will provide selected examples of one application of biostatistics: the collection and analysis of data on the utilization of mental hospitals and other psychiatric facilities (e.g. outpatient, inpatient, and transitional services). Other chapters of this volume will illustrate the uses of biostatistical and other quantitative methods in clinical, laboratory, and field research on mental disorders.

USES OF ADMINISTRATIVE STATISTICS ABOUT THE MENTAL HEALTH SERVICES

Statistics that describe the characteristics of mental health facilities and of the persons who use them provide the basis for an administrative epidemiology of mental disorders (Kramer 1975). They serve purposes similar to those described by Morris in his text on *Uses of Epidemiology* (1975).

Administrative statistics can be used for the following purposes:

1. to study historical changes in patterns of use of specific types of services; their staffing and financing, and to make projections for the future;
2. to assess the availability of specific types of services and the extent of their use, populations served, staffing, location, accessibility, costs, manpower, and quality, effectiveness, and efficiency of services rendered;
3. to study the working of health services with a view to their improvement;
4. to estimate chances of persons being admitted to a specific type of facility and their chances of being released alive from or dying in the facility;
5. to investigate the causes of institutionalization (for example, factors that determine pathways to care; behaviours and attitudes of consumers and providers of services; availability of community supports; and socio-economic factors).

In addition, the medical records of patients admitted to various types of facilities may be used in clinical, laboratory, and field research to carry out such other uses of epidemiology as:

6. to complete the clinical picture;
7. to identify syndromes;
8. to search for causes of health and disease.

Further elaboration and examples of specific uses may be found in various publications (World Health Organization 1963, 1969, 1971; Brooke 1963; Kramer 1969, 1977; Kramer *et al.* 1973; Kramer *et al.* 1973; Gruenberg 1968, 1986; National Institute of Mental Health 1983, 1985, 1987).

USES OF CENSUSES OF POPULATION AND VITAL STATISTICS

Population censuses provide basic statistics of a country and its geographical subdivisions by age, sex, race, socio-economic, marital status, household composition, educational level, and other characteristics of target populations. Such data are essential for computation of utilization rates of residents of a defined geographic area by specific demographic variables. Some national censuses provide basic data on the characteristics of their institutional population. Such data make it possible to compare characteristics of residents of mental institutions with those of residents of other institutions of interest to the mental health field. Vital statistics are also needed to provide birth, death, and migration rates of a target population and other indicators of the health situation of a population.

SELECTED ILLUSTRATIONS OF USES OF TREND DATA

The illustrations to be given in the following sections are derived from US Census Bureau publications on persons in institutions and from published analyses of data collected annually by the NIMH through its national reporting programme on the characteristics of the mental health services of the fifty states of the US and the characteristics of the persons using them (Redick *et al.* 1983). These data will illustrate only one of the uses of administrative statistics described earlier, namely, historical study of changes that have occurred in the utilization of mental hospitals and other types of institutions and of changes that have occurred in the use of specialty mental health services. Limitations of space do not permit other examples of applications of utilization statistics. The interested reader may find them in the references cited on p. 87.

These examples will be followed by three others to illustrate the potential effect on the prevalence of mental disorders of several important changes projected to occur in the US population by the year 2,000: (1) the increases in the numbers of persons 65–74, 75–84, 85+; (2) the increases in the Spanish-speaking population; and (3) the changes in the household composition and living arrangements of the population.

TRENDS OF THE INSTITUTIONAL POPULATION

At each decennial census the US Bureau of the Census enumerates inmates of the following institutions: correctional institutions; mental hospitals; residential treatment centres; tuberculosis hospitals; chronic disease hospitals; homes for the aged and dependent; homes and schools for the mentally handicapped; homes and schools for the physically handicapped; homes for dependent and neglected children; homes for unwed mothers; training schools for juvenile delinquents and detention homes (US Bureau of the Census 1953, 1973, 1984).

It is instructive to review the trends of number of persons resident in the

Table 7.1 Number, percentage distribution, and rate per 100,000 population of persons in mental institutions (mental hospitals and residential treatment centres), homes for aged and dependent, and correctional institutions: US 1950, 1960, 1970, and 1980.

Type of institution and total population of the US	1950	1960	1970	1980
	Number (000s)			
Total	1,566.8	1,887.0	2,126.7	2,492.1
Mental institutions	613.6	630.0	433.9	255.3
Homes for aged and dependent	296.8	469.7	927.5	1,426.4
Correctional institutions	264.6	346.0	328.0	466.4
All other	391.8	441.3	437.3	344.0
	Percentage of population in all institutions			
Total	100.0	100.	100.0	100.0
Mental institutions	39.2	33.4	20.4	10.2
Homes for aged and dependent	18.9	24.8	43.6	57.2
Correctional institutions	16.9	18.3	15.4	18.7
All other	25.0	23.5	20.6	13.9
	Number per 100,000 population of US			
Total	1,035.4	1,052.3	1,046.6	1,100.3
Mental institutions	405.5	351.3	213.5	112.7
Homes for aged and dependent	196.1	261.9	456.4	629.7
Correctional institutions	174.8	193.0	161.4	205.9
All other	259.0	246.1	215.3	152.0
Total resident population of US (000s)	151,326	179,323	203,302	226,546

Sources: US Bureau of the Census, 1953, 1973, 1984

total institutional population and their component parts for several reasons. First, factors that affect the use of any one type of institution, for example mental hospitals, can have both a direct and/or halo effect on the use of other institutions, such as nursing homes, and, in some instances, correctional institutions. Second, these trends reflect temporal changes in the many factors that determine the way a society uses the various institutions it has created. They have been created to serve various purposes. One type – the correctional institution – is for the incarceration of persons who have committed crimes against society. Other types provide a variety of services for persons who are mentally ill, mentally retarded, chronically ill or disabled, or have succumbed to problems that beset the aged. Still others provide services to persons who have manifested other kinds of behavioural and psychosocial problems – such as homes for unwed mothers and training schools for juvenile delinquents.

Table 7.1 provides the number and percentage of persons in all institutions

Figure 7.1 Distribution of persons in institutions per 100,000 population by type of institution, both sexes US, 1950, 1970 and 1980

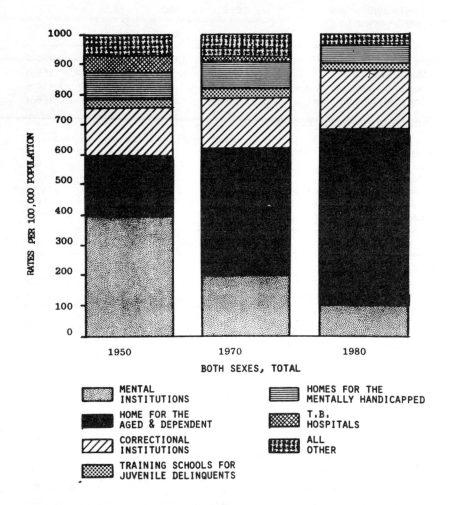

Sources: US Bureau of the Census, 1953, 1973, 1983

and the corresponding resident rates per 100,000 population for three major types of institutions for the years 1950, 1970, and 1980: mental institutions, homes for the aged and dependent, and correctional institutions. Figure 7.1 shows the changes in resident rates per 1,000 population.

Collectively, these three types of institutions have accounted for 75 per cent or more of the institutional population. However, striking changes occurred in the rank order of the number of persons resident in these institutions during this thirty-year period. In 1950 the mental institutions, which include mental hospitals and residential treatment centres, accounted for the largest number and percentage of all persons in institutions (613,600 or 39 per cent of the total), followed in order by homes for aged and dependent (296,800 or 19 per cent of the total), and correctional institutions (264,600 or 17 per cent of the total). All the other institutions accounted for 391,800 persons or 25 per cent of the total. By 1980 homes for the aged and dependent accounted for the largest number (1,426,400 or 57 per cent of the total), followed by the correctional institutions (466,400 or 19 per cent of the total) and mental institutions (255,300 or 10 per cent of the total). All other institutions accounted for 344,000 or 14 per cent of the total.

The percentage change in the numbers of persons in these three major categories of institutions as compared to that of the total population of the US is quite dramatic. Between 1950 and 1980 the total population of the US increased by 50 per cent (from 151.3 million to 226.5 million). The institutional population as a whole increased somewhat more rapidly, by 59 per cent. However, the population in homes for aged and dependent *increased* by 381 per cent and that in correctional institutions *increased* by 76 per cent, while that in the mental institutions *decreased* by 58 per cent.

Biostatisticians must not be content merely to collect data and to publish numbers. They must provide some insight into the factors operating in society that generate the data published in the statistical tables of a census volume or annual reports. The following is a conceptualization of several factors responsible for the trends just demonstrated.

The population trends for a specific type of the institution are governed by factors that determine the rate at which persons are admitted to the institution and other factors that determine their lengths of stay and the rates at which they are returned to the community or die in the institution. The following are broad classes of factors that have affected the size of the separate components of the institutional population: (1) social legislation that encourages and/or mandates programmes that affect the flow of people into and out of a specific type of institution; (2) discoveries of treatment for diseases that reduce or eliminate the need for institutional care or make possible shorter durations of stay in the institution; (3) demographic changes, particularly those that result in the creation of groups at high risk for institutional care; (4) skyrocketing costs of general hospital and domiciliary care for persons with chronic diseases that make it financially impossible to maintain a subject in the community; (5) societal conditions and problems that are associated with high risk for mental disorders, crime, delinquency, and other types of psychosocial problems; (6) racist and other discriminatory practices that determine who gets institutionalized in a specific type of facility; (7) insufficient and inadequate community programmes for preventing admission to an institution or for facilititating release of inmates to the community; and (8) inappropriate living arrangements in the community for persons with chronic and disabling conditions. These factors are discussed at some length in a paper by this author (Kramer 1977).

The next section provides a specific illustration of factors that accounted for the large, rapid decrease in the number of residents of mental hospitals.

CHANGES IN LOCUS OF CARE OF PERSONS WITH MENTAL DISORDER

The striking decrease in the number of persons in mental hospitals was the result of a series of actions that changed the primary locus of care of persons with mental disorders from the large state hospitals to community-based services (Kramer 1977; Regier and Taube 1981). These included:

- federal and state legislation that mandated the development of community-based programmes for diagnosis, treatment, and rehabilitation of persons with mental disorders;
- expansion of out-patient psychiatric services, psychiatric units in general hospitals, and community mental health centres;
- development and use of psychoactive drugs;
- development of procedures to prevent inappropriate placements of persons in state mental hospitals and other procedures to reduce length of stay of persons admitted to these hospitals;
- expansion of nursing homes and other facilities for the aged as a result of Title 19 of the Social Security Act in 1965 (Medicaid) and the 1965 amendments to the Act (Medicare).

As a result of these and other actions, the resident population of the state mental hospitals dropped from its maximum of 559,000 in 1955 to 140,355 in 1979, a decrease of 75 per cent (figure 7.2) (NIMH, 1983). While the mental hospital population was decreasing, the use of other mental health facilities was increasing. During the period 1955–77 the total number of patient care episodes in all facilities increased from 1.7 million to 6.9 million, an increase of 306 per cent; the number of episodes per 100,000 population increased from 1,028 to 2,964 or by 188 per cent. The shift from in-patient to out-patient care during this period is shown in figure 7.3 which demonstrates the changes that occurred in the percentage distribution of the patient-care episodes specific for type of facility (Witkin 1980).

Figure 7.2 Number of resident patients, total admissions, net releases[1] and deaths[1] in state and county mental hospitals, United States, 1950–1980

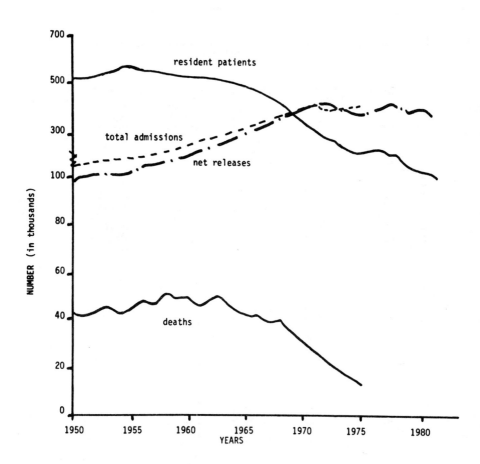

[1] Data available for the years 1950–1975.
Sources: Kramer, M. (1977); National Institute of Mental Health (1983)

93

Figure 7.3 Per cent distribution of inpatient and outpatient care episodes[1] in mental health facilities by type of facility: US, 1955, 1971, 1975, 1977

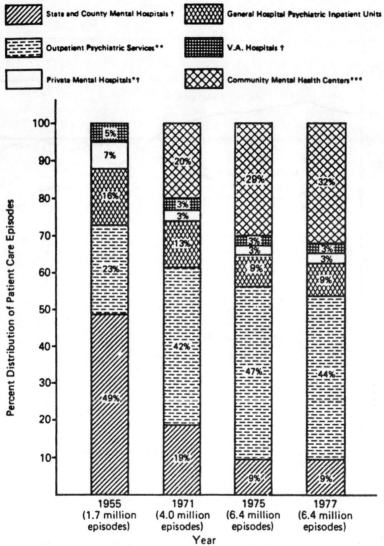

*Includes residential treatment centers for emotionally disturbed children.
†Inpatient services only.
**Includes freestanding outpatient services as well as those affiliated with psychiatric and general hospitals.
***Includes inpatient and outpatient services of federally funded CMHCs.
1/Excludes day treatment episodes and V.A. psychiatric outpatient services.

Source: Witkin, M.J. (1980)

TRENDS IN PATTERNS OF CARE FOR THE AGED

Mental hospitals

Of particular interest are changes that have occurred in the use of state mental hospitals for aged persons with mental disorders. Figure 7.4 shows the marked change in the age-specific first admission rates to these hospitals. In 1946 and 1955 these rates reached their maximum of about 240 per 100,000 in the age group 65+. By 1972, the rate for this age group dropped to about 75 per 100,000, 69 per cent lower than in 1955 and to 40 per 100,000 in 1975, 83 per cent lower than in 1955. Indeed the shape of the first admission rate curve for 1975 was similar to that of the curve for 1885. However, the characteristics of the communities, living arrangements, family composition, and related phenomena of the population of the US in 1885 were quite different from those that existed in 1975.

Between 1965 and 1979 the resident patient rate in state mental hospitals for person 65 years and over dropped from 773 per 100,000 to 164 per 100,000, a decrease of 79 per cent (Kramer 1977; NIMH 1983). The decrease was the result both of reductions in first admissions and of placement of aged residents in nursing homes and release of others to the community.

Nursing homes

The National Center for Health Statistics (NCHS) provides data which demonstrate the striking increase in the number of nursing homes and their residents (NCHS 1979, 1981, 1983). The number of these homes increased from about 13,000 in 1963 to about 18,900 in 1977, a 45 per cent increase. During the same period, the number of residents increased from 491,000 to 1,303,000, an increase of 165 per cent (NCHS 1981; US Bureau of the Census 1984). More recently, the NCHS (1983) reported that in 1980 there were 23,065 nursing homes in the US with 1,396,132 residents. These numbers represent a 22 per cent increase in the number of such homes and a 7 per cent increase in the number of residents since 1977.

Figure 7.5 shows the trend of the number of persons per 1,000 population in nursing home beds on a given day, specific for age for the years 1963, 1969, 1973–4, and 1977 (NCHS 1981).

For all persons 65 years of age and over, the rate increased from 25.4 per 1,000 population in the year 1963 to 47.9, an increase of 89 per cent (figure 7.5). However, the relatively low rate for this total group masks the dramatic increases that have occurred in the rates among persons in the age group 65–74, 75–84, and 85 and over, i.e., among the separate age groups that constitute the 65 years and over group. Increases have occurred steadily in these age specific rates. As of 1977, the rates of all races combined increased with advancing age from 14.5 per 1,000 persons 65–74 to 215.4 per 1,000 for persons 85 and over, a 15-fold increase. For the whites the

95

Figure 7.4 First admission rates per 100,000 population by age, state and county mental hospitals, US, 1946, 1955, and 1975 and Massachusetts, 1885

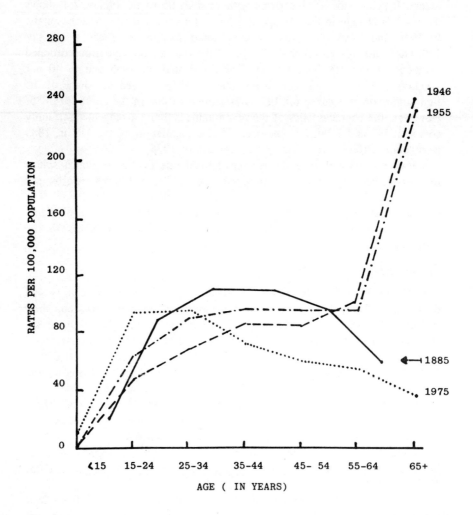

Sources: Kramer, M. (1977); Gruenberg, E.M. (1986)

Figure 7.5 Number of nursing home residents per 1,000 population by age for the years 1963, 1969, 1973–4 and 1977

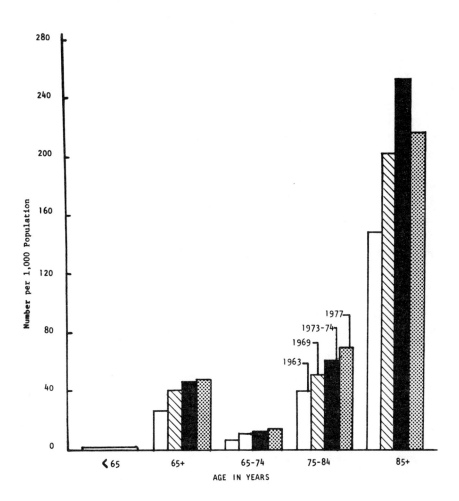

Source: National Center for Health Statistics (1981)

rates increased from 14.2 per 1,000 for persons 65–74 to 229.0 for persons 85 and over, a 16-fold increase. For the non-whites the corresponding rates increased from 16.8 per 1,000 to 102.0 per 1,000 (six-fold increase).

There are also considerable differences between the rates for males and females. The female rates are considerably higher than those for males. In the age group 65–74, the ratio is 1.25 increasing to 1.80 in the age group 85+. As a result of these higher female rates, females accounted for 74 per cent of the 1977 nursing home population 65 years and over and males, 26 per cent.

IMPLICATIONS OF PROJECTIONS OF THE US POPULATION TO THE YEAR 2000 FOR THE PREVALENCE OF MENTAL DISORDERS AND USE OF MENTAL HEALTH SERVICES

An important function of biostatisticians is to provide data required for the planning of mental health and related services. They must look ahead to determine what the future needs for facilities and services are likely to be. Accordingly they will require, *inter alia*, projections of the age and sex distribution of the population and a set of relevant rates to apply to them.

The following sections highlight the implications of: (1) projections of the aged population for beds in nursing homes; (2) projections of the age distribution of whites, blacks, and Hispanics for the prevalence of mental disorders in these populations; and (3) projections of the household composition of the population for community-based mental health programmes.

Projections of the population of the elderly

A crude estimate of the expected number of persons in nursing homes by the year 2005 can be obtained by applying the age, race, sex specific resident patient rates for the year 1977 to the corresponding age-race-sex specific groups of the population of the US in 1980 and the year 2005 (US Bureau of the Census 1979). The results of these computations are shown in table 7.2.

Between 1980 and 2005 the total number of nursing home residents would increase by 47.9 per cent, from 1,413,331 to 2,090,253. For the white population the numbers of residents would increase by 48 per cent, from 1,308,583 to 1,936,144 and for the black and others by 47.1 per cent, from 104,748 to 154,109.

These projections underscore the potential effect of the change in age composition of the population of the US between 1980 and 2005 on the need for additional nursing home beds. They also underscore the need for other data to assist administrators and planners to deal more effectively with problems currently encountered in providing adequate care for the elderly who require admission to these facilities and to develop alternate programmes of care.

Table 7.2 Illustration of the effect of population changes in the US between 1980 and 2005 on the number of residents of nursing homes, assuming 1977 resident patient rates applied to the projected population for 2005

Year	Total	White	Black/other
1980	1,413,331	1,308,583	104,748
2005	2,090,253	1,936,144	154,109
Increase	676,922	627,561	49,361
% increase	47.9	48.0	47.1

Projections of the white, black and Hispanic population

The Bureau of the Census publishes projections of the white, black, and Hispanic population of the US to the year 2080 (US Bureau of the Census 1986d). Table 7.3 shows the expected changes in these populations between 1985 and 2000 specific for age. The expected rate of growth of the Hispanic population exceeds by a considerable amount that of the white and black populations. The total white population is projected to increase by 9.6 per cent (from 203.1 to 222.6 millions) and the black by 23.0 per cent (from 29.1 to 35.8 millions). The Hispanic population is projected to increase by 45.9 per cent (from 17.3 to 25.2 millions). The expected increases in the numbers of persons in each of the age groups of the Hispanic population are quite extraordinary. Thus, the percentage increases specific for age are: under 18, 37 per cent; 18–24, 18 per cent; 25–44, 41 per cent; 45–64, 85 per cent; and 65 and over, 94 per cent.

Such changes will have a profound effect on the number of cases of mental disorder that will exist in this population group. The following computations, based on prevalence estimates from the Epidemiology Catchment Area Surveys, illustrate this effect (Regier *et al.* 1984).

The Epidemiologic Catchment Area Surveys, recently carried out in five catchment areas of the US, provide estimates of age specific one-month prevalence rates of mental disorders among whites, blacks, and Hispanics (Regier *et al.* in press). These estimates are based on computer analysis of responses to the Diagnostic Interview Schedule administered to a probability sample of respondents 18 years of age and over in each catchment area. Table 7.4 shows the results of the application of the age specific one-month prevalence rates in the age groups 18–24, 25–44, 45–64, and 65+ to the corresponding age groups of the populations of the whites, blacks, and Hispanics in 1985 and 2000. The expected number of cases among the whites would increase by 8.6 per cent (from 19.5 to 21.2 millions); among the blacks by 24.8 per cent (from 3.7 to 4.6 millions); and among the Hispanics by 48.0 per cent (from 1.6 to 2.4 millions). These projected increases in number of cases for the Hispanics plus those expected in the white and black

99

Table 7.3 Estimated population (in 000s) for whites, blacks, and Hispanics, US, 1985 to 2000

Age (years)	Year 1985	2000	Change in no. persons 1985–2000	Percentage change
		White		
Total	203,111	222,654	19,543	9.62
< 15	42,123	44,314	2,191	5.20
15–24	32,883	29,002	− 3,881	− 11.80
25–34	35,323	29,590	− 5,733	− 16.25
35–44	27,620	36,335	8,735	31.63
45–54	19,529	31,662	12,133	62.13
55–64	19,759	20,605	846	4.28
65–74	15,188	15,589	401	2.63
75+	10,686	15,537	4,851	45.40
		Black		
Total	29,078	35,754	6,676	22.97
< 15	8,061	9,500	1,439	17.85
15–24	5,732	5,672	− 60	− 1.05
25–34	5,212	5,316	104	2.00
35–44	3,404	5,811	2,407	70.71
45–54	2,336	4,124	1,788	76.54
55–64	2,003	2,355	352	17.57
65–74	1,410	1,589	179	12.70
75+	920	1,387	467	50.76
		Spanish origin		
Total	17,287	25,224	7,937	45.91
< 15	5,317	7,344	2,027	38.12
15–24	3,311	4,124	813	24.55
25–34	3,254	3,804	550	16.90
35–44	2,129	3,803	1,674	78.63
45–54	1,376	2,811	1,435	104.29
55–64	1,015	1,619	604	59.51
65–74	553	1,041	488	88.25
75+	332	678	346	104.22

Source: US Bureau of the Census, 1979, 1986d

Table 7.4 Estimated number of cases of any dis-disorder for whites, blacks, and Hispanics, US, 1985–2000

	1-month prevalence Rate (%)[1]	Population Number (000s) 1985	Population Number (000s) 2000	Percentage Change	Actual number 1985	Expected cases 2000	Percentage change
White							
18–24	15.14	23,817	19,816	−16.80	3,605,894	3,000,142	−16.80
25–44	14.73	62,943	65,945	4.77	9,271,503	9,713,699	4.77
45–64	9.96	39,288	52,267	33.03	3,913,084	5,205,793	33.03
65+	10.56	25,874	31,126	20.30	2,732,274	3,286,905	20.30
Total 18+		151,922	169,154	11.34	19,522,775	21,206,539	8.62
Black							
18–24	20.10	4,128	3,772	−8.62	829,728	758,172	−8.62
25–44	17.84	8,616	11,127	29.14	1,537,094	1,985,056	29.14
45–64	18.23	4,339	6,479	49.32	791,000	1,181,121	49.32
65+	23.50	2,330	2,976	27.73	547,550	699,360	27.73
Total 18+		19,413	24,354	25.45	3,705,372	4,623,709	24.78
Hispanic							
18–24	17.20	2,349	2,766	17.75	404,028	475,752	17.75
25–44	14.11	5,383	7,607	41.32	759,541	1,073,347	41.32
45–64	13.72	2,391	4,430	85.28	328,045	607,796	85.28
65+	12.50	885	1,719	94.24	110,625	214,875	94.24
Total 18+		11,008	16,522	50.09	1,602,239	2,371,770	48.03

[1] Based on weighted age specific rates for the five ECA areas specific for white, blacks, and Hispanics. (Regier *et al.* in press)

populations provide some indication of the increases in mental health, social, and related services that will be required to meet the needs of the diverse population groups in the US for mental health services.

Projections of household composition and living arrangements

Another demographic trend that will exacerbate the mental health problem in the US is that which is occurring in the family and household composition of its population (US Bureau of the Census 1985, 1986b). Between 1950, and 1985 married couple families increased by 48 per cent; families headed by a male without spouse (male householder families) by 91 per cent; families headed by a female without spouse (female householder families) by 182 per cent; and non-family households by 411 per cent. About 85 per cent of the non-family households consists of persons living alone (one-person households). The number of one-person households increased by 421 per cent during this period.

Projections between 1985 and 2000 of the number of households and their ratio per 1,000 population by type, shown in table 7.5, highlight the gradual decline in the number of married couple families per 1,000 population and accentuate the striking increases expected by 2000 in the numbers and ratios of the other types of family and non-family households (Kramer *et al.* 1987; US Bureau of the Census 1985, 1986c).

Several factors have brought about these changes in household and family structure: the increase in divorce rates; the increase in the number of widows and widowers; migration of workers to areas of the country with opportunities for employment; and trends in behaviour, life style, value systems, and aspirations of the members of the various social class strata of our society.

It is well known that persons who are separated, divorced, widowed, or never married, persons living alone or in non-family households and children living with one parent are at relatively high risk for developing a mental disorder. The US Census Bureau has recently published data on the changes in the living arrangements of several of these groups that have occurred between 1970 and 1985 (US Bureau of the Census 1986a). During this period the number of children who live in single-parent families increased by 78 per cent (from 8.2 millions to 14.6 millions); the number of divorced persons who live alone increased by 193 per cent (from 1.5 millions in 1970 to 4.4 millions); and the number of persons 65 and over who live alone increased by 59 per cent (from 5.1 millions in 1970 to 8.1 millions). Another characteristic of the female householder family with children is that a very large proportion of these families (about 35 per cent) live below the poverty level, a variable known to be a risk factor for mental disorder.

As a result of the continuing emphasis on community care, it is important to learn more about the living arrangements of persons in these high risk groups – who among them has a mental disorder; the role of this person in

Table 7.5 Type of households and family units, US, 1985–2000[1]

Type of household and family	1985	2000	Percentage change
	Number in 000s		
Total	86,789	105,933	22.1
Family households	62,706	72,277	15.3
Married couple	50,350	56,294	11.8
Other, male householder	2,228	3,282	47.3
Other, female householder	10,129	12,701	25.4
Non-family households	24,082	33,656	39.8
Male householder	10,114	15,452	52.8
Female householder	13,968	18,204	30.3
Living alone	20,602	28,944	40.5
Two or more persons	3,480	4,712	35.4
	Percentage of total		
Total	100.0	100.0	
Family households	72.3	68.2	− 5.7
Married couple	58.0	53.1	− 8.5
Other, male householder	2.6	3.1	19.2
Other, female householder	11.7	12.0	2.6
Non-family households	27.7	31.8	14.8
Male householder	11.7	14.6	24.8
Female householder	16.1	17.2	6.8
Living alone	23.7	27.3	15.2
Two or more persons	4.0	4.5	12.5
	No. of households per 1,000 population		
Total	363.7	395.3	8.7
Family households	262.8	269.7	2.6
Married couple	211.0	210.1	− 0.4
Other, male householder	9.3	12.2	31.2
Other, female householder	42.4	47.4	11.8
Non-family households	100.9	125.6	24.5
Male householder	42.4	57.7	36.1
Female householder	58.5	67.9	16.1
Living alone	86.3	108.0	25.1
Two or more persons	14.6	17.6	20.5
Population US (000s)	238,631	267,956	12.3

Source: US Bureau of the Census, 1987

103

the household (i.e., head of household, spouse of head, child, or other relative); the impact of the persons with a disorder on other persons in the household and vice versa – and to gather additional information about the familial aggregation of mental disorders and other disorders and disabling conditions (Downes and Simon 1954; Kellam and Ensminger 1980; Kellam *et al*. 1982; Rutter and Quinton 1984; WHO 1976). Indeed, more knowledge is needed about the family-household aggregation of mental and physical disorders in an era when the importance of primary health care and family-based preventive care is being increasingly emphasized.

The Eastern Baltimore Mental Health Survey provided a unique opportunity to collect data in a way that made it possible to allocate persons with a DIS disorder to the type of household in which they lived and to determine prevalence rates of specific DIS/DSM–III disorders among persons living in different types of households. Analyses of these data demonstrated that prevalence rates of mental disorders in male and female householder families, and non-family households are significantly higher than those found in married couple families (Kramer *et al*. 1987).

As a result of changes in the household composition of the nation during the past thirty years, results similar to those reported for Eastern Baltimore are likely to be quite general throughout the US and, probably, in other developed countries. This follows from the fact that female and male householder families and non-family households are heavily weighted with persons at high risk for mental disorder. As a result of the expected increases in the number of such households between 1985 and 2000, shown in table 7.5, and the high prevalence of mental disorders in these households, a marked increase can be expected in the number of US households in which one or more members will have a mental disorder.

CONCLUSIONS

Biostatistics plays an essential role in quantifying and evaluating community-wide mental health problems and in the design and implementation of clinical, laboratory, and field research on the mental disorders. This paper has illustrated only one of the many uses of biostatistics in the mental health field; namely, its use in the collection and analysis of data on utilization of mental health services. In particular, it has demonstrated how statistical data generated by the National Reporting Program for Mental Health Statistics in the US have been used to develop an administrative epidemiology of mental disorders based on systematically collected data on the characteristics of the mental health services and of persons who utilize these services. Illustrations have been given of how these data have been used to demonstrate changes in the locus of care of persons with mental disorders during the past twenty-five to thirty years. Other illustrations have been given of how demographic projections of a population, utilization rates of mental health services, and prevalence rates of mental disorder, derived from population-based epidemiologic surveys, can be used to provide quantitative estimates of future size of mental health problems and needs for mental health services.

Trends in use of mental health services similar to those in the US have occurred in many other countries (Freeman *et al.* 1985; International Journal of Mental Health 1983; World Health Organization 1980). As a result of population increases projected between 1985 and 2000 for age groups at high risk for mental disorder in all countries of the developed and developing regions of the world, it can be expected that there will be a large increase world-wide in the numbers of persons with mental disorder (Kramer and Anthony 1983; United Nations 1985). Administrators of mental health programmes will require statistical data on patterns of use of mental health services, epidemiologic data on the prevalence and incidence of mental disorders in their countries, projections of the age, sex, and other demographic features of their populations, to plan programmes to meet their needs for services. All of this emphasizes that the biostatistical approach will play an increasingly important role in planning, monitoring, and evaluating programmes for the prevention and control of mental disorders and their associated disabling conditions.

REFERENCES

Brooke, E.M. (1963) *A Longitudinal Study of Patients First Admitted to Mental Hospitals in 1954 and 1955* (Studies on Medical and Population Subjects No. 18), London: HM.

Downes, J. and Simon, S. (1954) 'Characteristics of psychoneurotic patients and their families as revealed in a general morbidity study', *Milbank Memorial Fund Quarterly* 32: 42–64.

Freeman, H.L., Fryers, T., and Henderson, J.H. (1985) *Mental Health Services in Europe: 10 Years On* (Public Health in Europe 25), Copenhagen: WHO, Regional Office for Europe.

Gruenberg, E.M. (1968) 'Epidemiology and medical care statistics', in M.M. Katz, J.O. Cole, and W.E. Barton (eds) *The Role and Methodology of Classification in Psychiatry and Psychopathology*, Washington, DC: US Government Printing Office.

Gruenberg, E.M. (1986) 'Mental disorders', in J.M. Last (ed.) *Maxey-Rosenau Public Health and Preventive Medicine*, 12th edn, Norwalk, Conn.: Appleton-Century-Crofts.

International Journal of Mental Health (1983) *International Perspectives on Deinstitutionalization* (guest editor, H. Goldman), Armonk, New York: M.E. Sharpe.

Kellam, S.G. and Ensminger, M.E. (1980) 'Theory and method in child psychiatric epidemiology studies in children', in F. Earls (ed.) *Monographs in Psychological Epidemiology*, New York: Prodist.

Kellam, S.G., Adams, R.G., Brown, C.H., and Ensminger, M.E. (1982) 'Long term evolution of the family structure of teen-age and older mothers', *Journal of Marriage and the Family*, August, 539–4.

Kramer, M. (1969) *Applications of Mental Health Statistics: Uses in Mental Health Programmes of Statistics Derived from Psychiatric Services and Selected Vital and Morbidity Records*, Geneva: World Health Organization.

Kramer, M. (1975) 'Diagnoses and classification in epidemiological and health services research', pp. 64–6, In N. Hobbs (ed) *Issues in the Classification of Children*, San Francisco: Jossey-Bass Publishers.

Kramer, M. (1977) *Psychiatric Services and the Changing Institutional Scene 1950–1985* (DHEW Publication No. (ADM) 77–433), Washington, DC: US Government Printing Office.

Kramer, M. and Anthony, J. (1983) 'Review of differences in mental health indicators used in national publications: recommendations for their standardization', *World Health Statistics Quarterly* 36: 256–338.

Kramer, M., Brown, H., Skinner, E.A., Anthony, J.C., and German, P. (1987) 'Changing living arrangements in the population and their potential effect on the prevalence of mental disorders: findings of the Eastern Baltimore Mental Health Survey', in B. Cooper (ed) *Psychiatric Epidemiology*, Bromley: Croom Helm.

Kramer, M., Rosen, B., and Willis, E.M. (1973) 'Definitions and distributions of mental disorders in a racist society', in C.V. Willie, B. Kramer, and B.S. Brown (eds) *Racism and Mental Health Essays*, Pittsburgh: University Pittsburgh Press.

Kramer, M., Taube, C.A., and Redick, R.W. (1973) 'Patterns of use of psychiatric facilities by the aged: past, present and future', in C. Eisdorfer and M. P. Lawson (eds) *The Psychology of Adult Development and Aging*, Washington, DC: American Psychological Association.

Milbank Memorial Fund Commission (1972) *Higher Education in Public Health*, New York: Prodist, p. 62.

Morris, J.N. (1975) *Uses of Epidemiology*, third edition, Edinburgh: Churchill Livingstone.

National Center for Health Statistics (1979) *The National Nursing Home Survey: Vital and Health Statistics* (Series 13, No. 43), Washington, DC: US Government Printing Office.

National Center for Health Statistics (1981) *Characteristics of Nursing Home Residents, Health Status and Care Received* (Vital and Health Statistics, Series 13, No. 27), Washington DC: US Government Printing Office.

National Center for Health Statistics (1983) 'An overview of the 1980 master facility inventory of nursing and related care homes', *Advance Data* 91.

National Institute of Mental Health (1983) *Mental Health: United States 1983*, edited by C.A. Taube and S.A. Barrett, (DHSS Pub. No. (ADM–83–1275)), Rockville, MD.

National Institute of Mental Health (1985) *Mental Health: United States 1985*, edited by C.A. Taube and S.A. Barrett, (DHSS Pub. No. (ADM–85–1378)), Washington, DC: Superintendent of Documents, US Government Printing Office.

National Institute of Mental Health (1987) *Mental Health: United States 1987*, edited by R.W. Manderscheid and S.A. Barrett, (DHSS Pub. No. (ADM–87–1518)), Washington, DC: Superintendent of Documents, US Government Printing Office.

Redick, R.W., Manderscheid, R.W., Witkin, M.J., and Rosenstein, M.J. 61983) *A History of the U.S. National Reporting Program for Mental Health Statistics, 1840–1983* (DHSS Pub. No. (ADM) 83–1296), Washington, DC: US Government Printing Office.

Regier, D. and Taube, C.A. (1981) 'The delivery of mental health services', in S. Arieti and H.R.K. Brodie (eds) *American Handbook of Psychiatry*, (2nd edn), New York: Basic Books Inc.

Regier, D.A., Meyers, J.K., Kramer, M., Robins, L.N., Blazer, D.G., Hough, R.L., Eaton, W.W., and Locke, B.Z. (1984) 'The NIMH Epidemiological Catchment Area

Program: historical context, major objectives and study population characteristics', *Archives of General Psychiatry* 44: 934–41.

Regier, D.A., Boyd, J.H., Burke, J.D., Rae, D.S., Meyers, J.K., Kramer, M., Robins, L.N. Gengl. L.K., Karno, M., and Locke, B.Z. (in press) 'One month prevalence of mental disorders in the U.S. – Based on five Epidemiological Catchment Area Sites', *Archives of General Psychiatry*.

Rutter, M. and Quinton, D. (1984) 'Parental psychiatric disorder: effects on children', *Psychological Medicine* 41: 853–80.

United Nations (1985) *World Population Prospects: Estimates and Projections as Assessed in 1982* (Department of International and Social Affairs, Population Studies No. 86 ST/FSA/SER a/86), New York: United Nations.

US Bureau of the Census (1953) *Census of Population 1950: Institutional Population* vol. IV, Special Reports part 2, Chapter C., Washington, DC: US Government Printing Office.

US Bureau of the Census (1973) *Census of Population 1970: Persons in Institutions and Other Group Quarters* (Final report PC (2) – 4E), Washington, DC: US Government Printing Office.

US Bureau of the Census (1979) *Projections of the Populations of the United States by Age, Sex and Race, 1983–2080* (Current Population Reports, Series P–25 No. 952), Washington, DC: US Government Printing Office.

US Bureau of the Census (1984) *Census of Population 1980: Persons in Institutions and Other Group Quarters* (Final Report PC–80–2–4D), Washington, DC: US Government Printing Office.

US Bureau of the Census (1985) *Households, Families, Marital Status and Living Arrangements* (March 1985, advance report, Series P–20 No. 402), Washington, DC: US Government Printing Office.

US Bureau of the Census (1986a) *Marital Status and Living Arrangements* (March 1985, Series P–20 No. 410), Washington, DC: US Government Printing Office.

US Bureau of the Census (1986b) *Households Families, Marital Status and Living Arrangements* (March 1986, Advance Report, Series P–20 No. 412), Washington, DC: US Government Printing Office.

US Bureau of the Census (1986c) *Projections of the Number of Households and Families, 1986–2000* (Series P–25 No. 986), Washington, DC: US Government Printing Office.

US Bureau of the Census; Gregory Spencer (1986d) *Projections of the Hispanic Population, 1983–2080* (Current Population Reports, Series P–25, No. 995), Washington, DC: US Government Printing Office.

Witkin, M.J. (1980). *Trends in Patient Care Episodes in Mental Health Facilities, 1955–1977* (Mental Health Statistical Note No. 154, DHSS Pub. No. (ADM–80–158) Sept. 1980), Rockville, MD: National Institute of Mental Health.

World Health Organization Expert Committee on Health Statistics (1963) *Hospital Statistics and Other Matters* (Eighth Report, Technical Report Series No. 261), Geneva: WHO.

World Health Organization, Expert Committee on Health Statistics (1969) *Statistics of Health Services and Their Activities* (Technical Report Series No. 429), Geneva: WHO.

World Health Organization, Expert Committee on Health Statistics (1971) *Statistical Indicators for the Planning and Evaluation of Public Health Programmes* (Fourteenth Report, Technical Report Series No. 172), Geneva: WHO.

World Health Organization (1976) *Statistical Indices of Family Health* (Report of a WHO Study Group, Technical Report Series No. 587), Geneva: WHO.

World Health Organization (1980) *The Work of WHO 1973–77* (Biennal Report of the Director General, chapter 4: 153–167), Geneva: WHO.

8

Screening for Psychiatric Disorder

David Goldberg

SCREENING VERSUS CASE FINDING

Many authors use the concept of a 'screening test' to mean no more than the use of an inexpensive test as the first part of a two-stage strategy of case identification, where the purpose of the first-stage is to enable those engaged in the more time-consuming task of administering the second-stage case-finding procedure to spend a greater proportion of their time interviewing subjects who will turn out to be cases. This procedure is properly referred to as *case finding*, and refers to 'the testing of patients who have sought health care for disorders which may be unrelated to their chief complaints . . . the execution of case-finding does not carry an implied guarantee that the patient will benefit, only that they will receive the highest standard of care available at that time and place' (Sackett and Holland 1975).

By contrast, *screening* is the testing of apparently healthy volunteers from the general population and separating them into groups with high and low probabilities of a given disorder. The objective of screening is the early detection of diseases whose treatment is either easier or more effective when undertaken at an earlier point in time, so that there is an implicit promise that those who volunteer to be screened will benefit. The requirement that application of the screening procedure will improve the prognosis is implicit in Wilson and Jungner's (1968) ten principles of screening and explicit in Grant's (1982) three conditions for screening.

Other requirements for screening tests are that the natural history of the condition should be understood and that there should be a latent or early symptomatic stage of the illness. We still know relatively little about the untreated course of minor illness, and the latter requirement cannot possibly be met by common mental disorders. However, Wilson (1986) has indicated that 'unreported illness' would be equally acceptable, and numerous surveys have shown that this requirement is easily satisfied.

Evidence that detection of psychiatric disturbance by screening test actually benefits the patient is hard to come by. An early study by Johnstone and Goldberg (1976) showed that detection of psychiatric disorder using the GHQ-60 caused patients to experience symptoms for an average of 2.1 months less than those in the undetected group, and presented suggestive evidence that this effect was especially marked for those with very high scores on their initial consultation. However, Hoeper *et al.* (1984) were unable to replicate this result, although there were a number of unsatisfactory features in the latter study (Goldberg 1984; Williams 1986; Burns 1986).

Before one could recommend that screening for mental illness should become health policy there would need to be uncontested evidence that patients benefit, so that previous reviewers of the field (Eastwood 1971; Goldberg 1974; Williams 1986) have all concluded that the time had not yet arrived. Until such evidence becomes available it should be clear that psychiatrists are in the business of case finding rather than screening, so that strictly speaking we should refer to 'case-finding tests' or 'putative screening tests'. However, both terms are clumsy, and in the remainder of the chapter we will follow common usage and call any inexpensive test or procedure that is applied to a sample in order to select probable cases for further examination a 'screening test'. All of them have been designed to form the first part of what is typically a two-stage research project.

It is still desirable to investigate possible benefits that may accrue to patients as a result of case-finding procedures, preferably using techniques of cost-benefit analysis described by Williams (1986). In addition to the kinds of mixed affective disorders detected by questionnaires such as the General Health Questionnaire (Goldberg 1978) or the Symptom Rating Questionnaire (Harding *et al.* 1980), it would be sensible to consider the costs and benefits of case finding for specific conditions such as alcohol dependence (King 1985; Saunders and Ausland 1987) or severe depressive illness. In the case of alcohol dependence, Kristenson *et al.* (1982) randomly assigned those with positive screening results to an intervention group and a no-treatment control: the former group were shown to have less disability and lower gamma-glutamyl transaminase relative to the latter at four-year follow-up.

In the remainder of chapter various aspects of two-stage survey designs will be considered, starting with the effects of refusals and going on to consider each stage in turn. Factors which affect the validity coefficients of a screening test will be reviewed with emphasis on data concerned with the GHQ, and the chapter will conclude with a short section on survey design.

THE EFFECTS OF REFUSALS

Condon (1986) has drawn attention to the variety of literary devices to which authors resort in order to give the impression that the sample reported upon is representative of the larger population at risk, and suggests that those who refuse are likely to be 'more paranoid, alienated and less compliant with treatment in general'. He points out that journals are likely to reject papers in which the non-representative nature of the sample is highlighted.

Williams and MacDonald (1986) have produced equations to model the effects of two kinds of bias that may arise in two-stage surveys due to refusal to participate: that due to illness and that due to defensiveness. Illness bias refers to the likelihood that psychiatrically ill individuals may be less likely to participate in case-finding surveys, and will, therefore, cause the sample studied to have rather too great a proportion of true normals. The authors show that this bias will have only a rather small effect on the estimated validity coefficients of the screening procedure, but will cause the investigators to underestimate prevalence of disorder.

Defensiveness bias refers to the tendency of those who wish to conceal their illness to refuse to co-operate with the survey. Such a bias will, of course, produce an underestimate of false negatives relative to true negatives, and thus sensitivity will be overestimated. The effect on specificity is negligible, and prevalence will be slightly underestimated.

If we assume that both types of bias are operating, the authors estimate that at a true prevalence of 25 per cent sensitivity will be overestimated and prevalence will be underestimated by between 5 and 6 per cent, while the effect on specificity is negligible. (These figures are derived by making the assumption that each type of bias reduces collaboration by 15 per cent at each stage of the case-finding procedure.)

CHARACTERISTICS OF THE SCREENING TEST

Type of screening procedure

Most screening procedures are pencil-and-paper tests, but other procedures include key informants, short structured interviews, and computer-administered tests. It is not known whether one kind of procedure is better than another, since it is unusual for researchers to compare different procedures during the same study. It has been usual for the type of procedure to be governed by available resources and the needs of a particular study: thus, computer-administered procedures are still relatively rare, while illiterate subjects must have a short structured interview by a research assistant.

Goldberg and Bridges (1987) compared the characteristics of screening by *key informant* (the family doctor) with screening by a *pencil-and-paper-test* (the GHQ-28). The criterion of illness was independent research interview by a psychiatrist using the DSM-III system. The family doctor was shown to be more specific than the GHQ (86 per cent vs. 75 per cent) but very much less sensitive (48 per cent vs. 87 per cent). Of those found to have psychiatric illnesses 41 per cent were detected by both screening procedures, a further 46 per cent by GHQ only, 7 per cent by family doctor only, while 5 per cent

Table 8.1 Validity indices for the DIS interview against research
assessments by psychiatrists (diagnoses with < 20 patients omitted)

	Number in sample	Sensitivity	PPV	Specificity	NPV
Major depressive episode	22	40%	0.20	98%	99%
Phobias	184	27%	0.52	93%	82%
Alcohol-use disorders	62	30%	0.55	98%	95%
Drug-use disorders	27	7%	0.21	99%	97%

were missed by both screening procedures. A broadly similar study by von
Korff *et al.* (1987) showed that the GHQ identified 39 per cent of the DSM-
III illnesses, the family doctor 33 per cent. In this study, a substantial proportion of patients were identified as cases by both GHQ and family doctor, but
not confirmed by the DIS interview.

Anthony *et al.* (1987) have considered the characteristics of the Diagnostic
Interview Schedule (DIS) administered by lay interviewers as a screening
test, when assessed against second-stage assessments by psychiatrists using a
research assessment capable of generating DSM-III diagnoses. Although
specificity and NPV were generally satisfactory, sensitivity and positive
predictive values were not (see table 8.1).

It can be seen that negative predictive values are generally high in conditions of low prevalence, but that the DIS interview is generally insensitive
for major diagnoses, and that the positive predictive value only exceeds 0.5
for alcohol-use disorder and phobias. The low sensitivity shown by the DIS
interview may account for findings in von Korff *et al.*'s paper referred to
earlier.

Computer-generated screening procedures have been described for both
Briquet's disorder (Woodruff *et al.* 1973; Reveley *et al.* 1977) and
alcoholism (Reich *et al.* 1975; Costello and Baillargeon 1978; Robins and
Marcus 1987). They have two advantages over other screening procedures.
The computer is able to incorporate precise decision trees for questions, and
it is able to adapt the questions asked to an individual's earlier responses.
This achieves great time savings without forfeiting accuracy. For example,
for alcohol-use disorder, the computer-generated interview asks on average
50 per cent fewer questions than are contained in the DIS, yet achieves a
sensitivity of 98 per cent and a positive predictive value (at an unstated
prevalence) of 93 per cent. Figures for other diagnoses are equally
impressive (Robins and Marcus 1987). It should be stressed that these coefficients are not comparable with those quoted in other work, since there is no
independent clinical assessment as a criterion: the screening procedure is
merely being compared with results of the whole interview.

A computer-administered version of the Clinical Interview Schedule has been shown to correlate highly with the same interview administered by a clinician (Lewis *et al.* 1988). There is no reason why such computer-administered screening procedures should not be targeted on specific disorders. These matters are discussed further by Hand and Glover in the next chapter.

Choice of screening test

There are now innumerable screening tests, some aimed at detecting a range of psychiatric disorders (for example, the Symptom Rating Questionnaire, the General Health Questionnaire or the Cornell Medical Inventory) while others purport to be diagnosis-specific (for example, the Zung Depression Inventory). Murphy (1981) covers six American screening tests and the GHQ in some detail, and shows that the similarities between them outweigh the differences. Langner's twenty-two-item screening instrument and the Center for Epidemiological Studies' Depression Scale (CES-D) both have unsatisfactory sensitivities, and the Hopkins SCL has somewhat lower specificity.

Those studies that have directly compared screening tests confirm this view. Thus Goldberg *et al.* (1974) compared the GHQ-30 with the Hopkins SCL-36, Maris and Williams (1985) compared the GHQ-12 with the WHO's SRQ, and Stefansson and Kristjansson (1985) compared the GHQ-30 with the CMI: all studies showed that the overall misclassification rates were within a few percentage points of one another. Choice of a particular instrument should, therefore, be determined by the availability of validity data for a comparable population, as well as the needs of a particular survey. Most information is available for the GHQ, and the factors which affect its validity will be considered later in this chapter.

It remains to ask whether it is reasonable to expect the design of screening tests to improve still further, or whether there is not some natural limit to what can be expected from a simple screening procedure. It is clear that any screening procedure which is merely a scaled-down version of the second-stage interview will produce optimal validity coefficients: this merely celebrates a tautology. However, there are indeed limits to what is likely to be achieved, for two reasons. The validity of any procedure cannot be higher than its own reliability, and in the present example both first- and second-stage assessments fall well short of perfect reliability even if the best examples of each are selected. The second reason is that screening procedures erect dichotomies on what are essentially continuously distributed dimensions: there are, therefore, natural limits to the validity coefficients that can be achieved.

Acceptability and ease of administration

Choice of a screening procedure will usually be determined by the available resources and the needs of the population being screened. Screening procedures which have been designed for patients attending general medical clinics (for example, the GHQ and the SRQ) may be more acceptable to respondents who do not see themselves as mentally ill than those whose items are entirely concerned with severe psychological malfunction.

When it is necessary to administer a screening procedure by research assistant (because of illitcracy or blindncss), it is obviously desirable that the interview should be as short as possible. In this connection it is of interest that the validity coefficients for the GHQ-12 are almost as good as those for the GHQ-60; the main advantage of the longer questionnaire being that its positive predictive value is somewhat better (see p. 115).

Reliability

The form of reliability that is most relevant to screening procedures is their internal consistency, usually measured by Cronbach's *alpha* coefficient or by split-half reliability. Shrout and Fleiss (1981) have shown that, provided a test has moderate reliability, sensitivity and specificity are little affected. There is, however, a strong relationship between positive predictive value (PPV) and reliability, which is especially marked for conditions of low prevalence. If, for example, we consider a disorder with a prevalence of 3 per cent which can be measured with a PPV of 72 per cent with a perfectly reliable instrument – then an instrument with a reliability of 0.9 would reduce the PPV to 67 per cent, while an instrument with a reliability of 0.5 would only achieve a PPV of 36 per cent.

The more carefully constructed scales have been shown to have high reliability: alpha for the Beck Depression Inventory is 0.87 (range 0.76 to 0.95), while median values for the GHQ are 0.92, 0.88 and 0.82 for the 60, 30 and 12 item versions respectively. Many screening questionnaires give no information about their reliability, and these should be avoided.

Three types of validity

The *specificity* of a screening test is the proportion of correctly identified normals, or the true negatives expressed as a percentage of the non-cases. The *sensitivity* of a test is the proportion of correctly identified cases, or the true positives expressed as a percentage of the cases. Both of these coefficients are independent of prevalence, and they are, therefore, the most usually quoted coefficients.

A third type of validity coefficient measures the ability of the screening test to respond to severity of disorder rather than merely to the presence or absence of disorder: this is usually measured by a rank-order *correlation coefficient* between scores on the instrument and total severity scores on some standardized research interview. It is thus a measure of concurrent validity.

There have now been over seventy validity studies conducted with the General Health Questionnaire in various parts of the world, of which forty-five give sufficiently detailed accounts of sampling procedures to allow direct

Table 8.2 Variance-weighted mean (VWM) validity coefficients from 43 validity studies of the GHQ

	Sensitivity	Specificity
GHQ-12	89% (85%, 92%)*	80% (77%, 83%)*
GHQ-28	84% (77%, 89%)	82% (78%, 85%)
GHQ-30	74% (70%, 77%)	82% (80%, 83%)
GHQ-60	78% (75%, 82%)	87% (86%, 89%)
All	76% (74%, 78%)*	85% (84%, 86%)*

Source: Goldberg and Williams 1988
* 95% confidence limits

comparisons to be made between them. Williams, Goldberg and Mari (1988) have carried out a meta-analysis of these studies, in which each estimate of validity is weighted by its own variance: so that studies which have used superior sampling strategies are given more weight, and large studies will inevitably count more than small studies. When this is done it is possible to compare estimates of sensitivity and specificity which are *variance weighted means* (VWMs) for each version of the GHQ, and these are shown as table 8.2.

It can be seen that, surprisingly, the best sensitivity has been obtained by the GHQ-12, partly because these studies have tended to use large samples and thus have more precise estimates. It is also noteworthy that the GHQ-28 out-performs the GHQ-30 as regards sensitivity. However, it can be seen that all versions of the questionnaire have very similar specificities.

Prevalence dependent measures of validity

Three other measures of the performance of a screening procedure are often quoted, but are in fact highly dependent upon the prevalence of disorder in a particular sample. The *positive predictive value* (PPV) is the probability that an individual with a high score on the test will be found to be a case at subsequent examination; the *negative predictive value* (NPV) is the probability that a low scorer will be found to be a non-case; while the *overall misclassification rate* (OMR) refers to the percentage of misclassified respondents.

To the working clinician, the PPV is the most important thing about a screening test. However, it is important to grasp that the PPV of any test is highly dependent upon prevalence: as prevalence becomes lower, the PPV must necessarily fall as well. All three measures can be readily calculated for any screening test at a stated prevalence, providing that the sensitivity and specificity are known. Positive predictive value is the number of true positives divided by the proportion with high scores. So:

$$\text{Positive Predictive Value} = \frac{\text{Prevalence} \times \text{sensitivity}}{\text{Percentage with high scores}}$$

Similarly, negative predictive value is the number of true negatives divided by the proportion with low scores. So:

$$\text{Negative Predictive Value} = \frac{\text{Prevalence of non-cases} \times \text{specificity}}{\text{Percentage with low scores}}$$

Similar arguments apply to the overall misclassification rate (OMR) as those described above for the predictive values. It is meaningless to quote an OMR for a particular screening test, since it varies directly with prevalence. However, the variation is not nearly so dramatic as that for the PPV, as it depends upon the difference between the sensitivity and specificity coefficients.

$$OMR = (1 - P) \cdot fp + P \cdot fn$$

Where

OMR = Overall misclassification rate
P $\quad$ = Prevalence
fp $\quad$ = false positive rate (= $1 - $specificity)
fn $\quad$ = false negative rate (= $1 - $sensitivity)

It is possible to calculate the PPVs for different versions of the GHQ scaled to a prevalence of 30 per cent (i.e., a level appropriate to attenders in general practice settings), using either median and variance-weighted mean validity coefficients obtained from public validity studies:

PPV_{30}:

	Using variance-weighted mean coefficients	Using median validity coefficients
GHQ-12	0.65	0.65
GHQ-28	0.67	0.67
GHQ-30	0.63	0.63
GHQ-60	0.73	0.72

Whichever set of coefficients is used, the GHQ-60 has the best performance as a screening instrument, while there is no appreciable difference between the other versions.

CHARACTERISTICS OF THE CRITERION INTERVIEW

Reliability

In general, the correlation between any two measures is attenuated by their unreliability, since the validity of a measure cannot be higher than the reliability of the measure. Lord and Novick (1968) showed the general relationship to be as follows:

$$R_T = \frac{R_0}{\sqrt{(r_1, r_2)}}$$

Where:

R_T = True relationship
R_0 = Observed relationship
r_1 = reliability of 1st stage assessment
r_2 = reliability of 2nd stage assessment

If the second-stage interview is assumed to be error-free, then validity coefficients for a screening test such as the GHQ can be calculated by taking the median values for correlations between the GHQ and research interviews for each version of the GHQ, taking Cronbach's alpha as a measure of 'r_1', and assuming 'r_2' to be unity. These are shown in the first column, and can be seen to be greater than the observed relationships.

However, it is unreasonable to assume that the criterion is free from error. If we use the value of $+0.92$ for the reliability of the CIS (see Goldberg *et al.* 1970) the the 'true correlation' between the GHQ and the criterion interview rises still further, as shown in the second column:

Version of GHQ:	Obtained median correlation	Assume perfect criterion	Assume criterion interview = +0.92
GHQ-12	0.70	0.77	0.81
GHQ-30	0.59	0.63	0.72
GHQ-60	0.72	0.75	0.78

What effects does unreliability of the criterion have on the conventional validity coefficients, sensitivity and specificity? Consider two raters, A and B, who are conducting a validity study of a screening test in a population whose 'true prevalence' is 20 per cent. Assume that rater A obtains values of 75 per cent and 85 per cent for the sensitivity and specificity of the test.

Suppose that the two raters now carry out an inter-rater reliability study, and are found to disagree about 'case/non-case' in a proportion of the cases. We can now examine the effects that this will have on validity coefficients between the GHQ and rater B's assessments – assuming that disagreement between the raters is randomly distributed.

Percentage disagreement	Sensitivity	Specificity
0%	75%	85%
1%	73.6%	84.7%
5%	68.1%	83.3%
10%	60%	81.3%
15%	52.4%	79.4%

It can be seen that unreliability of the criterion has a pronounced effect upon sensitivity, but a much smaller effect upon specificity. Now it is likely that clinical judgements made by investigators carrying out validity studies are indeed imperfect, and that the error in their estimates of sensitivity coefficients is greater than their error in estimating specificity.

Since most investigators are unaware of the asymmetry, they calculate a cut-off score by doing the best trade-off between sensitivity and specificity. In their efforts to increase sensitivity at the expense of specificity they, therefore, lower the threshold score, and will in general tend to produce cut-off scores that are too low. Thus, the less competent the investigator, the lower the threshold.

Validity

It might be supposed that different research interviews generate rather different validity coefficients for a particular screening test, since each incorporates somewhat different concepts of psychiatric 'caseness'. Curiously enough, this seems not to be the case.

The most commonly used structured psychiatric interview employed in validity studies of the GHQ is the Clinical Interview Schedule (CIS) of Goldberg *et al.* (1970). The Present State Examination (PSE) has been used in twelve of the validity studies, and in four others other standardized psychiatric interviews provided the criterion assessment. *The VWM sensitivities for these three groups are within 1 per cent of each other.* Similarly, the VWM specificities for the three groups are within 3 per cent of each other.

Duncan-Jones *et al.* (1986) provide a clue as to how this might come about. These workers used techniques of latent trait analysis to analyse a set

117

of over 6,000 responses to the GHQ-12, and demonstrated that the test can be shown to be providing maximum information over a fairly broad range of values on the underlying dimension of severity of disturbance, although the information provided tails off markedly at each extreme. Put another way, this means that the test will discriminate rather poorly between individuals in groups of respondents who are psychologically very healthy or between individuals within groups who are psychiatrically very ill; but that it provides maximum discrimination over the whole intermediate range of severities (Duncan-Jones *et al*. 1986: 399 figure 3).

Grayson *et al*. (1987) showed that three commonly used research criteria for psychiatric illness are all included within this range. Thus, even if, for example, a 'DSM-III case' is slightly less severe a concept than an 'ID-Catego 5+' case, both are within the optimal range of measurement of the screening test. Similar validity coefficients are thus obtained by finding the optimal trade-off for sensitivity against specificity for each 'criterion' of psychiatric illness. It can be seen that the obtained values are indeed likely to be similar providing that the criterion comes within the maximal range of information provided by the test on the underlying dimension of disturbance.

FACTORS WHICH AFFECT THE VALIDITY OF A SCREENING TEST

The General Health Questionnaire will be used as the example of a screening test in this section, since it has been possible to perform meta-analyses of the validity coefficients reported in studies conducted in a wide variety of settings. It has thus been possible to address possible influences on the validity of a well-known screening procedure in an objective way (described more fully in Goldberg and Williams 1988).

We have seen that the length of the screening test and the nature of the validating interview make rather small effects on validity coefficients, but that sensitivity is affected by non-response bias and by reliability of the criterion interview. In general terms, we have seen that the former tends to cause overestimates of sensitivity, while the latter may cause it to be severely underestimated. We shall now consider the effect of five further possible influences.

Socio-demographic characteristics of respondents

Goldberg *et al*. (1974) examined overall misclassification rates with respect to a variety of socio-demographic variables. They noted that GHQ performed better with men than with women and with whites than with blacks, but that the differences were small and not statistically significant. They found no effect of social class or age on misclassification.

Tarnopolsky *et al*. (1979) found that the positive predictive value of the GHQ was higher in women than in men. However, a direct comparison of

118

Table 8.3 The relationship between sex and the validity of the GHQ

| | Sensitivity | | Specificity | |
	Male	*Female*	*Male*	*Female*
Hobbs *et al.* (1983, 1984)	72	90	87	84
Jenkins (1985)	61	79	83	85
Vazquez-Barquero (1986)	48	67	86	86

the validity coefficients in men and women can be obtained from the studies of Jenkins (1985), Hobbs and his colleagues (1983, 1984) and Vazquez-Barquero *et al.* (1986). In each of the studies, the sensitivity was lower in the men than in the women, whereas this was not the case for the specificity (see table 8.3).

The finding is extended by the results of Williams *et al.*'s (1988) meta-analysis. The VWM sensitivity for the male data in table 8.3 is 64 per cent, the corresponding figure obtained from ten validity studies of female respondents was 80 per cent. As might be expected, the VWM sensitivity for thirty-one studies giving data for both sexes combined was exactly intermediate at 76 per cent! The table also shows that there was no substantial association between sex and specificity: a finding confirmed by the meta-analytic investigation.

Mari and Williams (1986) used ROC analysis to investigate the effects of five socio-demographic variables on misclassification by the GHQ-12 in their study in primary care in Brazil. While the pattern of results was complex, they found that, in general, men were more likely than women to be classified as false negative, while poorly educated respondents were more likely to be classified as false positive.

Language and culture

The GHQ has been translated into a wide variety of European, Asian, and other languages. Similarly, structured interviews such as the CIS and PSE have been translated and used in a wide variety of cultural settings. Many conceptual and practical problems arise when instruments designed and constructed in one culture are translated for use in another. Despite these problems, the GHQ appears to perform well in a variety of cultural settings, and has been translated into at least thirty-six languages.

Indeed, the VWM specificities for the English and the non-English studies in the meta-analysis were 85 per cent and 86 per cent respectively. The VWM sensitivity of the non-English studies was slightly higher than that for the English studies (78 per cent compared with 74 per cent), although the difference did not reach statistical significance ($Z = 1.68$). Cheng and Williams (1986) have shown that the addition of thirty specially designed

'Chinese' items to the GHQ-30 add a little to the validity of the GHQ: the overall misclassification rate with the GHQ-30 was 11.6 per cent, but this dropped to 9.6 per cent with the new 60-item 'Chinese GHQ'. This had the effect of improving the sensitivity of the revised instrument, and shows that taking local symptom patterns into account can slightly improve the overall discrimination obtainable.

However, in general it would appear that cultural factors make a rather small contribution to the identification of minor psychiatric illness, although it must be stressed that the research interviews used in these studies have all been designed in English-speaking countries. With this caveat, the item content of the GHQ identifies psychologically disordered people in a wide variety of cultures and languages.

Delay between stages

In a two-stage study it is desirable for the interview to take place as soon as possible after the questionnaire has been completed. Otherwise changes in the clinical state of respondents might be expected to result in lower validity coefficients than would otherwise be the case. Since the GHQ is designed to detect relatively acute changes in state, many of which are short-lived, the expected effect of delay is that a greater proportion of high-scoring respondents will be rated as non-cases on subsequent interview, i.e., will be regarded as false positives. A similar, but smaller, effect is to be expected from people becoming ill between questionnaire and interview.

The delay between stages is clearly stated in twenty-nine of the validity studies of the GHQ, and was one week or less in fourteen, and one month or less in a further ten. An effect in the predicted direction can be found for the sensitivity: the median values for the two groups of studies being 80 per cent and 70 per cent respectively. This was confirmed in Williams et al.'s meta-analysis, where the VWM sensitivities of the two groups of studies were 81 per cent for a delay between stages of up to one week, and 57 per cent for a delay of up to one month (Williams et al. 1988).

A similar effect was found for specificity, with VWM values of 86 per cent 62 per cent for the short and long delay respectively.

Interestingly, the values for the VWM sensitivity and specificity of twenty-four studies in which the interview was given at the same time as the questionnaire were 79 per cent and 83 per cent respectively – that is to say, no different from the values for a delay of up to one week. Even so, the implication for study design is clear: keep the delay between stages as short as possible.

Consulting setting

The validity of the GHQ has been investigated in a wide variety of settings, which can conveniently be considered in three categories according to their position on 'the pathway to specialist care' (Goldberg and Huxley 1980).

First are nineteen studies which have been conducted in a non-consulting setting, including community surveys and surveys of special groups such as students. Second are fourteen validity studies which have been located in the setting of primary medical care. Third are fourteen studies which have been conducted in the setting of secondary medical care. The VWM sensitivities and specificities are shown below:

Setting	VWM sensitivity	VWM specificity
Community	64%	85%
Primary care	83%	84%
Secondary care	81%	85%

Thus, it can be seen that the sensitivity is lower in studies in the community than in consulting settings, whereas the specificity appears not to differ between the settings.

Effects of physical ill-health

Since physically ill people score highly on screening tests it is not surprising that they are over-represented among those respondents classified as false positives. For example, Bridges and Goldberg (1986) had to raise the threshold score on the GHQ-28 as high as 11/12 in order to obtain optimal discrimination between cases and normals among neurological in-patients because of the very high levels of physical symptoms experienced by these patients.

If the GHQ is to be used with patients with severe physical illness, it may be necessary to raise the threshold in order to obtain an optimal trade-off between sensitivity and specificity.

Summary

It would appear that – when allowance is made for the size of the various samples – the sensitivities and specificities of the GHQ are fairly predictable, as shown by the fairly narrow confidence limits shown in table 8.2. The main reasons for carrying out further validity studies would be to establish the *optimal threshold* to be used in some new cultural or consulting situations, since the coefficients themselves appear to be relatively stable.

Table 8.4 gives a summary of the various factors which have been shown to have effects on screening procedures. It will be recalled that the nature of the second-stage case-finding interview, whether or not the study takes place in primary care or in a hospital setting, and factors relating to language and culture, all seem to have rather small effects.

Table 8.4 Summary of principal factors that affect the performance of screening procedures

	Sensitivity	Specificity	Correlation	PPV	Prevalence
for any screening procedure					
Illness bias	Little effect	Little effect			ca 6% under-estimated
Defensiveness bias	ca 6% over-estimated	Little effect			Slight under est.
Unreliability of screen	Little effect	Little effect	Attenuates	Attenuates at low prev.	
Unreliablity of criterion	Markedly depressed	Slightly depressed	Attenuates		
for GHQ:					
Length of screen	Little effect	Little effect		Increases steadily	
Delay between stages 1 week	Slightly depressed	No effect			
Delay between stages 1 month	Markedly depressed	Markedly depressed			
Sex	Males lower	No effect			
Community vs. consulting	Community lower	No effect			

SURVEY DESIGN

The main use of a case-finding test is to identify respondents who should be interviewed at greater length in order to identify true positives. Thus, an investigator may adopt a stratified sampling strategy in which as many as possible of those scoring above some arbitrary threshold are selected for interview, together with a probability sample of those with low scores. This is a perfectly legitimate use of a screening test, but it must be appreciated that it is not the optimal design for estimating validity coefficients.

To calculate the most precise validity coefficients in a new setting

If an investigator does not wish to rely on already published validity studies – either because none are available for the particular class of respondent, or because a new screening test is being studied – then the advice must depend on the estimated prevalence of disorder in the population to be examined.

If the estimated prevalence is between 25 and 35 per cent, it is best to select a random sample of respondents for the second-stage interview, since this will both allow the investigator to calculate a Relative Operating Characteristic (ROC) curve and provide the most precise estimates of validity coefficients.

An ROC curve is obtained by plotting sensitivity against false-positive rate (the complement of specificity) for all possible cut-off points of the screening procedure. ROC analysis was first developed in psychophysics to assess the ability of an observer to identify a signal against a background of noise (Swets 1964), and has been used in medical decision analysis by Weinstein and Feinberg 1980. Several investigators have applied ROC analysis to study the characteristics of screening procedures in psychiatry (Mari and Williams 1985, 1986; Bridges and Goldberg 1986; Bellantuono 1987; Surtees 1987; and Newman 1988). ROC analysis provides the best estimate of threshold score, and allows one screening procedure to be compared with another.

If, however, the estimated prevalence of disorder is low, then the use of a random sample of first-stage respondents for second-stage interview will result in the investigators spending most of their time interviewing non-cases. In such cases they may prefer to take either a truncated random sample (see p. 124) or a stratified sample.

Stratified sampling procedures have three disadvantages: it is essential to weight the data back to the original first-stage characteristics before calculating the validity cofficients; two strata models assume that the best threshold is known – whereas this is actually a most variable characteristic; and they produce less precise (in the sense of having larger variances) estimates of the validity coefficients (Williams *et al.* 1988).

Predicting prevalence from results of a screening test

This can readily be done by using known validity coefficients and substituting them in the formula shown below:

$$\frac{\text{pHS} + \text{Specificity} - 1}{\text{Sensitivity} + \text{Specificity} - 1}$$

Alternatively, it can be expressed as the sum of the true positives and the false negatives (both expressed as a proportion of the total sample), i.e.,

$$(\text{PPV} \cdot \text{pHS}) + (1 - \text{NPV}) \cdot \text{pLS}.$$

Where pHS, pLS denotes the proportion with high and low scores; PPV and NPV are the positive and negative predictive values.

To estimate the best threshold

The best threshold score is that which gives the best trade-off between sensitivity and specificity, and this is most easily calculated with an ROC curve. Sometimes researchers do not wish to take a random sample, since they do not wish to spend most of their time interviewing non-cases. An alternative strategy would be to take a *truncated random sample* in which all respondents with a score of zero are not selected for interview, but are assumed to be non-cases. A random sample of those with a score of one or more would be selected for interview. This strategy is considered in more detail by Goldberg and Williams (1988).

REFERENCES

Anthony, J., Folstein, M., Romanowski, A.J., von Korff, M., Nestadt, G., Chahal, R., Merchant, A., Brown, C., Shapiro, S., Kramer, M., and Gruenberg, E. (1987) 'Comparison of lay DIS and a standardised psychiatric diagnosis', *Archives of General Psychiatry*, in press.

Beck, T.A., Rial, W.Y., and Rickels, K. (1974) 'Short form of the Beck Depression Inventory: cross validation', *Psychological Reports* 34: 1184–6.

Bellantuono, C., Fiorio, R., Zanotelli, R., and Tansella, N. (1987) 'Psychiatric screening in general practice in Italy: a validity study of the GHQ', *Social Psychiatry* 22: 113–17.

Bridges, K.W. and Goldberg, D.P. (1986) 'The validation of the GHQ-28 and the use of the M.M.S.E. in neurological inpatients', *British Journal of Psychiatry* 148: 548–53.

Burns, B. (1986) 'General discussion: screening', in M. Shepherd, G. Wilkinson, and P. Williams (eds) *Mental Illness in Primary Care Settings*, London: Tavistock, 83.

Cheng, T.A. and Williams, P. (1986) 'The design and development of a screening questionnaire (GHQ) for use in community studies of marital disorders in Taiwan', *Psychological Medicine* 16: 415–22.

Condon, J.T. (1986) 'The unresearched: those who decline to participate', *Australian and New Zealand Journal of Psychiatry* 20: 87–9.

Costello, R.M. and Baillargeon, J.G. (1978) 'Alcoholism screening inventory: replication of Reich and extension', *British Journal of Addiction* 73: 399–405.

Duncan-Jones, P., Grayson, D., and Moran, P.A.P. (1986) 'The utility of latent trait models in psychiatric epidemiology', *Psychological Medicine* 16: 391–405.

Duncan-Jones, P. and Henderson, S. (1978) 'The use of a two-phase design in a prevalence survey', *Social Psychiatry* 13: 231–7.

Eastwood, M.R. (1971) 'Screening for psychiatric disorder', *Psychological Medicine* 1: 197–208.

Finlay-Jones, R.A. and Murphy, E. (1979) 'Severity of psychiatric disorder and the 30-item General Health Questionnaire', *British Journal of Psychiatry* 134: 609–16.

Gask, L., McGrath, G., Goldberg, D., and Millar, T. (1987) 'Improving the psychiatric skills of established general practitioners: evaluation of group teaching', *Medical Education*, in press.

Goldberg, D. (1974) 'Screening for disease – psychiatric disorders', *Lancet* ii: 1245–8.

Goldberg, D.P. (1978) *Manual of the General Health Questionnaire* Windsor: NFER/Nelson.

Goldberg, D. (1984) 'Screening for mental illness', letter, *Lancet* i: 224.

Goldberg, D. (1986) 'Use of the General Health Questionnaire in clinical work', *British Medical Journal* 293: 1188–9.

Goldberg, D. and Bridges, K. (1987) 'Screening for psychiatric illness in general practice: the general practitioner versus the screening questionnaire', *Journal of the Royal College of General Practitioners* 37: 15–18.

Goldberg, D.P., Cooper, A.B., Eastwood, M.R., Kedward, H.B., and Shepherd, M. (1970) 'A psychiatric interview suitable for use in community surveys', *British Journal of Social and Preventive Medicine* 24: 18–26.

Goldberg, D. and Huxley, P. (1980) *Mental Illness in the Community: The Pathway to Psychiatric Care*, London: Tavistock.

Goldberg, D.P., Rickels, K., Downing, R., and Hesbacher, P. (1974) 'A comparison of two psychiatric screening tests', *British Journal of Psychiatry* 129: 61–7.

Goldberg, D. and Williams, P. (1988) *The User's Guide to the General Health Questionnaire*, London: NFER/Nelson.

Goodchild, M.E. and Duncan-Jones, P. (1985) 'Chronicity and the General Health Questionnaire', *British Journal of Psychiatry* 146: 55–61.

Grant, I.W. (1982) 'Screening for lung cancer', *British Medical Journal* 284: 1209–10.

Grayson, D., Bridges, K., Duncan-Jones, P. and Goldberg, D.P. (1987) 'The relationship between symptoms and diagnoses of minor psychiatric disorder in general practice', *Psychological Medicine* 17, in press.

Harding, T.W., Arnago, M.V., Balthazar, J., Climent, C.E., Ibrahim, H.H.A., Ladrigo-Ignacio, L., Srivinatha Murthy, R., and Wig, N.N. (1980) 'Mental disorders in primary care: a study of their frequency and diagnosis in four developing countries', *Psychological Medicine* 10: 231–42.

Hobbs, P., Ballinger, C.B., and Smith, D.M.W. (1983) 'Factor analysis and validation of the General Health Questionnaire in women: and general practice surveys', *British Journal of Psychiatry* 142: 257–64.

Hobbs, P., Ballinger, C.V., Greenwood, C., Martin, B., and McClure, A. (1984) 'Factor analysis and validation of the General Health Questionnaire in men: a general practice survey', *British Journal of Psychiatry* 144: 270–5.

Hodiamont, P., Peer, N., and Syben, N. (1987) 'Epidemiological aspects of psychiatric disorder in a Dutch health area', *Psychological Medicine* 17: 495–505.

Hoeper, E., Nycz, G., Kessler, L., Burke, J., and Pierce, W. (1984) 'The usefulness of screening for mental health', *Lancet* i: 33–5.

Jenkins, R. (1985) 'Sex differences in minor psychiatric morbidity', *Psychological Medicine*, Supplement 7.

Johnstone, A. and Goldberg, D. (1976) 'Psychiatric screening in general practice', *Lancet* i: 605–8.

Johnstone, A. and Shepley, M. (1986) 'The outcome of hidden neurotic illness treated in general practice', *Journal of the Royal College of General Practitioners* 36: 413–15.

King, M. (1985) 'At risk drinking among general practice attenders: validation of the CAGE questionnaire', *Psychological Medicine* 16: 213–16.

Kristenson, H., Ohlin, H., Hulten-Nosslin, M., Trell, E., and Wood, B. (1983) 'Identification and intervention of heavy drinking in middle aged men: results and follow-up of 24–60 months of long term study with randomised controls', *Alcoholism: Clinical & Experimental Research* 7: 203–9.

Lewis, G., Pelosi, A.J., Glover, E., Wilkinson, G., Stansfeld, S.A., Williams, P., and Shepherd, M. (1988) 'The development of a computerised assessment for minor psychiatric disorder', *Psychological Medicine*, in press.

Lord, F.M. and Novick, M.R. (1968) *Statistical Theories of Mental Test Scores*, Reading, Mass.: Addison-Wesley.

Mari, J.J. and Williams, P. (1986) 'Misclassification by psychiatric screening

125

questionnaires', *Journal of Chronic Diseases* 39: 371–8.

Mari, J.J. and Williams, P. (1985) 'Comparison of the validity of two psychiatric screening questionnaires using ROC analysis', *Psychological Medicine* 15: 651–9.

Murphy, J.M. (1981) 'Psychiatric instrument development for primary care research: patient self-report questionnaire' (report to Division of Biometry and Epidemiology of the NIMH, Washington, on Contract No. SOMO14280101D), unpublished.

Newman, S.C., Bland, R., and Orn, H. 'General Health Questionnaire as a screening instrument in a community survey', *Psychological Medicine*, (submitted for publication).

Reich, T., Robins, L.N., Woodruff, R.A., Taibleson, M., Rich, C., and Cunningham, L. (1975) 'Computer-assisted derivation of a screening interview for alcoholism', *Archives of General Psychiatry* 32: 847–52.

Reveley, M.A., Woodruff, R.A., Robins, L.N., Taibleson, M., Reich, T., and Helzer, J. (1977) 'Evaluation of a screening programme for Briquet's syndrome', *Archives of General Psychiatry* 34: 145–50.

Robins, L.N. and Marcus, S.C. 'The diagnostic screening procedure writer', in press.

Sackett, D. and Holland, W. (1975) 'Controversy in the detection of disease', *Lancet* ii: 357–9.

Saunders, J.B. and Ausland, O.G. (1987) *WHO Collaborative Project on Identification and Treatment of Persons with Harmful Alcohol Consumption*, Geneva: WHO.

Shrout, P.E. and Fleiss, J.L. (1981) 'Reliability and case detection', in J.K. Wing, P. Bebbington, and L. Robins (eds) *What is a Case?*, London: Grant, McIntyre.

Stefansson, J.G. and Kristjansson, I. (1985) 'Comparison of the GHQ and the CMI', *Acta Psychiatrica Scandinavica* 72: 482–7.

Surtees, P.G. (1987) 'Psychiatric disorder in the community and the General Health Questionnaire', submitted to the *British Journal of Psychiatry* 150: 828–35.

Swets, J.A. (1964) *Signal Detection and Recognition by Human Observers*, New York: Wiley.

Tarnopolsky, A., Hand, D.J., McLean, E.K., Roberts, H., and Wiggins, R.D. (1979) 'Validity of uses of a screening questionnaire (GHQ) in the community', *British Journal of Psychiatry* 134: 508–15.

Vazquez-Barquero, J.L., Diez-Manrique, J.F., Pena, C., Quintanal, R.G., and Labrador Lopez, M. (1986) 'Two stage design in a community survey', *British Journal of Psychiatry* 149: 88–97.

von Korff, M., Shapiro, S., Burke, J., Teitlebaum, M., Skinner, E.A., German, P., Klein, L., and Burns, B.J. (1987) 'Mental disorders in primary care: assessment by the DIS, GHQ and practitioner', *Archives of General Psychiatry*, in press.

Weinstein, M.C. and Fineberg, H.V. (1980) *Clinical Decision Analysis*, Philadelphia: W.B. Saunders.

Williams, P. (1986) 'Mental illness and primary care: screening', in M. Shepherd, G. Wilkinson and P. Williams (eds) *Mental Illness in Primary Care Settings*, London: Tavistock.

Williams, P. and MacDonald, A. (1986) 'The effect of non-response bias on the results of two-stage screening surveys of psychiatric disorder', *Social Psychiatry* 21: 1–5.

Williams, P., Goldberg, D., and Mari, J.J. (1988) 'A method for comparing validity coefficients in two-stage screening studies', Institute of Psychiatry, unpublished.

Wilson, J.M. and Jungner, G. (1968) *The principles and practice of screening for disease* (WHO Public Health Papers No. 34), Geneva: World Health Organization.

Wilson, J.M. (1986) 'Screening: general discussion', in M. Shepherd, G. Wilkinson and P. Williams (eds) *Mental Illness in Primary Care Settings*, London, Tavistock, p. 79.

126

Woodruff, R.A., Robins, L.B., Taibleson, N., Reich, T., and Helzer, J. (1973) 'Evaluation of a screening interview for hysteria', *Archives of General Psychiatry* 29: 450–55.

9

The Impact of Information Technology

David Hand and Eric Glover

The nature of the effects that computers and information technology have upon everyday life can be classified according to a position on a continuum. At one extreme of this continuum lies the striking effect – the new development which makes one sit up and take notice. And at the other extreme lies the subtle effect – the development occurring in the background which serves to make everyday life easier in some way. In between these two extremes lies a range of developments with intermediate impact.

Precisely the same is true of the impact of computers and information technology on psychiatry. There are the novel and exciting breakthroughs and there are the subtle but nevertheless very influential background changes. In this article we shall look at this range, presenting examples from various points to demonstrate how computers are already beginning to influence the development and practice of epidemiological and social psychiatry. The four topics we have chosen to illustrate the effects are statistics, computerized interviewing, computerized diagnosis, and artificial intelligence. These range from developments extending the work of pre-computer days to developments which were completely infeasible prior to the computer.

Perhaps we should also remark that our four examples by no means exhaust the ways in which computers and information technology are changing psychiatry. Other examples include the different kinds of brain scanners, simulation models for teaching purposes, sophisticated graphics tools for exploring neurochemical phenomena, and so on.

STATISTICS

Statistical techniques are the fundamental tools of epidemiological research, and statistical techniques are experiencing an extraordinary era of development, driven in part by the computer. Anybody with a passing familiarity with epidemiological psychiatry will have encountered concepts such as that of relative risk, but a cursory glance at the literature now reveals that reports

128

of psychiatric research are liberally littered with the names of sophisticated new techniques. For example, in explicit recognition of the fact that it is not possible to characterize adequately the complexity of the human mind with just one or two scores, one sees increasing reference to multivariate techniques. Most readers will have seen accounts of cluster analysis (Everitt 1972, 1980) being used in attempts to clarify the typology of depression; accounts of factor analysis (Harman 1967; Tabachnik and Fidell 1983) being used in attempts to define personality more precisely (Eysenck 1981); and, more recently, accounts of multivariate analysis of variance (Hand and Taylor, 1987) being used to characterize the differences between groups of subjects. Other multivariate techniques which are beginning to appear in the psychiatric literature include correspondence analysis (Greenacre 1984; Dunn 1986) and linear structural relationship modelling (Everitt 1984).

The techniques listed above represent examples of methods which had their genesis in pre-computer days. For most of them it was possible to conduct such analysis by hand (or, at least, by mechanical calculator) although months rather than seconds would have been required. The fact that computers can perform the calculations very rapidly has had two effects. There is the obvious one that researchers now perform the analyses as a matter of course (a point to which we return below). Also there is the less obvious one that such computational facility has stimulated dramatic theoretical development of these techniques. Perhaps the prime example of this is the generalized linear model (McCullagh and Nelder 1983). This is a general structure, of which regression analysis and analysis of variance are special cases. Another very important special case is the log-linear model (Bishop, Fienberg and Holland 1975). This is particularly important in psychiatry because of the nature of psychiatric data (see below). A recent example of the use of this class of techniques in psychiatric research is given in Dunn (1986).

If the above represent theoretical and practical developments driven by the computer but having their origins in pre-computer-age methodology, then there are other developments which would have been inconceivable without modern computational power. Here, a perfect illustration is the bootstrap technique (Efron 1982). This permits one to assess the variation one would expect in an estimate, no matter how complex the estimator, by recalculating the estimate again and again using subsamples of the original data. The bootstrap idea is revolutionary – and very much a child of the computer age.

We referred above to the 'nature of psychiatric data'. Loosely, one might characterize it as involving mixed variable types, often ordinal and probably categorical. This poses particular challenges and, though it is by no means unique to psychiatry, it has led to a unique flavour to the class of statistical methods used in psychiatry. Similarly, the acknowledged difficulty of clearly defining many of the concepts has led to emphasis on exploring questions of reliability. Precise operational definitions have, therefore, been painstakingly

129

constructed and in many cases the results, involving carefully structured interviews and the like, have greater reliability than in other areas of medicine. Again, the computer, using statistical methods such as factor analysis, principal components analysis, discriminant analysis, and item analysis, has played a key role. Of course, many questions remain open, and it is a rich and exciting area for statisticians who wish to develop some practically relevant methodological theory.

Recent discussions of the relevance of statistics to psychiatry include Hand (1985a) and Everitt (1987).

All that we have said so far about the impact of computers on statistics in epidemiological psychiatry is to the good, but there is also a dark side. Statistical packages are designed to be easy to use, but they are also easy to misuse. The computer will do the calculations on whatever numbers are fed to it – regardless of their validity or meaningfulness. And, of course, the very sophistication of modern statistical packages makes things far worse. In many cases the user may have a weak grasp of the theory underlying a technique he is attempting to apply. He may not even understand the output. Several recent papers have drawn attention to the extent of misuse of statistical methods in medical and psychiatric research (e.g. White 1979; Gore *et al*. 1977). The ideal answer of more statistical education – both of researchers in psychiatry and of statistical consultants – is perhaps a forlorn hope. However, a more recent development, which makes the future look brighter, makes full use of the ideas of information technology. This is the advent of the statistical expert system – computer programs which help a user to apply statistical methods correctly without making errors. They will guide, monitor, and advise the researcher. Hand (1986) gives a recent review of this rapidly developing field.

COMPUTERIZED INTERVIEWING

Computers have been used sporadically in psychiatry for interviewing patients over the past twenty years. The term 'computerized interviewing' now seems to be common, although it must be borne in mind that in the systems currently being used it is really only multiple choice questionnaires which are being talked about. No system, yet, is capable of understanding and replying to a patient's typed or spoken utterance, nor will it be for the foreseeable future.

Typically, in current systems, a series of questions is presented to the patient on the visual display screen of a computer. To each question a series of answers is proposed by the computer and the patient has to choose the answer he or she feels is most appropriate for them by touching a certain key on the keyboard.

Among the many papers which report these systems in use we mention the following as a representative sample. Psychiatric case histories: Slack and Van

Cura (1968), Coddington and King (1972), Dove *et al.* (1977), Carr *et al.* (1983); depression and suicide: Greist *et al.* (1973), Carr *et al.* (1981); phobia: Carr and Ghosh (1983); general screening and assessment: Krynicki and Gould (1984), Comings (1984), Lewis *et al.* (1988).

These researchers (and others not mentioned) have established the viability of using computers in this way. On the whole, patients did not object to using them and the results obtained were satisfactory to the people involved. Most of the computerized interviewing projects have been confined to hospital settings (with both in-patients and out-patients) and the patients involved have sometimes been psychotic. A typical 'consultation' with a computer usually lasts between fifteen and thirty minutes, although one group (Dove *et al.* 1977) used a very long interview which took nearly two hours to complete. Unusually, this took place in a general practice health centre and the researchers claim that the easy-going nature of the computer-patient interview had a definite therapeutic effect.

A project to computerize the Clinical Interview Schedule is being undertaken at the General Practice Research Unit, Institute of Psychiatry. For this purpose, the existing CIS, which was not a questionnaire, has been transformed into one by expanding some questions and deleting others. The initial computer program has grown into a general purpose one enabling any questionnaire to be set up. The current system, called PROQSY (PROgrammable Questionnaire SYstem), which is still under development, has been used in a general practice setting with some degree of success (Lewis *et al* 1988). In addition to the CIS, it enables many different sorts of interview to be designed and then administered by psychiatrists.

A script of the desired questionnaire is prepared on a word processor and is then submitted to the PROQSY driver program for execution. This takes place according to the branching and scoring commands which the psychiatrist has specified within the script. The driver program automatically scores the patient as the interview proceeds and outputs a data file suitable for statistical analysis at the end. Alternatively, a brief clinical report of the interview can be prepared. A typical question, answer, and command set (called a frame) looks like

IRRIT_CHILDREN

Have you felt like hitting one of your children recently?

1 No
2 Yes, but I didn't hit out
3 Yes, and I did hit out

if IRRIT < answer then IRRIT: = answer − 1;

if IRRIT = = 0 then goto IRRIT_SPOUSE;

The answer is selected by typing the appropriate number key. Only the question and answer are displayed on the screen, but the Frame Label (first line) and the Frame Commands (last two lines) enable the psychiatrist to control the flow of the interview and to collect scores in a number of nominated variables (in this case IRRIT) according to the answers received. At the end of the interview the values of all the variables can be dumped to a file ready for inclusion as a record in a database or for clinical analysis.

From the experience gained in the GPRU and that reported by others, we can state that computerized interviews have the following advantages over human administered ones:

A1) Reliability is maximal. There is only one rater, the computer, and it is completely consistent. It never gets bored with patients and it never prejudges them. Patients can set their own pace and take as much time as they want.

A2) Interview structure can be more complex than is feasible for either self-report questionnaires or human administered interviews. Thus, complex branches may be set up to handle a large range of answering possibilities which a human interviewer would find difficult to cope with. Furthermore, questions can be tailored to suit specific social groupings.

A3) There is some evidence to suggest that people are more truthful to a computer than they are to other people in regard to certain areas of their lives (e.g. alcohol consumption, suicidal tendencies) which might concern deviant behaviour. This topic requires further research, however.

A4) Administering an interview by computer is cheap and easy (given the right facilities) when compared with the human method. Furthermore, most patients like it and some report beneficial effects.

A5) The computer method is thorough, and the multiple choice technique ensures that answers can't be fudged or skipped.

Against these must be set the disadvantages:

D1) The only communication between patient and interviewer is verbal and mostly one way, from computer to patient. Thus, possibly important auditory or visual clues emanating from the patient as to his or her mental state will be missed.

D2) The use of multiple choice questions makes the semantic range of answers discrete instead of continuous and thus suppresses any possible variation in meaning. Also, the interview designer may omit an important possibility from the answer set and the patient may be forced into giving a false answer. Moreover, the patient is not able to expand on the answer or to correct a misleading impression.

D3) Some patients cannot be interviewed by computer for a variety of reasons, such as timidity, illiteracy, poor eyesight, obesity, etc.

The chief uses of this form of interviewing for the psychiatrist would appear to be for epidemiological research and clinical screening, i.e., as an information gatherer, rather than for any therapeutic purpose. The assessment of psychiatric disorder by the various computer programs usually takes two forms. One is a numerical classification along one or more axes and the other is a brief verbal report based on the numerical score and possibly incorporating phrases excerpted from appropriate questions or answers. Mostly, the numerical scales, like the questionnaires themselves, are taken with minimal modification from existing questionnaires which have achieved some degree of acceptability among psychiatrists.

The prognosis for computerized interviews in general practice psychiatry is unclear at the moment. On the theoretical side, they will need to evolve away from the existing instruments if the advantages of computers are to be properly exploited, but in doing so they will become less acceptable for many researchers. On the practical side, it seems likely that, as computer hardware continues to fall in price and more and more general practices possess computers, greater use will be made of them by researchers in epidemiological psychiatry. However, practical difficulties and medical conservatism may delay or even prevent their widespread use in any clinical role.

COMPUTER-AIDED DIAGNOSIS

The possibility of using computers to assist in the diagnostic process is a very exciting one, and one which has attracted much interest in recent decades. For epidemiological and social psychiatry, the particular importance lies in the promise of replicable and reliable diagnoses as well as the potential for effective screening.

There are four basic types of approach, although naturally they overlap to some extent.

The *actuarial* approach begins with a large body of data describing patients with known diagnoses. From this, statistical methods are used to extract relevant information so that, when presented with a profile of symptoms for a new patient, one can calculate the probability that he belongs to each of the diagnostic categories.

A great many such schemes have been developed, many of them based on the ideas of statistical pattern recognition common to automatic EEG analysis and speech recognition. Hand (1981) describes such methods.

The second class of approaches is the *decision tree* approach. Here one progressively narrows down the diagnostic possibilities by answering a sequence of questions. The idea is an old one, but one which has grown with

133

the computer so that nowadays large decision trees require implementation on a computer.

The third kind of approach is illustrated by the CATEGO program. This is a hierarchical program which takes 500 items describing the patient and successively condenses them through a series of stages to arrive at a conclusion in terms of twenty-nine clinical categories. Sharp (1987) contains a brief description of the program.

The fourth approach to computer-assisted diagnosis is via *expert systems* technology. Basically such systems consist of a collection of 'rules' summarizing knowledge about (in this case) psychiatric illness. Each rule has the form 'IF (conditions) THEN (actions), where the 'conditions' describe some aspect of the patient and the 'actions' either represent some deduction about the patient or represent a diagnosis. (Sharp (1987) and Hand (1985b) give descriptions of rule-based systems.) More sophisticated expert systems contain complex causal models of the underlying disease process (e.g. Szolovits 1982).

ARTIFICIAL INTELLIGENCE

Artificial intelligence research impinges upon psychiatry in several ways. One is via expert systems for diagnosis and therapy, as outlined above. A second is via the recent revival in interest in neural networks. And the third is through attempts to model cognitive processes. We shall look at an example of the third here, one which has stimulated a considerable amount of controversy.

The basic idea underlying this use of artificial intelligence ideas is that the most effective way to test a theory of cognitive psychology is to attempt to build a working model. The supposition is that any gap in the theory will reflect itself in an inadequate performance for the model.

The most famous effort in this direction is undoubtedly that of the team led by K.M. Colby, a psychiatrist with an interest in paranoia. Over a period of years Colby and his co-workers created PARRY, a simulated twenty-eight-year-old paranoid man which, via a computer terminal, converses with interviewers in ordinary English. The theory under test was Colby's theory of paranoia – and the basic test method was to see if the simulation could be distinguished from a real paranoid patient. PARRY has internal representations of fear, anger, shame, and other affects and the strengths of these change during the course of the interview. The later versions of PARRY are intended to 'respond to treatment' by behaving in a less paranoid way if suitable therapeutic approaches are adopted by the interviewer. The challenge implicit in this is clear since normal behaviour is much less restricted than paranoid behaviour.

PARRY has attracted considerable interest – over 50,000 interviews have been conducted with various versions of it. However, it should be stated that PARRY has not yielded a definitive conclusion about Colby's paranoia theory. (But how much research in the behavioural sciences does yield a definitive conclusion?) What it has done is stimulate a tremendous amount of debate about the nature of scientific testing in behavioural research. Judging by this, PARRY is an important piece of work.

Colby (1981) provides a compact summary of the PARRY project, and the debate itself is encapsulated in the discussion following Colby (1981).

CONCLUSION

In an article as brief as this it is, of course, impossible to do more than scratch the surface of the way in which information technology is beginning to influence psychiatry. We mentioned a few 'striking' topics at the end of the first section which space would prevent us from discussing. There is also a whole host of subtle background topics which, likewise, we have been unable to discuss. These include such things as databases, word processors, and instrumentation. Schwartz (1984) discussed topics throughout the entire continuum of applications.

REFERENCES

Bishop, Y.M.M., Fienberg, S.E., and Holland, P.W. (1975) *Discrete Multivariate Analysis*, Cambridge, Mass.: MIT Press.

Carr, A.C., Ancill, R.J., Ghosh, A., and Margo, A. (1981) 'Direct assessment of depression by microcomputer', *Acta Psychiatrica Scandinavica* 64: 415–22.

Carr, A.C., and Ghosh, A. (1983) 'Response of phobic patients to direct computer assessment', *British Journal of Psychiatry* 142: 60–5.

Carr, A.C., Ghosh, A., and Ancill, R.J. (1983) 'Can a computer take a psychiatric history?', *Psychological Medicine* 13: 151–8.

Coddington, R.D., and King, T.L. (1972) 'Automated history taking in child psychiatry', *American Journal of Psychiatry* 129 (3): 52–8.

Colby, K.M. (1981) 'Modelling a paranoid mind,' *The Behavioural and Brain Sciences* 4: 515–60.

Comings, D.E. (1984) 'A computerized interview schedule (DIS) for psychiatric disorders', in M.D. Schwartz *Using Computers in Clinical Practice*, New York: The Hayworth Press, 195–203.

DeDombal, F.T., Leaper, D.J., Staniland, J.R., McCann, A.P., and Horrocks, J.C. (1972) 'Computer-aided diagnosis of acute abdominal pain', *British Medical Journal* ii: 9–13.

Dove, G.A.W., Wigg, P., Clarke, J.H.C., Constantinidou, M., Royapa, B.A., Evans, C.R., Milne, J., Goss, C., Gordon, M. and de Wardener, H.E. (1977) 'The therapeutic effect of taking a patient's history by computer', *Journal of the Royal College of General Practitioners*, 477–81.

Dunn, G. (1986) 'Patterns of psychiatric diagnosis in general practice: the second national morbidity survey', *Psychological Medicine* 16: 573–81.

135

Efron, B. (1982) *The Jackknife, The Bootstrap, and Other Resampling Plans*, Philadelphia: Society for Industrial and Applied Mathematics.

Everitt, B.S. (1972) 'Cluster analysis: a brief discussion of some of the problems', *British Journal of Psychiatry* 120: 143–5.

Everitt, B.S. (1980) *Cluster Analysis*, London: Heinemann.

Everitt, B.S. (1984) *An Introduction to Latent Variable Models*, London: Chapman and Hall.

Everitt, B.S. (1987) 'Statistics in psychiatry', *Statistical Science*, May.

Eysenck, H.J. (1981) *A Model for Personality*, New York: Springer.

Gore, S.M., Jones, I.G., and Rytter, E.C. (1977) 'Misuse of statistical methods: critical assessment of articles in *BMJ* from January to March 1976'. *British Medical Journal* i: 85–7.

Greenacre, M.J. (1984) *Theory and Applications of Correspondence Analysis*, London: Academic Press.

Greist, J.H., Gustafson, D.H., and Strauss, F. (1973) 'A computer interview for suicide risk prediction', *American Journal of Psychiatry* 130: 1327–32.

Hand, D.J. (1981) *Discrimination and Classification*, Chichester: Wiley.

Hand, D.J. (1985a) 'The role of statistics in psychiatry', *Psychological Medicine* 15: 471–6.

Hand, D.J. (1985b) *Artificial Intelligence and Psychiatry*, Cambridge, Cambridge University Press.

Hand, D.J. (1986) 'Expert systems in statistics', *The Knowledge Engineering Review* 1: 2–10

Hand, D.J. and Taylor, C.C. (1987) *Multivariate Analysis of Variance and Repeated Measures*, London: Chapman and Hall.

Harman, H.H. (1967) *Modern Factor Analysis*, Chicago: University of Chicago Press.

Krynicki, V. and Gould, R.C. (1984) 'A microcomputer program for scoring the SCL-90', in M.D. Schwartz *Using Computers in Clinical Practice*, New York: The Hayworth Press, 209–12.

Lewis, G., Pelosi, A.J., Glover, E., Wilkinson, G., Stansfeld, S., Williams, P., and Shepherd, M. (1988) 'The development of a computerized assessment for minor psychiatric disorder', *'Psychological Medicine*, in press.

McCullagh, P. and Nelder, J.A. (1983) *Generalized Linear Models*, London: Chapman and Hall.

Schwartz, M.D. (1984) *Using Computers in Clinical Practice: Psychotherapy and Mental Health Applications*, New York: The Hayworth Press.

Sharp, C.H. (1987) 'Expert systems and structured psychiatric assessment', MSc dissertation, Brunel University.

Slack, W.V, and Van Cura, L.J. (1968) 'Computer-based patient interviewing', *Postgraduate Medicine* 43: 68–74 and 115–20.

Szolovits, P. (1982) *Artificial Intelligence in Medicine*, Boulder, Colarado: Westview Press.

Tabachnik, B.G. and Fidell, L.S. (1983) *Using Multivariate Statistics*, New York: Harper & Row.

White, S.J. (1979) 'Statistical errors in papers in the British Journal of Psychiatry', *British Journal of Psychiatry* 135: 336–42.

Wing, J.K., Cooper, J.E., and Sartorious, N. (1974) *The Measurement and Classification of Psychiatric Syndromes*, Cambridge: Cambridge University Press.

Section Two

Epidemiological Studies of Mental Disorder

Introduction

This section, concerned with epidemiological studies of mental disorder, is divided into three subsections based on the *Uses of Epidemiology* as described by Jeremy Morris (1975). The structure serves to emphasize the link between epidemiological psychiatry and medical epidemiology.

The importance of the historical context for social and epidemiological psychiatry was discussed in section one. It is appropriate, therefore, that the first subsection here deals with the study of historical trends. As Morris points out, statements about such trends in medicine should be epidemiologically based, since they relate to the frequency of events among populations or samples at different points in time. The first paper, by Michael MacDonald, is based partly on work carried out while a Visiting Professor at the Institute of Psychiatry: it illustrates Bynum's (1983) conclusion that 'psychiatry must be, and must continue to be, a broadly based social enterprise with much to learn from its own past'.

The other two papers in this subsection are historical in a different sense. In them, history is taken to mean 'a course of events: a life story', rather than 'knowledge of past events' (*Chambers Twentieth Century Dictionary*, revised edition, 1972). Erik Strömgren's contribution illustrates the extensive Scandinavian tradition of longitudinal enquiry in psychiatry; then, Graham Dunn and Nigel Smeeton give an account of their studies of episodes of psychiatric disorder recorded by a sample of British general practitioners in the course of the Second National Morbidity Study. The contribution of longitudinal studies in psychiatry is well recognised and is difficult to overestimate (Leighton 1979).

The second subsection is essentially concerned with the intimate relationship between epidemiological enquiry and clinical psychiatry, which has been a consistent theme in Michael Shepherd's writings (e.g. Shepherd and Cooper 1964, Shepherd 1973, 1978, 1984, 1985). Morris's (1975) notion of epidemiology as being important in completing the clinical picture and the delineation of new syndromes is closely linked with this. This use of epidemiology was summarized by Morris as follows:

> The clinicians' experience of chronic disease is likely to be incomplete . . . numbers may be too few, with attendant troubles of chance variation. But even when numbers are large his experience may be peculiar and his patients unrepresentative, i.e. the picture may be biased. Such limitations apply also to the work of a hospital or any other clinical facility.
>
> The epidemiologist, who is concerned with the total of defined cases in a defined population and not merely with patients who present in particular hospitals, clinics or practices, can help to provide a fuller picture than is

obtainable in any or all of these. This fuller picture may prove to be a different one.

In psychiatry, Michael Shepherd's own enquiries have radically modified earlier views of the nature and distribution of mental illness in the population. For example, it is now generally accepted that psychiatric illness in the community is composed largely of minor affective disorders (Shepherd *et al.* 1966). From a large clinical perspective, it is apparent that this large pool of affective illness not only extends the spectrum of the concept of such disorders, but also bears pointedly on the aetiology of these illnesses and on the sterility of much work on their classification based on hospital cases (Shepherd 1978).

The use of epidemiological methods in the clarification of clinical psychiatric phenomena is addressed in the three chapters in this subsection. Gerald Klerman and Myrna Weissman concern themselves with anxiety disorders, Anthony Mann and Glyn Lewis deal with this theme in relation to personality disorders while Robin Eastwood explores the boundaries and relationships between physical and psychological morbidity.

Aetiology is the topic of the third and final subsection. John Wing examines causal factors and risks for schizophrenic psychoses; David Skuse considers influences on child development; Brian Cooper reviews the causes of psychiatric disorder in the elderly while Rachel Jenkins and Anthony Clare discuss mental health in women.

It is now generally accepted that the great majority of psychiatric disorders are multifactorial in origin: there is, in MacMahon and Pugh's (1970) words, a 'web of causality'. The problems associated with drawing causal inferences from epidemiological data have been discussed many times (e.g. Susser 1973). The best way to determine whether or not a statistical association is also a causal association is by means of experiment, a method not often available to epidemiologists. Despite a great deal of enquiry in recent years, the demonstration by Goldberger in 1914 of the aetiology of pellagra arguably 'remains the most elegant demonstration of the way in which the epidemiological method can be applied to elucidate the causes of a neuro-psychiatric disorder' (Shepherd 1978).

REFERENCES

Bynum, W.F. (1983) 'Psychiatry in its historical context', in M. Shepherd and O.L. Zangwill (eds) *Handbook of Psychiatry; Volume 1: General Psychopathology*, Cambridge: Cambridge University Press, 11–38.
Goldberger, J. (1914) 'The etiology of pellagra: the significance of certain epidemiological observations with respect thereto', *Public Health Reports* 29: 1683–5.

Leighton, A.H. (1979) 'Research directions in psychiatric epidemiology', *Psychological Medicine* 9: 235–47.

MacMahon, B. and Pugh, T.F. (1970) *Epidemiology: Principles and Methods*, Boston: Little & Brown.

Morris, J.N. (1975) *The Uses of Epidemiology*, third edition, Edinburgh: Churchill Livingstone.

Shepherd, M. (1973) 'Research report: the General Practice Research Unit at the Institute of Psychiatry', *Psychological Medicine* 3: 525–9.

Shepherd, M. (1978) 'Epidemiology and clinical psychiatry', *British Journal of Psychiatry* 133: 289–98.

Shepherd, M. (1984) 'The contribution of epidemiology to clinical psychiatry', *American Journal of Psychiatry* 141: 1574–6.

Shepherd, M. (1985) 'Psychiatric epidemiology and epidemiological psychiatry', *American Journal of Public Health* 75: 275–6.

Shepherd, M. and Cooper, B. (1964) 'Epidemiology and mental disorder: a review', *Journal of Neurology, Neurosurgery and Psychiatry* 27: 277–90.

Shepherd, M., Cooper, B., Brown, A.C. and Kalton, G. (1966) *Psychiatric Ilness in General Practice*, Oxford: Oxford Univesity Press.

Susser, M. (1973) *Causal Thinking in the Health Sciences*, New York: Oxford University Press.

Charting Historical Trends

10

Psychiatric Disorders in Early Modern England

Michael MacDonald

The two central questions in the history of mental illness before 1800 are almost certainly insoluble. What we really want to know is whether the kinds of mental disorders and their prevalence have changed over time. No matter how full our sources or rigorous our methodology, we shall never discover answers to these problems that are conclusive. We are utterly dependent on the observations of contemporaries for information about mentally ill people in the past. And since the records that normal people kept about the men and women they judged to be abnormal reflected the values of their own time, they cannot simply be translated into present-day language and analysed statistically. To psychiatrists with historical interests this may seem an unduly pessimistic assertion. It is, after all, not difficult to find descriptions of patients in the past who complained of symptoms that closely matched categories of illness described in current systems of classification. But, in fact, notions about the types of mental illnesses and their relative seriousness have varied quite markedly in succeeding ages in western history. There is, as Stanley G. Jackson recently remarked in an authoritative survey of the history of melancholia and depression, both a remarkable consistency in the core symptoms attributed to some disorders and an equally remarkable variation in others (Jackson 1986).

The aim of this brief paper is to explore some of the issues that are raised by the historical study of classifications of mental disorder. I shall focus mainly on sixteenth- and seventeenth-century England, the field I have studied most extensively. Thanks to the survival of a remarkable source, the practice notes of the astrological physician Richard Napier (1559–1637), it is possible to reconstruct on the basis of descriptions of actual patients the main stereotypes of mental illness that were recognized during the period. I shall, therefore, begin with a brief description of psychiatric ailments in Napier's practice. I shall turn then to assessing the typicality of the observations that he recorded, and discussing some of the ways that cultural and social factors influenced the classification of various signs of mental and spiritual disorders. And finally I shall return, in the conclusion, to some broader reflections on the methodology of psychiatric history. I hope to show that, although we cannot create a psychiatric epidemiology of the past that meets the scientific standards set by Michael Shepherd and by other contributors to this volume, we can pose new questions that are both significant and answerable.

MENTAL ILLNESS IN A GENERAL PRACTICE

Richard Napier was an astonishing man, whose manifold interests and activities make him look exotic to modern eyes. The rector of Great Linford in Buckinghamshire, Napier was trained in theology at Oxford. He developed strong interests in science and magic, especially alchemy, conjuring, and astrology, and after 1597 he built up a huge astrological practice, which was devoted chiefly to the diagnosis and treatment of disease. Astrological medicine was not unusual in seventeenth-century England, nor did it differ much in practice from orthodox medicine – at least not on the very high level of competence at which Napier worked. Napier was not a charlatan or a quack; he was no less scientific than his colleagues with medical degrees in his methods of diagnosis and treatments. His practice notes are atypical only in that they are remarkably specific and uniquely numerous. He summarized the complaints of every patient he saw (or heard about), often merely abbreviating their own words. And he saw a lot of patients, at least 60,000 of them between 1597 and 1634, drawn from every social class and complaining of almost every kind of mental and physical affliction (Sawyer 1986). Napier's medical practice and the reliability of his case notes as a historical source have been discussed by myself (MacDonald 1981) and more fully by Ronald C. Sawyer (Sawyer 1986).

Among the patients who consulted Napier, about 5 per cent suffered from symptoms that he and his contemporaries regarded as the signs of a psychiatric affliction of one kind or another (MacDonald 1981; Sawyer 1986). An examination of the entire corpus of his practice notes yielded descriptions of the symptons of 2,039 clients whose complaints were primarily psychological and whose cases were recorded in ways that could be studied more or less systematically. Since the same patient sometimes returned for more than one consultation, the total number of separate case notes on mental disorders was larger, 2,483. The words and phrases that Napier and his clients used to describe abnormal mental conditions were very numerous, there were over 150 of them, and after 300 years their meanings have become elusive. The most common ones he recorded were 'troubled in mind' (33 per cent of consultations), 'melancholy' (19.9 per cent), 'mopish' (15.2 per cent) and 'light-headed' (15.0 per cent). The words 'mad' and 'lunatic' appeared in 5.5 per cent of consultations and 'distracted' in 5.4 per cent. All of these words might appear together with one or more of the others, although the overlap between 'troubled in mind', 'melancholy', and 'mopish' on the one hand and 'mad' and 'lunatic' on the other was relatively slight. 'Light-headed' and 'distracted' were somewhat more elastic concepts.

Some of these words and phrases, notably 'troubled in mind', 'melancholy', 'mopish', 'mad', 'lunatic', and 'distracted', were both symptoms and names for disorders. (It would be overly precise to call them disease entities.) Linking these common complaints with the symptoms that were typically associated with them is the first step to identifying the types of mental disorder Napier and his clients implicitly recognized. The methods I have used to identify significant links are unashamedly unscientific although they are as systematic and as rigorous as the source itself permits. I have explained some of the obstacles to analysing Napier's records using rigorous statistical techniques elsewhere (MacDonald 1987). They are, above all, neither more nor less than the words thousands spoke and one man thought important enough to write down, sometimes verbatim but often in his own summary, not a research instrument designed for statistical analysis. They therefore employ language that is elusive and allusive, inconsistent and inexplicit. Different words were used to describe the same symptom; the same word connoted different symptoms in different contexts. Much was implied that was not explicitly stated. Key complaints were sometimes made in different consultations spaced days or weeks apart, for nothing required Napier to write down what he had already recorded and well remembered. I have, therefore, followed a two-stage procedure to discover what symptoms were characteristically associated with one another. First, I performed a series of simple cross-tabulations, counting the symptoms recorded together with the common words and phrases listed above, and compared the results with the frequency distribution of symptoms among consultations by all disturbed patients. (The results, which cannot be reproduced here for reasons of space, are given in MacDonald 1981.) Second, I then reviewed all of the case notes again, looking for instances in which symptoms that were found together relatively frequently in the cross-tabulations were linked by implication in a single consultation or appeared in a sequence of separate consultations.

This procedure revealed that Napier recognized two distinctive forms of severe disorder and two distinctive kinds of milder disturbance. He also recorded other maladies that were identified by their causes, namely supernatural powers, including the devil and evil spirits, witches and God himself. Many signs of mental abnormality were not associated more frequently with any particular kind of disorder, natural or supernatural, than with any other. Stark insanity was usually indicated by one of four words and phrases – 'mad', 'lunatic', 'light-headed', and 'distracted' – which actually described two distinct but overlapping categories. The patients who were called 'mad' and 'lunatic' were particularly prone to violence and rage. They were physically uncontrollable and very threatening. Napier described Thomas Bassington as a lunatic, noting that he 'rageth and talketh and will strive with three that hold him down' (Ashmole MS 224: 228). The violence and threats

147

of mad and lunatic people had a special quality, too – they were frequently directed at family members and neighbours. People who were 'light-headed' or 'distracted' were more given to idle talk – raving, incoherent speech – and less to violent rage. Both terms were a bit ambiguous. 'Distracted' sometimes indicated something very like violent madness; 'light-headed' shaded over into its modern meaning of mere vertigo. Significantly, the characteristics of the condition they usually described were virtually indistinguisable from the delirium caused by fevers and other life-threatening illnesses. 'Extreme sick', Napier wrote that Thomas Page was, 'like a distracted man. Calleth out on devils, raging, catching and pulling . . . Mind very much troubled; speaketh a little' (Ashmole MS 200: 237). The most severe kinds of mental illnesses were, as the listing above suggests, comparatively rare, comprising less than 15–20 per cent of all the consultations by disturbed patients. The precise figure is difficult to calculate because of the ambiguity of the phrase 'light-headed'.

An initial analysis was performed of the words denoting less severe kinds of mental disorder. 'Troubled in mind' was a generic phrase that could describe almost any psychological complaint short of madness, lunacy, and distraction. Except for the symptoms associated with those maladies, the distribution of symptoms in cases labelled 'troubled in mind' was much the same as it was in the general population of mentally disturbed patients. 'Melancholy' and 'mopish', in contrast, did exhibit some distinctive traits. The symptoms most conspicuously associated with patients Napier labelled as 'melancholy' were sadness, fearfulness, and 'fancies' and 'conceits'. Sadness and fear were the chief signs of melancholy. Here is how Napier described the condition of one Agnes Stiff:

> Troubled with melancholy, how to live for the death of her mother that died a quarter of a year since. Will weep and cry and wander abroad, she knoweth not whither, to her friends. Can follow no business. Yet can sensibly relate all things touching her infirmity as one that were wonderfully well. (Ashmole MS 238: 42)

The 'fancies' and 'conceits' that Napier linked with melancholy included the sorts of delusions of worthlessness that severely depressed patients display today, but they also embraced bizarre delusions and hallucinations. Of Michael Adams Napier wrote: 'Mind much troubled with false conceits and illusions. Melancholy false fears touching Satan's illusions. Fearfulness of sin . . . fearful dreams . . . . Supposeth that he seeth many things which he seeth not' (Ashmole MS 224: 231). Patients whom Napier described as 'mopish' were especially likely to have some sort of disturbance of the senses, but they were less likely to complain of 'fancies' and 'conceits' than melancholy folk or the mentally disturbed generally. Mopish folk were inactive and particularly liable to display conditions that Napier and his informants identified as 'senseless' or 'disturbed in his senses'. In most instances this seems merely to have indicated a passive, withdrawn state, disengaged from normal conversation and activities. 'Not mopish but of good senses and understanding', he wrote of one patient, 'not mopish but sensible and healthy' (Ashmole MS 233: 5–6). Melancholy and mopishness were very common, together accounting for 32 per cent of all consultations for mental disorder. (In seventy-five instances both words appeared in the same case history.)

Napier and his patients thought that other afflictions were caused by supernatural powers. The astrologer treated hundreds of disturbed people who attributed their mental distress to witches, the devil and evil spirits or to religious doubt. The symptoms they complained of were less distinctive than one might have expected. A great many such patients were described simply as 'troubled in mind'. The profiles of possessed, bewitched, or spiritually troubled patients differed from those of the disturbed generally in two respects only. First, persons who said they were vexed by the devil or by witches were far more likely to have been tempted to suicide than other troubled souls. Many of Napier's patients who said they were 'tempted' described actual encounters with Satan or some evil spirit who enticed them to commit suicide. The anguished Richard Lea, for example, told Napier that a malevolent spirit 'will speak often to him and appear in the likeness of a man, enticing him to kill himself (Ashmole MS 215: 298). Second, people who thought they were possessed or haunted were much more likely to report strange visions, sounds, and even sensations than others. One patient simply felt the presence of an evil spirit. 'She is haunted, as she thinketh, with an ill spirit, and feeleth some living thing roll up and down in her' (Ashmole MS 416: 329). Supernatural powers, in other words, might provoke any sort of mental illness, but they were especially likely to be blamed for suicidal impulses and hallucinations or delusions.

THE WIDER PICTURE

All four of the main types of mental illness that Napier recognized – violent madness, delirious insanity, melancholy and mopishness – may be found in contemporary medical works, popular literature, and other sources. The division of mental afflictions into two main types – stark madness and emotional disorders – had become a medical tradition by Napier's day. In fact analogues to all four of the kinds of disorder noticed by Napier can be found in the works of the ancients. In England the thirteenth-century encyclopedist Bartholomaeus Anglicus followed their lead in dividing mental illnesses into 'madness' or 'mania' (violent insanity), 'frensie' (delirium without an accompanying fever), 'melancholy' and 'gaurynge [staring] and forgetfulness' (dementia and stupor) (Hunter and Macalpine 1963). There are obvious parallels between his categories and the ones Napier used. This was partly due to the influence of Bartholomaeus himself. His work was hugely popular for centuries: it had been translated from Latin to English and reprinted twenty times by 1500, and it continued to be reissued for decades after then. Medical writers, reviving and elaborating classical texts, simply reinforced the basic scheme. This fourfold set of stereotypes of mental illness did not exhaust all the symptoms of psychiatric abnormality – far from it. Nor was it simply the residue of a learned tradition. Analogues to the main types of disorder Napier recorded may be found in a wide variety of popular literature as well. And it can never be emphasized too much that Napier was to a unique extent the amanuensis of the men and women whom he treated. He certainly edited and altered what they said to him, but he had neither the time nor the inclination to recast what they told him in terms of an elite scheme alien to their own way of thinking. There was, in other words, a strong congruence between this basic set of stereotypes and lay conceptions of mental illnesses and their signs. It could hardly have been otherwise. There were no specialized agencies, such as the police and psychiatric profession, to identify the insane. People who were diagnosed as mentally ill were singled out for treatment by their families or neighbours or they sought help for themselves.

Napier's notion of what symptoms might be attributed to various supernatural agencies was broader than that expounded by many medical authorities. Here, too, he was more sensitive to the beliefs of the common people than many doctors. Among physicians, who were by no means sceptics, there was a strong tendency to associate supernatural maladies with intractable cases, particularly when patients displayed very unusual symptoms. Medical tracts and judicial handbooks stressed the significance of highly uncharacteristic actions, convulsions, swooning, and behaviour that seemed impossible to account for naturally, speaking learned languages one had never been taught, for example (Thomas 1971; Kocher 1953; Walker 1981). Napier's clients certainly regarded such actions as evidence of possible possession, haunting, or bewitchment, but they also invoked those causes to explain a very wide range of mental abnormalities and physical disorders (Sawyer 1986). His notebooks embody the popular conception of supernatural afflictions that his patients conveyed to him – his fidelity as a recorder and his interest in the supernatural prevented him from dismissing their fears. Although he often subsequently dismissed their suspicions as groundless, he wrote down what his patient told him.

Both the elite and demotic conceptions of supernatural maladies, however, agreed that suicide was caused by the devil and that strange sights, sounds, and sensations might well be the work of Satan or some other evil spirit. Suicide had been condemned for centuries as a diabolical crime, and the posthumous persecution of people who killed themselves in England was more intense in the sixteenth and seventeenth centuries than ever before or afterwards. Almost everyone believed that suicides were murderers who killed themselves at the instigation of the devil. John Sym, the author of the first English treatise on the subject of suicide, claimed that 'strong impulse, powerful motions, and command of the Devil' was a chief cause of self-murder (Sym 1637: 246–7). There was a close chronological correspondence between the rise and fall of witchcraft trials and the rise and fall of the punishment of suicide. The Elizabethan and Jacobean age was perhaps more preoccupied with satanic powers than any other era (Thomas 1971). Few were prepared to dismiss reports of remarkable visions or sounds out of hand, for they might well be evidence of unseen forces. Even the most incredulous physicians granted that possibility. In fact, in the late seventeenth century, when the almost universal faith in the ubiquitous presence of supernatural powers began to wane among the upper classes, prominent authors gathered together tales of apparitions and strange cases of diseases that they offered as empirical proof of the existence of such forces (Thomas 1971; McKeon 1987).

The mix of natural and supernatural disorders in Napier's practice was somewhat unusual. He was less specialized than many practitioners. But it was not at odds with contemporary conceptions of the causes of and remedies for the maladies of the mind. The centuries prior to about 1700 were characterized by a profound conviction that events in this world might have natural or supernatural causes. The content of the ideas that explained how the two kinds of forces at work in the world might cause diseases varied, of course, but the faith in their existence never waned. As a consequence, there was a profusion of possible explanations for mental and physical maladies and a corresponding profusion of treatments available for them. It is often said that people in medieval or early modern England could not explain or understand illness. Nothing could be further from the truth. They possessed, if anything, too many explanations for illness, all of them logically coherent, none of them leading to therapies that were markedly superior or inferior to their alternatives. The sixteenth and seventeenth centuries were thus a period of medical eclecticism, during which most diseases, including mental illnesses, might be attributed to secular causes or supernatural ones or to both. Patients consulted healers who were experts in physical remedies or spiritual healing or, like Napier, both. The characteristics of the illness, the circumstances under which it first appeared, the religious convictions of the patient and his family and past experience with a particular affliction or healer all played a part in deciding how to respond to an illness. The perception of the important signs of alienation or sickness cannot be disentangled from this matrix of ideas and therapeutic traditions.

The influence of beliefs about the supernatural and existence of spiritual remedies for such maladies is perhaps most noticeable in the way suicidal despair and hallucinations and delusions were interpreted. Some medical authors attributed suicide to melancholy, but in spite of the fact that melancholy became the most fashionable diagnosis of the period, self-destructive urges were regarded as primarily a spiritual affliction. They might *also* have natural causes, for melancholy was, as a contemporary cliché put it, the devil's bath, but these were secondary. The force of this conviction may be seen in the pattern of the natural maladies Napier and his clients associated with suicidal feelings. They were never attributed to madness or lunacy and only once to distraction. None of other leading symptoms of mental illness was strongly associated with suicidal feelings – they were a little more common than usual among the 'troubled in mind' but they were a little less common among 'melancholy' patients. Suicide, in other words, was not associated with depression as strongly as it is today, for it had an alternative explanation. And although the link between suicide and melancholy was made more often in printed tracts, it is plain that religious convictions about the meaning of self-destruction shaped contemporary conceptions of its medical significance. They also reinforced legal interpretations of suicide, which treated it as a premeditated act of homicide rather than as the outcome of mental illness (MacDonald 1977).

Religious beliefs similarly influenced contemporary interpretations of the meaning and seriousness of hallucinations and delusions. These were characteristically attributed to melancholy or to maladies with a supernatural cause, as we have seen. To us it is striking that they were so seldom linked with madness, lunacy, or distraction. And this was not because the familiar delusions of extreme depression – convictions of worthlessness, guilt and helplessness – predominated. For the sort of experiences that were regarded as melancholy delusions and hallucinations included flagrant distortions of thought or perception. Medical authorities and popular lore blamed melancholy for the most spectacular delusions of identity, and in fact stories about melancholics who thought they were something other than themselves were commonly repeated. The attribution of hallucinations and delusions to melancholy and to supernatural forces were expressions of the same general notion, I think. Since everyone knew that supernatural foces could create illusions, introject unwelcome ideas into people's minds and even assume the palpable shape of human beings, there was always the possibility that even the most bizarre tale might be true – that is to say, a devilish illusion rather than a manifestation of mental illness. By the same token, while some stories might seem for various reasons doubtful, it was unreasonable to regard them as irrefutable evidence of severe insanity. When they were attributed to natural causes, they were instead linked with melancholy, an affliction that was supposed to have a paradoxical effect of heightening the imagination as it lowered the spirits. Melancholics thus might be either the victims of delusions or they might be clairvoyant, capable of grasping truths denied to men and women of less imagination (Babb 1951). The classification of delusions and hallucinations, in other words, expressed a profound cultural ambivalence about the ontological status of abnormal perceptions and convictions.

152

Both potential suicides and people suffering from visions or delusions might be treated with medical remedies or with religious and magical therapies. In fact many authorities, particularly churchmen, recommended both. But these maladies figured large in contemporary accounts of spiritual healing by religious counsel, prayer, and fasting, exorcism and magic. They were first and foremost spiritual afflictions. Ancient taboos in the case of suicide and metaphysical traditions in the case of hallucinations and delusions imbued those disorders with profound symbolic significance. And healers used a variety of rituals and objects, equally symbolic, to restore the victims of suicidal despair or people apparently possessed or bewitched to health. They were often strikingly successful, and spiritual healing became a matter of fierce political controversy among contending religious groups in the sixteenth and seventeenth centuries (Thomas 1971; MacDonald 1982; Walker 1981).

The emphasis that contemporaries placed on violence and delirium in their descriptions of people who were utterly insane was influenced by considerations that were (literally) more down to earth. Prior to the appearance of growing numbers of asylums, workhouses, and prisons in the eighteenth century, people possessed very few resources for managing aggressive madmen. Houses were not equipped to confine violent lunatics, and families could not for long devote themselves to the exhausting and frightening task of caring for such people. The stress that contemporaries placed on the violence and energy of madmen and lunatics reflected a quite understandable fear that they might not be able to protect themselves. Court records are full of examples of neighbours who were terrified by the insane. The Lancashire quarter sessions, for instance, learned in 1641 of a lunatic who had 'fallen by God's judgement and visitation into a lunatic frenzy and distraction of his wits and senses – he lying bound in chains and feathers [sic] – every [one] of the neighbours fearful to come near unto him' (Fessler 1956: 903). And such fears were justified often enough by acts of brutality to lend them credence. Small wonder that so many sources agree that madfolk were dangerous. 'Take heed of mad folks in a narrow place', warned a seventeenth-century proverb (Smith and Heseltine 1966: 396).

The other stereotype of severe insanity was reinforced by both cultural factors and social conditions. Raving insanity (insane light-headedness or distraction) was, we have seen, very similar to the delirium that was frequently the prelude to death. Everyone who fell ill in early modern England rightly worried that he might die. The most common killers were infectious diseases for which there were no effective remedies. Moreover, when a patient was not patently feverish, there were few means to discover whether delirium had organic causes or was a manifestation of insanity. Oliver Heywood, a nonconformist divine, described in his diary three young people in his neighbourhood who 'fell into a kind of frenzy', two of whom quickly died. Joshua Bates

153

was under deliration. At last it grew to a perfect distraction [so] that four men had much ado to hold him. He was bound, raved, raged, in a formidable manner, made rhymes, yea (which was sad) Satan used his tongue to swear many dreadful oaths, which he never did in all his life. In the morning I went to see him; he was a sad object. . . . That evening at ten o'clock he died. (Heywood 1885: 31–2)

People were especially terrified by the prospect of sudden death, for it forestalled the rituals in which dying persons and their families and neighbours normally participated. These rites were deemed essential both for the soul of the deceased and the consolation of his survivors, who were liable to feel especially distressed if they could not be performed. Thus, both contemporary patterns of mortality and the customs that enabled survivors to deal with ordinary deaths heightened the uncertainty and fear that assailed people who observed a delirious person. It is easy to see why stereotypes of mental illness emphasized the similarities between raving insanity and the symptoms of mortal illnesses.

Contemporary attitudes also reflected the way in which the various kinds of mental illness were diagnosed among different social groups. Reverence for rank was one of the fundamental social values of the age. And some maladies were thought to be more suitable for the genteel than for the rude masses. Melancholy was the badge of breeding, an intellectual's affliction to which men and women of fashion aspired. When a lowly barber in Lyly's *Midas* complains that he is 'melancholy as a cat', he is chided for his pretensions: 'Melancholy? Marry, gup, is melancholy a word for a barber's mouth? Thou shouldst say heavy, dull and doltish: melancholy is the crest of courtiers' arms, and now every base companion, being in his muble fubles, says he is melancholy' (Bamborough 1951: 108–9). When Napier saw base folk who were heavy, dull and doltish he called them 'mopish'. The contrast in the social statuses of those diagnosed as 'melancholy' and 'mopish' was striking. Almost half of his melancholy patients were members of the aristocracy or gentry; less than 15 per cent of his mopish patients were. The affiliation of melancholy and gentility was almost certainly more in the eye of the beholder than in the actual distribution of fear and sorrow in the population as a whole. And it was not just in Napier's eye, either. Many of his patients who were aristocrats or gentlemen diagnosed *themselves* as melancholy.

CONCLUSION

Even in this very compressed discussion, it should be evident that the recognition and classification of psychiatric disorders was strongly influenced by contemporary beliefs, customs, and social conditions. This should come as no surprise. Any system for classifying diseases is made for a purpose, and that purpose is not usually simply the objective study of illness – although it may be for that, too. In the sixteenth and seventeenth centuries people formed coherent stereotypes of mental illnesss that reflected their conceptions of the causes of psychiatric disorders and their recognition of the resources available for managing and treating them. The system that they devised deserves considerable respect. Its basic elements had lasted for several hundred years before it began to break down in the eighteenth century. Laymen and experts alike found it adequate to identify mentally ill people, and many suffering men and women were successfully treated with medical, religious, or magical remedies. For that reason alone we ought to study it in its own terms: simply to see how and why it seemed to contemporaries to provide a perfectly adequate account of mental disorder and a satisfactory array of responses to it.

It would not do, however, to adopt a kind of uncritical cultural relativism. Decoding the system of classifying mental disorders in the past is only the first step to understanding their nature and their prevalence. It is apparent that many of the disorders described in early modern sources are apparently identical to those that are recognized today. Indeed, Jackson has made the more sweeping claim that the core symptoms of depression can be identified in medical sources from ancient times until the present (Jackson 1986). It is possible to discover case histories in Napier's notebooks that satisfy all of DMS–III–R's criteria for major depressive episodes, schizophrenia, dementia, obsessive compulsive disorder, anorexia nervosa, delusional (paranoid) disorder, various phobias, and all kinds of anxiety disorders. Michael Shepherd has, in fact, annotated several hundred of my notes on Napier's case histories with such diagnoses. This is an important finding, for it confirms that there are many similarities between mental illnesses in the past and in the present. And it is a challenge as well, for it points up the need to explain why some maladies are evidently perdurable in western society.

But the very exercise that demonstrates the adamantine durability of some symptom clusters also raises some insurmountable limitations on the historical study of psychiatric epidemiology using modern categories. For, as Arthur Kleinman has pointed out in several forceful discussions of cross-cultural psychiatry, the translation of indigenous perceptions of mental illness into modern western terms may lead to a massive misunderstanding of the kinds and distribution of mental illnesses in the past (Kleinman 1977, 1986, 1987). The principal pitfall is what Kleinman calls a 'category fallacy', the mistake of presuming that symptom clusters that are identical to syndromes recognized in western psychiatric classifications have a superior ontological status to those that resist reclassification. The danger here is that by ignoring instances in which behaviours are identified in other cultures as mentally abnormal, one may overlook variations in the ways that maladies are manifested in different cultural contexts and misconstrue the significance of

155

afflictions that seem peculiar to particular cultures. For, as Kleinman argues, 'biological and cultural factors dialectically interact', to produce the patterns of symptoms that sufferers display and the frequencies with which various illnesses occur (Kleinman 1987: 450).

The perils that historians of mental illness in the west confront are somewhat less daunting than those facing psychiatric anthropologists. But they still place sharp limits on the conclusions we may legitimately draw. The prevalence of melancholy in Napier's practice and Shepherd's reclassification of a sample of his cases suggests that depression was very common. Evidence from other practice books and the relative frequency of suicide during the period reinforce the impression that depressive disorders were widespread in early modern England (Zell 1987). But the facts that melancholy was a fashionable affliction and that suicide was often not attributed to depression by contemporaries make it impossible to estimate with accuracy its prevalence among any practice or population. The same may be said for all of the other DSM–III–R categories I have mentioned. Every one of the clusters of symptoms associated with them was understood and explained differently three hundred years ago than it is now. All of them were liable to be recorded more or less often and in different contexts because of contemporary beliefs, customs, and institutions.

But if the study of the perception of mental illness in early modern England suggests that we need to moderate our aspirations, it also suggests a couple of new hypotheses that historians of psychiatry might consider. First, although the classification of various signs of mental abnormality has changed over time, there has been a very high degree of continuity in the *symptoms* themselves. Most of the actions and moods that seventeenth-century people regarded as evidence of insanity are still viewed as the tokens of mental illness today. The level at which cultural factors seem to have exerted their greatest influence therefore seems to have been at the stage of diagnosis – the point at which sufferers themselves, family members, and healers of various sorts recognized that someone was mentally ill and determined on a course of management and treatment. Second, the little that we know about how classifications of mental illnesses evolved indicates that changes occurred quite slowly prior to about 1750. This suggests that institutional changes in psychiatry in the eighteenth and nineteenth centuries affected the organization of mental abnormalities into stereotypes of disorder profoundly. Some promising beginnings have been made in the study of mental illness in this crucial period (Porter 1987), but a great deal more detailed work is necessary. Some crucial problems are the degree to which new nosologies were based on clinical observations, precisely how they altered older classifications and how well they matched popular conceptions of mental illness. By focusing on the units of analysis that seem most stable and tracing how and why they were combined to form more elaborate stereotypes, we may be able to see the dialectic between biology and culture at work over time.

156

REFERENCES

Ashmole MSS, Bodleian Library, Oxford (1597–1634) *Medical Practice of Richard Napier*, 60 vols.

Babb, L. (1951) *The Elizabethan Malady*, East Lansing, Mich.: Michigan State University Press.

Bamborough J.B. (1951) *Little World of Man*, London: Longmans, Green.

Fessler, A. (1956) 'The Management of Lunacy in Seventeenth Century England', *Proceedings of the Royal Society of Medicine* 49: 901–7

Heywood, O. (1885) *Oliver Heywood: His Autobiography, Diaries, Anecdote and Event Books*, vol. four, edited by J.H. Turner, Bingley: privately printed.

Hunter, R. and Macalpine, I. (1963) *Three Hundred Years of Psychiatry*, London: Oxford University Press.

Jackson, S.G. (1986) *Melancholia and Depression: From Hippocratic Times to Modern Times*, New Haven: Yale University Press.

Kleinman, A. (1977) *Patients and Healers in the Context of Culture*, Berkeley: University of California Press.

Kleinman, A. (1986) *Social Origins of Distress and Disease: Depression, Neurasthenia and Pain in Modern China*, New Haven: Yale University Press.

Kleinman, A. (1987) 'Anthropology and psychiatry: the role of culture in cross-cultural research on illness', *British Journal of Psychiatry* 151: 447–54.

Kocher, P.H. (1953) *Science and Religion in Elizabethan England*, San Marino, Calif.: Huntington Library Press.

McDonald, M. (1977) 'The inner side of wisdom: suicide in early modern England', *Psychological Medicine* 7: 565–82.

MacDonald, M. (1981) *Mystical Bedlam: Madness, Anxiety and Healing in Seventeenth-Century England*, Cambridge: Cambridge University Press.

MacDonald, M. (1982) 'Religion, social change and psychological healing in England, 1600–1800', in W.J. Sheils (ed.) *The Church and Healing* (Studies in Church History, 19), Oxford: Basil Blackwell.

MacDonald, M. (1987) 'Madness, suicide and the computer', in R. Porter and A. Wear (eds) *Problems and Methods in the History of Medicine*, London: Croom Helm.

McKeon, M. (1987) *The Origins of the English Novel, 1600–1740*, Baltimore: Johns Hopkins University Press.

Porter, R.S. (1987) *Mind Forg'd Manacles: A History of Madness in England from the Restoration to the Regency*, London: Athlone Press.

Sawyer, R.C. (1986) 'Patients, healers and disease in the Southeast Midlands, 1597–1634', unpublished Ph.D. thesis, University of Wisconsin-Madison.

Smith, W.G. and Heseltine J.G. (1966) *The Oxford Dictionary of English Proverbs*, second edition, edited by Paul Harvey.

Sym, J. (1637) *Lifes Preservative Against Self-Killing*, London.

Thomas, K. (1971) *Religion and the Decline of Magic*, New York: Scribner.

Walker, D.P. (1971) *Unclean Spirits: Possession and Exorcism in France and England in the Late Sixteenth and Early Seventeenth Centuries*, Philadelphia: University of Pennsylvania Press.

Zell, M. (1987) 'Suicide in pre-industrial England', *Social History* 11: 303–17.

11

Longitudinal Investigations in Psychiatric Epidemiology

Erik Strömgren

The goals of longitudinal studies can be of different kinds:

1) The purpose may be to study what happens to probands who can be characterized as belonging to a specific disease group, with the aim of describing the so-called 'natural history' of that disease.

2) The purpose may be to see if knowledge of the course and outcome of a disease can contribute to its delimitation.

3) If the course and outcome of a disease seem to be very variable, distinctions between cases with a favourable course and those with an unfavourable course may be studied separately with regard to initial symptomatology, premorbid characteristics, and environmental factors, with the aim of identifying traits which can make it possible to predict course and outcome at an early stage.

4) The main interest may be to see what happens to persons who are subjected to a certain kind of treatment. In such studies the establishment of comparison groups which receive no treatment, or some other treatment, is essential.

5) A number of studies have the aim of determining the incidence rates and life time expectancies, within certain population groups, for disorders and deviations of different kinds. Comparisons of the expectancies in the general population and among relatives of sick probands, respectively, are of basic importance for genetic studies.

Longitudinal studies can be performed either prospectively or retrospectively. Each of these methods has its merits and defects, as described with great clarity and realism by Robins (1979). It is often regarded as obvious that prospective studies are more trustworthy than retrospective studies, the probands being selected with a special purpose and described by well-defined criteria and then followed up continuously with regard to these criteria, whereas retrospective studies are supposed to suffer from insufficient accuracy and reliability of ascertainment of relevant criteria. Such drawbacks are of course of very different importance for different kinds of criteria. In retrospective studies it is usually clear which criteria to go for, whereas in prospective studies often a great number of criteria are registered which later on turn out to be irrelevant. The most serious drawback of prospective studies is the fact that it is often very difficult to keep them going on with unchanging intensity, not least because young researchers usually do not feel enthusiastic about investing too much of their time and energy in projects the results of which will be visible only decades later. The necessary patience is more likely to be provided by older researchers who are quite happy to leave the harvest to later generations. A realistic compromise is, therefore, a prospective study which, although the final results are far away, yields interesting results in a stepwise fashion during the whole period of investigation.

The population groups selected for longitudinal studies may be of two kinds: either cohorts or geographically determined population groups. One of the few studies which combined these approaches was the Lundby study, initiated by Essen-Möller (1956). All inhabitants in a Swedish community living there in 1947 have served as a cohort which has been followed up several times since, regardless of whether they are still in the community or have left it; in addition, all new inhabitants of the community have been investigated and followed up (Hagnell 1966, 1981; Hagnell et al. 1982, 1983).

Pure cohorts should preferably be birth cohorts, since all other kinds of cohorts constitute a selection of survivors. Birth cohorts investigated for psychiatric purposes were those of Klemperer (1933) and Fremming (1951), differing with regard to yield, Klemperer being able to identify only about 50 per cent of his probands, as compared to Fremming's 92 per cent. An even greater success was obtained by Helgason (1964) who retraced 99 per cent of his sample, all persons born in Iceland in the years 1895–7; this was not a true birth cohort since only those alive in 1910 were followed; excess mortality of mentally retarded children would make the sample less representative with regard to mental retardation, whereas it was unlikely that representativeness with regard to other mental disorders could be affected. A start with 12- to 15-year-old probands would reduce the amount of work to a considerable degree without loss of psychiatric information of any importance.

Cohort effects, in the sense that cohorts starting in different periods of time may differ as a consequence of environmental changes over time, can be useful for the distinction between genetic and environmental causes of mental disorders. It is, therefore, of great significance that the Helgason group is now engaged in a study of the spouses and children of the original probands. The results of this investigation will be a good opportunity to evaluate cohort effects.

It is not the purpose of the present chapter to give a comprehensive survey

159

of methods and results within longitudinal studies. Excellent surveys in this respect are available, e.g. the book edited by Mednick and Baert (1981), and, especially with regard to young probands, the review by Robins (1979). Instead, it seems appropriate to mention briefly some older studies which have played a great role in psychiatry and can serve as illustrations of the fact that longitudinal studies can contribute decisively to the understanding of psychiatric nosology. An outstanding example is the huge follow-up study performed by Mattauschek and Pilcz (1912, 1913) on syphilitics. The probands were 4,000 officers in the Austrian army who had acquired syphilis during the 1880s and 1890s. The follow-up was continued until 1911. The special conditions in the army made it possible to make a complete follow-up. At that time it was already well known that there was a connection between syphilis and General Paresis of the Insane (GPI); it had become increasingly clear that syphilis was a condition for the origin of GPI. It was an amazing result of the follow-up that only 5 per cent of the syphilitics acquired GPI. Mattauschek and Pilcz therefore studied what differences there were in the life histories of those who became paralytic and those who did not, and they found that all those who escaped GPI had had severe fevers during the first years after the syphilitic infection whereas those who did get the disease had not had similar infections. In this connection they mentioned the fact that in many tropical countries syphilis is practically endemic, but nevertheless GPI seems not to exist there. They stated expressly that these connections seemed to indicate new kinds of therapy in GPI. Peculiarly enough, there is no sign in the paper that they had any knowledge of what Wagner von Jauregg was doing in the same city, Vienna, at the same time – and had already been doing for several years – in the form of experiments with fever therapy in GPI.

The study of Mattauschek and Pilcz was a combined prospective and retrospective investigation carried out so systematically that important results must emerge. In contrast, some equally important findings might be mentioned which were obtained some fifty years earlier by pure serendipity (see Steenberg 1884) at a time when the aetiology of GPI was still the subject of great disagreement; syphilis was mentioned as one of the possible causes, but many other causes were seriously contemplated, and very few believed syphilis to be the *conditio sine qua non*. Already during the 1850s Esmarch and Jessen (1857) in Kiel had put forward the idea that GPI was caused by syphilis. The material on which they based this viewpoint was, however, very slight and not convincing. A few years later the following events occurred. A young doctor in Copenhagen, Valdemar Steenberg, who had worked for several years in a special hospital in Copenhagen which received all cases of venereal disease, paid a visit to one of his friends who worked in the mental hospital of Copenhagen, the Sct. Hans Hospital in Roskilde. His friend took him on ward rounds, and it turned out that Steenberg recognized a considerable number of the patients in the wards, because he had met them earlier in the department for venereal diseases in Copenhagen. It was obvious that all Steenberg's acquaintances among the psychiatric patients suffered from GPI as well. Immediately it became clear to him and his friend that the aetiology of GPI must be syphilitic. Starting with this observation, Steenberg continued to study the connection between the two diseases and wrote a thesis on it (1860) in which for the first time the connection between them was demonstrated quite convincingly. A few years later Steenberg started to work in the mental hospital in Schleswig. There he observed that cases of GPI were not nearly as frequent as among psychiatric patients in Copenhagen, and it turned out that all those in Schleswig who suffered from this disease had spent some time in Copenhagen, which was at that time within the Nordic countries the centre for culture, amusement, and venereal diseases.

GPI was the most frequent of those psychiatric disorders which, during the second half of the nineteenth century, was regarded as having an organic origin. A great number of severe mental disorders which could not be demonstrated to have an organic basis were still left, the functional psychoses. The epoch-making advance in the study of these psychoses was represented by the longitudinal studies of Kraepelin (1899) who demonstrated a high correlation between symptomatology and cause, thus contrasting dementia praecox and manic-depressive disorder. The correlation was, however, not complete; 13 per cent of dementia praecox cases turned out to recover completely. Manfred Bleuler's (1972) even more meticulous, indeed quite unique, longitudinal studies of schizophrenic probands, investigated by himself, showed a complete recovery of 20 per cent of the probands. Comparisons with older materials did not disclose any remarkable changes in the prognosis although advances with regard to therapy had of course modified symptomatology to a high degree in most cases.

Longitudinal follow-up studies of psychotic probands usually start with probands for whom the diagnosis has already been made. The search for possible causative factors must, therefore, be retrospective, and adequate control materials are very difficult to obtain. It is, therefore, difficult to say whether factors which are supposed to have a causative effect in the development of psychoses are indeed specific to the psychoses; in principle they may be more or less ubiquitous factors which are only noxious in persons who have a certain vulnerability. On the other hand, if cohorts, representative of the general population, are chosen for longitudinal studies, the number of psychoses arising in such samples will be so small that even if differences in their premorbid life histories are found, generalizations can usually not be made with any certainty. It is, therefore, an obvious advantage if for longitudinal studies a sample is selected which can be supposed to have an especially high risk of developing the disorder studied. No wonder that 'high risk' studies have become increasingly popular. One of the earliest and most well known is the Danish/American study on offspring of schizophrenic mothers, probands who can be supposed to have a risk of 10–15 per cent of developing schizophrenia. In such studies comparisons can be made between those probands who develop schizophrenia and those who do not, as well as with matched probands of 'neutral' origin. Such studies will have to be continued for several decades before the majority of questions raised can be answered. A follow-up of the probands of the Danish/American study when they were on average 23 years old (Parnas 1986) gave rise to the conclusion that a proportion of them had been subjected to early brain damage. The incidence of birth complications was significantly higher in those who suffered from schizophrenia or suspected schizophrenia than in those who did not. The results of CT scanning supported this distinction. Occurrence of schizophrenia-related abnormalities in the fathers increased the risk of developing schizophrenia in the children, a risk which was also connected with unstable home conditions during the first five years.

A special longitudinal study of schizophrenics was initiated by some observations made during the 1970s which seemed to indicate that cancer should be less frequent in schizophrenics than in the general population. A multinational study was organized by WHO with the aim of elucidating this problem. Studies were started in countries which had psychiatric registers as well as cancer registers. In Denmark the population studied consisted of 6,168 patients who had been diagnosed as schizophrenics during a nationwide census of hospitalized psychiatric patients in Denmark in September 1957. This population was linked with the Danish cancer registry. The patients were followed up until 1980. The follow-up was close to complete since only one patient could not be identified (Dupont et al. 1986). Among the males the incidence of malignant tumours was significantly lower than in the general population, due to a low incidence of lung and bladder cancer. In females the overall incidence of malignant tumours was lower than in the general population, but not significantly so, whereas the incidence of uterine cervical cancer was significantly lower. Mortensen (1987) tried to identify environmental factors modifying the cancer risk in schizophrenic patients. Whereas risk factors well known in other populations, such as occupation, sexual activity, and cigarette smoking, could also be demonstrated in the schizophrenic material, some factors special to the environment of schizophrenic patients, above all neuroleptic treatment, could be demonstrated to be of importance. Treatment with reserpine increased the risk of developing cancer whereas a number of neuroleptics, such as chlorprothixene, chlorpromazine and haloperidol, decreased the risk.

The cohort of schizophrenics which served as a basis for the cancer-schizophrenia study was, as mentioned, derived from a nationwide census in 1957 of hospitalized psychiatric patients in Denmark. Such census studies have been performed regularly with five-year intervals since 1957 (Weeke et al. 1986, Munk-Jørgensen et al. 1986), thus constituting a longitudinal study of hospital populations. The main feature was that the number of admissions remained nearly unchanged, while the total prevalence of in-patients and day-

Table 11.1 Census of patients in Danish psychiatric institutions in the years 1957, 1962, 1967, 1972, 1977, and 1982. Schizophrenia. Rates per 100,000

Age	1957	1962	1967	1972	1977	1982
			Males			
–14	0	0	0	0	0	0
15–24	18	28	34	50	41	31
25–34	96	76	67	85	91	106
35–44	167	129	102	98	89	107
45–54	253	203	156	121	96	91
55–64	363	300	225	186	132	95
65+	297	300	301	275	220	171
15+	132	118	101	97	83	78
			Females			
–14	0	0	0	0	0	0
15–24	12	11	14	22	12	11
25–34	51	41	33	36	42	41
45–54	134	75	57	57	54	51
55–64	378	290	207	167	106	70
65+	416	387	347	297	226	175
15+	140	117	96	86	69	66

patients showed only a slight decrease until 1982 (the increase of day-patients compensating for the decrease in in-patients), after which year changing policies caused a substantial and continuing decrease. The changes within the schizophrenia group are of special interest (table 11.1). During the period 1957–82 the prevalence (per 100,000) of schizophrenia had dropped from 132 to 78 in males and from 140 to 66 in females. This implies that whereas all other main diagnostic groups have showed increasing prevalences, the decreasing prevalence of schizophrenia has been able to compensate for this increase, thus leaving the total prevalence unchanged (until 1982). The changes within the schizophrenia group are, however, distributed very unevenly over the age groups. Within the age group 15–24 years there has been an unexpected increase during the years 1957–72, and since then a moderate drop. In female schizophrenics there have not been such remarkable changes, although, as in the males, the 1972 census showed a peak. It has been suggested that the increase in the prevalence of schizophrenic males in this age group could be due to misdiagnoses of drug psychoses which were mistaken for schizophrenia. The increase in drug abuse came, however, not until 1968, and in the males the increase in schizophrenia started long before that time.

163

Another striking feature is the conspicuous decrease of schizophrenia in females aged 45–64, much more expressed than in males of the same age group. A very probable explanation is the better response of female schizophrenics to combined drug and rehabilitation therapy which enables the greater proportion of these women to be discharged and stay in society.

More intriguing is the decrease in first admissions for schizophrenia which has taken place over the last fifteen years. In Denmark Munk-Jørgensen (1985, 1987) performed a longitudinal register study of all persons who had been admitted to psychiatric institutions in Denmark in 1972 and who during that year, or in connection with later admissions in the following decade, had received the diagnosis of schizophrenia. The annual statistics showed a conspicuous decrease in the rate of first admissions for schizophrenia, this diagnosis obviously being substituted to a considerable degree by diagnoses like borderline psychosis, reactive psychosis, etc. Many of those who ended up with a schizophrenia diagnosis did not receive it until the third or fourth admission or even later, sometimes several years after the first admission. Such sequences are of course well known, but they seem, at least in Denmark, to have acquired rapidly increasing importance in recent years. Different factors seem to contribute to this development. First there is, especially among younger psychiatrists, an increasing fear of 'labelling' patients with the diagnosis of schizophrenia, second, and partly as a consequence of this fear, the diagnosis of 'borderline state' has gained immense popularity.

These mechanisms seem to affect women more than men. It is, therefore, not only in the prevalence, but also in the incidence of hospitalized patients that the sex difference is conspicuous. In addition, there are some factors which may augment the difference which can be illustrated by findings made during a recent repeated survey study comprising the 'true' prevalence of schizophrenia on the Danish island of Bornholm in 1983, as compared with the prevalence in the year 1935 (Strömgren 1987, Bøjholm and Strömgren, to be published). The prevalence of schizophrenia was unchanged in males, but had decreased significantly in females. A tentative explanation for this difference between sexes is the following: Schizophrenia starts, on average later in females who have, therefore, more often obtained a more sheltered family and social position; in addition, the symptomatology is often more uncharacteristic initially in schizophrenic women. The mental health service on the island of Bornholm is well developed, so that a considerable number of females who would, if untreated, later develop definite schizophrenia are now taken on for efficient treatment with the result that clear-cut schizophrenic symptoms do not develop, and the diagnosis is never made.

It is obvious that similar mechanisms may be active also in male schizophrenics, but probably less frequently. The explanation for the fact that nevertheless the prevalence of schizophrenia has not decreased is no doubt that during the half century which has passed since the first census in 1937, the mortality of schizophrenics has decreased significantly.

Among the observations concerning (true or apparent) changes over time in the incidence of mental disorders, those of Hagnell *et al.* (1982, 1983) from the Lundby study deserve special attention, both from a theoretical and from a practical viewpoint: over a period of twenty-five years significant changes have occurred, an increase in the incidence of depressive disorders and a decrease in the incidence of organic brain disorders.

The small number of examples of longitudinal studies which have been mentioned in the preceding cannot, of course, allow any general conclusions, but they can serve as illustrations of some features characteristic of such studies. It is clear that prospective and retrospective studies each have their advantages and defects, that both of them can give rise to important conclusions, and that sometimes combinations of them are the best solutions. It is also clear that it is much easier to perform longitudinal studies in stable populations of moderate size which are well registered. Furthermore, the existence of special registers comprising individuals with diseases or other aberrations is particularly useful. This cannot be stressed too emphatically in a time when ill-founded aversion against all kinds of registers has become popular and even fashionable among influential politicians.

Some of the examples mentioned illustrate also that the dangers threatening the success of longitudinal studies do not all come from outside psychiatry. The increasing speed with which psychiatric concepts and terms are changing threaten to invalidate much serious and useful research.

REFERENCES

Bleuler, M. (1972) *Die schizophrenen Geistesstörungen im Lichte langjähriger Kranken- und Familiengeschichten*, Stuttgart: George Thieme Verlag.

Bøjholm, S. and Strömgren, E. 'Prevalence of schizophrenia on the island of Bornholm', to be published.

Dupont A., Jensen, O.M., Strömgren, E. and Jablensky, A. (1986) 'Incidence of cancer in patients diagnosed as schizophrenic in Denmark', in G.H.M.M. Ten Horn, R. Giel, W.H. Gulbinat and J.H. Henderson (eds) *Psychiatric Case Registers in Public Health*, Amsterdam: Elsevier Science Publishers.

Esmarch, F.R. and Jensen, W. (1857) 'Syphilis und Geistesstörung' *Allgemeine Zeitschrift für Psychiatrie und psychischgerichtliche Medicin* 14: 20–36.

Essen-Möller, E. (1956) *Individual Traits and Morbidity in a Swedish Rural Population*, Copenhagen: Ejnar Munksgaard.

Fremming, K.H. (1951) 'The expectation of mental infirmity in a sample of the Danish population (based on a biographical investigation of 5,500 persons born in the years 1883–1887)', *Occasional Papers on Eugenics, No. 7*, London: The Eugenics Society and Cassell.

Hagnell, O. (1966) *A Prospective Study of the Incidence of Mental Disorder* (Scandinavian University Books), Stockholm: Svenska Bokförlaget Norstedts-Bonniers.

Hagnell, O. (1981) 'The Lundby Study on psychiatric morbidity (Sweden)', in S.A. Mednick and A. Baert (eds) *Prospective Longitudinal Research: An Empirical*

Basis for the Primary Prevention of Psychosocial Disorders, Oxford, New York, Toronto, Melbourne: Oxford University Press.

Hagnell, O., Lanke, J., Rorsman, B., and Öjesjö, L. (1983) 'Current trends in the incidence of senile and multi-infarct dementia: a prospective study of a total population followed over 25 years; the Lundby Study', *Archiv für Psychiatrie und Nervenkrankheiten* 233: 423–38.

Helgason, T. (1964) *Epidemiology of Mental Disorders in Iceland: A Psychiatric and Demographic Investigation of 5,395 Icelanders* (*Acta Psychiatrica Scandinavica*, Supplement 173), Copenhagen: Munksgaard.

Klemperer, J. (1933) 'Zur Belastungsstatistik der Durchschnittsbevölkerung: Psychosenhäufigkeit unter 1000 stichprobenmässig aus den Geburtsregistern der Stadt München (Jahrgang 1881–1890) ausgelesenen probanden', *Zeitschrift für die gesamte Neurologie und Psychiatrie* 146: 277–316.

Kraepelin, E. (1899) 'Zur Diagnose und Prognose der Dementia praecox', *Allgemeine Zeitschrift für Psychiatrie und psychisch-gerichtliche Medicin* 56: 254–9.

Mattauschek, E. and Pilcz, A. (1912) 'Beitrag zur Lues-Paralyse-Frage (erste Mitteilung über 4,134 katamnestisch verfolgte Fälle von luetischer Infektion)', *Zeitschrift für die gesamte Neurologie und Psychiatrie* 8: 133–52.

Mattauschek, E. Pilcz, A. (1913) 'Zweite Mitteilung über 4,134 katamnestisch verfolgte Fälle von luetischer Infektion', *Zeitschrift für die gesamte Neurologie und Psychiatrie* 15: 608–30.

Mednick, S.A. and Baert, A.E. (eds) (1981) *Prospective Longitudinal Research: An Empirical Basis for the Primary Prevention of Psychosocial Disorders*, Oxford, New York, Toronto, Melbourne: Oxford University Press.

Mortensen, P.B. (1987) 'Neuroleptic treatment and other factors modifying cancer risk in schizophrenic patients', *Acta Psychiatrica Scandinavica* 75: 585–90.

Munk-Jørgensen, P. (1985) 'The schizophrenia diagnosis in Denmark: a register-based investigation', *Acta Psychiatrica Scandinavica* 72: 266–73.

Munk-Jørgensen, P. (1987) 'Why has the incidence of schizophrenia in Danish psychiatric institutions decreased since 1970?' *Acta Psychiatrica Scandinavica* 75: 62–8.

Munk-Jørgensen, P., Weeke A., Bach Jensen, E., Dupont, A., and Strömgren, E. (1986) 'Changes in utilization of Danish psychiatric institutions: II: census studies 1977 and 1982', *Comprehensive Psychiatry* 27: 416–29.

Parnas, J. (1986) *Risk Factors in the Development of Schizophrenia: Contributions from a Study of Children of Schizophrenic Mothers*, Copenhagen: Laegeforeningens Forlag.

Robins, L.N. (1979) 'Longitudinal methods in the study of normal and pathological development', in K.P. Kisker, J.E. Meyer, C. Müller and E. Strömgren (eds) *Forschung und Praxis: Grundlagen und Methoden der Psychiatrie*, Band I, 2, Auflage, Berlin, Heidelberg, New York: Springer-Verlag.

Steenberg, V. (1860) *Den syphilitiske Hjernelidelse*, København: Bianco Luno.

Steenberg, V. (1884) 'The role played by syphilis in the genesis of general paralysis: discussion' Congrés international des Sciences médicales, 8me Session, Copenhague 1884, X, Section de Psychiatrie et de Neurologie, 80–92.

Strömgren, E. (1987) 'Changes in the incidence of schizophrenia?' (The fifty-ninth Maudsley Lecture delivered before the Royal College of Psychiatrists, November 15, 1985), *British Journal of Psychiatry* 150: 1–7.

Weeke, A., Munk-Jørgensen, P., Strömgren, E., and Dupont, A. (1986) 'Changes in utilization of Danish psychiatric institutions: I: an outline of the period 1957–1982', *Comprehensive Psychiatry* 27: 407–15.

12

The Study of Episodes of Psychiatric Morbidity

Graham Dunn and Nigel Smeeton

It is well known that general practitioners (GPs) in Great Britain come into contact with, and are responsible for treating, the majority of patients with psychiatric disorders (Shepherd *et al.* 1966). It is not surprising, therefore, that one should look to records provided by GPs for important information about consultations and episodes of a wide variety of psychological problems. In particular, GPs are in a position to provide information on the natural history of these problems, on their patterns of incidence and recurrence, and on patterns of referral to other services. This information is rarely, if ever, available from other sources but the uncritical use of data provided by GPs, however, might be potentially misleading.

Unlike a psychiatrist, a GP cannot assume that a patient is consulting him because of psychological problems. Whether or not a psychiatric or psychological problem is detected is, of course, dependent on the state of the patient and what the patient is willing to reveal about this state. It is also dependent on the GP's background and beliefs as well as on the outcome of previous contacts that the patient has had with the GP. There is also the possibility that many people who suffer from various forms of psychological distress would never seek help from a GP. Those who do will have different 'thresholds'; many seeking help for relatively minor problems such as tension headaches or sleep loss, while others with psychotic symptoms such as paranoia or with dependencies on alcohol or other drugs might refuse to acknowledge that they need help.

Clearly, it is vital that the natural history of psychiatric disorders as seen in general practice be studied in depth. Small-scale, intensive, longitudinal studies (Kedward and Cooper 1966; Cooper *et al.* 1969; Mann *et al.* 1981; Dunn and Skuse 1981) are essential but, however detailed, they run the risk of being unrepresentative. Increasing their size and scope, however, would be a difficult and costly undertaking. Large-scale morbidity surveys, on the other hand, are comprehensive but the data obtained are, by necessity, relatively rather crude. The GPs taking part in the three UK National Morbidity Surveys (Logan and Cushion 1958; Logan 1960; GRO 1962;

HMSO 1974, 1979, 1986), for example, may not be representative of GPs in Britain as a whole; their diagnostic and case-finding criteria differ widely and have not been validated, and, when episodes rather than consultations are being recorded, there appears to be no clear-cut definition of what constitutes an episode of psychiatric disorder. Despite these criticisms, however, these morbidity surveys should provide some useful information, but much more work needs to be done on attempts to provide effective and valid ways of analysing and presenting the data (Dunn 1985).

It is the purpose of this chapter to review some of the problems encountered in these National Morbidity Surveys, with particular reference to the analysis of data provided by the longitudinal file of the Second Survey (HMSO 1979; RCGP 1980) and suggest some possibilities for solving them.

GENERAL PROBLEMS IN THE INTERPRETATION OF DATA FROM THE NATIONAL MORBIDITY SURVEYS

Case detection

The first problem in making any inferences concerning psychiatric morbidity from records provided by the Surveys is that they do not provide records of illness *per se*, but of consultations at which a psychiatric problem has been recognized. Many individuals suffer from various forms of psychological distress without ever seeking help from a GP. Others may not realize that there might be a psychological component to their physical ailments even though they do consult their GP for the latter problems. GPs, too, quite often fail to recognize the signs and symptoms of psychological distress in patients presenting with physical complaints (see Goldberg and Blackwell 1970, for example). For whatever reason, it must be acknowledged that surveys of this kind cannot, from their very nature, provide unbiased estimates of the incidence or prevalence of different types of disorder; they simply provide information on GPs' reported activities and may, in fact, be telling us more about the GPs than the patients themselves (Shepherd *et al.* 1966; Marks *et al.* 1979; RCGP 1980).

Episode definition

A serious flaw in the design of the Second National Morbidity Survey is its reliance on records of episodes of disorder in the absence of any clear operational definition of what constitutes an episode. It was simply left to the individual doctor to decide which consultations belonged to which episodes. In the second three years of the Survey only episodes were recorded, making it impossible to base any statistical analyses of the data on the consultations for which the episode patterns were inferred. Part of the problem has been summarized by Ashford:

> Often the episode pattern of patient contacts can be recognised only by a study of the medical history over a long period and it is not possible for the doctor to determine at the time whether a particular contact properly forms the beginning of a new episode or part of an existing episode.
>
> (Ashford 1972: 269)

Episode patterns can only be inferred from the data and decisions concerning the constitution of an episode should not be made at the time of data collection, particularly if the evidence used in making this inference is not itself summarized and recorded.

Another part of this problem is caused by apparent confusion concerning the concept of an episode. The National Morbidity Surveys fail to distinguish between episodes of *illness* and episodes of *care* (Ellis 1985; Hornbook *et al.* 1985; Keeler *et al.* 1986). Hornbook *et al.* (1985: 170) define an episode of illness as 'a single unbroken interval of time during which the patient suffers from a continuous spell of signs and/or symptoms that are perceived as sickness or ill-health'. They define an episode of care as 'a series of temporally contiguous health care services related to treatment of a given spell of illness or provided in reponse to a specific request by the patient or other relevant entity'. (Hornbrook *et al.* 1985: 171). Clearly, patterns of contact between a patient and a GP can be used to make inferences about both episodes of illness and episodes of care. It is not clear, however, which type of episode is being recorded by the GPs in the National Morbidity Surveys. Episodes of care are often easier to observe from medical records, but the possibility of multiple psychiatric diagnoses at a given consultation (see below) might imply that the GPs are attempting to record episodes of illness. Problems of case detection and diagnosis are relevant to inferences concerning episodes of illness. They are not, on the other hand, of paramount importance when considering episodes of care.

Diagnostic Practices

Another source of trouble, which is clearly related to the general problem of case detection, arises from the way in which GPs diagnose psychiatric disorders. Many GPs might not be interested in the use of formal diagnostic labels, but for the purposes of the National Morbidity Surveys they are required to use them. On the whole they appear to use labels for psychiatric disorders in a different way from psychiatrists. They have, for example, a tendency to miss many cases of depression and, instead, appear to give far too many patients a diagnosis of anxiety (Meyer-Gross 1954; Watts 1962; Clare 1982). The planners of the National Morbidity Surveys are aware of the difficulties of validating GPs' diagnostic practices but do not appear to be concerned by them. Logan and Cushion, for example, claim that a completely accurate identification is sometimes unnecessary and unwise, and they go on to state that 'To lay down standard diagnostic criteria is impossible and, in any event, the improvement in the records would probably be slight, particularly in large-scale enquiries, such as the present survey, where differences will to tend to cancel each other out' (Logan and Cushion 1958: 19). It is difficult to believe how anyone could possibly accept that this statement is true or that problems caused by confusion over the use of formal psychiatric diagnoses would not threaten the validity of the resulting 'morbidity' statistics.

To see why the lack of validation of diagnostic practices leads to serious difficulties in interpretation of the published statistics all one needs is to compare the First and Second National Morbidity Surveys. Consider, for example, the prevalence of 'depression'. There was a dramatic increase in the reported prevalence of depression between the First and Second Surveys. But does this represent a real increase in the prevalence of depression or does it reflect a change in the ways that GPs detect psychiatric disorders in general or, in particular, how they diagnose depression? In the absence of validation studies one cannot tell.

Immigration and Emigration

Clearly when one is calculating prevalence and incidence rates for any form of illness it is vital that one has a reasonably accurate knowledge of the number of people in the population at risk. Most people in Great Britain are registered with a GP but there are problems due to immigration and emigration. Many people, for example, will not register with a new GP when they move to a new area nor will they inform their former GP that they have moved from the area covered by his practice. A change in registration will often only occur when the patient falls ill and requires medical services.

In making inferences from longitudinal records (see below) one also has problems caused by incomplete data. Patients might leave the area or die before the study is completed. In addition, there are new patients entering the study population throughout the duration of the survey. If one chooses to study the psychiatric problems of the patients with complete records this might bias the results. Migrants, for example, might have different psychological problems from those who do not move.

THE SECOND NATIONAL MORBIDITY SURVEY

A general description of the Survey

The Second National Morbidity Survey was undertaken jointly by the Royal College of General Practitioners (RCGP), the Office of Population Censuses and Surveys (OPCS), and the Department of Health and Social Security (DHSS) (RCGP 1980). It was designed to yield information on episode and consultation patterns in a representative sample of general practices over a period of up to six years (1970–6). Sixty practices (115 GPs) took part in

170

1970–1, but only twenty-two contributed data for the whole of the six years of the Survey. The latter data comprise the longitudinal file of the Second National Morbidity Survey (RCGP 1980). The file contains complete six-year records of about 60,000 individuals, 43,000 of them providing details of psychiatric problems.

The work of the present authors has been based on patterns of episodes recorded in the longitudinal file of the Survey. This information was provided by the Medical Statistics Division of OPCS. The data file contains records of the number of episodes of psychiatric disorders (distinguished by a diagnostic code) for each of the six consecutive years. In each episode there is at least one consultation with the GP at which a relevant diagnosis has been made. The file also contains the numbers of consultations at which a psychiatric diagnosis was made for each of the first three years of the Survey. Details of some of the work done on analysing these data can be found in Dunn (1983, 1986) and in Smeeton (1986a, 1986b, 1987).

Since the Second Survey, a Third National Morbidity Survey has been undertaken, again jointly by the RCGP, OPCS, and DHSS (HMSO 1986). Its design was virtually identical to that of the Second Survey and most of the remarks made regarding the Second Survey apply to the Third. Conducted for one year from 1 July 1981, it involved forty-eight practices, 143 GPs, and 332,270 patients, including 282,253 with complete records for the twelve months. Diagnoses were additionally labelled as being serious, intermediate, or trivial. The main report (HMSO 1986) gives the episode distribution of all illness subdivided by age-group and sex but, as yet, no detailed analysis of the psychiatric data has been undertaken.

Variation Between Practices: Psychiatric Records

The results discussed here are based on preliminary investigations described by Dunn (1986). For the purpose of these analyses the data were simplified in the following way. For each of the patients, for the whole of the six years of the Survey, it was asked whether they had experienced one or more episodes (equivalent to one or more consultations with a GP) of, say, depression. If the answer was 'yes' the patient was coded as having a record of depression, but not otherwise. Similar codings were made for each of the other psychiatric disorders. These disorders are those defined by the College of General Practitioners' disease index (1963).

To summarize, each patient contributes a single record of a particular disorder if, and only if, he or she has received a diagnosis of that disorder at least once during the six years of the Survey. Taking all of the possible psychiatric problems, some patients will contribute no records at all, and others will contribute one, two, or even more records. Note that this simplification of the data avoids problems of episode definition but not those of case detection or diagnostic practices. Finally, only patients who were registered with the practices throughout the whole of the six-year Survey are

171

considered here. Those who joined or left the Survey population during the course of the study are ignored.

The practice sizes (indicated by the number of patients registered with the practice throughout the whole of the six years of the Survey) ranged from about 1,500 to approximately 6,500. The proportion of the registered patients having at least one psychiatric record ranged from 0.21 to 0.47, with a median value of 0.30. It is impossible to tell whether this variation in 'morbidity' is due to real differences in levels of psychiatric distress or to variation in the way in which GPs detect and diagnose psychiatric disorders.

Between-practice variation is much more marked if one considers individual diagnostic categories. Table 12.1 gives the proportions of those patients with at least one record of a psychiatric disorder who were given each of the eight most common diagnoses at least once during the Survey. There is great variability in these proportions, as summarized by the ratio of the highest to the lowest proportion, given at the foot of each column. The highest ratios relate to unclassified symptoms (code 150), physical disorders of psychogenic origin (code 135), affective psychosis (code 126), and neurasthenia (code 136).

Most GPs appear not to use the diagnostic category 'affective psychosis' (code 126). The GP or GPs in practice I, on the other hand, gave 20 per cent of the patients with at least one record of psychiatric illness this diagnostic label. As this is the practice in which 47 per cent of the registered patients received at least one record of psychiatric illness this finding implies that almost 10 per cent of the registered patients were thought to be suffering from psychotic symptoms at least once during the six years of the Survey! This is a particularly dramatic example of the problems to be faced in the interpretation of GPs' records. One is inclined to conclude that the records are revealing more about the GPs than they are about their patients.

Variation between practices: modelling episodes

This work, details of which are found in Smeeton (1986b), set out to investigate whether some individuals are more prone to episodes of mental illness than others. An analysis of the distribution of the number of episodes experienced by each individual with complete six-year records from the Second National Morbidity Survey was carried out. Only affective or possibly affective disorders were considered (affective psychoses, anxiety neuroses, phobic neurosis, depressive neurosis, physical disorders of presumably psychogenic origin, neurasthenia, insomnia, and tension headache), chronic disorders, such as mental retardation, with a single life-long episode not being deemed appropriate for study.

The psychiatric data file was subdivided by practice and sex, and theoretical statistical models were fitted to the forty-four subgroups. Under equality of proneness, the Poisson Distribution should provide a reasonable fit (Greenwood and Yule 1920). A flexible variable proneness model is the

Table 12.1 Proportion of psychiatric patients with each of the eight most common record types (× 100)

	Record type*							
Practice	130	134	150	135	146	147	126	136
A	41	13	15	20	13	7	11	0
B	63	41	2	1	16	4	0	0
C	38	33	18	9	17	10	0	4
D	39	50	3	33	13	9	0	0
E	15	51	35	32	5	8	1	6
F	68	25	2	3	20	16	0	0
G	49	32	9	19	4	7	14	8
H	35	68	8	2	2	6	1	0
I	32	22	41	13	9	4	20	18
J	35	48	12	6	7	4	2	0
K	10	21	60	17	8	17	0	0
L	52	28	11	16	7	9	0	1
M	56	48	1	1	9	7	0	0
N	57	40	8	10	23	7	2	2
O	43	31	11	16	21	12	2	2
P	25	21	36	22	19	8	5	10
Q	36	35	19	18	11	12	14	1
R	37	21	38	24	7	10	5	1
S	47	37	22	25	13	8	2	2
T	39	30	20	52	9	10	1	3
U	32	38	22	19	18	17	3	7
V	39	34	22	25	14	14	2	1
Mean	40	35	19	17	12	9	4	3
Ratio of highest to lowest	6.80	5.23	60.0	52.0	11.5	4.25	>50	>45

From Dunn 1986.
* Royal College Codes (in order of overall prevalence): 130, anxiety neurosis; 134, depressive neurosis; 150, unclassified symptoms; 135, physical disorders of presumably psychogenic origin; 146, insomnia; 147, tension headache; 126, affective psychosis; 136, neurasthenia.

Negative Binomial Distribution (NBD) (Greenwood and Yule 1920; Adelstein 1952). This model may also arise from formulations not dependent upon variable proneness (Irwin 1941). It is therefore necessary to check that individuals have consistent episode rates over time, by calculating the correlation between the numbers of episodes in the two halves of the six-year period.

The Poisson model turned out to be inadequate for all forty-four subgroups, suggesting some form of variable proneness model as an alternative. The NBD model provided a good fit in nearly all of the subgroups.

173

With correlations between the two halves of the six-year period ranging from 0.15 to 0.3 (statistically significant) there was some suggestion of a consistent pattern even though the correlation values were not impressive. Thus the variable proneness model explains the data observed reasonably well.

Looking at the forty-four subgroups, the variation across practices was considerable. The average number of episodes ranged from 0.134 to 0.555 for males and 0.327 to 1.125 for females. Thus, subdividing by sex, three to fourfold ratios between practices with the highest and lowest rates were observed.

The problems of collecting data from a number of practices have been highlighted once more. The question of episode definition is responsible for much of the between-practice variation. In addition, some practices used multiple diagnoses much more readily than others. In certain practices some individuals were given five or even six psychiatric labels over the six years. Even allowing for unrelated periods of illness, some of these patients must have been given several diagnoses at single consultations. With one episode recorded for each diagnosis at a consultation, practices which used multiple diagnoses frequently had far more individuals with large numbers of episodes (say ten or more). Thus, practices varied widely not only in *average* numbers of episodes but also in the *range* of values observed as seen in Smeeton (1986b).

Is it possible to salvage any results from this apparent mess? Although strongly influenced by the variation between the GPs, some clear findings about the patients nevertheless emerged. The females experienced about twice as many episodes as the males, on average, this being a consistent finding across all the practices. This sex difference was also found by Dunn (1983) in the stochastic modelling of anxiety and depression.

A consistent pattern related to age group and stability in the practice was also found (Smeeton 1987). Additional information on the numbers of entrants and leavers during each year of the Survey was provided by OPCS. Thus, entrants, leavers, and stayers were compared in the final year of the study, subdivided by age-group and sex, i.e., those with five years of records at the start of the final year and who stayed throughout that year were compared with those who joined or left during the final year. Transient individuals had, on average, six months' exposure. It was found that the average number of episodes experienced was highest among those aged 25 to 44 years. Entrants had a higher episode rate than stayers, above 15 years of age. Leavers tended to have similar episode rates to stayers.

The increased rate observed with the entrants could be due, in part, to a tendency for individuals to delay transfer to a local GP until one is needed. As leavers had similar rates to stayers, rather than reduced rates, it does seem that there may be some genuine increase among less stable individuals.

Thus, despite problems over between-practice variation, it is still possible to demonstrate the plausibility of the variable proneness theory, and indicate that females, the middle aged, and transient individuals are at increased risk of episodes of mental illness.

CONCLUSIONS

The results of these analyses have given us a broad overall picture of how GPs record the occurrence of episodes of mental illness in the community. How does this help the GP interested in local patterns of psychiatric morbidity? These findings are certainly not totally useless. The NBD model appears to act as an appropriate model independent of practice. However, due to the large between-practice variation, the exact results observed in one practice cannot be applied directly to another. Only general, rather than specific, statements can be made, such as about the apparent increase in risk among females, the middle aged, and individuals moving in and out of practices.

A more detailed understanding of episode patterns will only be gained by tackling the problem of between-practice variation. One approach would be to standardize the diagnoses of all GPs in the UK. This would be an extremely daunting task. Almost certainly, some GPs would see this as an attack on their independent judgement and would resist the implementation of any such attempt. Despite this, such an effort would be necessary in order to ensure that all morbidity statistics are reliable and meaningful.

A less ambitious approach would be the encouragement of studies in single practices. A GP seriously interested in looking at local patterns of psychiatric morbidity would certainly gain much from conducting a study of this type. Given the maintained interest of the GP, data can be collected over long periods of time (Dunn and Skuse 1981) and complex statistical models can be tailored to the experience of the individual practice. As a note of caution, such a model would clearly not be appropriate in other settings. Even in the practice for which it was designed it would need to be constantly checked, as changes in the staff at the practice might invalidate the model eventually. Indeed, the attitudes of the remaining staff might also change.

Finally, the National Morbidity Surveys themselves could provide a way of looking at individual practices over long periods of time. Sixteen practices were involved in both the Second and Third Surveys with records stretching from 1970 to 1982 (HMSO 1986). A comparison of data from the two surveys within these practices would be a useful first step. Further data collection from these practices would be far more useful than the future involvement of many more new practices. The problem of between-practice variation need not then make the results obtained totally meaningless.

What of the future? Training in the use of psychiatric labels needs to start at medical school and will take many years to implement. A medium-term solution might be the involvement of a modest number of GPs in the ongoing recording of episodes of psychiatric illness. An attempt to standardize the recording practices of these GPs would then be a more realistic possibility and the idea of obtaining meaningful statistics on episodes of psychiatric illness at some stage in the future may then be more than just an idle dream.

Acknowledgement: Nigel Smeeton is supported by the Department of Health and Social Security. Mrs P. Dixon of the Office of Population, Censuses and Surveys supplied the data on the new entrants and leavers.

REFERENCES

Adelstein, A.M. (1952) 'Accident proneness: a criticism of the concept based upon an analysis of shunters' accidents' (with discussion), *Journal of the Royal Statistical Society A* 115: 354–410.

Ashford, J.R. (1972) 'Patient contacts in general practice in the National Health Service', *The Statistician* 21: 265–89.

Clare, A.W. (1982) 'Problems of psychiatric classification in general practice', in A.W. Clare and M. Lader (eds) *Psychiatry and General Practice*, London: Academic Press, 15–25.

College of General Pracitioners Research Committee of Council (1963) 'A classification of disease: amended version', *Journal of the College of General Practitioners*, 6: 207–16.

Cooper, B., Fry, J., and Kalton, G. (1969) 'A longitudinal study of psychiatric morbidity in a general practice population', *British Journal of Preventive and Social Medicine* 23: 210–17.

Dunn, G. (1983) 'Longitudinal records of anxiety and depression in general practice: the Second National Morbidity Survey', *Psychological Medicine* 13: 987–906.

Dunn, G. (1985) 'Records of psychiatric morbidity in general practice: the National Morbidity Surveys', *Psychological Medicine* 15: 223–6.

Dunn, G. (1986) 'Patterns of psychiatric diagnosis in general pratice: the Second National Morbidity Survey', *Psychological Medicine* 16: 573–81.

Dunn, G., and Skuse, D. (1981) 'The natural history of depression in general practice: stochastic models', *Psychological Medicine* 11: 755–64.

Ellis, R.P. (1985) *Episodes in Mental Health: Issues and Literature Review*, Health Policy Center, Manuscript MH4, Hiller Graduate School, Brandeis University, Waltham, MA, USA.

General Register Office *Morbidity Statistics from General Practice, Volume III (Disease in General Practice)*, (Studies on Medical and Population Subjects No. 14), London: HMSO.

Goldberg, D. and Blackwell, B. (1970) 'Psychiatric illness in general practice: a detailed study using a new method of case identification', *British Medical Journal* ii: 439–43.

Greenwood, M., and Yule, G.U. (1920) 'An inquiry into the nature of frequency distributions representative of multiple happenings with special reference to the occurrence of multiple attacks of disease or repeated accidents', *Journal of the Royal Statistical Society* 83: 255–79.

Her Majesty's Stationery Office (1974) *Morbidity Statistics from General Practice, Second National Study 1970–1* (Studies on Medical and Population Subjects No. 26), London: HMSO.

Her Majesty's Stationery Office (1979) *Morbidity Statistics from General Practice 1971–2: Second National Study* (Studies on Medical and Population Subjects No. 36), London: HMSO.

Her Majesty's Stationery Office (1986) *Morbidity Statistics from General Practice, Third National Study 1981–82* (Series MB5, No. 1), London: HMSO.

Hornbrook, M.C., Hurtado, A.V., and Johnson, R.C. (1985), 'Health care episodes: definition, measurement and use', *Medical Care Review* 42: 163–218.

Irwin, J.O. (1941) 'Comments on the paper "Theory and observation in the investigation of accident causation" by Chambers, E.G. and Yule, G.U.', *Journal of the Royal Statistical Society (Supplement)* 7: 89–109.

Kedward, H.B., and Cooper, B. (1966) 'Neurotic disorders in urban practice: a three-year follow-up', *Journal of the Royal College of General Practitioners* 12: 148–63.

Keeler, E.B., Wells, K.B., Manning, W.G., Rumpel, J.D., and Hanley, J.M. (1986) *The Demand for Episodes of Mental Health Services*, The Rand Corporation, R-3432-NIMH, Santa Monica, California, USA.

Logan, W.P.D. (1960) *Morbidity Statistics from General Practice, Volume II (Occupation)* (General Register Office Studies on Medical and Population Subjects No. 14), London: HMSO.

Logan, W.P.D., and Cushion, A.A. (1958) *Morbidity Statistics from General Practice, Volume I (General)* (General Register Office Studies on Medical and Population Subjects No. 14), London, HMSO.

Mann, A.H., Jenkins, R., and Belsey, E. (1981) 'The twelve-month outcome of patients with neurotic illness in general practice', *Psychological Medicine* 11: 535–50.

Marks, J.N., Goldberg, D.P., and Hillier, V.F. (1979) 'Determinants of the ability of general practitioners to detect psychiatric illness', *Psychological Medicine* 9: 337–53.

Meyer-Gross, W. (1954) 'The diagnosis of depression', *British Medical Journal* II: 948–54.

Royal College of General Practitioners (1980) 'Second National Morbidity Survey', *Journal of the Royal College of General Practitioners* 30: 547–50.

Shepherd, M., Cooper, B., Brown, A.C., and Kalton, G.W. (1966) *Psychiatric Illness in General Practice*, London: Oxford University Press.

Smeeton, N.C. (1986a) 'Distribution of episodes of mental illness in general practice: results from the Second National Morbidity Survey', *Journal of Epidemiology and Community Health* 40: 130–3.

Smeeton, N.C. (1986b) 'Modelling episodes of mental illness: some results from the Second UK National Morbidity Survey', *The Statistician* 35: 55–63.

Smeeton, N.C. (1987) 'Surveys of mental illness in general practice', *The Professional Statistician* 6: 8–9.

Watts, C.A.H. (1962) 'Psychiatric disorders', in General Register Office *Morbidity Statistics from General Practice, Volume III (Disease in General Practice)*, London: HMSO, 35–52.

Completing the Clinical Picture of Disease
and the Delineation of New Syndromes

13

Continuities and Discontinuities in Anxiety Disorders

Gerald Klerman and Myrna Weissman

The role that epidemiology can play in helping to define a clinical disorder lies at the heart of the interface between epidemiology and clinical psychiatry. Historically, physicians have described and defined disorders based upon their experience with patients receiving medical attention. Subsequently, epidemiologists seek to determine the rates of these disorders in community samples independent of treatment-seeking and to quantify the risk factors associated with their incidence, prevalence, morbidity, disability, and mortality. Thus, clinical medicine and epidemiology are in a continuing dialogue, dependent upon each other, while, at the same time, engaged in a dynamic tension. In few areas of medical science is this tension as strong as between clinical and epidemiologic psychiatry. Shepherd has made this interchange a major focus of his efforts. He has emphasized the need for a dialogue between the psychiatric epidemiologist and the clinical psychiatrist and a public health perspective to clinical psychiatry (Shepherd 1978: 289–98).

In this essay, we apply these concepts to a particular clinical condition in psychiatry – anxiety – and reconstruct recent developments which illustrate the important interchange between clinical and epidemiological psychiatry.

Specifically, we will focus on the controversies concerning continuities and discontinuities in the anxiety disorders. Those who hold a continuity view emphasize the similarities between the normal emotional states, including fear and anxious response to stress, and regard clinical conditions as an intensification and quantitative exaggeration of otherwise normal responses. In contrast, clinicians and epidemiologists who hold discontinuous views, emphasize the uniqueness of certain diagnostic categories, particularly panic disorder, agoraphobia, and obsessive-compulsive disorder. They point to the qualitative differences between serious anxiety conditions and the milder and more 'normal' conditions seen in general practice and detected in community surveys.

UNDERSTANDING ANXIETY STATES THROUGH THE SECOND WORLD WAR

While concern for emotional states (called 'passions', 'moods', 'affects' at different times) has permeated the history of psychiatry, interest in anxiety and in anxiety disorders only emerged in the latter half of the nineteenth century. This interest was part of the growing attention to conditions which came to be called neuroses, and represented a convergence of interests within the profession and within the larger society, particularly in North America, the British Isles, and western Europe.

Psychiatry, as a medical speciality, had its origins in the late eighteenth century with growing concern for the insane. Special institutions for the insane were developed in North America, the British Isles, and western Europe. As Foucault pointed out, mental illness was an 'invention' of the Enlightenment. It is not that lunatics and the insane did not exist before Pinel and Tuke, but rather, that they were considered under the jurisdiction of the law and the Church rather than medical practitioners and public health authorities.

Medical physicians first became involved in the care of the insane in institutions, usually called asylums, or retreats. Thus, the founding of the American Psychiatric Association in 1844 was as the American Association of Medical Superintendents of Asylums for the Insane. The name was not changed until the beginning of the twentieth century.

Psychiatric writings through the nineteenth century were focused on conditions which today we would consider psychoses. At the end of the nineteenth century the focus began to change. A small but increasing number of psychiatric practitioners began to practise outside the mental institutions. A few served in the military in the First World War, and many more later became involved in general hospitals, out-patient services, and private consulting practice. In these settings they increasingly saw non-psychotic individuals, whose mental problems manifested themselves in conditions designated today as phobias, obsessions, compulsions, and disturbances of emotional state and bodily functions.

In the second half of the nineteenth century, a large medical literature developed in an attempt to understand the problems of an increasing number of patients, often female patients of middle- and upper-class background, seeking help from medical practitioners. Various terms were coined: 'neurasthenia' by Baird in 1871, 'psychasthenia' by Janet in France. The concept of hysteria was revived, particularly in the writings of Charcot. The term 'anxiety' did not appear prominently until 1895, when Freud wrote his paper 'Distinguishing anxiety neuroses from neurasthenia' (Freud 1894, 1957). The work of Kraepelin and his school focused mainly on psychoses, particularly on manic-depressive insanity, now called bipolar affective disorder, and on dementia praecox, now called schizophrenia (Kraepelin 1921).

Freud and others, practising outside mental hospitals or university clinics, were devoting increasing attention to conditions which came to be called neuroses. Prominent among them were anxiety states. States of fearfulness and nervousness were described throughout the medical literature, but the term 'anxiety' captured not only the psychiatric world, particularly up to the writings of Freud and the growing influence of psychoanalysis, but also the world of the philosopher and the existentialist.

The experience of psychiatrists in the military in the First World War focused attention on various kinds of war neuroses, or traumatic neuroses. Conditions of shell shock and neurocirculatory asthenia were given prominence. A large number of neuropsychiatrists who had served in the military, gained experience with the affects of trauma and the resulting non-psychotic conditions. They saw changes in bodily function and symptoms of cardiac and gastrointestinal nature without the impairments of higher mental functions usually seen by psychiatrists in the classic psychotic states in mental institutions.

By the end of the First World War, there was growing acceptance of a concept of a continuum of anxiety states (Klerman 1986: 3). Influenced by Darwinian concepts of evolution, anxiety was seen as the clinical equivalent of normal fear (Darwin 1872). Neurotic conditions were arrayed on a continuum of increasing severity, including obsessions and compulsions, phobias, and anxiety states. Gradually the classification of agoraphobia as the most disabling form of phobia was developed, particularly by English psychiatrists, including Roth and associates in Newcastle (Meyer-Gross *et al*. 1954), and by Marks and Gelder (Marks 1969).

In this respect, it is interesting that three divergent theories – biological, psychodynamic, and behavioural – emerged in the period between the First World War and the Second World War, all of which accepted the descriptive nature of anxiety and anxiety states and the continuum between normal fears and anxieties and severe clinical states, particularly phobias and anxiety neuroses.

Biological theories

The basis for biological theories for anxiety and anxiety neurosis is to be found in the theories of Darwin, particularly his volume on the expression of emotions in animals and humans (Darwin 1872). In his writing, Darwin laid down the premise that emotional expressions, like anatomical structures, changed with biological evolution and played an adaptive function in the relation between species and their environment. Darwin also postulated the universality of certain basic emotions and their expession through motor and postural changes, linking human emotional experience with animals.

Cannon identified the role of the adrenal medulla and epinephrine as involved in alleviating the 'flight-fight' response and the important function of the endocrine system in adaptation (Cannon 1936). Cannon's views were expanded by the work of Selye in the decade immediately preceding the First World War. Selye (Selye 1956) identified the important function of adrenal cortical substances, particularly cortisol, and the regulation of adrenal cortical function through the pituitary organ. In animal research, he investigated the role of stress in precipitating the general adaptation syndrome. During the First World War, the older concept of psychic trauma was generalized into the new concept of stress. Selye's work expanded the endocrine system to involve not only the adrenal medulla, but also the adrenal cortex and the important connections between CNS centres, particularly the hypothalamus, pituitary, and peripheral endocrine organs. This endocrine work paralleled the important work on neuropharmacotherapy of the autonomic nervous system – its role in regulating cardiovascular, gastrointestinal, and motor responses – and the sensitivity of the autonomic nervous system, particularly the sympathetic system, to environmental changes, including emotional states. All these biological investigations accepted the continuity between normal states of fear and the clinical disorders. It was assumed that the clinical states of anxiety, neurosis and phobias, were quantitative intensifications of normal physiologic and emotional processes.

The psychodynamic view

The psychodynamic view has its origins in the writings of Freud (Freud 1926). Freud was the first to describe anxiety neurosis as a separate nosologic condition in his 1894 paper (Freud 1894, 1957). He regarded anxiety neurosis as an 'actual' neurosis, based on biological causes. Later, he modified his theory, developing his concept of anxiety as 'signal anxiety' in 1923. Sigmund Freud postulated that anxiety was an unconscious signal of the threatened emergence into consciousness of ego-threatening material, mostly instinctual. In this theory, anxiety was the intra-psychic emotion parallel to fear, the threat of an external danger. All neurotic symptoms were explained by a unified theory of pathogenesis whereby symptoms were attempts to defend against and manage anxiety. Unconscious anxiety and its defences were postulated as the central pathogenic mechanisms for all neurotic symptom formation, including hysterical symptoms, obsessive-compulsive, neurotic depressions, and phobias. This point of view was increasingly accepted in US psychiatric centres during and after the Second World War and found its official expression in the APA DSM-III classification of disorders (APA DSM-III 1980).

Although most of psychiatry in the United Kingdom and western Europe did not accept the Freudian theory of the pathogenic role of unconscious anxiety and defenses, the psychotic-neurotic distinction was widely accepted. Neurotic conditions were characterized: (1) descriptively by the absence of impairment of higher mental functions and (2) aetiologically by a presumed non-constitutional environmental and psychosocial causation, which might involve personality maladaptations as well as responses to immediate or long-standing environmental changes.

184

Behavioural theories

The basic theoretical foundation of behavioural theories was found in the work of Pavlov and his theory of conditioned reflexes. The full expression of a behavioural theory was to follow the important work of B.F. Skinner on the role of instrumental conditioning. Skinner's theoretical work found expression in therapeutic endeavours, particularly for the treatment of phobias, using techniques, such as desensitization, relaxation, and, most notably, exposure (Marks 1969). Recently, the repertoire of behavioural techniques has been expanded to other neurotic conditions – particularly panic anxiety – and obsessive-compulsive states, as well as sexual dysfunctions.

Currently, the behavioural theories of anxiety are in a period of great research and therapeutic vigour. The development of behavioural observational scales and the application of psychophysiologic methods to clinical research have given increasing scientific validity to behavioural interpretations of anxiety. Moreover, these research investigations have been complemented by growing evidence for the therapeutic efficacy of behavioural techniques for the treatment of anxiety, phobias, obsessions, compulsions, and depressive states.

DEVELOPMENT SINCE THE SECOND WORLD WAR: CHALLENGES TO CONTINUITY THEORIES OF ANXIETY

By the end of the Second World War, the continuum theories of anxiety state were widely held. Categorical psychiatric diagnosis as the basis for clinical epidemiologic research was in disfavour. Critics called attention to the low reliability of diagnostic assessments and to the wide number of mixed and transient anxiety states, which occurred in individuals faced with external danger, as in combat, or during wartime air raids.

The 'Golden Era' of social epidemiology

The period after the Second World War ushered in a 'golden era' of social epidemiologic research (Weissman and Klerman 1977: 98; Robins 1978: 697). Selye's concept of stress proved useful to military psychiatry during the Second World War and the combat experience provided a paradigmatic basis for understanding medical disorders in civilian life. Psychiatrists in the military saw large numbers of men who had presumably been screened prior to induction and in whom the role of vulnerability and predisposition had been minimized.

A large number of community surveys were undertaken after the Second World War and they had a number of features in common. These features included: (1) careful attention to sampling methodology; (2) extensive use of questionnaires and scales for interviewing; (3) rejection of an explicit psychiatric diagnosis, e.g. a mental health/mental illness continuum; (4) focus on social factors as equivalent to military stress, e.g. poverty, low social class, migration, racial inequities, urbanization.

In these studies anxiety was conceived of as an important, if not the major, emotional reaction, mediating between the external environment (the stressor) and the internal reaction, whether it be mental illness or bodily change or physical illness. The writings of Sullivan and the interpersonal theorists had pointed out that in modern life the major threats to personal security were not external dangers – as had been true earlier in the history of the species, but were ongoing interpersonal events having to do with social status, personal role, and aspirations and frustrations in intimate and close relations.

Epidemiologic studies in general medical practice

In parallel with community samples, a number of investigators began intensive studies of psychiatric morbidity among patients seen in general medical settings, particularly in general practitioners' offices. The pioneering work in this endeavour was by Shepherd and his associates in their studies of London (Shepherd *et al.* 1966), out of which came the work of Goldberg (Goldberg 1978) in his various studies of psychiatric problems in general practice patients in Manchester. These studies demonstrated a high prevalence of psychiatric symptoms and morbidity in patients seeking medical assistance from general practitioners. As part of the methodologic advances in these investigations, Goldberg developed the General Health Questionnaire (GHQ) (Goldberg 1978). Previous work, mainly during the Second World War in the military, had made use of similar instruments, such as the Cornell Medical Index and the Health Opinion Surveys (HOS). These were extensively studied for reliability and discriminant validity using psychometric techniques; however, the Goldberg GHQ became the most widely used mode of assessing psychiatric morbidity in medical settings. Investigations using the GHQ and similar techniques documented high rates of psychiatric morbidity, often associated with symptoms of anxiety and depression. These symptoms were usually unrecognized and untreated by the general physician, who tended to see patients' complaints in terms of traditional medical disease categories. Theoretically, these studies, showing high degrees of association between symptoms of anxiety and depression, questioned the clinical value, as well as the epidemiologic validity, of traditional diagnostic efforts at identifying discrete syndromes.

Clinical research emphasizing discontinuities

A number of developments in the 1960s in clinical research came to challenge the continuity view. Some of this research made use of the availability of computers or multivariate statistical analyses. Other research began from clinical observations of the role of the new psychopharmacologic agents, particularly the MAO inhibitors or the tricyclic antidepressants and the benzodiazepines.

The development of multivariate statistical techniques and the availability of high-speed electronic computers made possible the application of these techniques to psychopathology in large samples. In the United Kingdom extensive controversy followed the use of multivariate techniques, particularly discriminate function and analysis, to identify subtypes within depression. In this work there was a controversy between the Newcastle group led by Roth and his associates (Meyer-Gross *et al.* 1954) and the London group, led by Lewis and his students (Shepherd 1986), notably Kendell (Kendell 1977: 3). Efforts were made to distinguish between anxiety states and depressive states. Factor analytic studies had identified separate anxiety and depression factors on many scales, particularly the Hopkins Symptom Checklist. Although these scales showed factorial independence, in clinical practice the anxiety and depression scales were almost highly correlated. Research in this area appeared to be unable to resolve the issues of the continuity or discontinuity between anxiety and depression.

More successful efforts were made with regard to the phobias. A combination of clinical research and factor analytic studies (Marks 1969) led to the proposal to separate phobias into three types – agoraphobia, social phobia, and simple phobia.

An important, and somewhat different line of investigation was under way in the 1960s and 1970s in the United States and the United Kingdom. Following the observations in the United Kingdom of the efficacy of MAO inhibitors for atypical depressions and many anxiety states, studies were undertaken to determine the possible efficacy of tricyclic antidepressants. Donald Klein noted the occurrence of panic attacks in the symptom picture of patients with severe agoraphobia who were often diagnosed pseudo-neurotic or borderline schizophrenic (Klein 1981). As part of a double blind randomized trial comparing imipramine to chlorpromazine, Klein observed the unexpected effect of imipramine in reducing panic attacks. Based upon this clinical observation, he pursued a number of studies refining the clinical syndrome of panic attacks and testing the therapeutic value of imipramine and other tricyclic antidepressants in their treatment.

Based on these findings, in the 1970s, anxiety neuroses were separated into two forms, generalized anxiety and panic anxiety. This separation was codified in the Research Diagnostic Criteria (RDC) and from the research in the NIMH Collaborative Programe in the Psychobiology of Depression, which used the SADS-RDC. The availability of standardized diagnostic criteria for distinguishing panic anxiety from generalized anxiety and linking panic anxiety to agoraphobia resulted in an increasing number of clinical studies on the validity of this distinction. Therapeutic studies indicated that two classes of antidepressant compounds, the tricyclic antidepressants and the MAO inhibitors, were useful in this condition (Klerman 1983: 3; Klerman *et al.* 1984: 539).

187

Thus, by the middle of the 1970s, an important line of investigation had challenged the continuity theory and emphasized the qualitative differences between panic anxiety and generalized anxiety and the differential efficacy of classes of psychopharmacologic agents in treating these disorders. Many of these nosologic and diagnostic concepts were embodied in the DSM-III, published by the American Psychiatric Association in 1980, embodying many of the features of the discontinuity point of view, but, at the same time, initiating many controversies and providing an important stimulus to empirical research.

CLINICAL AND EPIDEMIOLOGIC ASPECTS OF CURRENT CONTROVERSIES

The APA DSM-III, published in 1980, contained a number of important changes in the approach to anxiety and anxiety disorders. The previous continuity theory was abandoned, as well as the category of neurosis as a unifying and diagnostic classification. The previous category of neurotic conditions was broken down into a number of separate categories, in particular, affective disorders and anxiety disorders. Within the anxiety disorders two features were of note: the separation of panic anxiety from generalized anxiety and the linking of panic disorder and agoraphobia (APA DSM-III 1980).

These diagnostic distinctions were the focus of controversy among clinical and therapeutic researchers. Just at the time that the first large-scale epidemiologic studies of communities using clinical diagnostic approaches became possible, the integration of clinical and epidemiological research, described by Shepherd, became a real possibility in the US in the 1970s and 1980s (Shepherd 1978).

Recent epidemiologic research on anxiety disorders

In these new epidemiologic studies, structural interviews and diagnostic algorithms developed in the 1960s and 1970s were to be applied to probability samples of the communities in the United States. The diagnostic algorithms were initially developed in clinical settings by the group at Washington University in St Louis, led by Robins and Guze (Robins and Guze 1972), and were codified by Feighner. Similar developments were under way in the United Kingdom, where Wing developed the Present State Examination (PSE), which has been widely used in epidemiologic studies, e.g. the World Health Organization International Pilot Study on Schizophrenia (Wing et al. 1974).

Many of the features of these algorithms were incorporated in the SADS-RDC, developed by Spitzer, Endicott, and Robins in the NIMH Collaborative Program for the Psychobiology of Depression (Spitzer et al. 1978: 773). The

SADS-RDC came to be the most widely used diagnostic system in clinical, therapeutic, and family research in the United States (Endicott and Spitzer 1978: 837).

Since the 1980s, when the first multi-site community-based survey of psychiatric disorders in the United States was initiated by the National Institute of Mental Health, epidemiologic topics have been of increasing interest in psychiatry (Regier *et al.* 1984: 934; Klerman 1986b: 159). The data emerging from this survey have challenged the conventional view of the nature, frequency, risks, course, and co-morbidity of many psychiatric disorders, especially panic and agoraphobia.

There are four community surveys of treated and untreated persons which have incorporated the division of anxiety states into subtypes and used either RDC or DSM-III criteria.

(1) The New Haven Survey was the first application of the new structured diagnostic interview techniques (SADS-L and RDC) in a community sample of persons. The study was conducted in the New Haven, Connecticut, area in 1975, and included a sample of 511 probands (a follow-up of a probability community study) who were interviewed by clinically trained persons using the SADS-L which generated Research Diagnostic Criteria (RDC) (Weissman and Myers 1978: 1304).

(2) The National Survey of Psychotherapeutic Drug Use, conducted in 1979, was a survey of a probability sample of 3,161 adults living throughout the United States in which a symptom checklist, the SCL-90, was administered by survey interviewers. The primary interest was in drug use. However, based on an algorithm of symptoms, diagnostic counterparts of some DSM-III anxiety disorders, including panic and agoraphobia, were identified (Uhlenhuth *et al.* 1983: 1167).

(3) The Zurich Study, conducted by Angst and Dobler-Mikola (1984: 30), was a population study of 3,902 19-year-old men and 2,391 20-year-old women. Approximately 50 per cent of the population in this age group completed the SCL-90. Ten per cent of the total sample was selected to participate in a prospective interview study by having either high or low scores on the psychiatric self-rating instrument. Within one year of screening, about 500 persons were directly interviewed using a structured interview. DSM-III diagnoses were derived both from the checklist and the interview.

(4) The NIMH Epidemiologic Catchment Area Survey (ECA) (Klerman 1986b), by far the largest study, was conducted between 1980–4 and included a probability sample of over 18,000 adults using the Diagnostic Interview Schedule (DIS) which generated DSM-III diagnoses. The study was independently conducted at five United States sites: New Haven, Connecticut (Yale University); Baltimore, Maryland (Johns Hopkins University); St Louis, Missouri (Washington

University); Piedmont Area, North Carolina (Duke University); and Los Angeles, California (UCLA). This study provides the most comprehensive epidemiologic data available on panic and agoraphobia in large samples of adults (Myers *et al.* 1984: 959) (Regier *et al.* 1984: 934). This review will focus on the findings from the ECA data.

Panic symptoms

There is agreement that symptoms of panic are extremely common and that they occur in many psychiatric disorders. In an examination of panic attacks and panic disorder in the three ECA sites, von Korff *et al.* (1987: 152) found an increase in the onset of panic attacks in the 15–19-year-old group and rare onset in panic attacks after age 40. There was no clear demarcation between simple, severe, or recurrent panic attacks and DSM-III panic disorder in terms of autonomic systems, age of onset, and distribution of demographic factors. Panic attacks were quite common, with a six-month prevalence rate of 3/100. However, only 10 per cent of the population reported any history of panic attacks.

In a separate examination of the ECA five-site data, it was found that about 10 per cent of the sample (range 7.6 per cent to 11.6 per cent) answered positively to the question 'Have you ever had a spell when all of a sudden you felt frightened, anxious, very uneasy in situations, when most people wouldn't be afraid?'

The close association between current and lifetime rates of panic attacks noted by von Korff *et al.* (1985: 970) may be an artefact of reporting, or may suggest that a significant minority of individual persons have sporadic panic attacks, and that these are recurrent. Boyd and associates (1986: 983), in a separate examination of ECA data, also found a high prevalence of panic attacks in persons with other psychiatric disorders. The investigators recommend a flexible approach to classifying panic attacks until there is evidence from longitudinal studies or other data that indicates a clear separation of disorder from attacks.

Panic disorder

There is a convergence of findings concerning the epidemiology of panic disorder. The range of prevalence rates (one month to one year) was 0.4–1.6/100. The ECA study showed considerable consistency in six-month prevalence rates of panic disorder across the five sites: the rates were higher in women, in persons aged 25–44, and in the separated and the divorced. The increased risk in women as compared to men also has been found in family studies. The rates were lowest in persons over age 64. There was no consistent relationship to race or education. The mean age of onset was mid-to-late-thirties.

The relationship of panic disorder and agoraphobia

Of particular interest has been the relationship between panic disorder and agoraphobia. According to Klein's theory (Klein 1981), agoraphobia is a conditioned, learned reaction to unexplained panic attacks – a view that has been adopted by many clinicians and researchers who state that agoraphobia does not occur without panic disorder. At least two epidemiologic studies, however, have found cases of agoraphobia in the absence of current or past history of panic disorder. In a longitudinal study of young adults in Zurich, Angst and Dobler-Mikola (1984: 30) found that the one-year prevalence rate of agoraphobia without panic disorder was 1.6/100, while the rate for agoraphobia with panic disorder was 0.7/100. In the New Haven ECA site, the rate of agoraphobia with no history of panic disorder was 2.9/100, whereas the rate of agoraphobia plus panic was only 0.3/100 (Weissman, in press).

A more intensive investigation of the New Haven ECA findings revealed that of the 144 subjects with agoraphobia and no history of panic disorder, sixty-seven had experienced some panic symptoms. These attacks were often of insufficient number or magnitude to meet the criteria for the DSM-III. Furthermore, among the seventy-seven subjects with agoraphobia and no symptoms of panic, twenty-nine (38 per cent) had at least one other psychiatric disorder. Affective disorders were the most common diagnoses (Weissman, in press).

Although many subjects in the New Haven survey were identified by diagnostic criteria as having only agoraphobia and no panic disorder, one half did have panic symptoms. Of the other half with no symptoms of panic anxiety, more than one-third had another psychiatric disorder, usually major depression. Thus, only 33 per cent of the group diagnosed as having agoraphobia without panic disorder had neither panic anxiety nor other psychiatric disorders. If we consider only these forty-eight subjects as the cases of 'true' agoraphobia without panic, then the rate (1.0/100) is close to the rate 1.6/100 reported by Angst and Dobler-Mikola (1984: 30).

Co-morbidity

There is good evidence from epidemiologic studies for co-morbidity between disorders. Individuals who experience anxiety disorder tend to have other psychiatric disorders, including other anxiety disorders, over their lifetime. For example, in the 1975 survey, over 80 per cent of persons with generalized anxiety disorder had at least one other anxiety disorder; 30 per cent of persons with phobias had had panic disorder at some time. There was also an overlap between the anxiety disorders and major depression: over 7 per cent of persons with GAD, 2 per cent of persons with panic disorder, and 4 per cent with phobia had experienced major depression.

Similarly, on the basis of data from three ECA sites, Boyd *et al.* (1984: 983) found high co-morbidity between disorders. There was an 18.8-fold

191

increased risk of panic disorder and a 15.3-fold increased risk of agoraphobia, given a major depression. There was 4.3-fold increased risk of alcohol abuse, given a panic disorder, and an 18-fold increased risk of panic disorder, given agoraphobia. The risk of major depression, given panic disorder, could not be calculated, due to the exclusion criteria of DSM-III.

CONCLUSIONS: THE ONGOING DIALOGUE BETWEEN CLINICAL AND EPIDEMIOLOGICAL PSYCHIATRY

This review of current controversies in the investigation of anxiety and anxiety disorders points out the dynamic interplay and mutual dependence between clinical and epidemiologic psychiatry. The recent proposals for the separation of panic anxiety from generalized anxiety and the discontinuity of agoraphobia and panic disorder from other anxiety disorders which originated in clinical research and which were embodied in the DSM-III classification have provided the basis for controversy, not only among clinicians and therapists who are sceptical of these formulations, but also among epidemiologic investigators.

The development of structured interviews and diagnostic algorithms embody these descriptions. The PSE, DIS, SADS-RDC, and the DSN criteria have been applied in large-scale community and family surveys. The epidemiologic data give partial, but not complete, support to some of these revisionist ideas. Using structured interviews and diagnostic algorithms, it is possible to make distinctions between generalized anxiety and panic anxiety, and to assess agoraphobia. Although the diagnostic inquiries for agoraphobia, particularly at the DIS, do not fulfly mirror the clinical criteria, they, nevertheless, have provided a stimulus for investigation.

The new epidemiologic studies have clarified our thinking about the anxiety disorders.

(1) There is empirical basis for the separation of the anxiety disorders. These disorders have different epidemiologies; they have different rates and risk factors.

(2) The separation is best established for panic and agoraphobia.

(3) The high co-morbidity between the anxiety disorders and depression is *not* merely an artefact of sampling; i.e., persons with two disorders are more apt to seek health care. Community surveys, including both treated and untreated samples, also show high co-morbidity.

(4) There is a challenge to the concept that agoraphobia only occurs in the context of a history of panic disorder. There seem to be several diagnostic pathways to agoraphobia.

The discontinuity theorists have gained partial support from these recent epidemiologic studies. The epidemiologic research has confirmed the existence of a large number of adults, approximately 10–20 per cent, who experience sporadic or intermittent panic attacks, but who do not meet the full criteria of DSM-III panic disorder. Using techniques of genetic epidemiology, twin and adoption studies seem to lend partial support to evidence for familial aggregation of panic disorder and, to some extent, agoraphobia – but not for generalized anxiety disorder – supporting the discontinuity viewpoint.

In contrast, epidemiologic studies conducted in general practice and community health settings indicate a large reservoir of patients with symp-toms of anxiety, often combined with symptoms of depression, many of whom do not meet criteria for major mental disorders. Many of their condi-tions are associated with recent stress and appear to be attempts of the individual to cope with life events, difficult circumstances, and stress. Anxiety and related symptoms serve as a stimulus to seeking health care. Thus, the health care system increasingly has become part of the means by which individuals in society cope with change, particularly those changes which impact on the individuals' and family members' emotional situation. At this end of the spectrum, continuity theories are highly useful and valid. Clinicians working in general health care settings, such as consultants to health maintenance organizations or family practice groups, are more impressed with the lack of differentiation of clinical syndromes and the essen-tial continuity between normal adaptive functioning and psychopathology.

Looking to the future, it is likely that these trends will continue and that the continued interchange and dialogue between clinical and epidemiologic research in psychiatry will further clarify many issues. These issues involve a dynamic interplay, at times tense, conflictual, and disputatious, among groups of clinicians and between clinicians and epidemiologists. Neither group is of a single mind on these diagnostic or theoretical issues. As Shepherd has pointed out (Shepherd 1979: 191), these issues are of more than scientific and academic interest. Psychiatry has a uniquely social respon-sibility. The high prevalence and social disability associated with psychiatric disorders bring them into the centre of social concern.

REFERENCES

American Psychiatric Association (1980) *Diagnostic and Statistical Manual of Mental Disorders*, third edition (DSM-III), Washington, DC: AMA.
Angst, J. and Dobler-Mikola, A. (1984) 'The Zurich story: diagnosis of depression', *European Archives of Psychiatric Neurological Sciences* 234: 30–7.
Boyd, J.H., Burke, J.D., Gruenberg, E., Holzer, C.E., Rae, D.S., George, L.K., Karno, M., Stolzman, R., McEvoy, L. and Nestadt, G. (1984) 'Exclusion criteria of DSM-III: a study of co-occurrence of hierarchy-free syndromes', *Archives of General Psychiatry* 41: 983–9.

Cannon, W.B. (1936) *The Wisdom of the Body*, New York: W.W. Norton.

Darwin, C. (1872) *The Expression of the Emotions in Man and Animals*, London: John Murray.

Endicott, J. and Spitzer, R. (1978) 'A diagnostic interview: the schedule for affective disorder and schizophrenia', *Archives of General Psychiatry* 35: 837–44.

Freud, S. (1894, 1957) 'On the grounds for detaching a particular syndrome from neurasthenia under the description of "anxiety neurosis"', in J. Strachey (ed.) *The Complete Psychological Works of Sigmund Freud (Standard Edition) Volume III*, London: Hogarth Press.

Freud, S. (1926) 'Inhibitions, symptoms and anxiety', in J. Strachey (ed.) *The Complete Psychological Works of Sigmund Freud (Standard Edition) Volume XX*, London: Hogarth Press.

Goldberg, D.P. (1978) *Manual of the General Health Questionnaire*, Windsor: NFER/Nelson.

Kendell, R.E. (1977) 'The classification of depression: a review of contemporary confusion', in G.D. Burrows (ed.) *Handbook of Studies of Depression*, New York: Excerpta Medica, 3–19.

Klein, D.F. (1981) 'Anxiety reconceptualized', in D.F. Klein and J.G. Rabkin (eds) *Anxiety: New Research and Challenging Concepts*, New York: Raven Press.

Klerman, G.L. (1983) 'Significance of DSM-III in American psychiatry', in R.L. Spitzer, J.B.W. Wiliams, and A.E. Skodal (eds) *International Perspectives in DSM-III*, Washington, DC: American Psychiatric Press, 3–25.

Klerman, G.L. (1986a) 'Introduction', *The Journal of Clinical Psychiatry* (supplement) 47: 3.

Klerman, G.L. (1986b) 'The National Institute of Mental Health Environment Catchment Areas (NIMH-ECA) Program', *Social Psychiatry* 21: 159–66.

Klerman, G.L., Spitzer, R., Vaillant, G., and Michels, R. (1984) 'A debate on DSM-III', *American Journal of Psychiatry* 141: 53.

Kraepelin, E. (1921) *Manic-depressive Insanity and Paranoia*, translated by M. Barclay, Edinburgh: Livingstone.

Marks, I. (1969) *Fears and Phobias*, London: Heinemann.

Meyer-Gross, W., Slater, E., and Roth, M. (eds) (1954) *Clinical Psychiatry*, Baltimore, MD: Williams and Wilkins.

Myers, J.K., Weissman, M.M., Tischler, G.L., Holzer, C.E., Leaf, P.J., Orvaschel, H., Anthony, J.C., Boyd, J.H., Burke, J.D., Kramer, M. and Stoltzman, R. (1984) 'The prevalence of psychiatric disorders in three communities, 1980–1982', *Archives of General Psychiatry* 41: 959–67.

Regier, D.A., Myers, J.K., Kramer, M., Robins, L.N., Blazer, D.G., Hough, R.L., Eaton, W.W. and Locke, B.Z. (1984) 'The NIMH Epidemiological Catchment Area (ECA) Program: historical context, major objectives and study population characteristics', *Archives of General Psychiatry* 41: 934–41.

Robins, E. and Guze, S.B. (1972) *Classification of Affective Disorders: The Primary-Secondary Endogenous-Reactive and Neurotic-Psychotic Concepts in Psychobiology of Depressive Illness* (DEHW Publication (HSM) 79-9053), edited by T.A. Williams, M.M. Katz, and J.A. Shield Jr., Washington, DC: US Government Printing Office.

Robins, L. (1978) 'Psychiatric epidemiology', *Archives of General Psychiatry* 35: 697–702.

Selye, H. (1956) *The Stress of Life*, New York: McGraw-Hill.

Shepherd, M. (1978) 'Epidemiology and clinical psychiatry', *British Journal of Psychiatry* 133: 289–98.

Shepherd, M. (1979) 'From social medicine to social psychiatry: the achievement of

Sir Aubrey Lewis', in E.C. Rosenberg (ed.) *Healing and History Essays for George Rosen*, Folkestone: Dawson.

Shepherd, M. (1986) *A Representative Psychiatrist: The Career, Contributions and Legacies of Sir Aubrey Lewis* (A Psychological Medicine Monograph Supplement 10), Cambridge: Cambridge University Press.

Shepherd, M., Cooper, B., Brown, A.C., and Kalton, G.W. (1966) *Psychiatric Illness in General Practice*, London: Oxford University Press.

Spitzer, R.L., Endicott, J., and Robins, E. (1978) 'Research diagnostic criteria: rationale and reliability', *Archives of General Psychiatry* 35: 773–82.

Uhlenhuth, E.H., Balter, M.B., Mellinger, G.D., Cissin, I.H. and Clinthorne, J. (1983) 'Symptom checklist syndromes in the general population: correlation with psychotherapeutic drug use', *Archives of General Psychiatry* 40: 1167–73.

von Korff, M., Eaton, W., and Reyl, P. (1985) 'The epidemiology of panic attacks and disorder: results from three community surveys', *American Journal of Epidemiology* 122: 970–81.

von Korff, M., Shapiro, S., Burke, J.D., Teitelbaum, M., Skinner, E.A., German, P., Turner, R.W., Klein, L. and Burns, B. (1987) 'Anxiety and depression in a primary health care clinic: comparison of Diagnostic Interview Schedule, General Health Questionnaire, and practitioner assessments', *Archives of General Psychiatry* 44: 152–6.

Weissman, M.M. (in press) 'The epidemiology of panic disorders and agoraphobia', for Section 1, *Panic Disorders*, M.K. Shear and D. Barlow (section eds), *APA Annual Review of Psychiatry, Volume 7*, edited by A.J. Frances and R.E. Hales, Washington, DC: American Psychiatric Press.

Weissman, M.M. and Klerman, G.L. (1977) 'Sex differences and the epidemiology of depression', *Archives of General Psychiatry* 34: 98–111.

Weissman, M.M. and Myers, J.K. (1978) 'Affective disorders in a U.S. urban community: the use of research diagnostic criteria in a community survey', *Archives of General Psychiatry* 35: 1304–11.

Wing, J., Cooper, J., and Sartorius, N. (1974) *The Measurement and Classification of Psychiatric Symptoms*, Cambridge: Cambridge University Press.

14

Personality Disorder

Anthony Mann and Glyn Lewis

> Despite diagnostic imprecision and terminological confusion, the concept
> of personality disorder remains indispensable to clinical practice.
> > Shepherd and Sartorius (1974: 141).

So begins a brief review of the discussion concerning personality disorder
that preceded the publication of the ninth edition of the International
Classification of Diseases (ICD–9). It is timely to reconsider the position as
ICD–10 is being prepared. The intervening years have seen tentative efforts
in research and some standardization of the assessment of personality
disorder. However, personality remains one the most controversial and least
studied areas of psychiatry, and the quantity of work has been minuscule
compared to that on the symptomatology of psychiatric illness. The new
section on personality disorder in ICD–10 has been assembled by dint of
well-intentioned discussion rather than from research data. Comprehensive
epidemiological data, to complete the clinical picture on personality disorder,
is still some way away.

One reason for the lack of research must be the persisting doubts about
the validity of the diagnosis of personality disorder. To what extent is the
clinician using this term in a slipshod fashion to cover inadequate psychiatric
assessment, to convey a value judgement, or to justify therapeutic failure?
Behind such questions lie the doubts of those who believe that the concept
of personality inherent in ICD definitions is flawed.

In this chapter both points of view will be presented: firstly, the arguments
of those who aim to clarify 'the diagnostic imprecision and terminological
confusion' while working within the traditional concept of personality
disorder; and secondly, the point of view which criticizes the existing
concepts, so advocating alternative research strategies. The concepts of
personality will be discussed before recent research developments. The first
author holds the former viewpoint, while the second maintains the latter, and
this chapter has been written accordingly.

THE CONCEPT OF PERSONALITY AND PERSONALITY DISORDER

The traditional view

Personality is conceived by both ICD and DSM–III as a relatively fixed long-term collection of attitudes and behaviours by which one individual might be identified by another and into which the individual may have full or partial insight. These attributes are thought to become recognizable by adolescence, are generally stable throughout adult life, though they may modify with old age. Head injury is one of the few events that may alter this pattern. Against this background of personality, certain individuals may in clinical parlance be deemed as having a personality abnormality or personality disorder. To enter these categories the individual must posses certain types of attributes and behaviours without exclusion criteria that make them congruent with a particular description in ICD–9 or DSM–III.

The distinction between abnormal premorbid personality and personality disorder has never been defined formally. In practice, the first term is seen as a less marked variation and carries less suffering of handicap for the individual than the latter. Further, the former term is likely to be used if a diagnostic symptom state is also present as well as evidence of a personality abnormality. The latter is likely to be used if the personality attributes alone are the basis of diagnosis.

Clinical diagnosis of personality thus seems to require many arbitrary decisions based upon imprecise information. Where does the clinician derive data about personality attributes? How fixed through life do they have to be? How near a fit is necessary for a particular category to be chosen? How discrete and comprehensive are these taxonomic categories? Can stable personality traits be distinguished in a clinical setting from long-term neurotic symptoms? How much suffering and how much handicap is necessary for diagnosis of personality disorder? None of these questions is answered, yet the concept seems to remain 'indispensable to clinical practice'. Indeed, in 1974, 42 per cent of a consecutive series of Maudsley Hospital in-patient notes contained statements testifying to the significance of personality attributes to the understanding of the clinical picture (Mann et al. 1981a). However, clinicians still seem to use the concept of background personality for their practice despite its imprecision and operational difficulty.

Since 1974 the newer taxonomies have attempted to tackle some of the operational difficulties. DSM–III provides much more stringent inclusion and exclusion criteria for its diagnostic categories of personality; while ICD–10 has created parallel lists, one of personality accentuation, the other of personality disorder. Abnormal premorbid personality now can be classified, along with other diagnoses, rather than being omitted or subsumed under the more forbidding term of personality disorder. Both new systems have increased the range of personality types to try and make the total list more exhaustive. However, the fundamental questions about the clinician's concept

197

of personality, attitudes, behaviours, or self-concepts are not answered. Nor is the question of the persistence of such attributes. The justification for continuing with this imprecise term seems to have several roots. First, its history, for the concept of personality has been in use under one name or another for nearly 130 years. Second, there is the diagnostic imperative, for patients still present with complaints that seem similar to those with symptom states yet who have never developed symptoms. How are these to be labelled? Finally, much research into psychiatric illnesses, particularly into genetic linkage, uses the concept of spectrum which includes personality traits and is often necessary to provide an adequate model for the variable rates of expression of many psychiatric illnesses. It seems unlikely that personality abnormality will vanish from psychiatric parlance and, therefore, it seems relevant to pursue research in this area.

PROBLEMS WITH THE CONCEPT OF PERSONALITY AND PERSONALITY DISORDER

The nature of personality

The difficulty of defining personality and its use as a lay term have complicated discussion and added unnecessarily to the arguments over the nature of personality.

Personality can, therefore, mean different things to different people and can be defined in different ways. A very general definition might be: any psychological attribute of a person which varies between individuals. In the recent controversies over the nature of personality, no one doubts that people differ from one another in their psychological attributes. However, personality is also used in a much more specific way: personal attributes, as above (e.g. honesty), which are related to other attributes (e.g. conscientiousness) and endure over someone's whole lifetime. Within experimental psychology, this more specific view of personality is associated with those who conceptualize personality as 'traits' (e.g. Eysenck 1952; Cattell 1957) but a similar view of personality underlies psychodynamic personality theories (e.g. Storr 1979) and the categorical classification of personality disorders used in psychiatry.

Criticisms of trait theory have come from those experimental psychologists who emphasize the rational, cognitive determinants of social behaviour, who include both social learning theorists (Mischel 1968; Bandura 1977) and cognitive psychologists (Anderson 1980). Mischel (1968) in particular has argued that the trait theory of personality needs empirical support. One cannot begin to study personality if it is defined in a way which implies an unproven theory of personality.

Another point should be made before continuing. Personality can only be a description; it cannot explain or cause behaviour, though it is sometimes used as though it could. Gilbert Ryle (1949) has lucidly argued against this sort of 'explanatory' statement as creating a 'ghost in the machine'. Furthermore, personality traits are usually defined using behavioural measures so it is tautologous to say that a trait caused the behaviour which was used to define the trait in the first place. Wootton (1959) had made a similar point about the use of the terms psychopathic or antisocial personality disorder to explain criminal behaviour, when the criminal behaviour has been used as grounds for the diagnosis.

Lay personality theories

It is a truism to say that ordinary people have their own concept of personality. Allport (1937) found over 11,000 trait terms in English (e.g. outgoing, shy, nervous, intelligent, etc.), and in ordinary social interaction we often ask 'What sort of person is this?: a question that is often answered with a trait term. Allport's list, rooted in lay psychology, formed the basis of Cattell's (1957) and other trait theorists' way of measuring personality. Subjects were asked to rate themselves or others on a variety of trait terms and the results subjected to factor analysis. Cattell, Eysenck, and others interpreted such findings as revealing the underlying dimensions of personality but one can also interpret the results as reflecting the theory of personality used by ordinary people.

This interpretation is supported by the key experiment of Passini and Norman (1966). In the late 1950s and 1960s one group had shown that factor analysis of trait ratings from a variety of different studies all produced a similar five-factor result (Norman 1963). But Passini and Norman (1966) found an almost identical five-factor solution when raters who had only seen people for less than fifteen minutes and had not spoken to each other were asked to rate the subjects as they imagined they would be. This 'five-factor personality structure' therefore appeared to reflect the way ordinary people characterize each other, rather than representing the underlying structure of personality. Tyrer and Alexander (1979), though, argue that the similarity of the factor structure in those with and without personality disorders supports the idea that personality disorder is an extreme variant of normal, but it could merely reflect the 'personality theories' used by the informants and interviewers.

Situations

One of the key issues in the personality literature has been the assertion that behaviour is influenced by the situation as well as by personal factors. Trait-rating scales already imply cross-situational consistency and to examine whether people really do behave similarly in different situations needs direct behavioural measurement.

A number of such studies has been done and Mischel (1968), among others, has pointed out that the correlation coefficients in these studies (with the exception of that for intelligence) are usually very modest, less than 0.3 and account for less than 10 per cent of the variance. For instance, Hartshorne and May's (1928) study of school children found that the average correlations between cheating on four different tests was only 0.26, though the correlation between cheating on the same test on different occasions was 0.66. Mischel and Peake (1982) conducted two 'delay of reinforcement' studies on the same group of children which only differed in a single respect – in one group the experimenter remained in the room. The correlation coefficient between the two was only 0.22.

Mischel's conclusions have been challenged (e.g. Epstein 1979) but the data against substantial cross-situational consistency seem overwhelming. Broad behavioural consistencies must exist (a correlation coefficient of 0.3 is significant if the sample is large enough) but are too small to be of any use in predicting the behaviour of individual poeple.

When a thinking and reasoning person enters a situation it would be unlikely, indeed maladaptive, for broad personality traits to have a strong influence on behaviour. Perhaps cross-situational consistency should be regarded as a sign of an 'abnormal personality'? Indeed, Tyrer et al. (1979) have suggested that cross-situational consistency is more apparent in those classified as personality disordered.

The medical concept of personality disorder therefore rests on the rather shaky foundations of traditional personality theory.

State vs. Trait: can neurosis be distinguished from personality disorder?

Social learning theory does not need to make the distinction between state and trait. All behaviour, whether exhibited over a great length of time or only covering a short period, would have the same basis in beliefs and attitudes and their interaction with the environment (Mischel 1968; Beck 1976).

Many authors have shown that those with personality disorder experience neurotic symptoms (e.g. Lazare and Klerman 1968; Slavney and McHugh 1974; Gunn and Robertson 1976; Thompson and Goldberg 1987). Furthermore, some personality inventories, particularly the scales measuring 'neuroticism', appear to correlate markedly with measures of mental illness, and change with recovery from depression (Coppen and Metcalfe 1965; Kendell and DiScipio 1968; Hirschfeld et al. 1983). The distinction between trait and state may be an attractive simplification but there is still no way of distinguishing a neurotic trait from a neurotic state, nor a personality disorder from a chronic neurosis. Shepherd et al. (1968), in their international study of diagnostic habits, noted that personality disorder in one culture was neurosis in another.

Replacing the concept of personality disorder with the simpler and more comprehensive idea of chronic neurosis would fit the available evidence, but some features of personality disorder are not neurotic symptoms. For instance, the concept of antisocial personality disorder, at least in DSM–III, includes committing crimes. But many critics have pointed out the legal and philosophical difficulties of psychiatric explanations of crime (e.g. Wootton 1959). There are, therefore, definite advantages if psychiatrists abandon the impulse to explain all deviant behaviour.

Personality disorder and mental illness

Among all the controversy there is, surprisingly, one area of relative agreement: that personality disorder is not a mental illness (Lewis 1974). Though Henderson (1939) and Cleckley (1941) disagree, more recently personality disorder has increasingly been distinguished from illness.

Whatever mental illness means (Lewis 1953; Farrell 1979), it implies among other things a lack of control over behaviour and a lack of responsibility for action. The inference that an action is not under control has been linked with sympathy and willingness to help (Weiner 1980). In the contexts of a psychological abnormality, mental illness can be seen as a label conferring reduced responsibility for behaviour, legitimizing medical care, and encouraging sympathy.

Lewis and Appleby (1987) have thus argued that the assertion that personality disorder is used as a derogatory moral judgement (Gunn and Robertson 1976) results from the exclusion of personality disorder from the category of mental illness. Their study provided some evidence for this, based on questionnaire responses to case vignettes given the diagnosis of personality disorder. Compared with control vignettes, cases with personality disorder were seen as manipulative, attention-seeking, less sympathetic, not deserving NHS resources, and not being mentally ill. Someone who has a personality disorder is seen neither as normal nor as mentally ill; the worst of all possible worlds.

The claim that personality disorder is a derogatory moral judgement seriously questions the place of personality disorder in a scientific classification of mental disorder. Classifying these individuals as suffering from chronic neuroses would rely less on precarious theories of personality, would not be attempting to explain all deviant behaviour, and hopefully would eliminate a pejorative term from the psychiatric taxonomy.

CLINICAL RESEARCH INTO PERSONALITY DISORDER

The traditional view

Assuming the concept of personality disorder as reflected in ICD–9 or DSM–III can be tolerated, several basic research steps have to be taken before embarking on studies of prevalence and associations.

These general principles will be discussed before three published assessment schedules are described: the Standard Assessment of Personality (SAP, Mann *et al.* 1981a), the Personality Assessment Schedule (PAS, Tyrer and

Alexander 1979) and the Personality Disorder Examination (PDE) (Loranger *et al.* 1987).

a) *Standardizing data collection:* In clinical psychiatric practice it is usual to interview an informant for data on personality because most patients' abnormal mental states distort self concepts. However, self-report of habitual traits is possible in patients with a primary diagnosis of personality disorder. The difference between self-report and informant ratings was demonstrated in a study that assessed DSM–III personality disorder (Stangl *et al* 1985). Cases for whom there was an informant were almost twice as likely to be given a diagnosis of personality disorder. Thus, informants seem to provide more diagnostic information though they may not be available and they may be biased. This last point has been addressed to some extent in attempts to establish inter-informant agreement. This was poor, both when staff members were informants and when self and informant ratings were compared (Tyrer and Alexander 1979). However, in a study of obsessional patients, there was better agreement when both informants were relatives (McKeon *et al*, 1984). The best source of reliable personality information has not yet been resolved.

b) *Definition of the boundary:* The severity of personality abnormality necessary for inclusion in a diagnosis of personality disorder needs to be established. The ICD–9 definition, although imprecise, implies that for a disorder to be present the individual will be suffering, or others will, on account of personality. The DSM–III definition indicates inflexibility of trait, subjective distress, or social impairment. These definitions are intended to separate personality disorder from an intermediate state where a trait is present but there is no personal suffering. Frances (1982) argued for a dimensional approach to personality disorder, obviating the need for such arbitary boundaries.

The three diagnostic schedules contain different criteria for severity. The PAS emphasizes the need for impaired social adjustment for a diagnosis of personality disorder. Using the PDE, the clinicians can make a judgement on the basis of the responses to the standard questions in the schedule or can use a predetermined value of the total score. In the SAP the personality abnormality is called marked (Grade 2) and is equivalent to personality disorder if the informant reports the personality attribute either as extreme ('the most houseproud person I know') or handicapping social functioning. However, the SAP differs from the other two schedules as it recognizes an intermediate (Grade 1) category, similar to the concepts of Personality Accentuation defined by Leonhard (1968) and of abnormal premorbid personality used clinically and now recognized in ICD–10.

c) *Development of the taxonomy:* A descriptive typology of personality has evolved, based upon detailed clinical vignettes such as the sensitive personality disorder (Kretschmer 1918) and the psychopathic disorders described by Schneider (1950). Some personality types are similar in clinical features to a psychiatric symptom state, others have putative aetiological relationships to a psychiatric syndrome.

Even the existing typologies, however, are unable to categorize those personality abnormalities relevant to psychiatric practice. For example, only nineteen of a consecutive series of forty-two abnormal personalities among neurotic patients and twenty-nine of fifty-seven abnormal personalities discovered among psychotic patients could be matched to an ICD–9 category (Mann *et al*. 1981a, Cutting *et al*. 1986). The more recently derived DSM–III typography overlaps with that of ICD–9 but contains some categories that have roots in psychoanalytic theory (borderline, narcissistic, and passive aggressive personalities) which have not yet met universal acceptance.

The PAS and SAP have dealt with the inadequacy of ICD–9 in two separate ways. The SAP incorporates two new categories, not found in ICD–9, derived from case-note accounts of abnormal personalities. For the PAS, personality data were collected from a range of subjects with and without abnormal personality, and subjected to a factor analysis which defined four main categories: socio-pathic, passive-dependent, anhankastic and schizoid, with nine sub-groups. It is claimed to provide a better fit for clinical personality data than the historical derived descriptions (Tyrer and Ferguson 1987). The PDE, in contrast to these two, has been designed to fit the DSM–III typology without modifications.

d) *Achievement of reliability:* As with any standard measure for research, personality assessments must be capable of generating good inter-rater reliability among users. To this end, well-designed questionnaires with clear directions and definitions combined with preliminary training are needed. The three schedules have now published evidence of adequate inter-rater reliability for some of the personality categories, a considerable improvement on the more dismal reports based upon clinical assessment rather than standardized assessment schedules (Walton and Presley 1973, Mellsop *et al*. 1982).

e) *Evidence of validity:* Two further forms of reliability need consideration, inter-temporal reliability and, for the schedules that derive data from informants, inter-informant reliability. Adequate reliability of these forms will, in part, confirm the validity of the assessment. Demonstrable stability of personality categorization over time, preferably despite fluctuations of symptoms, conforms with the ICD–9 concept of 'persistently deeply ingrained traits' while satisfactory inter-informant reliability would help to overcome anxiety about informants' bias and show that the attribute is not confined to one relationship or setting. However, external validity must in time be demonstrated, for example by concurrent validity with other forms of personality assessment and predictive validity between a personality category and specific physiological, behavioural, or illness variables.

The three schedules

The Standard Assessment of Personality. This is a brief interview of an informant along clinical lines in which informant data are used to classify the

Table 14.1 Reliability of SAP: Weighted Kappa Values

	Inter-rater	Inter-temporal	Inter-informant
Self conscious	0.67, 0.47	0.41, 0.96	0.88
Schizoid			
Paranoid		0.41	
Cyclothymic	0.85, 0.78	0.13	
Anhankastic	0.60, 1.00	0.74, 0.76	0.93
Anxious	0.61	0.42, 0.96	0.96
Asthenic			
Sociopathic	1.00		
Explosive	0.90		
Hysterical	0.91		

patient's personality as normal or into one of ten abnormal categories. The severity of the abnormal personality can be graded as a result of the inter-view. This schedule has now been used to assess patients' personalities in various settings: general practice (Mann *et al*. 1981a), hospital admission unit (Cutting *et al*. 1986), mental handicap hospital (Ballinger and Reid 1987), and for research (McKeon *et al*. 1984). Each of these research groups examined some aspects of inter-rater, inter-temporal, or inter-informant reliability of the assessment of the SAP categories. The results from these papers are grouped together in table 14.1.

Some categories of personality have been so rare in the populations studied, that reliability calculations were not possible. For the remainder, the weighted Kappa (KW) value is always greater than 0.4, considered adequate agreement at a level just statistically significant. The failure of the cyclothymic category to reach a satisfactory level of inter-temporal reliability suggests that this label might not be appropriately placed in a section on personality.

Some data on the distribution of the abnormal personality categories are available from the published studies. Thirty-three per cent of general practice patients with neuroses were classed as having abnormal personality compared with 44 per cent of the hospital admission cohort (Mann *et al*. 1981b, Cutting *et al*. 1986). In contrast, 75 per cent of the mental handicap sample were so graded (Ballinger and Reid 1987).

The general practice study showed some predictive ability of the SAP personality categories (Mann *et al*. 1981b). Patients assessed as having marked personality abnormality at the outset of a twelve-month follow-up period were discovered to be over-represented among the frequent attenders. They were also more likely than the others to present with symptoms such as headache and dizziness, and personality classification predicted receipt of psychotropic medication more accurately than did the initial symptom state.

The Personality Assessment Schedule. Data for this schedule can be derived from an interview with the subject, with an informant, or by personal observation of the patient by the interviewer. While an interview with an informant should always be sought, the subject's mental state may preclude self-report information. Twenty-four personality variables are rated on a nine-point scale, the highest scores indicating increasing social dysfunction as well as possession of personality characteristics to a marked degree. There is satisfactory reliability between two interviewers (KW more than 0.5 for all twenty-four variables). Inter-temporal reliability however varied for the twenty-four variables, the KW ranging from 0 to +0.59. However, once these personality data had been grouped into the four major diagnostic categories, agreement between the two occasions was much higher (KW 0.64) (Tyrer *et al.* 1982).

Personality Disorder Examination. Designed systematically to survey the phenomenology and life experiences relevant to the diagnosis of personality disorder in DSM–III, this schedule is administered by an interviewer (Loranger *et al.* 1987). The personality disorder can be categorized either by using a computer algorithm or by the clinician interviewer making a clinical diagnosis. Good inter-rater reliability was reported both for individual items of the schedule and also for the diagnostic classification (KW 0.7–0.96) for the five DSM–III categories that were sufficiently common for statistical calculations to be made. Surprisingly, borderline personality was included in these categories despite being reported elsewhere as hard to distinguish from other DSM–III categories (Pope *et al.* 1983) and in need of improved definition. Such contradiction implies that the PDE may need further evaluation.

Conclusion

In conclusion, the proponent can claim modest advances by the creation of standardized schedules that psychiatrists can use reliably to assess the current clinical concept of personality. However, the data generated so far are limited and few of them specifically derived for the purpose of exploring the distribution and relationships of personality categories.

ALTERNATIVE APPROACHES TO STUDYING PERSONALITY DISORDER

Reliability

Trait ratings require global judgements based on ambiguous data. This vagueness must contribute towards the unreliability of personality assessment, and the trait ratings themselves can be very unreliable even in research settings (Gunn and Robertson 1976). There is now a striking contrast between the mental illness section of DSM–III or ICD–10, with its exactly specified operational criteria, and the section on personality disorder, with its rather vague trait descriptions. Antisocial personality disorder continues to be the most reliable of all the categories (Mellsop *et al.* 1982), possibly because the criteria include behavioural items (mostly about infringements of the law) as well as trait terms. It is ironic that the most reliable of all the personality disorder categories has also attracted the most controversy about its validity (Wootton 1959; Frances 1980).

Validity

Pre-existing beliefs or schemata can influence perception, memory, and social inferences (Anderson 1980) and in general the bias acts in order to confirm such beliefs (Nisbett and Ross 1980). Trait ratings are particularly suscept-ible, and such a confirmatory bias challenges the validity of trait ratings in assessing personality and in part explains why personality continues to make intuitive sense despite evidence to the contrary.

Cantor and Mischel (1979) illustrated a bias in recalling trait terms. They asked subjects (Ss) to remember a set of trait terms that applied to an imaginary person (e.g. that together described an extravert). When Ss were asked later to recognize these items they also recognized items that were related to the original trait (e.g. extravert) but which had not been originally presented. Once impressions are formed, they can have a powerful influence on memory. As Mischel (1968) has asserted, trait rating scales lead to infor-mation about what is in the mind of the rater, as well as, or even instead of, the behaviour of the rated.

These biases may also influence clinical assessment. For instance, suicidal thoughts in someone with a personality disorder could be seen as manipulative or histrionic, and therefore attract less sympathy and importance than the same complaints in someone regarded as 'ill'.

Alternative approaches to studying personality

What are the alternative strategies in attempting to study this difficult area? Personal attributes are probably important in determining vulnerability to mental illness; how can these attributes be assessed and studied?

Social learning theorists think of personality as a collection of personal attitudes and beliefs. Warr and his colleagues have developed a scale measur-ing commitment to work (including, for example, 'Even if I was given £1m I would still want to work') and have shown that those with a higher commit-ment to work have better mental health when in work and worse mental health when unemployed. Furthermore, they could demonstrate some predic-tive value for the scale, both when adolescents became unemployed (Jackson *et al.* 1983) and in predicting worsening of mental health in middle-aged men as unemployment continues (Warr and Jackson 1985).

This series of studies provides a model for studying personal attributes and their relationship with mental illness and shows an interaction between attitudes and the impact of a life event; a different approach to the personal meaning of life events (cf Brown and Harris 1978). It also illustrates the link between an individual's attitudes and societal norms, in this instance the social and economic importance of the 'work ethic' (Weber 1930).

This discussion may seem unrelated to the traditional preoccupations of personality disorder research. However, attitudes to work vary between people and are in all senses part of someone's personality, and part of the clinical assessment, particularly of the unemployed. The social learning approach to personality has many advantages; it does not use trait terms as a means of assessment nor imply a pre-existing theory of personality. It looks at the particular attitudes and beliefs of interest rather than trying to give a comprehensive description of the whole person, a Herculean task. Finally, the causes of mental as well as physical disorders must ultimately require social and economic explanations. Describing personality as a collection of attitudes may clarify the links between these socio-economic forces and the more proximate causes of mental illness.

This approach is more precise, less 'terminologically confused' than traditional approaches to personality and in time may become more indispensable to clinical practice than that unhappy ragbag of diagnosis, the personality disorders.

Acknowledgement: Glyn Lewis is supported by the Health Promotion Research Trust.

REFERENCES

Allport, G.W. (1937) *Personality: A Psychological Interpretation*, New York: Holt.

Anderson, J.R. (1980) *Cognitive Psychology and its Implications*, San Francisco. Freeman.

Ballinger, B.R. and Reid, A.H. (1987) 'A standardized assessment of personality in mental handicap', *British Journal of Psychiatry* 150: 108–9.

Bandura, A. (1977) *Social Learning Theory*, Englewood Cliffs, NJ: Prentice-Hall.

Beck, A.T. (1976) *Cognitive Therapy and the Emotional Disorders*, International University Press: New York.

Cantor, N. and Mischel, W. (1979) 'Traits as Prototypes: Effects on Recognition Memory', *Journal of Personality and Social Psychology* 35: 38–48.

Cattell, R.B. (1957) *Personality and Motivation: Structure & Measurement*, Yonkers-on-Hudson: World Books.

Chodoff, P. and Lyons, H (1958) 'Hysteria, the Hysterical Personality and "Hysterical" Conversion', *American Journal of Psychiatry* 114: 734–40.

Coppen, A. and Metcalfe, M. (1965) 'Effect of a depressive illness on MPI scores', *British Journal of Psychiatry* 111: 236–9.

Cutting, J., Cowan, P.J., Mann, A.H., and Jenkins, R. (1986) 'Personality and psychosis: use of the standard assessment', *Acta Psychiatrica Scandinavica* 73: 87–92.

Epstein, S. (1979) 'The stability of behaviour: 1: on predicting most of the people much of the time', *Journal of Personality and Social Psychology* 37: 1097–125.

Eysenck, J.J. (1952) *The Scientific Study of Personality*, London: Routledge & Kegan Paul.

Farrell, B.A. (1979) 'Mental illness: a conceptual analysis', *Psychological Medicine* 9: 21–35.

Frances, A. (1980) 'The DSM–III personality disorders: a commentary', *American Journal of Psychiatry* 137: 1050–4.

Frances, A. (1982) 'Categorial and dimensional systems of personality disorder', *Comprehensive Psychiatry* 23: 516–27.

Gunn, J. and Robertson, G. (1976) 'Psychopathic personality: a conceptual problem', *Psychological Medicine* 6: 631–34.

Hartshorne, H. and May, M.A. (1928) *Studies in the Nature of Character: Volume 1: Studies in Deceit*, New York: Macmillan.

Henderson, D.K. (1939) *Psychopathic States*, London.

Hirschfield, R.M.A., Klerman, G.L., Clayton, P.J., Keller, M.B., McDonald-Scott, P., and Larkin, B.H. (1983) 'Assessing personality: effects of the depressive state on trait measurement', *American Journal of Psychiatry* 140: 695–9.

Jackson, P.R., Stafford, E.M., Banks, M.H., and Warr, P.B. (1983) 'Unemployment and psychological distress in young people: the moderating role of employment commitment', *Journal of Applied Psychology* 68: 525–35.

Kendell, R.E. and DiScipio, W.J. (1968) 'Eysenck Personality Inventory Scores of patients with depressive illness', *British Journal of Psychiatry* 114: 767–70.

Kretschmer, E. (1918) *Die Sensitive Beziehungswan*, Berlin: Springer.

Lazare, A. and Klerman, G.L. (1968) 'Hysteria and depression: the frequency and significance of hysterical personality features in hospitalised depressed women', *American Journal of Psychiatry* 124: Supplement 48–56.

Leonard, K. (1967) *Kinder-neurosen und Kinder-persönlichkeiten* (3 Auflage), Berlin: Veb Verlag Volk und Gesundheit.

Lewis, A. (1953) 'Health as a social concept', *British Journal of Sociology* 4: 109–24.

Lewis, A. (1974) 'Psychopathic personality: a most elusive category', *Psychological Medicine* 4: 133–40.

Lewis, G.H. and Appleby, L.A. (in press) 'Personality disorder: the patients psychiatrists dislike', *British Journal of Psychiatry*.

Loranger, A.W., Susman, V.L., Oldham, J.M., and Russikoff, L.M. (1987) 'The personality disorder examination: a preliminary report', *Journal of Personality Disorders* 1(1).

McKeon, J., Roa, B., and Mann, A.H. (1984) 'Life events and personality traits in obsessive compulsive neurosis', *British Journal of Psychiatry* 144: 185–9.

Mann, A.H., Jenkins, R., Cutting, J.C., and Cowen, P.J. (1981a) 'The development and use of a standardised assessment of abnormal personality', *Psychological Medicine* 11: 839–47.

Mann, A.H., Jenkins, R., and Belsey, E. (1981b) 'The 12-month outcome of patients with neurotic illness in general practice', *Psychological Medicine* 11: 535–60.

Mellsop, G., Varghese, F., Joshua, A.S., and Hicks, A. (1982) 'Reliability of axis II of DSM–III', *American Journal of Psychiatry* 139: 1360–1.

Mischel, W. (1968) *Personality and Assessment*, New York: Wiley.

Mischel, W. and Peake, P.K. (1982) 'Some facets of consistency: replies to Epstein, Funder & Bem', *Psychological Reviews* 90: 394–402.

Nisbett, R. and Ross, L. (1980) *Human Inferences: Strategies and Shortcomings of Social Judgement*, Englewood Cliffs, NJ: Prentice-Hall.

Norman, W.T. (1963) 'Toward an adequate taxonomy of personality attributes: replicated factor structure in peer nomination personality ratings', *Journal of Abnormal and Social Psychology* 66: 574–83.

Passini, F.T. and Norman, W.T. (1966) 'A universal conception of personality structure?', *Journal of Personality and Social Psychology* 4: 44–9.

Pope, H.G., Jones, J.M., Hudson, J.I., Cohen, B.M., Gunderson, J.G. (1983) 'The validity of DSM–III personality disorders', *Archives of General Psychiatry* 40: 23–30.

Ryle, G. (1949) *The Concept of Mind* London, Hutchinson.

Schneider, K. (1950) *Psychopathic Personalities*, translated by M. Hamilton, London: Cassel.

Slavney, P.R. and McHugh, P.R. (1974) 'The hysterical personality: a controlled study', *Archives of General Psychiatry* 30: 325–9.

Shepherd, M., Brooke, E.M., Cooper, J.E., and Lin, T. (1968) 'An experimental approach to psychiatric diagnosis', *Acta Psychiatrica Scandinavica* Supplementum 201.

Shepherd, M. and Sartorius, N. (1974) 'Personality disorder and the classification of diseases', *Psychological Medicine* 4: 141–6.

Stangl, D., Pfohl, B., Zimmerman, M., Bowers, W., and Corenthal, C. (1985) 'A standardized interview for DSM–III personality disorders', *Archives of General Psychiatry* 42: 597–601.

Storr, A. (1979) *The Art of Psychotherapy*, London: Secker & Warburg.

Tyrer, P and Alexander, J. (1979) 'Classification of personality disorder', *British Journal of Psychiatry* 135: 163–7.

Tyrer, P., Alexander, M.S., Cicchetti, D., Cohen, M.S., and Remington, M. (1979) 'Reliability of a schedule for rating personality disorders', *British Journal of Psychiatry* 135: 168–74.

Tyrer, P. and Ferguson, B. (1987) 'Problems in the classification of personality disorders', *Psychological Medicine* 17: 15–20.

Tyrer, P., Strauss, J., and Cicchetti, D. (1982) 'Temporal reliability of a schedule for rating personality disorders', *Psychological Medicine* 13: 393–8.

Thompson, D.J. and Goldberg, D. (1987) 'Hysterical personality disorder: the process of diagnosis in clinical & experimental settings', *British Journal of Psychiatry* 150: 241–5.

Walton, H.J. and Presley, A.S. (1973) 'Use of a categoric system in diagnosis of abnormal personality', *British Journal of Psychiatry* 122: 259–68.

Warr, P.B. and Jackson, P.R. (1985) 'Factors influencing the psychological impact of prolonged unemployment and of re-employment', *Psychological Medicine* 15: 795–807.

Weber, M. (1930) *The Protestant Ethic and the Spirit of Capitalism* London: Allen and Unwin.

Weiner, B. (1980) 'A cognitive (attribution) – emotion – action model of motivated behaviour: an analysis of judgements of help giving', *Journal of Personality and Social Psychology* 39: 186–200

Wootton, B. (1959) *Social Science and Social Pathology* London: George Allen.

15

The Relationship Between Physical and Psychological Morbidity

Robin Eastwood

The work done at the General Practice Research Unit at the Institute of Psychiatry has led to a better understanding of the role of the general practitioner in treating mental illness. The gain in knowledge has been significant in several areas, including the prevalence of mental illness in the community, the chronicity of this illness, the difficulties of diagnosis, and the realization of the important associations with physical illness and social factors. The early findings were summarized by Shepherd et al. (1966: 169). They made the following points:

> Emotional disorder in the survey sample was found to be related to a high demand for medical care. Those patients identified as suffering from psychiatric illness attended more frequently and exhibited higher rates of general morbidity and more categories of illness per head than the remainder of the patients consulting their doctors. Furthermore, patients with chronic psychiatric illness were particularly frequent attenders and appeared to constitute a highly vulnerable group from the point of view of loss of work and permanent incapacity.

Sub-studies further supported these main findings and enabled the group to take the view that 'chronic psychiatric disturbance is positively associated with other forms of chronic ill-health' (Shepherd et al. 1966: 170); and that the high illness-expectation could be seen as 'illness-proneness' (Hinkle and Wolff 1957) which might be further examined by longitudinal studies.

The stage was then set for the group to elaborate the findings by enhancing the methodology and further testing the relationships. The General Health Questionnaire was developed as a screening instrument (Goldberg 1972) and the Clinical Interview Schedule (Goldberg et al. 1970) as a diagnostic instrument. Mental illness appeared to have associations with both social factors (Kedward and Sylph 1974; Cooper 1972) and physical illness and I had the task of confirming the latter. The initial design and method problems were:

(1) To obtain a random sample of the general population;
(2) To screen and further examine for mental illness;
(3) To screen and further examine for physical disorder;
(4) To test the association between psychiatric and physical disorder.

SAMPLING

The need for a random sample of the general population was obvious and critical. Psychosocial factors influence illness presentation. Thus, clinicians presume that a biological component determines a consultation, but 'illness behaviour' is important, being a composite of the way in which an individual perceives, evaluates, and acts upon his symptoms in his particular social setting (Mechanic 1966).

There are those who are ill and fail to consult and, conversely, those who make a habit of consulting, whatever their state of health. Genuine illness has to be teased out from other factors in a medical consultation. This problem has been elegantly discussed by Goldberg and Huxley (1980). In their extensive review they particularly mention the work of Mechanic and his considerable contributions to our understanding of the determinants of perceived health status.

SCREENING

Screening for disease was in vogue in the 1950s and 1960s. Multiple screening surveys started in the United States and the proposed definition of the Commission on Chronic Illness (1957) was that screening was 'the presumptive identification of unrecognized disease or defect by the application of the tests, examination or other procedures which can be applied rapidly.' The World Health Organization monograph by Wilson and Jungner (1968) said that the purpose was to discover and cure disease in its early stages before medical help was sought and to make the best economic use of the available medical manpower. Screening for psychiatric disorder, in my study, has been discussed at length (Eastwood 1971, Eastwood 1975) and the utility of psychiatric screening has been dealt with elsewhere (Goldberg 1974; Goldberg and Huxley 1980; Goldberg 1986; Williams 1986). Suffice to make three brief points in regard to screening: first, apart from phenylketonuria, hardly any diseases have satisfied general screening criteria; second, psychiatric disorder has not been approved generally for screening; and third, this fortunately has not stopped psychiatric case finding for research purposes with a variety of screening instruments and clinical interview schedules. In the St Paul's Cray Study screening was done with the modified version of the Cornell Medical Index and the second stage with the Clinical Interview

211

Schedule. Today, the General Health Questionnaire would replace the Cornell Medical Index and the choice for the second stage would be between such instruments as the Clinical Interview Schedule, the Present State Examination (Wing *et al.* 1967) and the Schedule for Affective Disorders and Schizophrenia (Endicott and Spitzer 1978).

Screening for physical disease was the main intention of the St Paul's Cray study. Early assessments of screening (McKeown 1968) suggested that the evidence was deficient for most chronic disorders, particularly cost-effectiveness and natural history. Although screening for disease has not been found generally acceptable (South-East London Screening Study Group 1977), the St Paul's Cray screening protocol (Eastwood 1975) was adequate for testing the relationship between physical and psychiatric disorder.

RESULTS

Results of the St Paul's Cray study were as follows:

(1) A 71 per cent response rate was obtained with a fairly homogeneous population made up of persons between the ages of 40 and 64, largely married and of the skilled artisan class.

(2) From 369 clinical interviews, 124 matched pairs, consisting of a psychiatric patient and a normal control, were derived.

(3) The psychiatric cases were largely the minor, neurotic cases seen in general practice, although some were of moderate severity, with the men having more personality disorders and the women more hypochrondiacal neuroses. A substantial number of the cases, the less severe variety, had not been recognized by the general practitioners prior to the survey. Thus, 19 per cent of the men and 27.5 per cent of the women had a psychiatric disturbance unknown to the general practitioner and a further 21.6 per cent of the men and 25.2 per cent of the women were similarly unknown but had had a recognized psychiatric illness in the past. The more serious disorders were known to the general practitioners.

(4) Both male and female psychiatric cases had more major physical and major psychosomatic conditions than normal controls, and the males more minor physical conditions and minor psychosomatic conditions.

(5) Multiple physical disorders occurred more among the psychiatric cases and these increased with the severity of psychiatric disorder, especially major physical conditions.

(6) The findings confirmed a positive association between physical and psychiatric disorder with a tendency for clustering of illnesses to occur in some individuals (Eastwood 1975).

SUBSEQUENT WORK IN THE NEXT TWO DECADES

Since this study was mounted there has been a variety of investigations and commentaries. A literature search showed these to be legion and it would be impossible and invidious to attempt to include them all. What is done here is to describe several studies which have been seminal or accounts which have collated contemporary wisdom in this area (other publications are frequently cited in these works).

In the ensuing years several studies have fleshed out the findings. Goldberg and Blackwell (1970) undertook a unique study. Both were psychiatrists, with a common training, but it so happened that Goldberg was working, at that time, as a research psychiatrist and Blackwell as a general practitioner.

Some 200 attenders at the general practice survey were interviewed by both, with complete agreement upon diagnosis for two-thirds of the patients. Presenting symptoms were classified along a spectrum between entirely physical complaints and those entirely psychiatric. Least agreement occurred with physical illness in a neurotic personality, physical illness with associated psychiatric disturbance, psychiatric disturbance with somatic symptoms and unrelated physical and psychiatric disorder. 'Conspicuous psychiatric morbidity' was found in two-thirds and 'hidden psychiatric morbidity' in one-third, with the latter differing in both attitude toward illness and presenting physical symptoms.

What is unique about this study is that both physicians were trained psychiatrists from the same post-graduate school but functioning in different roles at that time. Their failure to agree in one-third of psychiatric cases, given their level of training, must indicate the inchoate nature of much morbidity at the general practice level. If difficult for these newly trained and enthusiastic specialists, then a most complicated clinical mosaic for the average generalist.

Goldberg *et al.* (1976) repeated the study in Philadelphia with similar findings. In *Mental Illness in the Community* (Goldberg and Huxley 1980), Goldberg points out how common it is for psychiatric patients, in all sorts of settings, to present with nonspecific physical symptoms. Later Bridges and Goldberg (1985) spelt out this somatic manifestation of psychiatric disorder, 'somatization', in general practice in DSM-III terms. In this study patients had to satisfy certain criteria: these were seeking help for somatic manifestations of psychiatric illness (these had to be considered by the patient to be caused by a physical problem when seeing their general practitioner); having a psychiatric diagnosis when seen by the research psychiatrist and a condition assumed to be treatable by a psychiatric means producing symptom relief. Some 417 inceptions were classified and in a subsequent analysis the following information emerged. The initial analysis showed that of patients presenting to their general practitioner 54 per cent had a physical disease, 13 per cent an adjustment disorder, and 33 per cent a psychiatric disorder. Subsequent analyses showed the relationship of these three presentations to each other and to somatization. Finally, the types of psychiatric presentation were presented. Thirty-two per cent had pure somatization disorder, 27 per cent a psychiatric disorder with co-existing physical illness, 17 per cent with a purely psychological presentation, and 24 per cent with facultative somatization. (Although these patients somatized to the general practitioner, they did not do so to the research psychiatrist.) Thus over 50 per cent of cases consulting general practitioners with a psychiatric disorder had a somatic presentation. Finally, while the general practitioners were good at recognizing purely psychiatric disorder, they tended to be misled by somatization. The rest of the undetected cases had a physical illness. In this important paper the authors discuss the implications of psychiatric illness in primary care presenting so frequently with somatic symptoms. They point out that the failure to detect and treat will be a burden to the patient, it may affect an accompanying physical illness, and could lead to a great deal of extra subsequent consulting behaviour. The authors wondered why the majority of patients with diagnosable psychiatric disorders only present somatically to their family doctor.

In a recent review of depression in primary care, Blacker and Clare (1987) argue for a reciprocal connection between mental and physical illness, but question any direct aetiology because of such factors as skewed consulting patterns and threshold effects by patients in primary care, possible age effects and physical illness delaying recovery from mental illness.

Corresponding work has been undertaken in Australia and the United States. Andrews et al. (1977, 1978) confirmed the relationship between physical and mental illness in a random sample in Sydney, and also looked at social factors. All illness was assessed by questionnaire. Twenty-four per cent had psychiatric and 46 per cent one or more physical conditions, with 15 per cent having an overlap. Psychiatric illness was independent of age and more common among females; physical illness was also more common, but to a lesser extent, among females and increased with age. All illness was predicted by life events, poor upbringing and poor social support, and, separately, low occupational status to physical illness and poor coping style to mental illness. Social factors accounted for some variance in physical illness (20 per cent) and mental illness (37 per cent).

The US findings come from the Epidemiologic Catchment Area studies (ECA). Shepherd (1987), in an editorial in the *American Journal of Public Health*, pointed out that his 1960s British study, identifying a 14 per cent period prevalence for psychiatric disorder in the community and largely treated by primary care physicians, had been subsequently confirmed and supported in Europe and the US. The ECA studies were set up in the late 1970s and have been described in detail (Eaton and Kessler 1985). The programme was set up to collect incidence and prevalence data for mental

214

illness in several cities across the United States; and to assess the need for and utilization by both health and mental health services per person in community samples. The most recent paper by Kessler *et al.* (1987) from five of these cities found medical users to have a prevalence rate of 21.7 per cent, compared with 16.7 per cent for non-users, for DIS disorders. This confirms significant rates of psychiatric disorder among medical service users and reiterates that much psychiatric disorder is seen and treated by those in primary care.

Several authors cited in this paper have suggested that age has a bearing upon the connection between physical and mental illness. However, Eastwood and Corbin (1986) have pointed out that, based on empirical evidence, few conclusions regarding a generalized relationship between physical illness and depression in old age can be drawn. For a start, physical illness increases in old age and depression does not. Associations appear to be nonspecific, heterogeneous, likely multiple and require multi-variate analysis. In other words, 'the heterogeneity of evidence appears to support the concept of multiple etiology in chronic disease, both physical and psychological, and multiple responses by aged individuals to health-threatening agents across variable situations.' (Eastwood and Corbin 1986: 184)

LONGITUDINAL STUDIES

Another way of looking at the relationship between physical and mental disorder is the longitudinal method, which may be prospective or case control. This approach has been adopted many times in past decades with, perhaps, the most recent publication being from the Stirling County Group under the directorship of Professor Alexander Leighton. The authors point out that the gist of the previous findings has been a definite association between psychiatric disorder and premature death, with the trend being for death to be increasingly due to unnatural causes, suicide and accident, rather than natural ones. Some recent studies failed to show any excess of natural deaths in psychiatric patients, including such community surveys as the Midtown Manhattan.

The Stirling County study paper (Murphy *et al.* 1987) examined the association between affective disorders and mortality in a sixteen-year follow-up, 1952–68, from a general population in Nova Scotia. In 1952 there were 456 men and 547 women in the survey; 5 per cent of the men and 10 per cent of the women had co-existing affective and physical disorder. By 1968, 24 per cent of the subjects were dead. Depression, not age or anxiety, was significantly associated with excess mortality. (The Standardized Mortality Ratio (SMR) was 2.1 for men and 1.2 for women.) The association was striking in such groups as both sexes under 50 years of age, both with circulatory diseases and cancer in women. Most of the depressive illnesses

215

and about half the anxiety states had a poor outcome. Physical disorders by themselves were at the outset not associated with excess mortality. The authors point out the familiar finding that women have more physical ailments than men but live longer and quote the Almeda County study to the effect that it is not physical health problems that bear on mortality but rather health practices such as diet, fitness, and alcohol consumption. The Stirling County Study suggests that psychiatric rather than physical problems predicate mortality. This means depression, rather than anxiety, with the paradox that men have higher mortality rates and less depression. The Stirling County Study differs from other studies in finding similar rates of depression for the sexes, which the authors think may be due to 'sexually neutral' questionnaires. Nevertheless, they suggest that, if the usual finding of an excess of depressed females is true, this may be because males die from depression while women survive disabled. They go on to say that, conversely, anxiety may make people vigilant and health conscious and thus make the women, who had more of this disorder, protected and, thereby, live longer. Finally, the study was undertaken when antidepressants were in their infancy and so it is unlikely that much of the depression was treated. It remains to be seen, therefore, whether chronically depressed people can avoid premature death through adequate treatment; and whether depression is aetiological to premature death by directly affecting the circulatory and immunological systems, or acts indirectly by producing dependency syndromes, slothful habits, and unfitness.

Vaillant (1979) examined the effects of mental health on physical health. An educationally homogeneous sample of white males from Harvard University, born around 1921, was followed for over thirty years and given serial examinations. Some 188 men were included in the sample. Poor adult adjustment was strongly associated with deterioration of physical health. Curiously, obesity, alcohol use, and cigarette smoking had a relatively weak association with health deterioration. Psychosocial factors explained 23 per cent of the health deterioration while longevity of ancestors, capacity to work hard, and freedom from physical disease explained 2 per cent of the remaining variance. Thus in the sample 'chronic anxiety, depression, and emotional maladjustment, measured in a variety of ways, predicted early aging, defined by irreversible deterioration of health' and 'positive mental health significantly retards irreversible midlife decline in physical health' (Vaillant 1979: 1253). The author says that, although previous research has attempted to link stressful life events and poor social supports in the development of chronic illness, it has ignored alcoholism, psychopathology, and maladaptive coping mechanisms. Finally, Vaillant speculates that 'stress does not kill us so much as ingenious adaptation to stress (call it good mental health or mature coping mechanisms) facilitates our survival' (Vaillant 1979: 1253).

PSYCHIATRIC MORBIDITY IN THE GENERAL HOSPITAL

Proceeding through what Goldberg and Huxley (1980) have termed a 'series of filters', it is possible to see the relationship between physical and mental illness at different levels of care. In a detailed review, Mayou and Hawton (1986) looked at psychiatric disorder in the general hospital. They point out that surveys of general hospitals, compared with those described for general practice by Goldberg and Huxley, have been of poor quality and that the research instruments have been found wanting. Nevertheless, they take the view that there is considerable psychiatric morbidity at all levels in general hospitals, much of it unknown to the hospital doctors.

Lipowski has written extensively in the areas of psychosomatic medicine and consultation-liaison psychiatry. Some selected papers were collated in a volume entitled *Psychosomatic Medicine and Liaison Psychiatry* (Lipowski 1985). In a paper entitled 'Physical illness and mental disorder – epidemiology' he sees four reasons for the increased attention to the relationship between physical and mental illness. First, consultation-liaison developments have brought psychiatrists in contact with physical illness on a considerable scale, second, the aging population brings with it increased risk of both mental and physical illness; third, chronic diseases have a high prevalence and may cause much psychiatric disorder although this needs documenting; and, finally, new medications and procedures have psychiatric sequelae.

He sees psychiatric disorders, judged to be causally related to physical illness, as being of three major classes: organic brain syndromes, reactive functional disorders, and deviant illness behaviour. Organic brain syndromes occur as a result of demonstrable or presumed cerebral pathology; 'reactive' functional disorders, mainly affective disorders, occur as a consequence of the meaning for a patient of a physical illness or injury. The term 'deviant illness behaviour' refers to a physically ill patient's behaviour that militates against recovery or optimal attainable health.

Lipowski, like Mayou and Hawton, underscores the poor hospital epidemiological information due to unreliable terms and methods. He indicates that existing epidemiological data indicate only concurrence and not a causal relationship between physical and psychiatric disorder. He accepts that such a concurrence has been reasonably well documented by community studies but concludes that hospital data are less satisfactory. While it is widely accepted that organic brain syndromes and affective disorders make up much of psychiatric morbidity in the medical population, Cavanaugh and Wettstein (1984: 203) assert that the 'medical inpatient studies to date permit few inferences about the prevalence of psychiatric distress, symptoms, or diagnoses.'

In a further paper entitled 'Physical illness and psychiatric disorder-pathogenesis', Lipowski indicates that specific agent models of causality do not apply and the concept of vulnerability is better. Obviously, physical illness may be independent, causal, or caused by psychiatric disorder. Lipowski makes an attempt to spell out multifactorial psychopathogenesis and suggests that the following psychosocial and psychobiological factors can influence a patient's response to physical illness in the direction of psychopathology:

(1) frustration of drives and needs;
(2) increased intensity of intra-psychic conflicts;
(3) failure of defence mechanisms;
(4) loss of self-esteem;
(5) alteration of body image;
(6) disruption of normal sleep-wake cycle;
(7) social isolation and alienation.

Elsewhere, Lipowski discusses somatization in 'Somatization: a borderline between medicine and psychiatry' (Lipowski 1986). He defines somatization as 'a tendency to experience and communicate psychologic distress in the form of physical symptoms and to seek medical help, [which] constitutes a very common and often exasperating problem' (Lipowski 1986: 609). He points out that more than half of the patients in primary care, given one of these diagnoses, present primarily with somatic symptoms, and somatization constitutes a major medical and economic problem.

DISCUSSION

It is quite clear that the epidemiological work in primary care carried out by Michael Shepherd and his group was seminal and heralded important work in that sphere. It pinpointed that the prevalence of psychiatric disorder in the community was considerable, that such disorders were largely managed by the general practitioner, and that they tended to be associated with physical illness and social difficulties. In the St Paul's Cray study, when every effort was made to exclude diagnostic, method, and sampling problems, physical and mental disorder were significantly related. Later work by Goldberg and his group showed how complex the presentations of psychiatric disorder are in primary care and how difficult it is for the general practitioners to treat the total person. Elsewhere, in Australia and the United States, the community findings were corroborated. (Epidemiology in the community now seems to have a primacy over that in general hospitals, since the research in the latter has been described as being inadequate.)

Subsequent work has shown that psychiatric patients frequently present with somatic complaints and are excessive attenders of medical facilities. So the conundrum is that psychiatric patients both appear to be physically ill often when psychiatrically disturbed and yet bear excessive risk of physical illness. They present mainly to general practitioners and, by dint of their symptoms, also to medical specialists. As a result they are often investigated for sundry medical conditions with exposure to medical hazards, such as radiation and drug toxicity, and their *actual* psychiatric conditions may be ignored. If they are bracketed as 'psychiatric', the patience of their medical attendants may wear thin and their *actual* physical conditions may be overlooked. Thus, 'illness behaviour', 'illness proneness', and 'clustering' of physical and psychiatric disorder may well not be incompatible and it behoves the generalist to take due note.

Nevertheless, according to MacMahon's criteria (1960), the relationship between physical and mental illness is still largely descriptive and correlational rather than causal. Putative causal mechanisms are discussed in psychosomatic journals but tend to be speculative. Epidemiology, however, deals with the mass aspects of disease. Hypotheses should be tested as to whether affective disorders, particularly depression, in a longitudinal sense, cause physical illness and premature death directly or indirectly via bad habits such as dependency syndromes and general unfitness.

Behavioural science and epidemiology, so often Cinderella topics in the medical school curriculum, will, in all likelihood, provide a part of the understanding of chronic morbidity and mortality rates.

REFERENCES

Andrews, G., Schonell, M., and Tennant, C. (1977) 'The relationship between physical, psychological and social morbidity in a suburban community', *American Journal of Epidemiology* 106: 324–9.
Andrews, G., Tennant, C., Hewson, D., and Schonell, M. (1978) 'The relation of social factors to physical and psychiatric illness', *American Journal of Epidemiology* 108: 27–35.
Blacker, C.V.R. and Clare, A.W. (1987) 'Depressive disorders in primary care', *British Journal of Psychiatry* 150: 737–51.
Bridges, K.W. and Goldberg, D.P. (1985) 'Somatic presentation of DSM III psychiatric disorders in primary care', *Journal of Psychosomatic Research* 29: 563–9.
Cavanaugh, S. and Wettstein, R.M. (1984) 'Prevalence of psychiatric morbidity in medical populations', in L. Grinspoon (ed.) *Psychiatry Update: The American Psychiatric Association Annual Review, Volume III*, Washington, DC: American Psychiatric Press.
Commission on Chronic Illness (1957) *Chronic Illness in the US: Volume 1: Prevention of Chronic Illness*, Cambridge, Mass.: Harvard University Press.
Cooper, B. (1972) 'Social correlates of psychiatric illness in the community', in G. McLachlan (ed.) *Approaches to Action: A Symposium on Services for the Mentally Ill and Handicapped*, London: Oxford University Press.
Eastwood, M.R. (1971) 'Screening for psychiatric disorder', *Psychological Medicine* 1: 197–208.

Eastwood, M.R. (1975) *The Relation Between Physical and Mental Illness*, Toronto: University of Toronto Press.

Eastwood, M.R. and Corbin, S.L. (1986) 'The relationship between physical illness and depression in old age', in E. Murphy (ed.) *Affective Disorders in the Elderly*, Edinburgh: Churchill Livingstone.

Eaton, W.W. and Kessler, L.G. (eds) (1985) *Epidemiologic Field Methods in Psychiatry: The NIMH Epidemiologic Catchment Area Program*, New York: Academic Press.

Endicott, J. and Spitzer, R.C. (1978) 'A diagnostic interview: the schedule for affective disorders and schizophrenia', *Archives of General Psychiatry* 35: 837–44.

Goldberg, D.P. (1972) *The Detection of Psychiatric Illness by Questionnaire* (Maudsley Monograph No. 21), London: Oxford University Press.

Goldberg, D.P. (1974) 'Psychiatric disorders', *Lancet* 2: 1245–7.

Goldberg, D.P. (1986) 'Discussant on screening, part 2,', in M. Shepherd, G. Wilkinson, and P. Williams (eds) *Mental Illness in Primary Care Settings*, London: Tavistock.

Goldberg, D.P. and Blackwell, B. (1970) 'Psychiatric illness in general practice: a detailed study using a new method of case identification', *British Medical Journal* 2: 439–43.

Goldberg, D.P., Cooper, B., Eastwood, M.R., Kedward, H., and Shepherd, M. (1970) 'Psychiatric interview suitable for using in community surveys', *British Journal of the Society of Preventive Medicine* 24: 18–26.

Goldberg, D.P. and Huxley, P. (1980) *Mental Illness in the Community: The Pathway to Psychiatric Care*, London: Tavistock Publications.

Goldberg, D.P., Rickels, K., Downing, R., and Hesbacher, P. (1976) 'A comparison of two psychiatric screening tests', *British Journal of Psychiatry* 129: 61–7.

Hinkle, L.E. and Wolff, H.G. (1957) 'The nature of man's adaptation to his total environment and the relation of this to illness', *Archives of Internal Medicine* 99: 442–60.

Kedward, H.B. and Sylph, J. (1974) 'The social correlates of chronic neurotic disorder', *Social Psychiatry* 9: 91–8.

Kessler, L.G., Burns, B.J., Shapiro, S., Tischler, G.L., George, L.K., Hough, R.L., Bodison, D., and Miller, R.H. (1987) 'Psychiatric diagnosis of medical service users: evidence from the Epidemiologic Catchment Area Program', *American Journal of Public Health* 77: 18–24.

Lipowski, Z. (1985) *Psychosomatic Medicine and Liaison Psychiatry: Selected Papers*, New York: Plenum Medical Book Co.

Lipowski, Z. (1986) 'Somatization: a borderland between medicine and psychiatry', *Canadian Medical Association Journal* 135: 609–14.

McKeown, T. (1968) 'Validation of screening procedures', in *Screening for Medical Care* (Nuffield Provincial Hospitals Trust), London: Oxford University Press.

MacMahon, B., Pugh, T.F., and Ipsen, J. (1960) *Epidemiologic Methods*, Boston: Little, Brown.

Mayou, R. and Hawton, K. (1986) 'Psychiatric disorder in the general hospital', *British Journal of Psychiatry* 149: 172–90.

Mechanic, D. (1966) 'Response factors in illness: the study of illness behaviour', *Social Psychiatry* 1: 11–20.

Murphy, J.M., Monson, R.R., Olivier, D., Sobol, A., and Leighton, A.H. (1987) 'Affective disorders and mortality', *Archives of General Psychiatry* 44: 473–9.

Shepherd, M. (1987) 'Mental illness and primary care', *American Journal of Public Health* 77: 12–13.

Shepherd, M., Cooper, B., Brown, A.C., and Kalton, G. (1966) *Psychiatric*

Illness in General Practice, London: Oxford University Press.

South-East London Screening Study Group (1977) 'A controlled trial of multiphasic screening: results of the South-East London screening study', *International Journal of Epidemiology* 6: 257–63.

Vaillant, G.E. (1979) 'Natural history of male psychologic health: effects of mental health on physical health', *New England Journal of Medicine* 301: 1249–54.

Williams, P. (1986) 'Mental illness and primary care: screening', in M. Shepherd, G. Wilkinson, and P. Williams (eds) *Mental Illness in Primary Care Settings*, London: Tavistock.

Wilson, J.M.G. and Jungner, G. (1968) 'Principles and practice of screening for disease' (WHO Public Health Papers, No. 34), Geneva: WHO.

Wing, J.K., Birley, J.L.T., Cooper, J.E., Graham, P., and Isaacs, A.D. (1967) 'Reliability of a procedure for measuring and classifying "Present Psychiatric State"', *British Journal of Psychiatry* 113: 499–515.

Identification of Causal Factors and the Computation of Individual Morbid Risks

16

Schizophrenic Psychoses: Causal Factors and Risks

John Wing

The scientific literature on causal and risk factors in schizophrenia is now so immense that even a summary based only on studies whose design and methods are adequate by the standards of their time would run into volumes. Michael Shepherd (1987) has recommended Warner's schema (1985), modified from that of Strauss and Carpenter (1981), which lists risk factors under four headings, depending on the period during which they first operate: pre- and peri-natal, infancy and childhood, immediate pre-onset, and long-term 'career'. Each item in the four lists has its own substantial literature and, as soon as one tries to use the schema, it becomes clear that theories of pathology, causation, precipitation, and exacerbation tend to interact without respect for its categories. Nevertheless, with further modification, it is convenient for exposition.

Since much of the relevant research uses the epidemiological method, it is appropriate to begin with the two principal terms in the calculation of the rate of incidence of schizophrenia. In the numerator is placed the number of cases of schizophrenia or of some specified subgroup of it, with an onset in a given period, usually a year. In the denominator is placed the number of people in the population at risk, subdivided according to the risk factor under investigation. If proper epidemiological principles are followed, the relative risk associated with each factor can be calculated by comparing the resulting incidence (or in some cases, with great caution, the prevalence) rates. Since schizophrenia can rarely be confidently diagnosed until adolescence or adult life, estimating the effect of potential risk factors occurring in childhood requires a longitudinal design. Relative risks can also be assessed by using less demanding research designs, for example, case-control studies.

One of the chief sources of difficulty in comparing the results of research into risk factors is variation in the criteria used for diagnosis, a problem compounded by the fact that diagnostic concepts are often tied to theories of aetiology. The US-UK Diagnostic Project (Cooper et al. 1972) and the International Pilot Study of Schizophrenia (WHO 1973) demonstrated the problem and indicated one way to tackle it by using standardized techniques of data

225

collection and applying standard classifying rules (Wing *et al.* 1974). Since then, the American Psychiatric Association has accepted the need to specify the criteria for diagnosis and the third and revised third editions of its *Diagnostic and Statistical Manual*, DSM–III (1980) and DSM–IIIR (1987), have provided explicit criteria. The tenth edition of the *International Classification of Diseases* will adopt a similar approach (WHO 1987).

These rule-based systems are 'top-down', in the sense that they begin with the need to specify the criteria for each diagnosis. After prolonged negotiation between parties representing various conceptual approaches, a compromise set of rules is published that both achieves a degree of consensus and imposes a degree of uniformity on those who use it. A 'bottom-up' system begins with the phenomena, ideally with a glossary of differential definitions of symptoms and signs (Wing 1983). The item-pool can be sufficiently broadly based to allow the application of rules from a variety of classifications. If agreement on the phenomena can be obtained, diagnostic disagreement is reduced even without the application of standard rules (Cooper *et al.* 1972; Shepherd *et al.* 1968).

The 'bottom-up' approach also allows an examination of the contribution of specified symptoms or syndromes to any variation found in incidence rates. In the case of schizophrenia several such syndromes are evident, each having some claim to a partially independent status. These include: the positive syndrome, chiefly composed of symptoms regarded by Kurt Schneider as 'of the first rank', which is almost always accompanied by other psychotic phenomena; the paranoid syndrome, comprising other delusions not congruent with affect; the 'negative' syndrome of slowness, underactivity, flattening of affect, lack of motivation, poverty of quantity or content of speech and poor use of non-verbal means of communication; and thought disorder, manifested in various degrees of incoherence of speech and neologisms. It is only recently that such syndromes have been examined in their own right, as distinct from their contribution to an overall diagnosis. Other syndromes of relevance are those of the autistic spectrum (Wing, L. 1982) and motor syndromes of various kinds. Manic and severe depressive syndromes may also modify the diagnosis. Most studies exclude schizophrenia that appears in a context of recognizable cerebral disease.

Problems in comparing incidence rates arising from variations between the denominators are most clearly demonstrated in studies involving countries whose population statistics are of doubtful reliability, and where estimates of the population size and indices such as birth and death rates may be seriously inaccurate. Even in countries with well-developed population censuses, the numbers and characteristics of recently arrived migrants and of people who are not part of a well-recognized household must be estimated with caution. Prevalence rates are even more susceptible to errors in estimating the denominator since the number of active cases during any recent period of time will have accumulated over a much longer period, during which population criteria might have changed (Der and Wooff 1986).

All studies of schizophrenia that use rates must, therefore, be scrutinized carefully before use is made of the figures for comparative purposes. Rates of first admission to hospital, for example, long provided a mainstay for epidemiological research, on the fairly reasonable assumption (Ødegaard 1952) that most of those afflicted are eventually admitted. The life-time expectancy rate was regarded as stable at about one per cent. Recent trends in first admission rates, however, have shown a decrease in England (Annual Reports of Mental Health Statistics), Scotland (Eagles and Whalley 1985) and Denmark (Munk-Jørgensen 1987). Against this must be set the fact that 'first contact' rates, which cover contacts with services other than hospital wards, have shown no such decline. In Camberwell, they remained steady at about 12–15 per 100,000 population per year between 1964 and 1984 (Wing and Der 1984). In Nottingham, the rate is similar when ICD–9 criteria are used (Cooper et al. 1987). A multinational study of the incidence of schizophrenia found similar first contact rates in all the centres involved, whether in developed or developing countries (WHO 1986).

Two decades of studies, principally in Scandinavia, suggested that the lifetime risk of schizophrenia was remarkably similar at just under one per cent. Shields (1978), using Camberwell Register data, estimated it at 0.90 per cent to age 65. Nevertheless, the question of whether the rate has fluctuated over time has received far from unanimous answers and still remains unresolved (Cooper and Sartorius 1977; Goldhamer and Marshall 1953; Hare 1983; Scull 1979, 1984; Torrey 1980; Warner 1985). In former times, rates tended to be higher in the USA than in the UK (Kramer 1961), and high rates were reported in Eire, Finland, Iceland, and the Federal Republic of Germany. A consensus on lower rates may be due, in part, to the use of standardized methods of data collection and classification but the requirement, in DSM–III, for the course to be taken into account, means that even lower rates must be expected, as a recent study in Nottingham has suggested (Cooper et al. 1987). A report on schizophrenia research commissioned by the Neurosciences and Mental Health Board of the Medical Research Council suggests that a standard data base should always be collected and the rules at least of ICD–10 and DSM–IIIR applied, in addition to any local diagnostic system (MRC 1987). In the longer term, robust research results will, in turn, refine the diagnostic criteria.

In spite of these introductory reservations, a few risk factors have emerged with a degree of solidity and stability that encourages confidence and several others deserve, at the least, substantial further attention.

PRE- AND POST-NATAL RISK FACTORS

The risk factor most securely associated with schizophrenia is genetic. The disorder, whether broadly or narrowly defined, occurs more commonly among the first degree relatives of those afflicted than in control groups or the general population. It is more frequent in the adopted-away children of schizophrenic mothers than in other adoptees. And in twins, if one member of a pair has schizophrenia the other is two or three times more likely to be similarly affected when the twins are monozygotic than when they are dizygotic. (For a review of the complexities associated with these simple facts, see Part III of the volume edited by Häfner, Gattaz and Janzarik, published in 1987, and the MRC report referred to above.)

Increased risks of this order do not suggest straightforward mechanisms of inheritance. Only about a fifth of sufferers have a close relative with the disorder and the concordance in identical twins falls well short of the total agreement needed for full genetic determination. There have been many attempts, both in purely genetic and in a combination of genetic and environmental terms, to unravel the mystery. (For the moment, *purely* environmental theories are in disorderly retreat.) The most prominent of the competing theories are: (a) that there are inherited and non-inherited forms of schizophrenia, (b) that the genetic contribution (or contributions, since more than one gene may be involved) determines a predisposition which can become manifest following environmental insults of various kinds, and (c) that some or all of the various schizophrenia syndromes have their own particular risk factors. These ideas are not mutually exclusive.

A second pre-natally determined risk factor is sex, which is most conveniently discussed in terms of age of onset. While the lifetime risk has been shown to be approximately equal in most studies, it has long been observed that the onset is earlier in men than in women (Noreik and Ødegaard 1967; Lindelius 1970; Watt, Katz and Shepherd 1983; Wing and Fryers 1976). It is well known that communication disorders of many varieties, including aphasia, dyslexia, and disorders in the autistic spectrum, are commoner at birth in boys than girls. With rare exceptions, however, schizophrenia is not manifested frankly until after puberty. Nevertheless, the possibility that it is also a developmental disorder, with possible 'premorbid' or subclinical manifestations, must be considered. This would be true whether risk factors that were not genetic in nature had or had not contributed during the pre-natal period. In fact there is evidence that what Pasamanick called 'the continuum of reproductive casualty' includes, as one of its possible consequences, schizophrenia developing later in life.

The most consistent part of the evidence concerns season of birth. The excess of winter births in both hemispheres of the world, though small, can hardly be a matter of chance. A critical review of more than twenty studies, carried out in fourteen countries, suggested that the results were not artefacts of methodology or design but could best be explained as due to brain damage by a seasonal risk factor such as viral infection, nutritional deficiency, or perinatal complication. Moreover, affected individuals were likely to have an early onset, less genetic loading, and better prognoses (Boyd *et al*. 1986). Mednick and colleagues (1987) refer to a follow-up study of young adults who had been at the second trimester of foetal development during the serious A2 influenza virus epidemic in Copenhagen in October/November 1957. They had a higher rate of admission with a diagnosis of schizophrenia compared with controls.

The recent reporting of high rates of schizophrenia in patients admitted to hospital for the first time, or making first-ever contact with psychiatric services, among Afro-Caribbean residents in the UK, raises a further question as to whether environmental risk factors are responsible. Not only is the incidence three or more times greater in those born in the West Indies than in native-born residents (Dean *et al*. 1981; Harrison *et al*. 1988), but it appears to be substantially higher still among the second generation, who were born in the UK (Harrison *et al*. 1987). Studies of early childhood autism in immigrant populations suggest that viral infection during an immigrant mother's pregnancy, while she has not developed antibodies, or some other environmental insult, might explain the excess in immigrant groups (Akinsola and Fryers 1986; Gillberg *et al*. 1987; Wing, L. 1979).

Genetic studies of schizophrenia have not been carried out as thoroughly, or to the same extent, in Third World compared with developed countries. The similar incidence across countries reported in the latest WHO report, mentioned earlier, does not eliminate genetic variations because there could be a differential incidence of subtypes. However, there is little evidence of variation due to 'ethnicity'. The apparently better course in developing countries (see below) could be interpreted as due to a higher proportion of environmentally precipitated acute schizophrenias, appearing without long-term 'personality' precursors, although there is little systematic evidence one way or the other. The very high risk in children of first-generation immigrants would then require explanation; consideration being given to the risk factors, including infection, occuring perinatally, as well as during later life.

McNeil and Kaij (1978), in a thorough review of the risks of obstetric complications, investigated using a variety of designs and methods, concluded that they 'are a risk-increasing factor to be taken seriously in the etiology of schizophrenia'. Murray and colleagues have linked this conclusion to the fact that nearly all studies that have collected data on the presence or absence of peri-natal abnormalities in those who subsequently developed schizophrenia and had CT scans performed showed that early hazards were significantly associated with increased ventricular size in adulthood. Moreover, the relationship was particularly noticeable in those without a family history of schizophrenia (Murray *et al*. 1987).

229

RISK FACTORS DURING CHILDHOOD

Genetic, intra-uterine, and perinatal risk factors, if present, combine to form a predisposition to schizophrenia that may or may not be sufficient for its later manifestation. Other risk factors may operate during childhood to increase this vulnerability. For example, a substantial literature has accumulated around the subject of parental rearing patterns. Empirical tests of hypotheses derived from such theories have been more than usually plagued by poor design and methodology and have rarely, in fact, been concerned directly with parent-infant interaction and its subsequent effects in adulthood. Such evidence as exists, derived mainly from studies of communication patterns in the parents of adult offspring diagnosed schizophrenic (Singer et al. 1978), is unconvincing. One of the most obvious problems, diagnosis (Rutter 1978; Hirsch and Leff 1975), is illustrated by data from a current longitudinal study (Wynne et al. 1987) in which, of sixty-three index parents diagnosed as schizophrenic according to DSM–II (much used in earlier research), only eighteeen were so diagnosed according to DSM–III. At the moment, there is little evidence to suggest that the parents of those who later develop schizophrenia have any specific characteristics, other than genetic, that constitute additional risk factors.

More general factors in child-rearing must also be considered. If relevant, they should show up in studies of adopted-away children of mothers afflicted by schizophrenia. A research project with this design, not yet completed, is being carried out by Tienari and colleagues (1987), who have examined all such offspring born in Finland in the years 1928 to 1979, together with matched controls. Preliminary results suggest an interaction between genetic and environmental factors, in that schizophrenia appears more frequently in children with a genetic loading but is also concentrated and more severe in the most disturbed adoptive families. The latest results from the Copenhagen high-risk project (Mednick et al. 1987), which began with a cohort of adolescents, one or both of whose parents had suffered from schizophrenia, also point to an interaction between genetic, perinatal, and environmental factors in probands compared to controls.

Since criteria for schizotypal personality disorder were laid down in DSM–III, several studies have been undertaken to determine their relationship to schizophrenia. Kendler (1981, 1987) has argued that the criteria can be divided into two groups: one closer to the negative symptoms of schizophrenia (social isolation, odd speech, aloofness, and suspicion), one closer to the positive (magical thinking, ideas of reference and recurrent illusions). Whether the DSM–III items are well chosen, and whether Kendler's division of them makes clinical sense, is not here the point. The 'negative' items are said to be commoner among the biological relatives of people with schizophrenia, but so (Kendler and Gruenberg 1982) is paranoid personality disorder. Whether any of the three predict the later manifestation of schizophrenia is a moot point.

230

Schizophrenic and paranoid psychoses can begin during childhood, usually in the immediately pre-pubertal years. The symptoms are typical except for the obvious pathoplastic effects of age. There should be no confusion with psychoses having an onset in early childhood, usually on the basis of a global language disorder (Ricks and Wing 1975), since the symptoms of the latter are quite distinct, the children do not develop schizophrenic psychoses in later life, and there is no increase in the frequency of schizophrenia in first-degree relatives (Kolvin 1971; Wing, L. 1982). One other possible confusing condition (in fact, a variant of early childhood autism) is Asperger's syndrome (Asperger 1944, 1968; Wing, L. 1981). Like Kanner's syndrome, it has often been misdiagnosed as schizophrenia, and may account for a proportion of the cases labelled as 'simple schizophrenia' or schizoid personality.

Retrospective studies of the childhood years of those who have already developed schizophrenia tend to show a higher frequency of disturbed or withdrawn behaviour compared with controls (Robins 1970; Bower *et al* 1960; Watt 1978). As part of any predisposition manifested in personality disorder such as 'schizotypy' (DSM–III). or schizoid personality (ICD–10), the clinical observation that people presenting with frank schizophrenia for the first time have often become withdrawn and odd over quite long periods, sometimes reaching back into childhood, suggests that cognitive abnormalities may already have been present. Such results as are available indicate a global intellectual deficit (though verbal skills are better preserved than non-verbal) before clinical onset in a proportion of cases, usually correlated with a poor prognosis (Lane and Albee 1965; Offord 1974; Watt and Lubensky 1976). The IPSS two-year follow-up (WHO 1979) indicated that socially isolated or underperforming patients had the worst outcome. In general, negative impairments manifested before clinical onset are the best predictors of later outcome (Wing 1987 and in press).

Such considerations suggest that a proportion of those who later become frankly schizophrenic are likely to show a range of other characteristics: single status, poor employment record, domicile in a socially isolated area, recent migration, and relative poverty. This will particularly be true of males. These results of classical epidemiology are well known and properly attributed mainly to 'drift' rather than to causal factors (Cooper 1978). (The study by Dunham in Detroit, published in 1965, is a useful reference, since he had earlier been associated with a causal hypothesis.) There is, however, a further consideration. A high intelligence, a helpful and supportive family and educational background, occupational skills that are in demand, an economic environment that provides plenty of opportunities for employment, a society that is not highly competitive – these and other factors may protect against the development of schizophrenia even in someone who is already at higher than average risk (Warner 1985). On the other hand, as Cooper (1961) pointed out, someone who is deprived of such benefits is likely to become more vulnerable: an example of disability amplification operating long before clinical presentation.

THE IMMEDIATE PRECURSORS OF ACUTE 'POSITIVE' EPISODES

The positive syndrome of schizophrenia is more dramatic and publicly visible than the negative, or than any pre-clinical manifestations of eccentricity or social withdrawal. In a proportion of cases the clinical onset is, or appears to be, relatively sudden. Putative precipitating factors are more likely to have been present in such cases. (They are nearly always determined retrospectively.) An acute schizophrenic syndrome can follow the misuse of amphetamine, and 'alcoholic hallucinosis' is a well-known diagnosis, although not represented as such in ICD–10. The account of Evelyn Waugh's own experience, in *The Ordeal of Gilbert Pinfold*, puts it down to over-indulgence in port and potassium bromide, the tranquillisers of the time, in addition to family, religious, and occupational problems. Such disorders may be accompanied by disorientation in minor degree. They usually clear up fairly quickly and rarely follow a chronic course with a negative impairment. Schizophrenic symptoms accompanying cerebral disease such as temporal lobe epilepsy are also well documented.

Such cases account for only a small proportion of acute onsets. Commoner environmental precipitants are psychosocial in nature. One of the first to be demonstrated was iatrogenic, relapse after years without positive symptoms of long-stay patients suddenly exposed to unrealistic expectations of social performance during a course of rehabilitation, followed by recovery (to the previous level of functioning) when sheltered conditions were reinstated (Stone and Eldred 1959; Goldberg *et al.* 1977; Wing *et al.* 1964: Wing, L *et al.*, 1972).

Since then, attention has focused chiefly on other 'life events', usually adverse and stressful, that put stress upon an individual (Brown and Birley 1968; Steinberg and Durrell 1968). There is no suggestion that such events are in any way specific in their effect; they operate through an existing vulnerability. The most recent replication of such a result was in six of seven centres taking part in a WHO collaborative study (Leff 1987). However, Dohrenwend and colleagues (1987) and Tennant (1985) are cautious in their assessment of the significance of the effects. Certainly, there is a paucity of properly conducted studies and a failure to distinguish clearly between precipitation of first florid onset and precipitation of florid relapse as part of a chronic course. The problem of the course criterion indroduced into DSM–III also complicates intepretation of the many studies carried out using its rules and exacerbates the difficulty of defining 'onset'. The status of 'stress' as a risk factor for the onset of schizophrenia remains uncertain. Much of the evidence so far concerns course rather than first onset (Wing 1986).

A third non-specific factor that has attracted considerable attention has become reified under the label 'emotional expression' (EE), although the concept is wider than that (Brown *et al.* 1962; Brown *et al.* 1972; Vaughn and Leff 1976). High EE does not occur in all relatives and it does occur in the relatives of people with many other (including physical) diseases. Leff (1987) has recently discussed the interactions between life events, EE, and prophylactic medication as they affect the course of schizophrenia. The first evidence that intervention based on such theories can improve the course has been provided by Leff and colleagues (1985). All three environmental factors, unrealistic expectations, life events, and EE, can be summed up as environmental intrusions on people whose capacities for social communication are impaired, whether by 'premorbid' factors or as part of the clinical condition. It is somewhat artificial to theorize about them in isolation from each other. Each has a supportive as well as a toxic aspect. Low EE relatives, for example, seem to exert a beneficial influence.

FACTORS INFLUENCING THE COURSE AND OUTCOME OF SCHIZOPHRENIA

Manfred Bleuler (1978) has suggested that about 25 per cent of patients in a first episode of schizophrenia are likely to have a good outcome after about five years. About 10 per cent never improve. These two proportions have not, he thinks, changed much during his long lifetime. Between the two extremes, the outcome depends quite substantially, in his view, on the influence for good or ill of environmental factors. Some of these, for example the precipitants of acute episodes, and the protective effects of medication and social support, have been considered earlier. Others, such as factors that influence the severity of the negative impairment, are usually considered in the context of the long-term course, although there is no obvious reason why they should not operate at any time, including before clinical onset, if an underlying vulnerability is present.

The environmental factors likely to increase negative impairment are social under-stimulation (Wing and Brown 1970; Wing and Freudenberg 1961) and over-medication. It has been argued, therefore, that people with chronic schizophrenia have to walk a tightrope, balanced between twin dangers; unrealistic expectation on one side and a strong temptation to withdraw from efforts at social adjustment on the other. These dangers arise from a common source. A reduced ability to communicate freely with others, which is 'intrinsic' in the sense of being based in biological impairments, depends (if it is not so severe as to be incapacitating), as much on his or her lifestyle and self-attitudes, and on the toxicity or benevolence of the environment, as it does on the intrinsic deficits (Wing, 1975, 1977, 1987b).

These arguments suggest that the more favourable course of schizophrenia found in developing countries (Murphy and Raman 1971; WHO 1979), if not due to the predominance of a relatively benign subtype, differential mortality, etc., may be found to be associated with a less 'stressful' environment. Some preliminary evidence concerning the family environment already suggests this (Leff *et al.* 1987).

CONCLUDING COMMENT

This very broad and brief summary of risk factors in schizophrenia began with a discussion of the daunting methodological problems that must be overcome if the results of risk research are to be taken as seriously as those of genetics. One or more of these problems, notably diagnosis, the calculation of rates, the selection of case controls, and the conduct of longitudinal surveys, is likely to prove a substantial obstacle so far as comparison between the results of different studies is concerned.

The classification of risks as though they operate in a cumulative hierarchy, from conception to death in old age, is misleading. Most factors, apart from those operating at conception or during the period of maturation of the nervous system, could exert their effects at any period. Theories of interactive causation need not recognize such artificial boundaries. Although it is sometimes dispiriting, when trying to review the enormous literature on risk factors, to note how frequently theories come into favour, then disfavour, with possible repetitions of the cycle, often in association with the advocacy of different 'product champions', several lines of real progress are discernible.

The idea that a few interlinked pathologies underlie the phenomena of schizophrenia, leading to vulnerability to a variety of environmental risk factors, remains highly plausible and eminently suited to the opportunities for interactive host-and-environment research presented by the new non-invasive methods of investigating brain structure and function. It is important to remember, however, that the eventual end-point of such investigations is to develop better theories of how such physical mechanisms can produce symptoms that take the form both of abnormal subjective experiences and of abnormalities of behaviour, each of which can be modified through environmental action. The relationship between the positive and the negative syndromes remains at the heart of the mystery.

REFERENCES

Akinsola, H.A. and Fryers, T. (1986) 'A comparison of patterns of disability in severely mental handicapped children of different ethnic origins', *Psychological Medicine* 16: 127–33.

American Psychiatric Association (1980) *Diagnostic and Statistical Manual of Mental Disorders*, third edition, Washington, DC: APA.

American Psychiatric Association (1987) *Diagnostic and Statistical Manual of Mental Disorders*, third edition, revised, Washington, DC: APA.

Asperger, H. (1944) 'Die autistischen Psychopathen im Kindesalter', *Archiv für Psychiatrie und Nervenkrankheiten.* 117: 76–137.

Asperger, H. (1968) 'Zur Differentialdiagnose des kindlichen Autismus', *Acta Paedopsychiatrica* 35: 136–45.

Bleuler, M. (1978) *The Schizophrenic Disorders: Long-term Patient and Family Studies*, translated by S.M. Clemens, New Haven: Yale University Press.

Bower, E., Shellhamer, T., and Daily, J. (1960) 'School characteristics of male adolescents who later became schizophrenic', *American Journal of Orthopsychiatry* 30: 712–29.

Boyd, J.H., Pulver, A.E., and Steward, W. (1986) 'Season of birth: schizophrenia and bipolar disorder', *Schizophrenia Bulletin* 12: 173–86.

Brown, G.W. and Birley, J.L.T. (1968) 'Crisis and life changes and the onset of schizophrenia', *Health and Social Behaviour* 9: 203–14.

Brown, G.W., Birley, J.L.T., and Wing, J.K. (1972) 'Influence of family life on the course of schizophrenic disorders: a replication', *British Journal of Psychiatry* 121: 241–58.

Brown, G.W., Monck. E., Carstairs, G.M., and Wing, J.K. (1962) 'Influence of family life on the course of schizophrenic disorders', *British Journal of Preventive and Social Medicine* 16: 55–68.

Cooper, B. (1961) 'Social class and prognosis in schizophrenia', *British Journal of Preventive and Social Medicine* 15: 17–41.

Cooper, B. (1978) 'Epidemiology' in J.K. Wing (ed.) *Schizophrenia: Towards a New Synthesis*, London, Academic Press.

Cooper, J.E., Goodhead, D., Craig, T., Harris, M., Howat, J., and Korer, J. (1987) 'The incidence of schizophrenia in Nottingham', *British Journal of Psychiatry* 151: 619–26.

Cooper, J.E., Kendell R.E., Gurland, B.J., Sharpe, L., Copeland, J.R.M., and Simon, R. (1972) *Psychiatric Diagnosis in New York and London. A comprehensive study of mental hospital admissions. Maudsley Monograph No. 20*, London: Oxford University Press.

Cooper, J.E. and Sartorius, N. (1977) 'Cultural and temporal variations in schizophrenia: a speculation on the importance of industrialisation', *British Journal of Psychiatry* 130: 50–5.

Crow, T.J. (1985) 'The two syndrome concept: origins and current status', *Schizophrenia Bulletin* 11: 471–86.

Dean, G., Walsh, D., Downing, H., and Shelley, E. (1981) 'First admissions of native-born and immigrants to psychiatric hospitals in south-east England, 1971', *British Journal of Psychiatry* 139: 506–12.

Der, G. (1987) 'The effect of population changes on long-stay in-patient rates', in J.K. Wing (eds.) *Contributions to Health Service Planning and Research*, London; DHSS.

Der, G. and Wooff, K. (1986) in G.H. ten Horn, R. Giel, W.H. Gulbinat, and J.H. Henderson (eds) *Psychiatric Case Registers in Public Health*, Amsterdam: Elsevire, pp. 338–42.

Dohrenwend, B.P., Shrout, O.E., Link, B.G., and Skodoe, A.E. (1987) 'Social and psychological risk factors for episodes of schizophrenia', in H. Häfner, W.F. Gattaz, and W. Janzarik (eds) *Search for the Causes of Schizophrenia*, Heidelberg: Springer-Verlag, pp. 275–96.

235

Dunham, W.H. (1965) *Community and Schizophrenia: An Epidemiological Analysis*, Detroit: Wayne State University Press.

Eagles, J.M. and Whalley, L.J. (1985) 'Decline in the diagnosis of schizophrenia among first admissions to Scottish mental hospitals from 1969–78' *British Journal of Psychiatry* 146: 151–4.

Frith, C.D. (1987) 'The positive and negative symptoms of schizophrenia reflect impairments in the perception and initiation of action', *Psychological Medicine* 17: 631–8.

Gillberg, C., Steffenburg, S., Börjesson, B., and Anderson, L. (1987) 'Infantile autism in children of immigrant parents: a population based study from Göteborg', *British Journal of Psychiatry* 150: 856–8.

Goldberg, S.C., Schooler, N.R., Hogarty, G.E., and Roper, M. (1977) 'Prediction of relapse in schizophrenic patients treated by drug and sociotherapy', *Archives of General Psychiatry* 34: 171–84.

Goldhamer, H. and Marshall, A. (1953) *Psychosis and Civilisation*, Glencoe Ill.: Free Press.

Häfner, H., Gattaz, W.F. and Janzarik, W. (eds) (1987) *Search for the Causes of Schizophrenia*, Heidelberg: Springer-Verlag.

Hare, E.H. (1983) 'Was insanity on the increase?' *British Journal of Psychiatry* 142: 439–55.

Harrison, G., Owens, D., Holton, A., Neilson, D., and Best, D. (1988) 'A prospective study of severe mental disorder in Afro-Caribbean patients', to be published.

Hirsch, S.R. and Leff, J.P. (1975) *Abnormalities in Parents of Schizophrenics: A Review of the Literature and an Investigation of Communication Defects and Deviances*, London: Oxford University Press.

Kendler, K.S. (1987) 'Diagnostic approaches to schizotypal personality disorder: an historical perspective', *Schizophrenia Bulletin* 11: 538–53.

Kendler, K.S. and Gruenberg, E.M. (1982) 'Genetic relationship between paranoid personality and the "schizophrenic spectrum" disorders', *American Journal of Psychiatry* 139: 1185–6..

Kendler, K.S., Gruenberg, E.M., and Strauss, J.J. (1981) 'An independent analysis of the Copenhagen sample of the Danish Adoption Study of Schizophrenia: II: the relationship between schizotypal personality disorder and schizophrenia', *Archives of General Pscyhiatry* 38: 982–4.

Kolvin, I. (1971) 'Studies in the childhood psychoses: I: Diagnostic criteria and classification', *British Journal of Psychiatry* 118: 381–4.

Kramer, M. (1961) 'Some problems for international research suggested by observations on differences in first admission rates to the mental hospitals of England and Wales and of the United States', in *Proceedings of the Third World Congress of Psychiatry*, volume three, 153–60.

Lane, E. and Albee, G. (1965) 'Childhood intellectual differences between schizophrenic adults and their siblings', *American Journal of Orthopsychiatry* 35: 747–53.

Leff, J. (1987) 'A model of schizophrenic vulnerability to environmental factors', in H. Häfner, W.F. Gattaz, and W. Janarik (eds) *Search for the Causes of Schizophrenia*, Heidelberg: Springer-Verlag, 317–30.

Leff, J., Wig, N., Ghosh, A., Bedi, H., Menon, D.K., Kuipers, L., Korten, A., Ernberg, G., Day, R., Sartorius, N., and Jablensky, A. (1987) 'Influence of relatives' expressed emotion on the course of schizophrenia in Chandigarh', no. 3, *British Journal of Psychiatry* 151: 166–73.

Leff, J., Kuipers, L., Berkowitz, R., and Sturgeon, D. (1985) 'A controlled trial of social intervention in the families of schizophrenic patients: two-year follow-up', *British Journal of Psychiatry* 146: 594–600.

Lindelius, R. (1970) 'A study of schizophrenia', *Acta Psychiatria Scandinavia*, Supplement 216.

McNeil, T.F. and Kaij, L. (1978) 'Obstetric factors in the development of schizophrenia', in L.C. Wynne, R.L. Cromwell, and S. Matthysse (eds) *The Nature of Schizophrenia*, New York: Wiley, 401–29.

Medical Research Council (1987) *Research into Schizophrenia* (Report of the Schizophrenia and Allied Conditions Committee), London: MRC.

Mednick, S.A., Parnas, J., and Schulsinger, F. (1987) 'The Copenhagen High-Risk Project, 1962–86', *Schizophrenic Bulletin* 13: 485–95.

Munk-Jørgensen, P. (1987) 'Why has the incidence of schizophrenia in Danish psychiatric institutions decreased since 1970?' *Acta Psychiatrica Scandinavia* 75: 62–8.

Murphy, H.B.M. and Raman, A.C. (1971) 'The chronicity of schizophrenia in indigenous tropical peoples', *British Journal of Psychiatry* 117: 489–97.

Murray, R.M., Lewis, S.W., Owen, M.J., and Forster, A. (in press) 'The neurodevelopmental origins of dementia praecox', in P. McGuffin and P. Bebbington (eds) *Schizophrenia: The Major Issues*, London: Heinemann.

Noreik, K. and Ødegaard, Ø. (1967) 'Age of onset of schizophrenia in relation to socio-economic factors', *British Journal of Psychiatry* 1: 243–9.

Offord, D. (1974) 'School performance of adult schizophrenics, their siblings and age mates', *British Journal of Psychiatry* 125: 12–19.

Ricks, D.M. and Wing, L. (1975) 'Language, communication and the use of symbols in normal and autistic children' *Journal of Autism and Childhood Schizophrenia* 5: 191–221.

Robins, L.N. (1970) 'Follow-up studies investigating childhood disorders', in E.H. Hare and J.K. Wing (eds) *Psychiatric Epidemiology*, London: Oxford University Press.

Rutter, M. (1978) 'Communication deviance and diagnostic differences', in L.C. Wynne, R.L. Cromwell, and S. Matthysse (eds) *The Nature of Schizophrenia*, New York: Wiley.

Scull, A. (1979) *Museums of Madness: The Social Organization of Insanity in Nineteenth Century England*, London: Allen Lane.

Scull, A. (1984) 'Was insanity increasing? a response to Edward Hare', *British Journal of Psychiatry* 144: 432–6.

Shepherd, M. (1987) 'Formulation of new research strategies on schizophrenia', in H. Häfner, W.F. Gattaz, and W. Janzarik (eds) *Search for the Causes of Schizophrenia*, Heidelberg: Springer-Verlag.

Shepherd, M., Brooke, E.M., Cooper, J.E., and Lin, T.Y. (1968) 'An experimental approach to psychiatric diagnosis', *Acta Psychiatrica Scandinavica*, Supplement 201, Copenhagen: Munksgaard.

Shields, J. (1978) 'Genetics of schizophrenia', in J.K. Wing (ed.) *Schizophrenia: Towards a New Synthesis*, London: Academic Press, 56.

Singer, M.T., Wynne, L.C., and Toohey, M.L. (1978) 'Communication disorders and the families of schizophrenics', in L.C. Wynne, R.L. Cromwell, and S. Matthhysse (eds) *The Nature of Schizophrenia*, New York: Wiley.

Steinberg, H.R. and Durell, J. (1968) 'A stressful social situation as a precipitant of schizophrenic symptoms: an epidemiological study', *British Journal of Psychiatry* 114: 1097–105.

Stone, A.A. and Eldred, S.H. (1959) 'Delusion formation during the activation of chronic schizophrenic patients', *Archives of General Psychiatry* 1: 177–9.

Strauss, J.S. and Carpenter, W.T. (1981) *Schizophrenia*, New York: Plenum, chapter 2.

Tennant, C.C. (1985) 'Stress and schizophrenia: a review', *Integrative Psychiatry* 3: 248–61.

Tienarie, P., Sorri, A, Lahti, I., Naerala, M., Wahlberg, K., Moring, J., Pohjola, J., and Wynne, L.C. (1987) 'Genetic and psychosocial factors in schizophrenia: the Finnish Adoptive Family Study', *Schizophrenia Bulletin* 13: 477–95.

Torrey, E.F. (1980) *Schizophrenia and Civilisation*, New York: Aronson.

Vaughn, C. and Leff, J.P. (1976) 'The influence of family and social factors on the course of psychiatric illness', *British Journal of Psychiatry* 129: 125–37.

Watt, D.C., Katz, K., and Shepherd, M. (1983) 'The natural history of schizophrenia: a five-year prospective follow-up of a representative sample of schizophrenics by means of a standardized clinical and social assessment', *Psychological Medicine* 13: 663–70.

Watt, N.F. (1978) 'Patterns of childhood social development in adult schizophrenics', *Archives of General Psychiatry* 35: 160–5.

Watt, N. and Lubensky, A. (1976) 'Childhood roots of schizophrenia', *Journal of Consulting and Clinical Psychology* 44: 363–75.

Warner, R. (1985) *Recovery from Schizophrenia: Psychiatry and Political Economy*, London: Routledge & Kegan Paul, 24.

Wig, N., Menon, D.K., Bedi, H., Ghosh, A., Kuipers, L., Leff, J.P., Korten, A., Day, R., Sartorius, N., Eernberg, G., and Jablensky, A. (1987) 'Expressed emotion and schizophrenia in North India: I: the cross-cultural transfer of ratings and relatives' expressed emotion', *British Journal of Psychiatry* 151: 156–73.

Wing, J.K. (1975) 'Impairments in schizophrenia: a rational basis for social treatment', in R.D. Wirt, G. Winokur, and M. Roff (eds) *Life History Research in Psychopathology, Volume 4*, Minneapolis: University of Minnesota Press.

Wing, J.K. (1977) 'The management of schizophrenia in the community', in G. Usdin (ed.) *Psychiatric Medicine*, New York: Brunner Mazel.

Wing, J.K. (1983) 'Use and misuse of the PSE', *British Journal of Psychiatry* 143: 111–17.

Wing, J.K. (1986) 'Commentary on "Stress and Schizophrenia" by C.C. Tennant', *Integrative Psychiatry* 4: 57–8.

Wing, J.K. (1987) 'Has the outcome of schizophrenia changed?' in T.J. Crow (ed.) 'Recurrent and Chronic Psychoses', *British Medical Bulletin* 43: 741–53.

Wing, J.K. (1987) 'Long-term adaptation in schizophrenia', in N.E. Miller, and G.D. Cohen (eds) *Schizophrenia and Aging*, New York: Guilford Press, 183–6.

Wing, J.K. (in press) 'The nature of negative symptoms', in T. Barnes (ed.) *Negative Symptoms in Schizophrenia*, London: Gaskell Press.

Wing, J.K., Bennett, D.H., and Denham, J. (1964) *The Industrial Rehabilitation of Long-Stay Schizophrenic Patients* (Medical Research Council Memorandum No. 42), London: HMSO.

Wing, J.K., and Brown, G.W. (1970) *Institutionalism and Schizophrenia*, London: Cambridge University Press.

Wing, J.K., Cooper, J.E., and Sartorius, N. (1974) *The Description and Classification of Psychiatric Symptoms: An Instruction Manual for the PSE and CATEGO System*, London: Cambridge University Press.

Wing, J.K., and Der. G. (1984) 'Report of the Camberwell Psychiatric Register, 1964–1984', Medical Research Council Social Psychiatry Unit, mimeo.

Wing, J.K., and Freudenberg, R.K. (1961) 'The response of severely ill chronic schizophrenic patients to social stimulation', *American Journal of Psychiatry* 118: 311.

Wing, J.K., and Fryers, T. (1976) *Psychiatric Services in Camberwell and Salford, 1964–1975*, London: MRC Social Psychiatry Unit.

Wing, L. (1979) 'Mentally retarded children in Camberwell', in H. Häfner (ed.) *Estimating Needs for Mental Health Care*, Heidelberg: Springer-Verlag.

Wing, L. (1981) 'Asperger's syndrome', *Psychological Medicine* 11: 115–29.

Wing, L. (1982), chapters 29, 30, and 34, in J.K. Wing and L. Wing (eds) *Psychoses of Uncertain Aetiology*, Cambridge: Cambridge University Press.

Wing, L., Wing, J.K., Griffiths, D., and Stevens, B. (1972) 'An epidemiological and experimental evaluation of industrial rehabilitation of chronic psychotic patients in the community', in J.K. Wing and A.M. Hailey (eds) *Evaluating a Community Psychiatric Service*, London: Oxford University Press, 283–308.

World Health Organization (1973) *The International Pilot Study of Schizophrenia*, Geneva: WHO.

World Health Organization (1979) *Schizophrenia: An International Follow-up Study*, New York: Wiley.

World Health Organization (1986) 'Early manifestations and first-contact incidence of schizophrenia in different cultures: a preliminary report', *Psychological Medicine*, 16: 909–28.

World Health Organization (1987), chapter five on 'Mental, behavioural and development disorders, FOO–99', in *ICD-10 Research Diagnostic Criteria*, Geneva: WHO.

Wynne, L.C., Cole, R.E., and Perkins, P. (1987) 'University of Rochester Child and Family Study: risk research in progress', *Schizophrenia Bulletin*, 13: 463–76.

17

Psychosocial Adversity and Impaired Growth in Children: In Search of Causal Mechanisms

David Skuse

In 1976 the Committee on Child Health Services, chaired by Professor Donald Court, reported to the Secretaries of State (DHSS 1976). Three years of 'unremitting enquiry' had led, *inter alia*, to the conclusion that a significant correlation between social class and the prevalence of ill-health and disability among children persisted in our society. The effect of the environment could also be seen in growth. The Committee commented (p. 50) 'short stature can be normal; it can also be a disease of the social environment and an important pointer to a group of socially deprived children'. These comments are echoed in the recent report *Investing in the Future*, produced by the Policy and Practice Review Group at the National Children's Bureau (NCB 1987).

The key phrase 'an adverse family and social environment can retard physical . . . growth' (p. 50) begs the question 'How?' What are the mechanisms by which social disadvantage results in stunted children in a relatively prosperous, developed society such as our own? If there is to be provision of assistance to those in the community whose children are at risk, what form of intervention is most likely to be effective in ameliorating the consequences of that social deprivation?

The aim of this contribution is, first, to discuss the evidence that there is an undoubted association between certain indices of social deprivation and the impaired growth of many children raised in those conditions; second, to review critically the evidence for some of the mechanisms that have been proposed, emphasizing the often contradictory nature of that evidence; third, to propose a unifying hypothesis about the mechanisms by which 'psychosocial adversity' may affect growth and development, drawing upon findings from work of myself and colleagues with deprived families living in conditions of socio-economic disadvantage in the inner city. Emphasis will be placed upon the use of epidemiological research designs to generate hypotheses about causal mechanisms, which may then be tested in complementary case-control studies.

I propose to examine the association between 'poor home conditions' or 'psychosocial adversity' and short stature by discussing briefly genetic influences on growth, then certain broad environmental variables, such as social class, which are known to differentiate children with retarded growth from those who are fulfilling their genetic potential. Finally, I shall consider a number of specific mechanisms by which these broad environmental variables may exert their effect.

GENETIC INFLUENCES ON GROWTH

The correlation between parent and child heights increases during the first two years of the child's life, and then changes little until puberty. During adolescence the correlation decreases, corresponding to differences between children in the timing of the adolescent growth spurt – but eventually the correlation reaches levels slightly above the prepubertal values. Values of 0.5 to 0.6 are usually found for sample sizes above 500 pairs. The question arises, to what extent do such correlations result from genetic influences, and to what extent do they reflect a common environment or assortative mating?

This is a complex issue, and one which is not answered by an observation such as the fact that parent-child correlations (mother's, father's, and mid-parental height correlated with child's height at 5–11 years) are on the whole very similar across all social classes in England and Scotland (Rona 1981). The interesting question here remains unanswered; viz, are the correlations higher when the two generations remain in the same social class, and are they lower when there has been upward or downward movement between generations?

A normal curve of distribution of a quantitative character in a population may be generated entirely by its genetic determination. Normally, however, the total phenotypic variance is divided into a) additive polygenic effects; b) environmental effects; c) other sources (Roberts 1985). The additive genetic contribution expressed as a proportion of the total variance is the hereditability: a variable that may be estimated in a number of different ways. Genetic analyses of adult height are complicated because, besides being subject to environmental variation, stature changes with age and differs between the sexes. Furthermore, in European populations parent-child correlations may reflect an appreciable degree of assortative mating, which in a recent British survey (Mascie-Taylor 1987) was found to be largely *independent* of age or social and regional background, being related more closely to stature. That is rather a surprising finding, for there is certainly a tendency for people to marry those similar to themselves in terms of educational and social background, a major part also being played by geographical propinquity.

Both environmental and genetic hypotheses have been advanced to explain secular trends (Martorell 1985). For example, that they reflect an improved standard of living, especially in nutrition and sanitation. Also, that a potential contributory factor is genetic heterosis, or hybrid vigour, resulting from the breakdown of breeding isolation brought about by increased social and geographical mobility. Whatever the explanation, ultimately, secular changes in growth must depend upon systematic phenotypic deviation in the stature of offspring from their parents, and trends towards greater adult height in new generations must result from the fact that children outgrow their like-sexed parent (Bielicki 1986).

ENVIRONMENTAL INFLUENCES

Social class

Since the Second World War there have been numerous large-scale epidemiological surveys on the effect of the socio-cultural environment in England and Scotland upon child development (e.g. the National Study of Health and Growth, Rona *et al.* 1978; and the Preschool Child Survey, Fox *et al.* 1981). The NSHG was set up to provide surveillance of primary schoolchildren, concentrating on height as the main measure of nutritional status.

Analysis of data on the 1946 birth cohort (comprising children born in the UK during one week, see Douglas and Simpson 1964) revealed that the difference in the height of infants between the two extremes of the social-class distribution was 2 cm by the age of 2 years. This finding was confirmed by the later NSHG survey and various other surveys, both national and regional, have reported similar values (e.g. Fox *et al.* 1981). There has been almost no change in the last thirty years in terms of the relative differences between the most and least advantaged (top and bottom) social groups in the United Kingdom. However, the proportion of the population in the lowest social class (V – unskilled manual workers) is decreasing.

In both the 1946 and 1958 national birth cohorts (the latter also known as the National Child Development Study, Goldstein 1971) there was a tendency for a gradient of stature within the non-manual classes (i.e., from social class I–IIIa), but this was not observed in the NSHG, whose first cohort was born in 1976. At present, differences in height in children of primary school age are mainly due to the short stature of those in social class V. The absolute differences in mean height between social class increase with age. At age 2 the difference between the two extremes of the social class spectrum is about 0.33 standard deviation units, but this increases to 0.5 standard deviation units by age 4. Eventually, the difference reaches 0.6–0.7 standard deviation units by the time children enter primary school. Rona *et al.* (1978) report a study of 9–11 year-old English boys and girls measured in 1972. When the groups were classified according to their father's occupation it was found, as in previous surveys, that the children of fathers in non-manual occupations were taller than those of manual workers at most ages.

242

It is important to note that no association was found by the NSHG between the rate of growth in a year and father's social class in school-age children, once dependency of height gain on initial height was accounted for. In other words, the gap between the two extreme social class groups increases with age, but most of the increase (about 90 per cent) occurs before the child enters school. Thereafter, the child enters a stable trajectory of growth velocity.

There is an interaction between the effects of social class and the number of siblings in the family (Rona *et al.* 1978). Expressed as standard deviation scores from the median, there is little evidence of any effect of sibship size upon the height of English children in the non-manual groups, unless that figure is greater than five. However, there is a marked reduction in the height of children of manual workers for sibship groups of two or more. Of course, a distinction ought really to be made between sibship size and ordinal position. For example, it is unlikely the adversity of being in a large sibship group (e.g. of five) will be as marked on the first as on the fifth-born child. 'Number of younger siblings' is a wise modification to ordinal position status (Goldstein 1971), when undertaking data analysis of this nature.

Profile of social distribution of stature

A very important observation has been made about the *profile* of the distribution of stature among the children of manual workers. As has already been discussed, this is usually approximately normally distributed. At any particular age 50 per cent of the population will be above or below the 50th centile (median) of what is an approximately Normal or Gaussian distribution, although the absolute position of the median (the 50th centile) will vary between populations of children from different countries, or between relatively homogeneous sub-populations within countries (defined, for example, in socio-economic terms). In their recent survey of English schoolchildren Rona *et al.* (1978) found that the distribution of heights is not merely shifted downwards, but is 'spaced out' at the lower extremes of social class. The difference in stature between the children of manual and non-manual workers, of primary school age, is about 2 cm at the 50th centile, but is nearly 4 cm at the 3rd centile. This finding suggests that there is an excess of very small children of manual workers, which ties in with the reports from epidemiological surveys by both Lacey and Parkin (1974a, 1974b) and Vimpani *et al.* (1981).

Stability of growth patterns and secular trends

When one considers the growth rates of different social groups the absolute differences (measured in, for example, centimetres) in actual height gains are not a very satisfactory indicator of the period when the maximal effect of the social environment is operative. Taller children grow faster than shorter children, therefore the variance about the median increases with age. There

243

is also a strong tendency for individual children to remain in the approximately same centile of the height distribution after the first year or so of life (Smith *et al.* 1976; Smith *et al.* 1980; Elwood *et al.* 1987; Moar and Ounsted 1982).

As I have already emphasized, in the UK, social-class differences in height begin to emerge around two years of age. From this age onwards there is a consistent tendency for children from social class I to outgrow those from the lower social classes (Elwood *et al.* 1987). There is also some tendency for the head circumference of children from social classes I and II to grow more rapidly than those from social class V – although this difference achieves statistical significance only after 3 years of age (Elwood *et al.* 1987). The distribution of reduced stature is related more closely to social factors than to geographical differentiation (Mascie-Taylor and Boldsen 1985), although in England Caucasian children living in poor inner-city areas are approximately 1 cm shorter than the national average at 5–11 years of age (Rona and Chinn 1986). There was a tendency for the height of children studied by the NSHG (Rona *et al.* 1978) to be *less* in more densely populated areas than in less densely populated areas.

Secular trends in stature might be expected to *diminish* the differences between the growth of children from upper and lower social classes. One example that is often quoted is that of Sweden where obliteration of social-class gradient in stature was demonstrated by Lindgren (1976). Subsequently, a similar picture was found in Norway (Brundtland *et al.* 1980; see Bielicki 1986). It is, however, important to note that this finding should not be taken to mean that *social class* differences no longer exist in Scandinavian society. The lower classes have to some extent caught up with the upper ones but there are *still* significant differences in economic control, political influence, incomes, education, and social prestige (Bielicki 1986). Lindgren (1976) followed the course of growth of a large urban epidemiological sample of schoolchildren from 1964 to 1973. She concluded that differences in height had been eradicated by a relatively larger gain in the lower social groups than the higher.

The Dunedin birth cohort study, in New Zealand, has reported statistically significant but relatively small correlations between socio-economic status and stature (0.11 and 0.12 for boys and girls respectively) (Silva *et al.* 1985). However, the difference in mean stature between those at the top and bottom of the socio-economic scale is just two-thirds the magnitude of the corresponding British values as reported by Goldstein (1971).

Compared with other European and North American growth statistics, British 7 year olds are among the smallest, the median stature of boys of this age being nearly 0.7 s.d. below that of the tallest North American groups (Waterlow 1985). There has been a great deal of debate about the significance of such international comparisons (see, for example, Graitcer and Gentry 1981; Goldstein and Tanner 1980) but the weight of current opinion seems to be that mean sizes of children from different populations are, on the whole, due more to environmental factors than to genetic ones, at least up until puberty, excepting for certain races in the Far East (Martorell 1985; Martorell and Habicht 1986).

But even in the Far East there have been marked secular trends in the direction of increased stature over the past thirty years. Between 1957 and 1977 almost all the secular change in the height of young adults has been due to change in leg length. Final sitting height has changed little, if at all (Martorell and Habicht 1986). Incidentally, the *tempo* of change has affected both sitting height and leg length, both body segments reaching their pubertal growth spurt nearly a year earlier in 1977 than in 1957.

The relevance of this observation, an aspect of differential growth rarely commented on in reports of secular trends, is that there is evidence that 'psychosocial adversity' exerts its main effect upon leg length (Meredith 1984). It might be thought that under-nutrition would be a prime candidate as an explanatory variable, but Tanner (1978) believes under-nutrition in man does not alter body shape significantly; a malnourished European child 'by no means acquires the short legs of the Asiatic'. One is nevertheless tempted to draw an analogy between the chronically undernourished short-legged Asiatics and the clinical findings of western doctors, faced with children who have been subject to severe emotional deprivation and neglect, who report subischial lengths (stature minus sitting height) to be less than 70 per cent of the population mean (McCarthy 1981).

The best explanation for secular trends of this nature is thought to be an improvement in some aspect of the social and material conditions for the population concerned (Rona 1981). In the *most* advantaged strata of society the trend is *least* marked, a point neatly made by an observation by Bakwin and McLaughlin (1964) who found the height of students from modest social backgrounds entering Harvard university had increased nearly 4 cm between 1930 and 1958, whereas entrants from wealthy backgrounds did not change at all in height over that period. There is no evidence that the secular trend of growth has persisted since the mid-1950s in the United States but it *has* done so in Britain (Chinn and Rona 1984).

Unemployment

There has been much dispute over the interpretation of the findings that there are significant differences in stature between the children of employed and unemployed fathers, even within the same social class. For instance, Tanner (1987) has commented that there is unlikely to be any causal connection through a process of sub-optimal nutrition that might accompany a brief period of unemployment.

Unfortunately, most studies of the association between unemployment and children's growth have failed to take account of the differences between short- and long-term unemployment, asking only (for example) if the head of household has been out of work in the previous four weeks (Rona and Chinn 1984). Differences in height between children of the employed and unemployed have been found *within* each social class but the effect is largest in social class V where it is reported to be as large as 0.6 s.d. at school age (Rona and Chinn 1984). Nevertheless, the evidence points to the fact that such differences in stature are associated with long-term cultural and material hardships, rather than single brief episodes of unemployment.

Psychosocial adversity

In a small proportion of the population, maybe 5 to 10 per cent, many adverse social circumstances are linked (Rona 1981). It seems to be especially among that subgroup that socio-economic factors are in some way associated with a threat to the normal growth of children. These effects can be detected very early in a child's life. A recent Swedish study, longitudinal in design, examined the social circumstances of a group of thirty-four infants with abnormally low rates of weight gain in the first eighteen months of life (Kristiansson and Fallstrom 1981). An excess of 'psychosocial' risk factors was found more commonly in the families of these infants than in a comparison group. Such factors included unemployment, paternal ill health, dependence on social welfare, abuse of alcohol and drugs, single parenthood, and a history of criminal offences. Kristiansson concluded that 'psychosocial stress' was in some way a causal factor. However, he made no attempt to ascertain by direct observation how such stress might be affecting the *parenting* of the infants concerned.

A somewhat similar conclusion was reached by Lacey and Parkin (1974a, 1974b) who conducted a well-known epidemiological study of the growth of a cohort of children born in 1960 in Newcastle-upon-Tyne. The children were examined at 10 years of age. Their stature at that age was compared with standards for height at successive ages in UK children (Tanner 1978).

The study is often quoted as being of 'all' children born in 1960 (of Newcastle-upon-Tyne mothers), who were below the 3rd height centile at 10 years of age. In fact, only approximately 45 per cent of the original cohort were examined. Of those actually measured, 3.63 per cent were considered 'short normal' and 0.71 per cent had an organic disease or disorder to account for their short stature. An additional 0.58 per cent of children under the 3rd centile for height (total 4.92 per cent) were not investigated because of parental refusal. Social-class distribution of the sample was skew in comparison with the 1961 and 1962 cohorts of the Newcastle Survey of Child Development, with nearly twice as many parents of short normal children in social classes IV and V. Parents of short children were smaller than adults in the general population, an average about 1 standard deviation below the median.

The authors rated the care of their short normal sample from observations made at home visits, in terms of 'good, average or poor'. No details are given about how those ratings were derived, nor indeed about how a similar 'social score' was arrived at. Nevertheless, the important conclusion was reached that an adverse score on both variables was found far more frequently among the families of short normal children than among even the most disadvantaged in the general population (viz. social class V). They state 'poor home conditions have been of importance in causing the short stature of at least 30 per cent of the children under the 3rd height centile in Newcastle-upon-Tyne'.

Maternal care

This has rarely been assessed directly, but is usually discussed in the context of proxy measures such as maternal age or single parenthood. Children whose mothers were less than 25 years of age when they gave birth are on average 0.6 cm smaller than those whose mothers were older than 25 years (Goldstein 1971). Maternal age does not seem to affect birthweight, but this small but significant difference in their children's stature seems to persist even after allowance is made for other relevant biological factors (such as parity). Goldstein concludes, 'This effect [may represent] residual social factors associated with the mother's age, for example, illegitimacy'. Certainly the NSHG (Garman *et al.* 1982) reported that children from two-parent families are usually taller than those from one-parent families, but the difference is very small. When adjustments have been made for birthweight, number of sibs, mother's and father's stature, and mother's educational background, *statistically significant* differences were found only in respect of girls from Scotland. Interestingly, persons in one-parent families are on average shorter than those in two-parent families, and their children have on average lower birthweights.

Apart from the survey of Lacey and Parkin (1974a, 1974b) and the recent work conducted by myself and colleagues (*vide infra*), direct measures of maternal care and growth have not been done, except in a study of thirty years ago by Douglas and Blomfield (1958). They found a very small association between standard of maternal care, as reported by health visitors, and children's height at 4.25 years. Only in children from intermediate social classes was there a tendency towards shorter stature in those children whose mothers were given the poorest ratings.

The inconclusive findings of former studies should not be taken to imply that caretaking quality is not a relevant variable. As Rona (1981) emphasizes, all the operational variables that have been used to measure the standard of maternal care have been unsatisfactory.

Thus, we may conclude, with regard to broad environmental influences on children's growth:

1. There is *no* inevitable difference between the stature of children in the upper and lower social classes – even though many inequalities in the

247

distribution of resources to those classes continue to exist.

2. Since the Second World War in the UK the absolute difference in stature between upper and lower classes persists but the proportion of the population in the lower range of the social-class distribution is decreasing. The finding is largely accounted for by an *excess* of very small children, mainly from social class V. The magnitude of the statural difference is exacerbated when there is associated unemployment.

3. By far the greater part of the growth retardation in disadvantaged groups, relative to national norms, is evident by the time the child enters primary school at age 5 years. Substantial differences are initially seen within the first year or two of life.

SPECIFIC INFLUENCES

I shall now consider some of the relatively specific factors that are known to be intervening variables between general environmental influences and rates of physical development.

Birthweight

During infancy a reassortment of relative sizes among children comes about, those who are larger at birth tending to grow more slowly and those who are smaller often growing more quickly. The correlation between length at birth and adult height is low – about 0.3. By six months it has risen to 0.5 and by one year to 0.7. By two years a stable pre-pubertal level of 0.8 is reached (Tanner 1986). Nevertheless, small-for-dates babies often stay small (Smith *et al.* 1976). There is now good evidence that those who are born relatively long, but of low weight (type II) will tend to catch up in weight, length, and head circumference by the age of one year. But those who are of low birthweight for their statistical age and who are also short (type I) will tend to stay small (Holmes *et al.* 1977). In view of the difference in prognosis of the two conditions, it is obviously crucial to distinguish between them in epidemiological research, especially in view of the fact that some intra-uterine insults – such as chronic maternal under-nutrition associated with socio-economic deprivation (Lin and Evans 1984), alcohol abuse (Smithells and Smith 1984) or smoking (D'Souza *et al.* 1981) – may be associated with type I rather than type II intra-uterine growth. Unfortunately, such data are rarely reported.

For many years a difference in the birthweight of infants born to mothers from different social classes has been recognized, both in developing as well as more socio-economically advantaged countries (e.g. Rosa and Turshen 1970). However, the broad association between social class and birthweight conceals a complex web of other associated variables. Recent evidence suggests that the finding may be accounted for entirely by specific factors such as poor weight gain during pregnancy, smoking, inadequate ante-natal care, use of alcohol, etc.

A large epidemiological survey at the University of Kansas Medical Center (e.g. Miller *et al.* 1976), on more than 2,700 white women and their singleton infants, found *no* differences in the incidence of low birthweight babies (defined as weighing < 2500g but over thirty-seven weeks gestation) across four socio-economic groups, once indices such as cigarette smoking during pregnancy, alcohol or drug abuse, and maternal malnutrition were taken into account. These data accord with smaller-scale surveys in this country (e.g. Ounsted and Scott 1982). In a recent careful investigation of 483 women living in the city of Oxford, Stein *et al.* (1987) found no association between social class and birthweight (once factors such as smoking were controlled for) but he did discover low income to be an independent predictor of birthweight, over and above unemployment. He also measured the expectant mother's psychiatric state using the Present State Examination (Wing *et al.* 1974) but found *no* evidence of an association between psychiatric morbidity, adverse life events, or long-term social difficulties and birthweight.

Smoking

There is substantial evidence that smoking during pregnancy results in newborn infants who are both lighter and shorter than those born to women who do not smoke, even after gestational age differences are taken into account (Meredith 1975). Smoking is significantly more common among parents from a poor social environment or limited educational background (59 per cent of social class V mothers, 15 per cent of social class I) (Rona *et al.* 1985).

Analyses of data from the National Study of Health and Growth (NSHG) in England and Scotland have shown that the number of cigarettes smoked by parents at home is significantly associated with the attained height of their children aged 5 to 11 years. This relationship is statistically significant, *even after* allowing for parental height, child's birthweight, mother's smoking during pregnancy, overcrowding, and number of siblings (Rona *et al.* 1985). Passive smoking therefore seems to have an effect on the linear growth of the child, *independent* of genetic factors, the social environment, and mother's smoking in pregnancy.

The mechanisms by which parental smoking and the linear growth of their children are linked have not been clarified. There are a number of potential aetiological processes. One possibility is that the infants of such parents have an excess of respiratory illnesses in infancy (e.g. Chen *et al.* 1986). Accordingly, it may be these recurrent illnesses that lead to a diminution of linear growth. However, there does not in general seem to be any close correlation between the number of *minor* respiratory illnesses during this period and an infant's rate of growth (Elwood *et al.* 1987).

249

An alternative hypothesis is that the food intake of children from families who smoke is diminished, perhaps because there is direct suppression of their appetite. Alternatively, families of smokers may provide smaller portions (Bergen 1981). This may be due either to the parents' own diminished appetite or, perhaps, the lower allocation of the families' resources for food purchase (Rona *et al.* 1985).

Third, cigarette smoke may contain components that have a directly harmful effect upon growth outside the uterus (e.g. Richardson *et al.* 1975). If that is the case, it has been postulated that the aetiological factor is likely to be the level of carbon monoxide in the child's environment. Perhaps an intermittent moderate increase in carbon monoxide, resulting in carboxyhaemoglobin formation, leads to a significant decrease in the amount of oxygen released at tissue level and a lowering of the efficiency of the cytochrome chain (Hamosh *et al.* 1979).

Fourth, passive cigarette smoking may be associated with an excess of digestive disorders in infants, including post-prandial colic (Said *et al.* 1984). A dose-response relationship between the number of cigarettes smoked by parents and the frequency of post-prandial colic has been reported. This association has also been investigated by an epidemiological survey of infants born in Tayside during 1980 (Ogston *et al.* 1987). Parental smoking was found to be associated with a higher frequency of reported alimentary disorders (as well as respiratory illnesses) in the first year of the child's life. It was hypothesized that there might be a link between parental smoking and reflex intestinal activity. The component of cigarette smoke responsible has not yet been identified.

Finally, a longitudinal study of children between 6 and 11 years of age demonstrated a dose-response relationship between the amount of current maternal cigarette smoking and attained height (Berkey *et al.* 1984). Analyses indicated that the observed association at that age was almost certainly due either to *former* exposure in utero and/or during *early* infancy. In light of Rona *et al.*'s (1981) conclusion that the association between the number of smokers in the home and their children's height could not be explained by maternal smoking during *pregnancy*, the authors hypothesize that it was sustained exposure to the products of smoking during the *first year of life* that produced an effect still observable in 6 year olds.

Illnesses

It has been known for many years that illness in childhood can have a significant effect upon the rate of growth, although a slowing of that rate is more likely to be found as a result of a relatively severe illness or in children who have a chronic condition such as recurrent respiratory illness or asthma (Elwood *et al.* 1987).

Recent evidence (Rogers 1984; Tanner 1986) has shown that during periods of acute illness children of school age grow more slowly than during corresponding periods without illness, but that on recovery from that illness they grow more rapidly, demonstrating 'catch-up' growth provided their nutrition at this time is good. There is no evidence that recurrent minor illnesses are associated with lower eventual heights nor even with reduced velocities over a period of one year or more (Elwood *et al.* 1987; Tanner 1986).

Nutrition

Children have higher requirements for energy, per unit body weight, than adults. This is due partly to a need to cover their higher metabolic rate per unit weight, which is twice that of an adult during infancy, but also to provide energy for the purposes of growth (Widdowson 1985). The energy cost of growth is highest in the first few months after birth. It then falls rapidly throughout the first year, from 30 per cent of normal energy intake at 1–2 months to 3 per cent at 9–12 months and only 1 per cent by 18–24 months (Bergmann and Bergmann 1986). Per unit body weight, energy intake has been reported to be greatest in normal healthy infants during the interval fourteen through twenty-seven days of age, decreasing thereafter. The correlation between weight gain and caloric intake is statistically significant (between 0.4 and 0.7) for both sexes during the first ten months of life. The ratio of dietary energy contributed by carbohydrates and fat does not seem to affect growth rates (Fomon *et al.* 1976). In the developed world, protein intake is rarely a limiting factor in determining rates of linear growth (Tanner 1978).

When energy availability is deficient, growth and maintenance become competitive, and growth disorders, as well as reduced activity levels, may ensue. Infants eat mainly for energy (Bergmann and Bergmann 1986).

Many studies have attempted to demonstrate an association between deficient nutritional intake, social deprivation, and retarded physical growth of children in the developed world. Most of these investigations have been of children of school age. For example, Hackett *et al.* (1984) conducted a two-year longitudinal survey of dietary intake and growth in height and weight of 11- and 12-year-old English schoolchildren. The expected differences in height and weight were found between the social classes, but there was no significant correlation between energy or protein intake and height and weight increments during the period of the study, even within social classes.

A careful prospective survey of ninety-one families with children under 4 years of age found that the energy intake of children from families headed by a manual worker was higher than those from children of non-manual workers (Black *et al.* 1976). This finding not only replicated the results of earlier investigations (e.g. Widdowson 1947) but also anticipated the results of later epidemiological surveys in other settings. For example, Jones *et al.* (1985) in the USA examined associations between various measures of child growth, dietary variables, and an index of poverty status in a sample of 13,750 black and white children aged 1–17 years. Differences in growth were not consistently associated with differences in the dietary intake of energy between poverty groups. and in the 1–5 year age range poor children seemed to have a higher energy intake than comparisons from families above the poverty level. Differences *did* however exist in child growth variables, in the expected direction.

Nevertheless, we know from innumerable studies in the developing world that, when children are faced with chronic but moderate deficiencies of nutrients, they will grow less in weight and height, but will manage to maintain *normal proportions* of weight to height so long as the severity of nutritional deficiency does not increase dramatically (e.g. Martorell 1985; Martorell and Habicht 1986). They will, therefore, be stunted. Stunting refers to retardation in linear growth, as measured by total body length or height. Wasting, in contrast, has to do with the relationship of body weight to length, and is usually seen when either severe food shortages or infections impair the body's ability to regulate growth and sustain adaptation to adverse circumstances (Waterlow 1985). It is important to note that, when faced with chronic but moderate deficiency of nutrients, the child will grow less in height and weight, but will manage to maintain fairly normal proportions of weight to height (i.e. will not be extraordinarily skinny) (Alvear *et al.* 1986).

In the developing world, the mean length of infants at birth is usually near the 50th centile of growth charts applicable to relatively affluent societies. Then, in societies where chronic under-nourishment is endemic, between the second and sixth months (when energy needs for growth are relatively high) supine length begins to fall precipitously relative to western standards as rates of linear growth begin to be affected (see Martorell and Habicht 1986).

A similar profile of growth trajectories has been reported in clinical populations of infants aged 2 to 28 months who were failing to thrive in a western society. The important observation was made that in those who were *proportionately small* for their age, or stunted (i.e. > 80 per cent ideal body weight for length), there was no significant correlation between caloric intake and weight gain in hospital (Schaffer Bell and Woolston 1985). Even high intakes of energy were often associated with little percentage weight change. There was, however, a slight tendency for the highest percentage change to occur in the youngest subjects (i.e. under 9 months). In contrast, those who were relatively underweight for their length gained weight in proportion to their ingestion of energy-rich nutrition.

Catch-up growth

In favourable environmental conditions the trajectory of growth in height of children is so constant that it may be represented by a relatively simple mathematical curve (Preece and Baines 1978). Should adverse circumstances supervene, the rate of growth starts temporarily to slow down, whether because of acute malnutrition, or in association with organic disorders such as growth hormone deficiency or coeliac disease. After rectifying the disorder a phase of more rapid or accelerated growth is seen which persists until the child's growth is back on the pre-existing trajectory (Tanner 1986). Some children will catch up very quickly, but others may take relatively longer, yet eventually end up on the predicted trajectory. In general, the more severe the growth-retarding influence, the longer it acts, and the earlier in life it occurs, the worse the ultimate outcome.

The completeness and speed of catch-up may depend upon the nature of the growth-retarding influence (e.g. growth hormone deficiency seems to be more devastating than hypothyroidism). Somehow, the growth-retarded child recognizes that it is small, but it also recognizes when it is restored to normal size – since, when approaching the normal curve, the rate of growth slows down and settles back on to it, no overshoot occurring in stature.

There is no general agreement about whether growth retardation caused by malnutrition in early infancy is a reversible or an irreversible phenomenon (Alvear *et al.* 1986). However, there is evidence that the possibilities for catch-up growth are very limited once the child reaches 3–5 years of age. If he or she is already small the probability is that they will remain small throughout the growing years, eventually becoming a small adult (Martorell 1985).

First year as sensitive period

There is a long-established view, based upon work both with animals (e.g. McCance and Widdowson 1962) and with humans (e.g. Eid 1971) that early infancy represents in some way a sensitive period with regard to growth. There are relatively few studies that have specifically examined this issue. One such investigation by Eid (1971) examined 132 infants who were failing to thrive during the first year, 88.5 per cent of whom had a physical disease or disorder to account for the pattern of growth. Subjects were followed up to 5 years of age, by which time 16 per cent of those who had received active treatment were still significantly growth retarded (height and weight < 3rd centile) as were 37 per cent of those who had not received active treatment. The authors concluded that, if the failure to thrive had not been corrected during the first year, there was a significantly greater retardation in subsequent height, weight, and head circumference. Unfortunately, there is little discussion of the fact that half of the children in the treatment group were small-for-dates babies, as were all of those in the untreated group, i.e. this was an example of poor study design because the small-for-dates babies might have had a limited capacity for catch-up growth. Both groups had birthweights significantly lower than a comparison group. Waterlow *et al.* (1980), among others, have reported that the rate of weight gain in infants in the developing world begins to fall off sharply, when compared to a reference population, as early as 3–4 months. The pattern of growth thenceforth is very similar to that seen in Eid's sample (Eid 1971).

Additional data on these questions are provided by an intriguing case comparison study of the Bedouin in the Negev desert (Dagan *et al.* 1983). The growth and feeding practices of 353 Bedouin infants were studied; they were fed irregularly whenever they expressed hunger, but as soon as the baby stopped eating mother would stop feeding. Breast feeding was prolonged (63 per cent at 12 months) and there was little supplementary nutrition with animal products. Fruit and vegetables were introduced later (to only 50 per cent of infants by the seventh month of life) than for the comparison group of Jewish children living in the same area. Rice, the most important supplementary food, was introduced only after six months. During the first half of the first year the mean weight of Bedouin infants progressively approached the 3rd centile of the NCHS curves (WHO 1983), and there was also progressive stunting of supine length. The infants did seem to be malnourished relative to the comparison population, because of poor feeding practices. Yet, weight for length remained approximately normally distributed about the median (50th) NCHS percentile, and triceps skinfold thickness was only slightly diminished. Catch-up growth did not subsequently occur to any great extent, the adult height of Bedouin men and women being between the 10th and 15th centiles for a western population (Groen *et al.* 1964).

In a totally different setting, Pollitt and Leibel (1980) studied a sample of nineteen children between 12–59 months of age from one out-patient department in the urban United States whose heights and weights were below the 3rd centile. These children had failed to thrive without organic disease or disorder, yet had not been premature or small for dates. No significant differences between the degrees of thinness or obesity were found between the groups, although there had been a downward drift in weight-gain rates since birth. Although the children in a comparison group, growing well, had a statistically higher intake of calories, in both groups the value for virtually all nutrients was very close to or above the recommended dietary allowance (NAS 1974). The index children had a history of poor feeding *within the first year of life*, and the pattern of growth exhibited by several of the cases was very similar to that seen in malnourished infants and pre-schoolers in developing countries (Waterlow *et al.* 1980). The authors conclude that *current* malnutrition seemed an unlikely explanation for the poor growth rates of their case sample, although the measures of intake were crude. The implicit corollary is that malnutrition occurred at an *earlier* age and the children had not 'caught up', but continued growing at a steady low average velocity.

Thus we may conclude:

1. Although the lower social classes tend to have children who are of lower birthweight, due either to shorter periods of gestation or because they are lighter for dates, these differences alone are *not* sufficient to account for persisting growth retardation. Comparable light birthweight children from the upper social classes show catch-up growth to

trajectories within the normal range within two years.

2. Growth trajectories are largely established within the first year or so of life. This is a time when the developing organism is especially vulnerable to environmental insults, because a small diminution in rate of growth for relatively briefer times will have a more devastating effect. If the growth trajectory diverges drastically from the ideal population median during this period there is probably a *limited opportunity* for full catch-up growth, even if circumstances later improve.

3. When all the specific postulated aetiological factors are considered the final common denominator seems likely to be nutritional deficiencies. Given the evidence that a close correlation between energy intake and growth has been demonstrated in western infants only within the first year and given the findings on the timing of growth delays in disadvantaged populations, it seems a reasonable working hypothesis that growth delay attributed to so-called 'psychosocial deprivation' may ultimately be due to under-nourishment at a *very early stage* in an infant's life. Such under-nourishment is likely to be linked to inadequate parenting, exemplified by poor feeding practices. It may be exacerbated by an infant's persistent exposure to cigarette smoke and associated relatively high carbon monoxide levels.

PARENTING STYLES AND GROWTH DELAY AMONG INNER-CITY INFANTS

Research by myself and colleagues over the past five years has sought to provide some answers to the questions raised by a consideration of the nature of social adversity and its relation to children's growth. An epidemiological approach has been taken, and all assessments of parenting have been done blind to the children's case/comparison status. The population under investigation has comprised the inhabitants of a geographically delimited, racially heterogeneous inner-city area (population 140,000) in which there are approximately 2,500 births each year. In socio-economic terms the district is relatively homogeneous and quite severely disadvantaged (South East Thames Regional Health Authority 1984). Two whole population surveys have been conducted. The first centred on a cohort of 1980 births (the 1980 birth cohort) for whom limited longitudinal data were available between birth and four years of age. At one year of age, nearly 5 per cent of full-term Caucasian singletons were found to have weights below the 3rd population centile on national charts (Skuse 1987). Their profile of growth since birth, at near normal birthweights, was virtually identical to undernourished infants from less developed countries (Waterlow *et al.* 1980).

The great majority had no organic disease or disorder that could account for their condition. Few (28 per cent) had received hospital referral, investigation, or treatment; of these who had been seen, most cases of growth retardation did not recover.

The 1980 birth cohort survey aimed to examine, at four years of age, those children in the community with the *poorest* rates of growth, in terms of weight gain, since infancy. A case-comparison design was used, full details of which are given in Dowdney *et al.* (1987). The case group were stunted, with heights and weights in proportion but on average below the 3rd population centile on national charts, even when their parents' stature was taken into account.

In view of the strong evidence that, although the origins of such growth problems seem to lie in a complex interaction between child and family variables, the proximal cause is inadequate nutrition for the infant's needs (Skuse 1985), a particular emphasis was placed on nutritional assessment. Direct observations were made of family interactions during meal-times when the children were four years of age. Detailed dietary information was obtained, and a history of feeding practices and problems was taken from the mother (Heptinstall *et al.* 1987). Findings indicated that neither quantity of food intake (calorie/protein) nor gross environmental variables distinguished the case and comparison groups. However, the meal-time observations revealed considerably more disorganization and negative attitudes in case-group families, the number of instructions and negative comments to the index child being significantly higher than in comparison families. Interview data revealed that the observed pattern of lack of supervision, coupled with a somewhat arbitrary and insensitive approach to control of feeding, seemed to have characterized the case mothers' parenting style from the earliest days. For example, 35 per cent of the case group had frequently been fed as infants by bottles propped in their mouths, nearly four times as many in the comparison group. Incidentally, one in every three mothers of growth-retarded 4-year-olds reported that their children stole food, whereas only one comparison mother made this complaint.

When the data on feeding practices had been analysed, there was compelling evidence that a period of chronic and severe under-nourishment was likely to have occurred in early infancy. All case children had begun to fail to thrive *within the first year of life*. The design of the 1980 birth cohort 'catch-up' prospective study generated challenging hypotheses on the factors associated with a poor prognosis, but it was not possible adequately to test them.

A second, truly prospective, epidemiological study was therefore designed, with the intention of examining postulated causal mechanisms, derived from analysis of the original data. Again a whole population survey technique was used, in exactly the same geographical area as before. The sampling frame comprised all 1986 births in the district (the '1986' birth cohort). Cohort infants have been monitored since birth, cases and comparisons being examined at approximately 12 to 15 months of age. Data collection on this investigation is still in progress but a substantial pilot survey, using a case-comparison design, has been completed. Semi-structured interview and direct observation techniques within subject's homes were employed. The research design anticipated the hypothesis that growth delay among inner-city infants is usually the outcome of a subtle interaction between the individual biological and psychological characteristics of the child and features of the caretaking environment which fail to meet that child's specific and particular needs (Skuse 1985). Inappropriate management can exacerbate pre-existing delays or disorders in age-dependent processes (such as the acquisition of oral-motor skills). Disruption in normal processes of adaptation and change may result in poorly regulated and unpredictable children who fail to signal their needs clearly and unambiguously.

The results of the pilot survey showed case infants possessed characteristics of behavioural style, communication skills, oral-motor behaviour, and attentional processes in line with the above hypotheses. Such features were found in association with mothers who expressed more negative emotion, showed less reciprocity, and were poorer managers of their infant's behaviour (Wolke *et al.* 1987). No significant differences were found between the groups in terms of the quantities of nutrition *presented* to the infants by their mothers, but case infants did possess characteristics that rendered them more difficult to feed successfully, therefore their actual *intake* was probably deficient due to food loss, refusal, etc. (Subsequent data collected on the 1986 birth cohort, using multi-method assessments of nutritional status, have confirmed this impression.) Their behavioural style was either irritable and fussy *or* apathetic and undemanding. The latter picture characterized infants who were most seriously underweight and was reminiscent of the 'reductive adaptation' described by Jackson and Golden (1987) in which energy resources are conserved during conditions of severe shortage, by a reduction in energy expenditure. Case mothers' style of feeding and associated contextual features (such as positioning and ambient noise) accentuated the problem (Mathisen *et al.* 1987). None of the case subjects in the pilot survey had an organic aetiology of their failure to thrive. Little indication was found of overt child abuse, rejection, or deliberate neglect of case infants.

In conclusion, there is substantial evidence that the small size of children from developing countries is not due, on the whole, to ethnic variations but rather to the effects of environmental factors. Among these, poor nutrition seems to be the most important. Growth patterns of a significant minority of infants from deprived inner-city areas in western countries seem to be very similar to those of their stunted brethren overseas. A parsimonious hypothesis about mechanisms states that the proximal aetiological factors are also similar, and evidence has been adduced which supports that view. Following failure to thrive in early infancy, affected children do *not* completely catch-up in their growth rates, at least so long as they continue to live in the same

257

family unit. Early poor rates of weight gain probably precede a similar pattern of retardation in the development of stature.

One further test of the proposed causal chain would be a trial to alter feeding practices among mothers of infants believed to be at risk. Such studies have already been undertaken in poor, under-privileged communities in South and Central America, and elsewhere (see Martorell and Habicht 1986).

Of course, those interventions aimed to provide additional nutrients to impoverished communities. There is no suggestion from our work that poverty among inner-city families is the determining factor leading to under-nourishment of case infants. Adequate food *is* available, in quantity if not in quality. The essential problem seems to be that some mothers do not recognize, or adapt to, the special qualities of 'at risk' infants, especially the characteristics of their neuromotor development and behavioural style. Such mothers may, in contrast, have coped perfectly well with other children, who lack such characteristics and whose growth has been correspondingly unremarkable.

Further pilot work has demonstrated that it is possible and indeed relatively easy to alert many such mothers to the problem. Video-feedback techniques are used, based upon the thesis that an intervention aimed at changing *maternal* responsivity and emotional expression is likely to be followed by a rapid change in child behaviour, leading to greater reinforcement for the mother (Crittenden 1985). Interactions are videotaped in the home and immediately played back, with a commentary by the observer. Dramatic results have been documented after a relatively few sessions with this technique.

A parent health education study along these lines is now planned, using a novel case-comparison factorial design to assess the impact of such an intervention upon *all* families containing a growth- retarded infant, who live within the geographical boundaries of an inner-city health district.

REFERENCES

Alvear, J., Arjaza, C., Vial, M., Guerrero, S., and Muzzo, S. (1986) 'Physical growth and bone age of survivors of protein energy malnutrition', *Archives of Disease in Childhood* 61: 257–62.

Bakwin, H. and McLaughlin, S.M. (1964) 'Secular increase in height: is the end in sight?' *Lancet* 2: 1195–6.

Bergen, S. (1981) 'Parental smoking at home and height of children (correspondence)', *British Medical Journal* 282: 1612.

Bergmann, R.L. and Bergmann, K.E. (1986) 'Nutrition and growth in infancy', in F. Falkner and J.M. Tanner (eds) *Human Growth: A Comprehensive Treatise: Volume 3: Methodology: Ecological, Genetic, and Nutritional Effects on Growth*, London: Plenum Press, 389–413.

Berkey, C.S., Ware, J.H., Speizer, F.E., and Ferris, B.G. (1984) 'Passive smoking and height growth of preadolescent children', *International Journal of Epidemiology* 13 (4): 454–8.

Bielicki, T. (1986) 'Physical growth as a measure of the economic well-being of populations: the twentieth century', in F. Falkner and J.M. Tanner (eds) *Human Growth: A Comprehensive Treatise: Volume 3: Methodology: Ecological, Genetic, and Nutritional Effects on Growth*, London: Plenum Press, 283–305.

Black, A.E., Billewicz, W.Z., and Thomson, A.M. (1976) 'The diets of preschool children in Newcastle upon Tyne, 1968–71', *British Journal of Nutrition* 35: 105–13.

Brundtland, G.H., Liestøl, K., and Walløe, L. (1980 'Height weight and menarcheal age of Oslo schoolchildren during the last 60 years', *Annals of Human Biology* 7: 307–22.

Chen, Y., Li, W., and Yu, S. (1986) 'Influence of passive smoking on admissions for respiratory illness in early childhood', *British Medical Journal* 293: 303–6.

Chinn, S. and Rona, R.J. (1984) 'The secular trend in the height of primary school children in England and Scotland from 1972–1980', *Annals of Human Biology* 11(1): 1–16.

Crittenden, P.M. (1985) 'Maltreated infants: vulnerability and resilience', *Journal of Child Psychology & Psychiatry* 26: 85–96.

Dagan, R., Sofer, S., Klish, W.J., Hundet, G., Saltz, H., and Moses, S.W. (1983) 'Growth & nutritional status of Bedouin infants in the Negev desert Israel: evidence for marked stunting in the presence of only mild malnutrition', *American Journal of Clinical Nutrition* 38: 747–56.

Department of Health & Social Security, Department of Education & Science, & Welsh Office (1976) *Fit for the Future* (Report of the Committee on Child Health Services, Chairman Professor S.D.M. Court), London: HMSO.

Douglas, J.W.B. and Blomfield J.M. (1958) *Children Under Five*, London: Allen & Unwin.

Douglas, J.W.B. and Simpson, H. (1964) 'Height in relation to puberty family size and social class', *Millbank Memorial Fund Quarterly* 42: 20–35.

Dowdney, L., Skuse, D., Heptinstall, E., Puckering, C., and Zur-Szpiro, S. (1987) 'Growth retardation and developmental delay among inner city children'. *Journal of Child Psychology & Psychiatry* 28(4): 529–41.

D'Souza, K., Black, P., and Richards, B. (1981) 'Smoking in pregnancy: associations with skinfold thickness, maternal weight gain, and fetal size at birth', *British Medical Journal* 282: 1661–3.

Eid, E.E. (1971) 'A follow-up study of physical growth following failure to thrive with special reference to a critical period in the first year of life', *Acta Paediatrica Scandinavica* 60: 39–48.

Elwood, P.C., Sweetman, P.M., Gray, O.P., Davies, D.F., and Wood, P.D.Q. (1987) 'Growth of children from 0–5 years: with special reference to mother's smoking in pregnancy', *Annals of Human Biology* 14(6): 543–57.

Fomon, S.J., Thomas, L.N., Filer, L.J.Jr., Anderson, T.A., and Nelson, S.E. (1976) 'Influence of fat and carbohydrate content of diet on food intake and growth of male infants', *Acta Paediatrica Scandinavica* 65: 136.

Fox, P.T., Elston, M.E., and Waterlow, J.C. (1981) *Preschool Child Survey* (DHSS Report of Health & Social Subjects no. 21), London: HMSO, 64–84.

Garman, A.R., Chinn, S., and Rona, R.J. (1982) 'Comparative growth of primary schoolchildren from one and two parent families', *Archives of Disease in Childhood* 57: 453–8.

Goldstein, H. (1971) 'Factors influencing the height of seven year old children – results from the national child development study', *Human Biology* 43: 92–111.

259

Goldstein, H. and Tanner, J.M. (1980) 'Ecological considerations in the creation and use of child growth standards', *Lancet* i: 582–5.

Graitcer, P.L. and Gentry, E.M. (1981) 'Measuring children: one reference for all', *Lancet* ii: 297–9.

Groen, J.J., Balogh, M., Levy, M., and Yaron, E. (1964) 'Nutrition of the Bedouins in the Negev Desert', *American Journal of Clinical Nutrition* 74: 33–46.

Hackett, A.F., Rugg-Gunn, A.J., Appleton, D.R., Parkin, J.M., and Eastoe, J.E. (1984) 'Two-year longitudinal study of dietary intake in relation to the growth of 405 English children initially aged 11–12 years', *Annals of Human Biology* 11(6): 545–53.

Hamosh, M., Simon, M.R., and Hamosh, T. (1979) 'Effect of nicotine on the development of fetal and suckling rats', *Biology of the Neonate* 35: 290–7.

Heptinstall, E., Puckering, C., Skuse, D., Dowdney, L., and Zur-Szpiro, S. (1987) 'Nutrition and mealtime behaviour in families of growth retarded children', *Human Nutrition: Applied Nutrition* 41a(6): 390–402.

Holmes, G.E., Miller, H.C., Hassanein, K., Lansky, S.B., and Goggin, J.E. (1977) 'Postnatal somatic growth in infants with atypical fetal growth patterns', *American Journal of Diseases of Children* 131: 1078–83.

Jackson, A.A. and Golden, H.M.W. (1987) 'Severe malnutrition', in D.J. Weatherall, J.G.G. Ledingham, and D.A. Warrell, (eds) *Oxford Textbook of Medicine*, second edition, Oxford: Oxford Univerisity Press, pp. 812–28.

Jones, D.Y., Nesheim, M.C., and Habicht, J.P. (1985) 'Influences in child growth associated with poverty in the 1970s', *American Journal of Clinical Nutrition* 42: 714–24.

Kristiansson, B. and Fallstrom, S.P. (1981) 'Infants with low rates of weight gain: II: a study of environmental factors', *Acta Paediatrica Scandinavica* 70: 663–68.

Lacey, K.A. and Parkin, J.M. (1974a) 'Causes of short stature: a community study of children in Newcastle-upon-Tyne', *Lancet* 1: 42–5.

Lacey, K.A. and Parkin, J.M. (1974b) 'The normal short child: a community study of children in Newcastle-upon-Tyne', *Archives of Disease in Childhood* 49: 417–24.

Lin, C.C. and Evans, M.I. (1984) *Intrauterine Growth Retardation: Pathophysiology and Clinical Management*, New York: McGraw-Hill.

Lindgren, G. (1976) 'Height weight and menarche in Swedish urban school children in relation to socioeconomic and regional factors', *Annals of Human Biology* 3: 501–28.

McCance, R.A. and Widdowson, E.M. (1962) 'Nutrition and growth', *Proceedings of the Royal Society B* 156: 326–37.

McCarthy, D. (1981) 'The effects of emotional disturbance and deprivation on somatic growth', in J.A. Davis and J. Dobbing (eds) *Scientific Foundations of Paediatrics*, London: Heinemann.

Martorell, R. (1985) 'Child growth retardation: a discussion of its causes and its relationship to health', in K. Blaxter and J.C. Waterlow (eds) *Nutritional Adaptation in Man*, London and Paris: John Libbey, 13–29.

Martorell, R. and Habicht, J.P. (1986) 'Growth in early childhood in developing countries', in F. Falkner and J.M. Tanner (eds) *Human Growth: A Comprehensive Treatise: Volume 3: Methodology Ecological Genetic and Nutritional Effects on Growth*, London: Plenum Press, 241–62.

Martorell, R., Yarborough, C., Klein, R.E., and Lechtig, A. (1979) 'Malnutrition body size and skeletal maturation: interrelationships and implications for catch-up growth', *Human Biology* 51(3): 371–89.

Mascie-Taylor, C.G.N. (1987) 'Assortative mating in a contemporary British population', *Annals of Human Biology* 14(1): 59–68.

Mascie-Taylor, C.G.N. and Boldsen, J.L. (1985) 'Regional and social analysis of height variations in a contemporary British sample', *Annals of Human Biology* 12(4): 315–24.

Mathisen, B., Skuse, D., and Wolke, D. (1987) 'Oral-motor dysfunction and growth retardation amongst inner-city children', *Developmental Medicine & Child Neurology* (in press).

Meredith, H.V. (1975) 'Relation between tobacco smoking of pregnant women and body size of their progeny: a compilation of published studies', *Human Biology* 47: 451–72.

Meredith, H.V. (1984) 'Body size of infants and children around the world in relation to socioeconomic status', *Advances in Child Development and Behaviour* 18: 81–146.

Miller, H.C., Hassanein, K., Chin, T.D.Y., and Hensleigh, P. (1976) 'Socioeconomic factors in relation to fetal growth in white infants', *Journal of Pediatrics* 89: 638.

Moar, V.A. and Ounsted, M.K. (1982) 'Growth in the first year of life: how early can one predict size at twelve months among small-for-dates & large-for-dates babies?' *Early Human Development* 6: 65–9.

National Academy of Sciences, National Research Council (1980) *Recommended Dietary Allowances* 9th edition, Washington, DC: National Academy of Sciences.

National Children's Bureau (1987) *Investing in the Future: Child Health Ten Years after the Court Report* (A report of the Policy and Practice Review Group National Children's Bureau), London: NCB.

Ogston, S.A., Du V. Florey, C., and Walker, C.H.M. (1987) 'Association of infant alimentary and respiratory illness with parental smoking and other environmental factors, *Journal of Epidemiological Community Health* 41: 21–5.

Ounsted, M. and Scott, A. (1982) 'Social class and birthweight: a new look', *Early Human Development* 6: 83–7.

Pollitt, E. and Leibel, R.L. (1980) 'Biological and social correlates of failure to thrive', in L. Green and F.S. Johnston (eds) *Social and Biological Predictors of Nutritional Status, Physical Growth, and Neurological Development*, New York: Academic Press.

Preece, M.A. and Baines, M.J. (1978) 'A new family of mathematical models describing the human growth curve', *Annals of Human Biology* 5: 1.

Richardson, D., Coates, F., and Morton, R. (1975) 'Early effects of tobacco smoke exposure on vascular dynamics in the microcirculation', *Journal of Applied Physiology* 39: 119–23.

Roberts, D.F. (1985) 'Genetics and nutritional adaptation', in K. Blaxter and J.C. Waterlow (eds) *Nutritional Adaptation in Man*, London and Paris: John Libbey, 45–59.

Rogers, A. (1984) *The Effects of Illness on Growth During Childhood and Adolescence*, M.Phil. thesis, Oxford: Oxford University Press.

Rona, R.J. (1981) 'Genetic and environmental factors in the control of growth in childhood', *British Medical Bulletin* 37(3): 265–72.

Rona, R.J. and Chinn, S. (1984) 'The National Study of Health and Growth: nutritional surveillance of primary school children from 1976–1981 with special reference to unemployment and social class', *Annals of Human Biology* 11(1): 17–28.

Rona, R.J. and Chinn, S. (1986) 'The National Study of Health and Growth: social and biological factors associated with height of children from ethnic groups living in England', *Annals of Human Biology* 13(5): 453–71.

261

Rona, R.J., Chinn, S. and Du V. Florey, C. (1985) 'Exposure to cigarette smoking and children's growth', *International Journal of Epidemiology* 14(3): 402–9.

Rona, R.J., Du V. Florey, C., Clarke, G.C., and Chinn, S. (1981) 'Parental smoking at home and height of children', *British Medical Journal* 283: 1363.

Rona, R.J., Swan, A.V., and Altman, D.G. (1978) 'Social factors and height of primary schoolchildren in England and Scotland', *Journal of Epidemiological & Community Health* 32: 147–54.

Rosa, F.W. and Turshen, M. (1970) 'Fetal nutrition', *WHO Bulletin* 43: 785–95, Geneva: WHO.

Said, G., Patois, E., and Lellouch, J. (1984) 'Infantile colic and parental smoking', *British Medical Journal* 289: 658–60.

Schaffer Bell, L. and Woolston, J.L. (1985) 'The relationship of weight gain and caloric intake in infants with organic and nonorganic failure to thrive syndrome', *Journal of the American Academy of Child Psychiatry* 24(4): 447–52.

Silva, P.A., Birkbeck, J., and Williams, S. (1985) 'Some factors influencing the stature of Dunedin 7 year old children', *Australian Paediatric Journal* 21: 27–30.

Skuse, D. (1985) 'Non-organic failure to thrive: a reappraisal', *Archives of Disease in Childhood* 60(2): 173–8.

Skuse, D. (1987) 'Social deprivation and early intervention: research to practice', in G. Hosking and G. Murphy (eds) *Prevention of Mental Handicap: A World View.* (Proceedings of the RSM Forum on Mental Retardation), London: RSM.

Smith, A.M., Chinn, A., and Rona, R.J. (1980) 'Social factors and height gain of primary schoolchildren in England and Scotland', *Annals of Human Biology* 7: 115–24.

Smith, D.W., Truog, W., Rogers, J.E., Greitzer, L.J., Skinner, A.L., McCann, J.J., and Harvey, M.A.S. (1976) 'Shifting linear growth during infancy: illustration of genetic factors in growth from fetal life through infancy', *Journal of Pediatrics* 89(2): 225–30.

Smithells, R.W. and Smith, I.J. (1984) 'Alcohol and the fetus', *Archives of Disease in Childhood* 59: 1113–4.

South East Thames Regional Health Authority (1984) *Statistics and Operational Research Department* (District Health Authority A.C.O.R.N. populations), unpublished..

Stein, A., Campbell, E.A., Day, A., McPherson, K., and Cooper, P.J. (1987) 'Social adversity, low birthweight and preterm delivery', *British Medical Journal* 295(ii): 291–93.

Tanner, J.M. (1978) *Foetus into Man: Physical Growth from Conception to Maturity,* London: Open Books.

Tanner, J.M. (1986) 'Growth as a target-seeking function: catch-up and catch-down growth in man', in F. Falkner and J.M. Tanner (eds) *Human Growth: A Comprehensive Treatise: Volume 1: Developmental Biology Prenatal Growth,* London: Plenum Press, 167–79.

Tanner, J.M. (1987) 'Growth as a mirror of the condition of society: secular trends and class distinction', *Acta Paediatrica Japonica* 29: 96–103.

Vimpani, C.N., Vimpani, A.F., Pocock, S.J., and Farquhar, J.W. (1981) 'Differences in physical characteristics, perinatal histories, and social backgrounds between children with growth hormone deficiency and constitutional short stature', *Archives of Disease in Childhood* 56: 922–8.

Waterlow, J.C. (1985) 'What do we mean by adaptation?' in K. Blaxter and J.C. Waterlow (eds) *Nutritional Adaptation in Man,* London and Paris: John Libbey, 1–11.

Waterlow, J.C., Ashworth, A., and Griffiths, M. (1980) 'Faltering in infant growth in less-developed countries', *Lancet* ii: 1176–8.

Widdowson, E.M. (1947) *A Study of individual children's diets* (Medical Research Council Special Report Series 257), London: HMSO.

Widdowson, E.M. (1985) 'Responses to deficits of dietary energy', in K. Blaxter and J.C. Waterlow (eds) *Nutritional Adaptation in Man*, London and Paris: John Libbey, 97–104.

Wing, J.K., Cooper, J.E., and Sartorius, N. (1974) *The Measurement and Classification of Psychiatric Symptoms*, London: Cambridge University Press.

Wolke, D., Skuse, D., and Mathisen, B. (1987) 'Behavioural style in failure to thrive infants: a preliminary communication', *Journal of Pediatric Psychology* (in press).

World Health Organization (1983) *Measuring Change in Nutritional Status*, Geneva: WHO.

18

The Epidemiological Contribution to Research on Late-life Dementia

Brian Cooper

Epidemiological research on dementia is currently in a highly frustrating phase. Hardly a month goes by without reports of new, challenging findings in neuro-pathology, biochemistry, or molecular biology, which seem to offer the promise of scientific advance in this field. Yet the epidemiologist remains uncomfortably aware that primary degenerative dementia is essentially a diagnosis of exclusion, which cannot be definitely confirmed during life and, indeed, not always *post mortem*; that no biological marker is available for use in case identification and, finally, that neither for dementia of Alzheimer type (DAT) nor for multi-infarct dementia (MID) is it yet clear whether we are dealing with a single disease entity or with the final common pathway of a number of different morbid processes. Until these issues have been resolved, the pace of epidemiological progress is unlikely to accelerate.

While brain-imaging and electrophysiological techniques play an increasing role in hospital-based investigation (McGreer 1986; Fenton 1986) each has so far found only limited application in field studies, for obvious practical reasons. Here the most pressing need is for the establishment of differential-diagnostic criteria, based on the phenomena of disease and validated against autopsy findings. Diagnostic guidelines for dementing illness are incorporated in the manuals both for the standard American psychiatric classification DSM–III (APA 1980) and for the current draft form of the International Classification of Diseases, Tenth Revision – ICD–10 (WHO 1987); in addition, more detailed criteria have been proposed by a multi-disciplinary work group in the USA (McKhann *et al.* 1984). These various systems of classification, which are said to be mutually compatible, can undoubtedly help clinicians to arrive at a more accurate diagnosis; so far, however, they have not been made fully operational for research purposes.

Reports on the accuracy of differential diagnosis by clinical methods have varied a good deal in their conclusions. In the more careful of recent studies, the efficiency of clinical diagnosis, judged as a screening procedure, has been of the order of 70 per cent, while its positive predictive value – i.e. the probability that it will be confirmed at autopsy – has ranged from 55 per cent to 80 per cent (Rocca *et al.* 1986). These results pose a question as to whether the diagnostic accuracy in field studies is yet high enough to permit the testing of aetiological hypotheses in relation to specific disease entities (Liston and La Rue 1983).

DESCRIPTIVE EPIDEMIOLOGY

Prevalence and incidence studies

A recent meta-analytical study (Jorm *et al.* 1987) examined data on the prevalence of late-life dementia from forty-seven field studies, carried out during the forty-year period 1945–85. The estimates were found to vary widely both between countries and between individual studies, largely as a function of the research methods employed. Nevertheless, two general trends could be discerned. To begin with, there was a relative excess of DAT among women and of MID among men. Second, there was a consistent relationship between the estimates for successive five-year age-groups above 60, the age-specific prevalence ratio doubling on average for each additional 5.1 years of age.

In figure 18.1 the smooth age-curve is based on pooled data from the twenty-two field studies analysed by Jorm *et al.* (1987) which give age-specific prevalence estimates for dementia or closely related diagnoses (senile psychoses, organic psychoses, or chronic brain syndromes). Since not all these studies achieved full population coverage, the pooled estimates are somewhat lower than those derived from the individual field studies also represented in figure 18.1, each of which was fairly comprehensive in coverage. Nonetheless, the age-related curves appear to be similar in all the studies, once allowance is made for random fluctuation, This degree of uniformity suggests that the different investigators were studying the same phenomenon. Any more far-reaching interpretation of the data can only be speculative, since prevalence ratios are a function of the course and outcome of a disease, as well as of its incidence in a population, and in the case of dementia too little is known about the range of variation around each of these axes.

For the same reason, prevalence estimates make an unsatisfactory basis for aetiological research. In this context incidence rates – i.e., rates of occurrence of new cases in defined populations – must be established, and any variation compared with the distribution of suspected risk factors. The basic practical difficulty resides in monitoring the onset of new cases and making a reliable diagnostic assessment. Psychiatric first-admission rates are sometimes used to estimate the so-called 'treated incidence', but in respect of dementia this index tells more about the utilization of treatment agencies than it does about the frequency of occurrence in the elderly population. Most cases of late-life dementia are not referred to psychiatrists, and those

265

Figure 18.1 Age-specific prevalence of late-life dementia (findings of field studies)

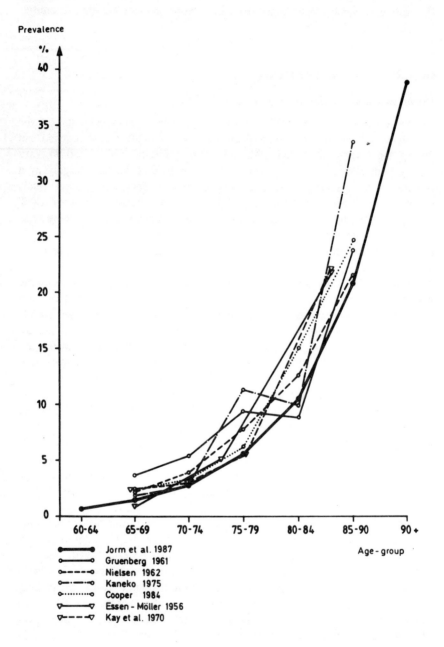

Table 18.1a Treated incidence of organic mental disorder in the elderly population, reported from hospital-census and case-register studies. Annual age-specific rates per 1,000 population

Author(s)	Survey area & period	Sample size	Age-group			
			60-69	70-79	80+	Total (60+)
Adelstein *et al.* 1968	Salford, UK, 1959-63	M 9,228 F 15,581	1.1 0.8	2.4 2.8	6.9 6.7	1.9 2.1
Akesson 1969	Swedish islands, 1964-7	M 2,071 F 2,127	0.3 1.2	4.8 3.6	8.6 13.7	2.6 3.5
Helgason 1977	Iceland, 1966-7	M 22,206 F 25,130	0.8 0.7	2.6 2.8	9.4 8.3	2.3 2.5
Mölsä *et al.* 1982[1,2]	Turku, Finland, 1966-76	M 6,378 F 13,104	0.8 1.4	4.0 7.7	15.6 21.0	1.9 4.1

[1] Age-groups 65-74; 75-84; 85+
[2] Nursing home and community nursing cases included

Table 18.1b Incidence of organic mental disorder (severe or moderately severe) in the elderly population, reported from area field surveys. Annual age-specific rates per 1,000 population

Author(s)	Survey area & period	Sample size[1] (persons aged over 60)	Age-group			
			60-69	70-79	80+	Total (60+)
Bergmann *et al.* 1971	Newcastle, UK (a) 1960-4; (b) 1964-7	760 (2,000)	–	–	–	15.0
Hagnell *et al.* 1981	'Lundby', Sweden, 1947-57	655 (4,224)	5.1	18.8	57.3	16.3
	dto. 1957-72	696 (7,959)	2.9	14.8	33.7	10.7
Nielsen *et al.* 1982	Samsø Island, Denmark 1972-7	1,564 (6,580)	2.8	22.7	34.6	12.0
Nilsson 1984	Gothenburg, Sweden 1971-81	364 (2,665)	–	16.2	–	–
Bickel and Cooper 1988	Mannheim, F.R.G. 1978-86[2]	314 (1,912)	4.8	12.2	34.1	17.8[3]

[1] Figures in brackets refer to numbers of 'person-years' at risk
[2] Age-groups 65-69; 70-79; 80+
[3] Total for age-group 65+

267

admitted to institutional care tend to be at a relatively advanced stage of the disease.

In tables 18.1a and 18.1b estimates of the incidence of dementia derived from hospital and case-register studies are juxtaposed to others reported from a number of area field surveys; all the studies were carried out in European countries. The rates for 'treated incidence' vary between 1.9 and 2.6 per 1,000 for men and between 2.1 and 4.1 per 1,000 for women, based on the age-range above 60 years. The true incidence on the other hand, as indicated by field-survey findings, is of the order of 10 to 16 per 1,000 for both sexes combined, or about four times as high as the treated rates. It need scarcely be added that analogous studies of populations which have fewer hospital facilities, e.g. in developing Third World countries, would reveal much bigger disparities. Both for aetiological research and in the estimation of service needs, therefore, community-based surveys must be regarded as indispensable.

Studies of incidence may help to throw light on the nature of the relationship between pre-senile and senile dementia. If these categories indeed represent different nosological entities, one would expect the corresponding age-specific incidence rates to show evidence of bimodality; whereas, if they are sub-groups of a single disease, separated only by an artificial age limit, a unimodal distribution could be anticipated. Incidence rates for pre-senile dementia are difficult to estimate with any accuracy, because cases are rare in the general population. Data from the Israeli National Register of Neurological Disease (Treves et al. 1986) permit treated incidence rates to be computed for the age-range 40–60 years, using this age group of the national population as the denominator. The rate for both sexes combined increases steeply with age, from 0.3 per 100,000 at 40–44 years to 5.8 per 100,000 at 55–59 years. If the age-related curve, which corresponds to a doubling in incidence rate with each three to four additional years of age, is extrapolated beyond 60 years, it conforms quite well to the estimates derived from hospital census and case-register studies in a number of other countries (Rocca et al. 1986). To this extent the empirical data provide support for the view that DAT is a single pathological process, and that age alone is unsatisfactory as a basis for division into specific sub-categories. The findings are, however, far from being definitive, because of the qualifications surrounding treated-case data.

Prediction of individual risk

Can descriptive surveys help towards achieving a better prediction of individual risk? The evidence for some degree of familial aggregation suggests that dementia does not strike randomly, but this in itself is not of much help in prediction. Prospectively designed cytogenetic and immunologic studies, which may eventually throw light on the question, are so far wanting. More immediate promise is offered by evidence that the cognitive performance of 'young-old' persons may be useful as a pointer in identifying those of them who, given survival into later old age, will become clinically demented. La Rue and Jarvik (1986) were able to examine this issue in their longitudinal study of elderly twins. Those subjects who developed the clinical features of dementia were found to have had lower mean scores than other persons on tests of cognition administered some twenty years earlier. The authors did not, however, calculate the positive predictive value of these tests.

More recently, a preliminary report from a community-based study has suggested independently that premorbid cognitive performance may be an important indicator of risk for dementia. Bickel and Cooper (1988), in an eight-year follow-up of a representative sample of old people in Mannheim, noted a raised incidence of dementing illness among those who, at the first interview, had manifested mild memory defects, though without functional disability at that time. Once the influence of subclinical deficits was partialled out by statistical analysis, age ceased to be of predictive significance: in other words, the risk appeared to be no greater for the aged than for the young-old, given the same standard of cognitive performance. Of thirty-four new cases of dementia developing in the follow-up period, fourteen had been rated initially as subclinically impaired in cognitive performance.

If this tentative finding is confirmed, the way may be open to an earlier identification of persons at high risk for dementia, and hence for secondary preventive measures. Whether the cognitive deficits should be regarded as early signs of an incipient dementing illness, or as premorbid attributes of the individual which increase his susceptibility to the disease, must remain for the present an open question.

ANALYTICAL EPIDEMIOLOGY: COMPARATIVE AND CONTROL STUDIES

Analytical epidemiology is a logical extension and development of the descriptive population survey. It proceeds by exploring differences in the occurrence of disease by person, time, and place, and relating these to the strength of exposure to suspected risk factors. Because of a dearth of suitable research, little is known as yet about differences in the incidence of dementia by time and place. The repeated field studies in 'Lundby' have suggested a possible decline in the frequency of senile dementia (Hagnell et al. 1983), while a direct comparison of samples of old people in London and New York, based on a standard interview technique, has indicated large disparities in this respect, which are unlikely to have a genetic explanation (Copeland and Gurland 1985); but these are both isolated findings, which await replication.

Leaving aside the possible significance of exotic neuropsychiatric disorders, such as kuru (Gajdusek 1977) and the Guam-Parkinsonism syndrome (Hirano et al. 1966), such epidemiological clues as we have to the aetiology of DAT have been derived from case-control studies, in which samples of clinically diagnosed cases have been matched with control groups drawn either from among other hospital patients, or from the local community, or both. Only a handful of such studies have been reported (Bharucha *et al.* 1983; Heyman *et al.* 1984; French *et al.* 1985; English and Cohen 1985; Amaducci *et al.* 1986), although others are currently in progress. This research strategy, while currently the most favoured by epidemiologists, presents formidable difficulties. Quite apart from the problems of differential diagnosis, already referred to, the degree of exposure to individual risk factors cannot as a rule be ascertained accurately. All the studies so far have had to employ a retrospective design, which is notoriously weak for aetiological inquiry, and especially so when the affected persons tend to be unreliable as informants about their own medical history and life course. While the research findings have pointed tentatively to a number of possible causal links, the nature and strength of associations vary from one study to another and, indeed, within a single study according to the type of control group used as a standard of comparison. Since the evidence has been ably reviewed by others (Rocca *et al.* 1986; Henderson 1987), only a brief resumé of the more promising causal hypotheses will be given here.

Genetic determinants

Though it is now generally accepted that genetic factors play some part in determining the incidence of DAT, their precise role and importance remain matters for debate. The earlier population-genetic studies reporting familial aggregation displayed serious faults of method and tended to exaggerate the excess of risk in affected families, in that they underestimated the frequency of dementing illness in the elderly population as a whole. The kind of large-scale twin study required to assess the strength of genetic determination poses great practical difficulties in the field of geriatric research. Hence the contribution of population-based studies to this question has been a modest one (Bergmann and Cooper 1986).

In view of recent progress in molecular biology, which has again thrown up the possibility of a major gene locus for DAT (Kang *et al.* 1987), there has been a recent renewal of interest in this field, and studies are now being undertaken which avoid at least some of the earlier methodological weaknesses.

A recent multi-centred case-control study in Italy (Amaducci *et al.* 1986) reported a significant increase in the frequency of dementing illness among the first- and second-degree relatives of patients with diagnosed DAT. The results are summarized in table 18.2. But this, like most genetically oriented inquiries, was focused primarily on pre-senile or early-onset dementing illness; i.e., on cases becoming manifest before the age of 70. That the age of onset may be of critical importance in this context is suggested by the widely cited findings of Heston and his co-workers (Heston *et al.* 1981).

Heston's study, based on a sample of cases confirmed at autopsy,

Table 18.2 Associations between DAT in probands and a family history of dementing illness: case-control comparisons

Affected family members	Relative risk (odds ratio)	
	Hospital-patient control-group	Community control-group
Mother	2.20	3.33*
Father	3.50	1.00
Siblings	11.00**	5.50*
First-degree relatives	5.00**	2.56*
First- or second-degree relatives	6.67***	3.44***

Source: Amaducci *et al.* (1986)
 * significant at 5% level
 ** significant at 1% level
*** significant at 0.1% level

demonstrated a familial predisposition among the siblings of early-onset dementia patients, who revealed an increased risk for dementing illness, especially when one or both parents had also manifested the condition. In cases of clinical dementia first apparent after the age of 70, no increase in morbid risk was detected among other family members. It appears that cases of early-onset dementia tend to cluster in certain families, possibly because the influence of a genetic or other risk factor to which they are exposed advances the age at which cognitive decline commences and accelerates its progress. Even of the early-onset cases in this study, however, three-fifths showed no evidence of familial aggregation. To what extent deviation from a Mendelian pattern of inheritance can be explained in terms of mortality (Folstein and Powell 1984) is not yet established.

The role of environmental toxins

A number of research findings have pointed to possible associations between DAT and exposure to a range of chemical products, including metallic salts, organic solvents, pesticides, and pharmaceutical products. For some time aluminium seemed a promising candidate, because of its implication in secondary dementia among patients on long-term haemodialytic treatment (Dunea *et al.* 1978). The neuropathology of this condition is, however, quite distinct from that of DAT and, moreover, after some fifteen years of research no firm evidence of a causal link has yet been identified. Although in case-control studies it has not been possible to measure directly the strength of exposure to aluminium, such indirect methods as assessment of the intake of aluminium-containing antacid preparations, as a palliative for peptic ulcer or chronic indigestion, have been employed without confirming the association.

The most challenging evidence to date for a possible toxic factor has

Figure 18.2 Cumulative risk of DAT among siblings of DAT patients

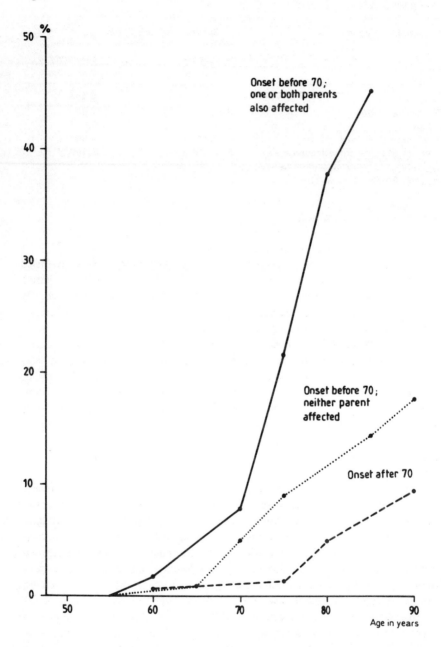

Source Heston et al. (1981)

Table 18.3 Associations between DAT and earlier viral infections: case-control studies

Authors	Relative risk (odds ratio)	Significance level
Heyman *et al.* 1984		
– Influenza		
(1918 pandemic)	3.65	NS
– Herpes zoster	3.33	NS
Amaducci *et al.* 1986		
– Encephalitis	1.00	NS
– Herpes zoster	0.62	NS

Table 18.4 Associations between DAT and reported contacts with animals: case-control comparisons

Type of animal	Relative risk (odds ratio)	
	Hospital-patient control-group	Community control-group
Dogs	2.83*	0.67
Cats	1.75	1.29
Cagebirds	0.87	0.68
Any kind of domestic animal	2.36**	0.95
Cattle	1.63	1.22
Game	1.00	1.25

Source: Amaducci *et al.* (1986)
 * significant at 5% level
** significant at 1% level

come, not from case-control studies but from investigation of the exotic neuropsychiatric syndromes which have been found in local endemic pockets. The Guam-Parkinsonism syndrome, in which some features of an Alzheimer-type pathological process are found, has long been suspected of having a dietary cause because of the steady fall in incidence which was observed as more and more foodstuffs were imported into Guam and other affected areas, replacing the traditional diet. Earlier causal hypotheses focused on an excess or deficiency of trace elements, but recently suspicion has also lighted on neuro-excitatory amino-acids found in a local plant from which formerly sago flour was extracted in large quantities (*Lancet* 1987). The relevance for dementia research of neurotoxic amino-acids found in various plant species seems destined to be a subject of increasing epidemiological scrutiny in the next decade.

The relevance of earlier viral infections

Demonstration of the transmissibility of kuru and Creutzfeld-Jakob disease sparked off a train of investigations of DAT, all of which have yielded negative findings (Corsellis 1986). Case-control studies have been used to test for a possible viral aetiology by estimating the relative frequency of earlier viral infections affecting the central nervous system. Apart from enquiries about meningitis, encephalitis, and Herpes zoster infection, such indirect evidence as a history of skin grafting, ingestion of animal brains, contact with animals, and travel in endemic areas has also been examined, but so far with no consistently positive results. The study by Amaducci and others (1986) reported some suggestive evidence of an association with exposure to domestic animals, especially dogs, which would seem to merit further inquiry, but this finding has yet to be replicated by other workers.

Dementia as an auto-immune disease

To place DAT in the broad category of auto-immune diseases postulates a pathogenetic process rather than an aetiology, and relegates empirical causal inquiry one stage further. Nevertheless, findings from the laboratory suggesting a source of immunoglobulins in the central nervous system (Williams *et al.* 1980) have stimulated epidemiologists to examine associations within families between DAT and diseases believed to be mediated by auto-immune reactions. Interest in this possibility was reinforced when an increase in myelo-proliferative disorders (lymphoma, lymphosarcoma, and Hodgkin's disease), and more generally of diseases considered to be 'related to the immune system' were reported to have a raised incidence among first-degree relatives of probands with DAT (Heston *et al.* 1981). However sound the underlying theoretical assumptions, this finding has not been confirmed by other workers and, moreover, no relative excess of allergies, asthma, or rheumatoid arthritis has been detected in the medical records of old people with DAT, as compared with controls (Heyman *et al.* 1984; French *et al.* 1985; Amaducci *et al.* 1986). The increased incidence of thyroid disease – a disorder also linked to the auto-immune system – noted by Heyman *et al.* (1984) in the medical records of DAT patients, also lacks confirmation from other studies. Once again we are confronted by intriguing but isolated findings, whose significance it is not yet possible to assess.

Head injury as a predisposing factor

Because of individual case reports, head injury has long been suspected as one possible risk factor of DAT. Studies of former professional boxers have confirmed the presence of Alzheimer-type changes, notably formation of neuro-fibrillary tangles, in persons with Dementia pugilistica whose mental deterioration may have begun many years after retirement from the ring (Corsellis *et al.* 1973). Inquiry after a history of earlier head injury, severe enough to cause loss of consciousness, has therefore been included in a

Table 18.5 Associations between DAT and a history of earlier head injury: case-control comparisons

Authors	Relative risk (odds ratio)	Significance level
Heyman *et al.* 1984	5.31	0.05
Mortimer *et al.* 1985		
– Patient control group	4.50	0.05
– Community control group	2.80	NS
Amaducci *et al.* 1986		
– Patient control group	3.50	NS
– Community control group	2.00	NS

number of case-control studies, but with no consistent findings. In the light of present evidence it seems improbable that a single episode of cerebral contusion in earlier life is often of aetiological significance, though severe or repeated trauma may be so. Few people are subjected to repeated head injury to an extent comparable to professional boxers, so that this particular risk factor is intrinsically implausible as a major determinant of the incidence of DAT in elderly populations.

Towards an integrated model: shared and cumulative effects

Attempts have not been wanting to combine the various hypotheses in a single aetiological and pathogenetic model. It has been postulated that a number of different risk factors may share some mediating pathogenetic effect in common. Thus, different noxae could pick out a *locus minoris resistentiae* in hippocampus or basal nuclei, leading to diffuse secondary degenerative changes in the neocortex (Ball *et al.* 1985). A biochemical abnormality, such as abnormal peroxidation with production of free oxygen radicals, could be the missing pathogenetic link if, as is suspected, this abnormality is present in the brain following a number of different kinds of insult (Henderson 1987). Such models must, however, be tested in the laboratory and have as yet no direct significance for epidemiological research.

More immediately relevant in this context is the notion of a clinical 'threshold' for dementia (Roth 1982), according to which the effect of earlier brain insults combines with age-related degenerative changes to overstep the line at which functional decompensation occurs and mental impairment becomes manifest. Earlier head injury, viral encephalitis, or exposure to one or more neurotoxins can all serve, according to this concept, to advance the point in time at which decompensation occurs. The dementing disorder then represents the end result, not of a single specific aetiology, but rather of a variety or combination of types of brain insult to which individuals are exposed over the life span. This of course does not preclude the possibility that in any given society one form of insult may predominate and act as the main determinant of incidence over prolonged periods of time, much as alcohol abuse has done with respect to hepatic cirrhosis.

Such a general model would help to explain the prolonged latent period that often elapses between exposure to a risk factor and the onset of clinical dementia, as well as the positive association between Alzheimer-type and cerebrovascular dementia, which is suggested by the relative frequency of mixed forms in the elderly population (Tomlinson *et al.* 1970). It has obvious implications for the methodology of case-control studies and for analytical epidemiology more generally.

STUDIES OF THE COURSE AND OUTCOME OF DEMENTING ILLNESS

Hospital-based studies

Our knowledge of the course and outcome of late-life mental disorders is remarkably limited, the firmest information being still that derived from the study of psychiatric hospital patients. This has consistently revealed a large excess of mortality in association with organic mental disorders (Bickel 1987). In particular, mortality among patients with a diagnosis of senile dementia is of the order of four times that for the elderly population as a whole. The recorded causes of death suggest a general tendency towards multi-morbidity, rather than specific associations with somatic disease.

Up to the 1960s, patients suffering from dementia had a mortality rate of around 50 per cent in the first six months following hospital admission. More recently the rate has fallen to around 30 per cent, while at the same time the proportion of patients discharged from hospital has increased. The trend towards an improved prognosis is, however, much less pronounced after two years, at which point in time the mortality rate is still above 60 per cent. The research findings summarized in figure 18.4 provide little indication of a significant increase in survival rates at this stage.

It must also be remembered that most hospital-based studies give no information concerning the fate of patients once they have been discharged from hospital care. Probably in a high proportion of cases no more than a change of institution, from hospital to geriatric home, is involved. In some countries a large-scale shift in the locus of care for mentally impaired old people has occurred within the past two or three decades, from clinical to non-clinical residential care (Jaeger 1987), a transition more readily explained in socio-political terms than by any real improvement in the outcome of illness.

Community-based studies of course and outcome

Anamnestic data suggest that dementing conditions have as a rule been clinically apparent for some years by the time the affected persons are

Figure 18.3 Outcome after six months, elderly psychiatric patients with organic mental disorders

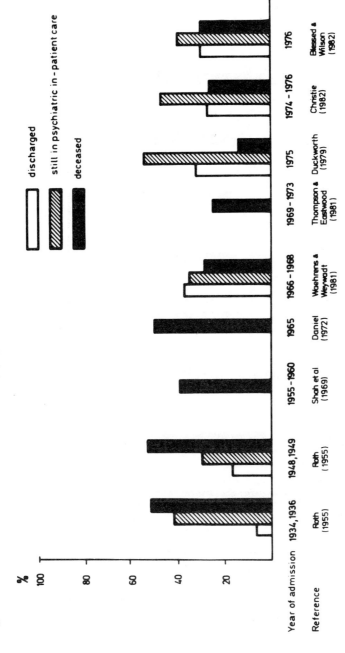

Source Bickel (1988)

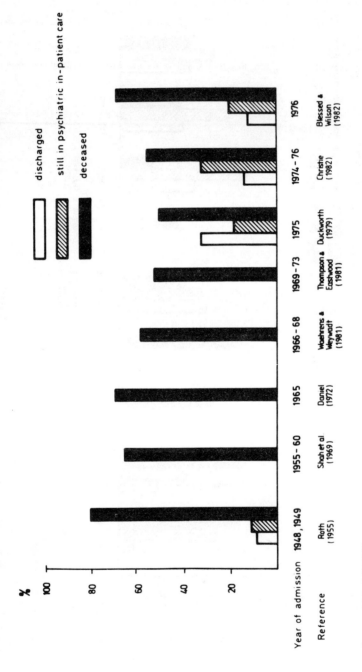

Figure 18.4 Outcome after two years, elderly psychiatric patients with organic mental disorders

☐ discharged

▨ still in psychiatric in-patient care

■ deceased

Year of admission 1948,1949 1955-60 1965 1966-68 1969-73 1975 1974-76 1976

Reference Roth (1955) Shah et al (1969) Daniel (1972) Waehrens & Weywadt (1981) Thompson & Eastwood (1981) Duckworth (1979) Christie (1982) Blessed & Wilson (1982)

Source Bickel (1988)

admitted to hospital care (Wang and Whanger 1971). Furthermore, it can be inferred from field-survey findings that most old people with dementia never enter psychiatric institutions (Bergmann and Cooper 1986). One would expect cases identified in the community to be on average clinically milder, or at an earlier stage of deterioration, than those studied in hospital. The few community-based longitudinal studies so far undertaken confirm that this is broadly the case, and lend some support to the view that there has been a limited improvement in medical prognosis in recent decades. Nevertheless, a diagnosis of organic mental disorder continues to have serious implications, in terms of mortality risk, admission to institutional care, and dependency on others.

These issues were examined in some detail in the recently completed longitudinal study of old people in Mannheim. After four years, the mortality rate among those with organic mental impairments was 46 per cent, compared with 20 per cent in the cohort as a whole (Bickel 1987). By means of an events-analytical technique, it was possible to estimate the influence of psychiatric status on the survival time, while holding constant other factors such as sex, age, and degree of physical impairment. The presence of an organic mental disorder was found to predict a reduction of 54 per cent in survival time, and that of functional mental illness a reduction of 47 per cent, once these other factors had been partialled out.

When the status of the elderly cohort was again reviewed after eight years, differences between the diagnostic groups emerged more clearly. By this time mortality among those with organic mental disorders was 81 per cent, compared with 42 per cent in the remainder of the sample. The findings of a survival analysis using the Kaplan-Meier method of estimation (Chase et al. 1983) are shown in figure 18.5. Persons initially diagnosed as having a 'functional' mental illness and those categorized as cases of 'mild dementia' shared a similar mortality curve in the earlier follow-up years, but the survival curves then diverged. The risk for the 'mild dementia' group began to approach that for the clinically demented, whereas that for the group with functional mental disorders approximated increasingly to the level of risk for the mentally normal group. Over the follow-up period as a whole, the mortality curves for organic and functional mental disorders differed markedly, underlining the importance of this basic diagnostic distinction in community surveys of the elderly.

Longitudinal studies of old people have shown a greatly increased frequency of long-stay institutional care among those with organic mental impairment (Bergmann 1977; Teresi et al. 1984; Campbell et al. 1985). While the findings in Mannheim were at first inspection broadly consistent with those of earlier studies, detailed analysis revealed a more complex picture. In order to control for the effects of age, physical health status, and differing survival times, a regression analysis was undertaken, which permitted simultaneous assessment of a number of independent variables in the

279

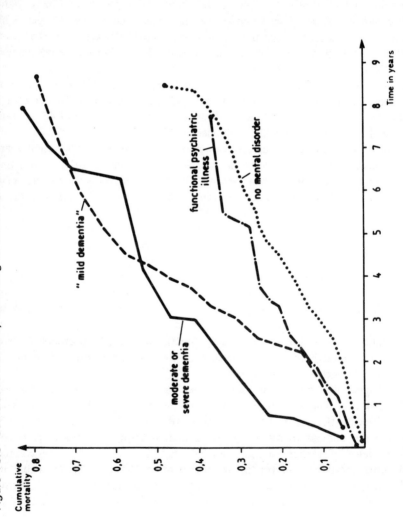

Figure 18.5 Cumulative mortality according to initial mental status (Kaplan-Meier estimation)

presence of 'censored' data (Allgulander and Fisher 1986). Against expectation, the initial diagnostic category was found to have no influence on the interval from first interview to geriatric home admission: this despite the fact that dementing disorders are found frequently among geriatric home residents and, indeed, are often the immediate reason for admission. A possible explanation is that old people with clinically manifest dementia are more likely to remain in the community if they have good family support. Provision of care by other members of the family, once commenced, tends to be continued for long periods. Hence the decision for or against institutional admission is often taken relatively early in the course of the illness. Cases of dementia identified in community surveys therefore tend to be found disproportionately among those old people who enjoy some measure of family support. This is a selective factor which should be borne in mind when interpreting the findings of cross-sectional surveys.

Table 18.6 Influence of selected predictor variables on the probability of geriatric home admission

Predictor variable	Coefficient[1]	Effect on rate of geriatric-home admission[2]
Each additional year of age	0.083** (0.029)	+8.6%
Onset of clinical dementia	1.825*** (0.345)	+520.0%
Admission to any hospital	1.322* (0.541)	+275.0%

[1] Standard errors shown in brackets
[2] Percentage increase or decrease for a unit change in each variable
  * significant at 5% level
  ** significant at 1% level
  *** significant at 0.1% level

In keeping with this hypothesis is the finding that occurrence of a new case of dementing illness increased the probability of admission to a geriatric home more than fivefold and appeared, indeed, to be the single most important determinant of the demand for institutional care (cf. table 18.6).

CONCLUSION

These research findings underline the need for a more systematic and intensive approach to the epidemiological aspects of late-life dementia, on two main grounds. First, it seems improbable that laboratory investigation alone can elucidate the nature of the causal nexus for a group of disorders which, on present evidence, must be to some extent environmentally determined. The causal research of recent years has been largely concentrated, as the above review indicates, on Alzheimer-type dementia. There are, however, no rational grounds for neglecting the cerebrovascular group of dementias, which in the short term may well afford greater opportunities for preventive action. The search for causes of both these broad disease-categories will call for prospectively planned longitudinal and case-control studies, and for an increasing emphasis on international collaborative projects.

Second, even if a major scientific breakthrough in neurobiological research can be anticipated within the next one or two decades – and this must still be regarded as an optimistic assumption (Besson 1986) – translation of the aetiological findings into large-scale therapeutic or preventive programmes, calling in all probability for a massive and sustained investment, could not be expected to yield rapid returns. World demographic projections leave no room for doubt that, over the next generation, the absolute numbers of cases of late-life dementia will continue to increase rapidly, or that the additional burden of disability and dependency will fall disproportionately on those poor developing countries of the Third World whose care facilities are least adequate to meet the growth in demand (Jablensky 1979; Kramer 1980). It is, therefore, vital to start planning ahead now for the next half-century, and epidemiological research can help to provide the necessary rational basis for doing so.

Acknowledgement: I am grateful to Dr Horst Bickel for much valuable assistance with the preparation of this review.

REFERENCES

Adelstein, A.M., Downham, D.Y., Stein, Z., and Susser, M. (1968) 'The epidemiology of mental illness in an English city', *Social Psychiatry* 3: 47–59.
Akesson, H.O. (1969) 'A population study of senile and arteriosclerotic psychosis', *Human Heredity* 19: 546–66.
Allgulander, C., and Fisher, L.B. (1986) 'Survival analysis (or time to an event analysis) and the Cox regression model: methods for longitudinal psychiatric research', *Acta Psychiatrica Scandinavica* 74: 529–35.
Amaducci, L.A., Fratiglioni, L., Rocca, W.A., *et al.* (1986) 'Risk factors for clinically diagnosed Alzheimer's disease: a case-control study of an Italian population', *Neurology* 36: 922–31.
American Psychiatric Association (1986) *Diagnostic and Statistical Manual of Mental Disorders*, third edition, Washington, DC: APA.
Ball, M.J., Hachinski, V., Fox, A., *et al.* (1986) 'A new definition of Alzheimer's disease: a hippocampal dementia', *Lancet* i: 14–16.

Bergmann, K. (1977) 'Prognosis in chronic brain failure', *Age and Ageing* 6 (supplement): 61-6.

Bergmann, K. and Cooper, B. (1986) 'Epidemiological and public health aspects of senile dementia', in A.B. Sørensen, F.E. Weinert, and L.R. Sherrod (eds) *Human Development and the Life Course: Multi-Disciplinary Perspectives*, Hillsdale, NJ: Erlbaum, 71-97.

Bergmann, K., Kay, D.W.K., Foster, E.M., *et al.* (1971) 'A follow-up study of randomly selected community residents to assess the effects of chronic brain syndrome and cerebrovascular disease', *Psychiatry II: Proceedings of the 5th World Congress of Psychiatry, Mexico*, Amsterdam: Excerpta Medica, 856-65.

Besson, J. (1983) 'Dementia: biological solution still a long way off', *British Medical Journal* 287: 926-7.

Bharucha, N.E., Schoenberg, B.S., and Kokmen, E. (1983) 'Dementia of Alzheimer's type (DAT): a case-control study of associations with medical conditions and surgical procedures', *Neurology* (NY, supplement 2) 33: 85.

Bickel, H. (1987) 'Psychiatric illness and mortality among the elderly: findings of an epidemiological study', in B. Cooper (ed.) *Psychiatric Epidemiology: Progress and Prospects*, London: Croom Helm, pp. 192-211.

Bickel, H. (1988) 'Verlauf und Ausgang psychischer Storungen im Alter', in R.K. Olbrich (ed.) *Prospektive Verlaufsforschung in der Psychiatrie*, Berlin: Springer, pp. 83-98.

Bickel, H. and Cooper, B. (1988, in press) 'Incidence of dementing disorders in an elderly population cohort', in B. Cooper and T. Helgason (eds) *Epidemiology and Prevention of Mental Disorders*, London: Routledge.

Blessed, G. and Wilson, I.D. (1982) 'The contemporary natural history of mental disorder in old age', *British Journal of Psychiatry* 141: 59-67.

Campbell, A.J., McCosh, L.M., Reinken, J., and Allan, B.C. (1983) 'Dementia in old age and the need for services', *Age and Ageing* 12: 11-16.

Chase, G.A., Folstein, M.F., Breitner, J.C.S., *et al.* (1983) 'The use of life-tables and survival analysis in testing genetic hypotheses, with an application to Alzheimer's disease', *American Journal of Epidemiology* 117: 590-7.

Christie, A.B. (1982) 'Changing patterns in mental illness in the elderly', *British Journal of Psychiatry* 140: 154-9.

Cooper, B (1984) 'Home and away; the disposition of mentally ill old people in an urban population', *Social Psychiatry* 19: 187-96.

Copeland, J.R.M. and Gurland, B.J. (1985) 'International comparative studies', in T Arie (ed.) *Recent Advances in Psychogeriatrics*, Edinburgh: Churchill Livingstone, pp. 175-95.

Corsellis, J.A.N. (1986) 'The transmissibility of dementia', *British Medical Bulletin* 42: 111-14.

Corsellis, J.A.N., Bruton, C.J., and Freeman-Browne, D. (1973) 'The aftermath of boxing', *Psychological Medicine* 3: 270-303.

Daniel, R. (1972) 'A 5-year study of 693 psychogeriatric admissions in Queensland', *Geriatrics* 27: 132-58.

Duckworth, G.S., Kedward, H.B., and Bailey, W.F. (1979) 'Prognosis of mental illness in old age: a four-year follow-up study', *Canadian Journal of Psychiatry* 24: 674-82.

Dunea, G., Mahurka, S.D., Mamdani, B., and Smith, E.C. (1978) 'Role of aluminium in dialysis dementia', *Annals of International Medicine* 88: 502-4.

English, D. and Cohen, D. (1985) 'A case-control study of maternal age in Alzheimer's disease', *Journal of the American Geriatric Society* 33: 167-9.

Essen-Möller, E. (1956) 'Individual traits and morbidity in Swedish rural population', *Acta Psychiatrica Scandinavica*, supplement 100.

Fenton, G.W. (1986) 'Electrophysiology of Alzheimer's disease', *British Medical Bulletin* 42 (1): 29–33.

Folstein, M.F. and Powell, D. (1984) 'Is Alzheimer's disease inherited? a methodological review', *Integrative Psychiatry* (September-October), Amsterdam: Elsevier, 163–70.

French, L.R., Schuman, L.M., Mortimer, J.A., *et al.* (1985) 'A case-control study of dementia of the Alzheimer type', *American Journal of Epidemiology* 121: 414–21.

Gajdusek, D.C. (1977) 'Unconventional viruses and the origin and disappearance of kuru', *Science* 197: 943–60.

Gruenberg, E.M. (1961) 'A mental health survey of older persons', in P.H. Hoch and J. Zubin (eds) *Comparative Epidemiology of the Mental disorders*, New York: Grune & Stratton, pp. 13–23.

Hagnell, P., Lanke, J., Rorsman, B., and Ojesjo, L. (1981) 'Does the incidence of age psychosis decrease? a prospective longitudinal study of a complete population investigated during the 25-year period 1947–1972: the Lundby study', *Neuropsychobiology* 7: 201–11.

Hagnell, O., Lanke, J., Rorsman, B., *et al.* (1983) 'Current trends in the incidence of senile and multi-infarct dementia', *Acta Psychiatrica Nervenkr* 233: 423–38.

Helgason, T. (1977) 'Psychiatric services and mental illness in Iceland', *Acta Psychiatrica Scandinavica*, supplement 268.

Henderson, A.S. (1988, in press) 'The aetiology of Alzheimer's disease: can epidemiology contribute?', in B. Cooper and T. Helgason (eds) *Epidemiology and Prevention of Mental Disorder*, London: Routledge.

Heston L.L., Mastri, A.R., Anderson, E., and White, J. (1981) 'Dementia of the Alzheimer type: clinical genetics, natural history and associated conditions', *Archives of General Psychiatry* 38: 1085–90.

Heyman, A., Wilkinson, W.E., Stafford, J.A., *et al.* (1984) 'Alzheimer's disease: a study of epidemiological aspects', *Annals of Neurology* 15: 335–41.

Hirano, A., Malamud, N., Elizan, T.S., Kurland, L.T. (1966) 'Amyotrophic lateral sclerosis and parkinsonism-dementia complex on Guam: further pathologic studies', *Arch. Neurol.* 15: 35–51.

Jablensky, A. (1979) 'Priorities for cross-cultural mental health research in old age', in World Health Organization *Psychogeriatric Care in the Community* (Public Health in Europe, 10), Copenhagen: WHO Regional Office for Europe, pp. 103–12.

Jaeger, J. (1986) 'Trends in der stationaren gerontopsychiatrischen Versorgung in der Bundesrepublik Deutschland', *Z. Gerontol.* 20: 187–94.

Jorm, A.F., Korten, A.E., and Henderson, A.S. (1987) 'The prevalence of dementia: a quantitative integration of the literature', submitted for publication.

Kaneko, Z. (1975) 'Care in Japan', in J.G. Howells (ed.) *Modern Perspectives in the Psychiatry of Old Age*, New York: Brunner Mazel, 519–39.

Kang, J., Lemaire, H.G., Unterbeck, A., *et al.* 'The precursor of Alzheimer's disease, amyloid A4 protein, resembles a cell-surface receptor', *Nature* 325: 733–6.

Kay, D.W.K., Bergmann, K., Foster, E.M., *et al.* (1970) 'Mental illness and hospital usage in the elderly: a random sample followed up', *Comprehensive Psychiatry* 11: 26–35.

Kramer, M. (1980) 'The rising pandemic of mental disorders and associated chronic diseases and disabilities', in E. Strömgren, A. Dupont, and J.A. Nielsen (eds) 'Epidemiological research as a basis for the organisation of extramural psychiatry', *Acta Psychiatrica Scandinavica*, supplement 285, 62: 382–97.

Lancet (1987) 'A poison tree', editorial, *Lancet* ii: 947–8.

La Rue, A. and Jarvik, L.F. (1986) 'Towards the prediction of dementias arising in the senium', in L. Erlenmeyer-Kimling and N.E. Miller (eds) *Life-Span Research on the Prediction of Psychopathology*, Hillsdale, NJ: Erlbaum, 261–74.

Liston, E.H. and La Rue, A. (1983) 'Clinical differentiation of primary degenerative and multi-infarct dementia: a critical review of the evidence: Part I: clinical studies', *Biological Psychiatry* 18: 1451–65.

McGreer, P.L. (1986) 'Brain imaging in Alzheimer's disease', in M. Roth and L.L. Iversen (eds) 'Alzheimer's disease and related disorders', *British Medical Bulletin* 42 (1): 24–28.

McKhann, G., Drachman, D., Folstein, M., et al. (1984) 'Clinical diagnosis of Alzheimer's disease: report of the NINCDS-ADRDA Work Group', *Neurology* 34: 939–44.

Mölsä, P.K., Marttila, R.J., and Rinne, U.K. (1982) 'Epidemiology of dementia in a Finnish population', *Acta Neurologica Scandinavica* 65: 541–52.

Mortimer, J.A., French, L.R., Hutton, J.T., and Schuman, L.M. (1985) 'Head injury as a risk factor for Alzheimer's disease', *Neurology* (Cleveland) 35: 264–7.

Nielsen, J. (1962) 'Gerontopsychiatric period-prevalence investigation in a geographically delimited population', *Acta Psychiatrica Scandinavica* 38: 307–30.

Nielsen, J.A., Biörn-Henriksen, T., and Bork, B.R. (1982) 'Incidence and disease expectancy for senile and arteriosclerotic dementia in a geographically delimited Danish rural population', in G. Magnussen, J. Nielsen, and J. Buch (eds) *Epidemiology and Prevention of Mental Illness in Old Age*, Hellerup, Denmark: EGV.

Nilsson, L.V. (1984) 'Incidence of severe dementia in an urban sample followed up from 70 to 79 years of age', *Acta Psychiatrica Scandinavica* 70: 478–86.

Rocca, W.A., Amaducci, L.A., and Schoenberg, B.S. (1986) 'Epidemiology of clinically diagnosed Alzheimer's disease' *Annals of Neurology* 19: 415–24.

Roth, M. (1955) 'The natural history of mental disorder in old age', *Journal of Mental Sciences* 102: 281–301.

Roth, M. (1982) 'Some strategies for tackling the problems of senile dementia and related disorders within the next decade', WHO Working Paper IRP/ADR 117 (01)/6, unpublished.

Shah, K.V., Banks, G.D., and Merskey, H. (1969) 'Survival in atherosclerotic and senile dementia', *British Journal of Psychiatry* 115: 1283–6.

Teresi, J.A., Golden, R.R., and Gurland, B.J. (1984) 'Concurrent and predictive validity of indicator scales developed for the Comprehensive Assessment and Referral Evaluation Interview Schedule', *Journal of Geronotology* 39: 158–65.

Thompson, E.G. and Eastwood, M.R. (1981) 'Survival rates and causes of death in geriatric psychiatric patients', *Canadian Psychiatric Association Journal* 17: 17–22.

Tomlinson, B.E., Blessed, G., and Roth, M. (1970) 'Observations on the brains of demented old people', *Journal of Neurological Science* 11: 205–42.

Treves, T., Korczyn, A., Zilber, N., et al. (1986) 'Presenile dementia in Israel', *Arch. Neurologica* 43: 26–9..

Waehrens, J. and Weywadt, B. (1982) 'Prognosen for förstegangsindlagte geronto-psykiatriske patienter', in G. Magnussen, J. Nielsen, and J. Buch (eds) *Epidemiology and Prevention of Mental Illness in Old Age*, Hellerup, Denmark: EGV, 81–3.

Wang, J.A. and Whanger, A. (1971) 'Brain impairment and longevity', in E. Palmore and F.L. Jeffers (eds) *Prediction of Life Span*, Lexington, Mass.: Heath, 95–101.

Williams, A., Papadopoulos, N., and Chase, T.N. (1980) 'Demonstration of CSF gamma-globulin banding in senile dementia', *Neurology* 30: 882–4.

World Health Organization (1987) Chapter V (F) on mental, behavioural and developmental disorders, in *Tenth Revision of the International Classification of Diseases*, draft for field trials, Geneva: WHO.

19

Women and Mental Illness

Rachel Jenkins and Anthony Clare

One of the more consistent findings of epidemiological research is that women report symptoms of both physical and mental illness and utilize physicians and hospital services at higher rates than men. This chapter sets out to explore this phenomenon, in relation to mental illness, from a detailed examination of the current epidemiological evidence in the light of potential explanations of the sex differences.

Sex differences in morbidity and mortality have attracted considerable attention for several centuries. In the seventeenth century, John Graunt, the founder of demography, noted that, while women attend doctors more frequently than do men, their life expectancy is no less than that of men. Graunt took the view that either women were generally cured by their physicians or that the men suffered from untreated morbidity (Graunt 1667). This paradox between apparent morbidity and actual mortality still exists today, and is illustrated in table 19.1 with figures from current UK sources.

Is the apparent excess of women's mental illness more artefactual rather than real? Is it due to social and environmental pressures or is it inherent in biology? If biological, is it hormonal and as closely linked to women's reproductive systems as has so long been assumed? It behoves us to examine the evidence carefully.

EVIDENCE FOR SEX DIFFERENCES IN AFFECTIVE DISORDERS

Sex differences in hospital admissions

Among the statistics reviewed by Weissman and Klerman (1979) for treated cases of depression, western countries such as the United States and England report higher rates of treated depression in women than in men. This accords with the figures in table 19.2 for episodes of psychoneuroses and affective psychoses treated in England in 1982.

However, Weissman and Klerman note exceptions in studies arising from several developing countries such as India, Iraq, New Guinea, and Rhodesia,

Table 19.1 A comparison of life expectancy, certified sickness absence and use of health services for all disorders (physical and mental)

	Males	Females
Life expectancy[1] (years at age 0) England and Wales 1983–5	71.8	77.6
Hospital discharges[2] (rates per 1,000) England and Wales 1985	101	110
Persons making use of out-patient[3] facilities (rates per 1,000) GB 1984 in 3 months reference period	130	130
Persons making physician[4] visits in a 14-day reference period (rates per 1,000) GB 1984	110	150
% of persons consulting a doctor[5] in last 14 days who obtained a prescription from the doctor GB 1984	74%	74%
% of persons absent from work[6] because of sickness in a 7 day reference period GB 1984	4.5%	5.1%

[1] *Health and Personal Social Services Statistics for England 1987*, p. 14
[2] *Health and Personal Social Services Statistics for England 1987*, p. 74
[3] *General Household Survey*, p. 135
[4] *General Household Survey*, p. 139
[5] *General Household Survey*, p. 140
[6] Central Statistical Office (1988) *Social Trends 18*, London: HMSO: 74.

where rates are either equal in men and women, or higher in men. Two further exceptions have been reported by Haavio Manilla (1976) and Ananth (1978) for Finland and India respectively. Thus, it seems that the sex ratio of treatment indices for depression and the psychoneuroses is not an invariable finding but one that varies from culture to culture. A female excess of treated cases is usually although not always found in western countries, but not always found in studies of developing countries.

Sex differences in general practice consultations

The evidence from both national and primary care surveys in the US supports the view that women seek help from doctors at a greater rate than men (Gurin, *et al.* 1960: Dohrenwend and Dohrenwend 1976; Horowitz 1977; Veroff 1981). Data for the UK may be obtained from the Third National Morbidity Survey of General Practice (see table 19.3 OPCS 1987).

It can be seen that general practitioners, taken as a whole, record more consultations in women than in men for 'all diseases and conditions', 'all mental disorders', and for the psychoneuroses. General practitioners also record more episodes of these conditions in women than in men but this does not account for the excess consultation rate in women for the psychoneuroses,

288

Table 19.2 Comparison of recorded episode rates of psychiatric illness in general practice and admission rates to psychiatric hospitals for the year 1982 in men and women (rates quoted per 100,000 population England and Wales)

ICD category	Episode rate recorded in general practice		All psychiatric admissions	
	M	F	M	F
All mental disorders 290–319	5,540	11,270	330	451
Senile and presenile dementia 290	10	30	27	46
Organic psychosis 291	10	10	2	1
Schizophrenia, schizoaffective and paranoid states 295–297	170	210	60	58
Affective psychosis 296	140	280	32	67
Other, and unspecified psychoses 292–4, 298, 299	60	100	24	35
Psychoneuroses 300	3,210	8,390	25	51
Personality disorders and sexual deviation 301–2, 307–9, 312–5	260	250	29	33
Alcoholism and drug dependency 303–4	260	140	17	41
Other psychiatric conditions 306, 310, 316	1,750	3,450	1	1
Mental retardation 317–9	40	40	1	1

where women consult, on average, 4.3 times per illness episode, compared with a rate of 2.5 times per illness episode for men. There is no particular sex difference in the average number of consultations per episode for 'all diseases and conditions' or for 'all mental disorders'.

Sex differences in prescriptions

Examining data from the General Household Survey (OPCS 1985), more women than men report taking prescribed medication, but there is no sex difference in the percentage of persons consulting a doctor who obtained a prescription from the doctor (see table 19.1).

Where psychotropic drugs are considered, women are higher users than

Table 19.3 A comparison of certified sickness absence and use of health services for mental disorders in men and women

		Males	*Females*
Hospital admissions per[1] 100,000 background population England and Wales		364	482
General practice episode rates[2] per 100,000 population England and Wales 1981–2		3,540	11,270
Certified incapacity[3] for mental	days	292,000	198,000
disorder 1985	spells	4,512	3,877

[1] *Health and Personal Social Services Statistics, 1987*, p. 130
[2] *Morbidity Statistics from General Practice – Third National Morbidity Survey 1987*, p. 196
[3] Personal communication, Robert Chew, OHE, 1987
Not all employed women are contributing to national insurance and hence included in the DHSS incapacity figures

men (Parrish 1971) and this holds across all age groups (Murray *et al.* 1981). This topic is dealt with in the chapter by Williams and Gabe elsewhere in this book.

Sex differences in community surveys

Rates of treated illness are underestimates of rates of illness in the general population since they are affected by individuals' readiness to recognize illness in themselves and to seek medical care for their symptoms, by the availability of medical services, by the primary care physician's ability to diagnose illness and treat it, and to refer on to the specialist service if necessary (Goldberg and Huxley 1980). In order to further our research into sex differences in depression it is important to look at community studies where it is hoped that the sex-biasing effects of the different filters into medical care should cease to influence reported rates of illness. However, close examination of the methodology of reported community studies shows that this is not always the case. For example, some 'community' studies actually ascertain prevalence rates from counts of individuals reported by all the primary care physicians in a given area (Sorenson and Strömgren 1961), or by the case reports of individuals in a given area (Weeke *et al.* 1975). It is readily apparent that such rates are affected by the readiness to acknowledge symptomatology in oneself and to seek medical care, and the readiness of the physician to recognize illness and act upon it by referral to specialist institutions, and the ease with which the individual may be admitted to in-patient care.

Jenkins (1983, 1985) has reviewed community surveys for the US, UK, Australia, and the developing countries from a methodological standpoint, in relation to sex differences, and found that those studies with adequate sampling, appropriate case-finding techniques, adequate data on the characteristics of respondents and the reasons for non-response do not provide nearly such a clear picture of excessive depression in women. Comstock and Helsing (1976) found a sex difference in whites but not in blacks; Linn *et al.* (1979) in a survey of elderly whites found no sex differences at all. Finlay-Jones and Burvill (1977) found no sex differences in adults aged from 30 to 39, persons born in Britain and emigrated to Australia, and in married persons in social class V. Bash and Bash-Liechti (1969, 1974) found a sex difference in urban areas but not among the rural population in Iraq; Dube and Kumar (1973) found that mental illness was more frequent in females in rural areas, but predominated in males in urban areas. In the rural areas, the female excess was almost entirely due to the category of hysteria, found largely among the uneducated. Orley and Wing (1979) found no sex differences in overall psychiatric morbidity nor in depression among Ugandan villagers. Bebbington *et al.* (1981) did find a sex difference in Camberwell.

Sex differences in surveys of homogeneous populations

Parker (1979) and Jenkins (1983, 1985) have pointed out the methodological significance of choosing a homogeneous sample of men and women to examine sex differences in prevalence of depression. If social variables are controlled or reduced and no sex difference is found in a homogeneous sample then one must consider the possibility that those social factors account for the sex differences found by other workers in non-homogeneous samples.

Parker (1979) reported a study of 242 students undertaking the one-year postgraduate Diploma of Education at Sydney Teachers' College. The sexes were equally represented and the response rate was high. No sex difference was found on the measures of trait depression, self-esteem, duration of episodes, or frequency of depressive episodes. This study provides support for the findings of two other comparable groups. Golin and Hartz (1977) gave the Beck Depressive Inventory to 446 college students and found that 25 per cent of the males and 25 per cent of the females scored as depressed. Hammen and Padesky (1977) also gave the Beck Depression Inventory to 2,272 male and female college students enrolled in introductory psychology courses. No sex differences were found in the degree of depression experienced by students.

It is important to assess how far groups of university students form homogeneous groups suitable for examining sex differences in prevalence. First, homogeneity is probably not achieved within some specialities, such as medicine where, until recently, fewer women were accepted into training than men. Second, the age range found amongst university students is predominantly 18–21, which is not the age group where sex differences are usually reported, but rather in the age group 25–44. Thus, there is still a need to seek and study homogeneous groups older than university students.

291

Third, there is evidence that students are exposed to special risk in that their suicide rate is many times that for the equivalent age group in the general population (Carpenter 1959). The risk of being exposed to the competitive and demanding world of higher education may differ between the two sexes (Horner 1972).

It is interesting at this stage to look briefly at sex differences in psychiatric illness in children. The Isle of Wight studies formed a useful source of data for this purpose (Rutter et al. 1976). In the age group of 10 to 12-year-olds, the researchers found that emotional disorders were slightly more common in girls, while conduct disorders were very much commoner in boys. No sex difference in outcome existed. In the age group of 14 to 15, emotional disorders were equally common in the two sexes, while males exhibited a much higher risk of conduct disorders, resulting in the overall prevalence of psychiatric disorder being twice as common in boys as in girls (Graham and Rutter 1973).

Unfortunately, many so-called surveys of homogeneous populations are, in fact, surveys of primary care attenders. Therefore, they are not suitable for prevalence estimates since they are affected by readiness to consult doctors, which differs between the two sexes (Hinkle et al. 1960; Kidd et al. 1966; O'Mahoney and O'Brien 1980). In addition, close scrutiny reveals that some are not in fact homogeneous for occupation or marital status (e.g. Hinkle's (1960) study of female telephone operators and male craftsmen). In others, the two sexes occur in differing proportions and, therefore, perhaps under different environmental constraints (e.g. Farmer and Harvey's (1975) survey of medical students). Here it is interesting to note that Lloyd and Gartrell (1981) found no initial sex difference in adjustment in first-year medical students, but sex differences were found by mid-year and at the end of the first year. Those surveys which come closer to satisfying the criterion of homogeneity and which survey the base population rather than those who consult medical services are not able to demonstrate any sex difference in the prevalence of depression (Golin and Hartz 1977; Hammen and Padesky 1977; Parker 1979). Studies of schoolchildren provide further evidence of no overall sex differences in the prevalence of psychiatric disorder (Rutter et al. 1976). There is a notable shortage of adequate surveys of homogeneous populations in the age groups over 25, probably at least partly due to the lack of occupations in western countries without some degree of sexual differentiation by task, grade, or pay.

It was in order to fill this gap that Jenkins carried out a study of a homogeneous population, selected to minimise occupational, social and role differences between the sexes (Jenkins, 1983, 1985). This study, of executive officers aged 20–35 in the Civil Service, found no significant sex difference in the prevalence of minor psychiatric morbidity, its symptom profile, or its outcome after twelve months, in a relatively homogeneous group of men and women of similar age, education, and occupation, and subject to similar levels of social stress and support. These findings are of interest because they suggest that there can be little or no overall contribution from biological factors or from sex differences in upbringing to the commonly reported excess of depression in women, since, if there were such a contribution, an excess of depression in women would be visible even in homogeneous populations. Therefore, there is a need for studies of the homogeneous populations, both in older age groups, and in different social settings to see if these findings are replicated. Any such study should measure the degree of heterogeneity remaining in relevant environmental and personal variables, so that it is possible to make comparisons between studies.

EXPLANATIONS OF REPORTED SEX DIFFERENCES

Constitutional

Genetic theories. While there is little doubt that there is a significant genetic contribution to the aetiology of major affective disorders (Price 1968; Gershon *et al.* 1971; Rosenthal 1971), the evidence concerning the genetic contribution to neurotic affective disorders is conflicting. Here, twin studies reveal divergent results which may in part be due to differences in selection procedures applied to twin pairs. Early studies were often based on samples drawn from a single hospital or consisting of twins detected in an uncontrolled way. Shields and Slater (1971) found a concordance rate which was almost three times higher in monozygotic (MZ) than in dizygotic (DZ) twin pairs (40 per cent v. 15 per cent). Schepank (1973) summed the results of thirteen studies, finding a concordance rate in MZ twins more than double that of DZ twins (59 per cent v. 28 per cent). Torgersen (1983), recognizing the importance of using a complete nationwide sample of neurotic twin patients, examined all twins admitted to any in-patient or out-patient psychiatric institution in Norway for a diagnosis of neurosis, and their co-twins.

He analysed his data separately for anxiety and depressive neuroses, and found a proband concordance rate for neurotic depression of 21 per cent in MZ twins and 27 per cent in DZ twins, indicating no genetic contribution to depressive neurosis.

Despite these persuasive findings that heredity does not contribute to non-hospitalized depressive neurosis, it has nonetheless been suggested that either X-linkage or autosomal inheritance with sex-related liability thresholds accounts for the female preponderance of depressive illness in general. For X-linkage to explain the usual male-female differences in community studies one would have to postulate a dominant X-linkage gene which produced liability to non-psychotic depression and which played a role in the majority of minor depressions affecting women (i.e. it would be a common gene). The evidence is against this because even in bipolar affective illness, X-linkage,

293

if it exists, is responsible for only a small proportion of genetic depressions (Gershon and Bunney 1976), and there is no evidence of X-linkage in unipolar mild depressions. The hypothesis of autosomal linkage with sex-related liability thresholds receives no support from the reported data for bipolar illness or unipolar illness. Autosomal linkage remains the most likely hypothesis for depressive psychosis, but not with sex-related thresholds. Again, there is no evidence for autosomal linkage in unipolar mild depression. Indeed, there is no evidence that heredity has a major effect on depression in non-psychotic female psychiatric patients. Since non-patient samples are less severe, there is even less chance of heredity playing a major role here.

The evidence from genetic studies indicates that the influence of sex on liability to affective disorders is therefore likely to be environmental rather than genetic.

Hormone theories. Sex differences in hormones have been invoked to explain behavioural and psychological differences between men and women. Frankenhauser and her colleagues have examined the physiological and psychological response to stress in men and women (Frankenhauser *et al.* 1976, 1978). They demonstrated that females are less prone than males to respond with increased adrenaline release and with increased cortisol release when exposed to various challenging and demanding influences in the psychological and social environment such as a matriculation examination. Despite both sexes performing equally well in the examination, the females reported more intense negative feelings than did the males and none of the sense of success and satisfaction that was a rather common feeling among the males. These results suggest an interesting potential mechanism whereby, under stress, women may perform as well as men, yet nonetheless experience worse self-esteem.

While these studies have succeeded in correlating catecholamine metabolite levels with a measure of self-esteem under stress conditions in men and women, no studies have yet succeeded in definitely correlating clinical state in men and women with levels of gonadal hormones (Weissman and Klerman 1979). The evidence that mood changes may be caused by cyclical changes in female hormones therefore remains circumstantial, from observations that depression tends to occur in association with events in the female reproductive cycle, including menstruation, use of contraceptive drugs, childbirth, and the menopause.

There is strong evidence of an increase in depression in the post-partum period, although the evidence that the hormonal and other metabolic changes taking place during and after childbirth in women who develop either mild mood disturbances or fully fledged psychoses are any different from those of normal women is weak and inconclusive (Nott *et al.* 1976; Ballinger *et al.* 1979; Handley *et al.* 1980). However, there remain a number of potent circumstantial arguments that hormonal and other metabolic changes may be important in puerperal illness, which were recently summarized by Kendall *et al.* (1981).

The menopause is not associated with an increased risk of depression (Green and Cook 1980) and the balance of evidence at the present time suggests that where depression does occur at the time of the menopause, environmental factors are still more important in its aetiology than the menopause itself (Slater and Roth, 1969; Ballinger 1975, 1976; Green and Cook 1980). There is evidence that premenstrual tension is associated with depression, but the evidence relating this association to specific hormonal changes remains conflicting (Clare 1980).

Environmental explanations of the reported sex differences in minor psychiatric morbidity. Research on mental illness in the community has provided evidence that life events, such as the death of a spouse or job loss, and chronic social stresses, such as financial hardship, social isolation, migration, and low social class, are implicated in the aetiology of depression (Dohrenwend and Dohrenwend 1974; Liem and Liem 1978). Furthermore, social supports may ameliorate or buffer the effect of social stresses (Cobb 1976; Gore 1978) on health and reduce the liability to depression. It has been argued that women, by virtue of the roles they occupy, experience more life events and chronic social stresses, and less social support than men, and that this differential exposure to risk factors explains women's greater vulnerability to depression.

Social stress. The empirical data available so far suggest that there is no difference in the rates at which men and women experience acute life events or adversity (Myers *et al.* 1971; Dekker and Webb 1974; Newman 1975; Henderson *et al.* 1980). However, the possibility remains to be tested that women in general may experience more undesirable life events by virtue of their lower socio-economic status overall (Myers *et al.* 1975), since there is much evidence that women still have less overall status than men, both at home and at work, and frequently earn less even when in comparable jobs (General Household Survey 1987). There is no evidence that life events have more impact on women than men (Paykel *et al.* 1971: Personn 1980). However, there is evidence that women experience more chronic social stress than men. Radloff and Rae (1979) reported that women were more exposed than men to low education, low income, low occupational status, fewer leisure activities, and more current and recent physical illness.

Social supports. There are few studies which specifically address the question of whether women experience less social support than men. Miller and Ingham (1976) found that casual, less intimate friends as well as intimates afforded protection from developing illness, and that 'Psychological symptom

295

levels probably vary with social support even when there is no serious life event present'. It is, therefore, apparent that contacts with colleagues at work may also be supportive to the individual, and it may be that the housewife experiences relative isolation in the home, having less frequent daily verbal exchanges with other individuals than does her counterpart in the office.

Henderson *et al.* (1979) found that males reported more availability of social integration than females, while females scored higher on the quality or adequacy of the social integration. Females scored more availability of attachment than males, but there was no sex difference on the quality or adequacy of the attachment. It was the authors' view that special attention should be paid to those social bonds which promote self-esteem – both the esteem of self in terms of appearance, abilities, competence, and position in a dominance hierarchy, as well as the degree to which one believes one is lovable by others. The question is, therefore, whether such self-esteem is more likely to be derived from a close intimate attachment or the more loose social integration within a group. The esteem of self in terms of appearance, abilities, competence, and position are probably more likely to be derived from social integration within a group, while the extent to which one believes one is lovable by others may be obtained from both kinds of social bond. If the important attributes of self-esteem are more likely to be derived from social integration, then Henderson's finding, that males reported quantitatively more availability of social integration than females, may be of crucial significance to the question of whether women experience less social support than men. While females report a better quality of social integration, in terms of self-esteem thus engendered, quality may not make up for quantity. Henderson found that for minor psychiatric morbidity social integration has a stronger association with symptom level than does attachment for women. For men, the strength of the association of symptom level with social integration and with attachment was the same. Henderson concluded that 'social bonds appear to be related to morbidity in a manner independent of the challenge of adversity'. While these primary questions afford some hope of elucidating the nature of the sex difference in prevalence of minor psychiatric morbidity, it is clear that as yet little research attention has focused on them and further work is required. In the meantime, the evidence suggests that women in general do experience more chronic social stresses – such as lower occupational status and lower income – than men, and women also experience less availability of social integration – a factor with a strong negative association with minor psychiatric morbidity.

Sex roles. Some considerable attention has been paid in the literature to the elaboration of complex hypotheses, based upon interpretations of western sex roles, which are intended to provide explanations for women's greater prevalence of reported mental illness. Sex role hypotheses have proved difficult to test convincingly and this may be attributed partly to their inadequate specification and partly to the lack of directly measurable social indicators which might be used to assess their explanatory power.

Interaction with constitution. It has been suggested that sex differences in the early upbringing and social environment of males and females place a permanent stamp on the phenotype of the individual, thus affecting constitutional vulnerability to psychiatric illness in adult life (Chesler 1971, 1972; Chodorow 1974). The learned helplessness model proposes that helplessness is the salient characteristic of depression and that it results from learning that one's actions do not produce predictable responses (Seligman 1975). Cochrane and Stopes-Roe (1980) argue that girls are traditionally more sheltered than boys, women have less initiative in selecting their spouses than do men, their life styles face more disruption with the advent of children, and they have to follow their husbands geographically and socially. This relatively low ability to influence their environment may make females more prone to 'learned helplessness' than males.

Evidence certainly exists to support the notion of sex stereotypic belief about male and female abilities (Williams and Best 1982), and also supports the view that such stereotypes are influential in the development of male and female abilities (Rheingold and Cook 1975). There is some evidence that stereotypic female abilities encourage low self-esteem, but how far this phenomenon accounts for the reported sex differences in illness rate has yet to be assessed.

Interaction with environment. Regardless of the influence of early environment, it has been suggested that sex differences in adult sex roles lead to men and women being differentially exposed to environmental risk factors. Gove (1972) argues that if women are biologically more susceptible to mental illness than men, we would expect women to have higher rates of mental illness in each marital category. His literature review concluded that married women do indeed have higher rates than married men, but single women, the divorced, and the widowed do not have higher rates than their male counterparts – indeed the reverse is true. Gove asserts that a role explanation accounts for these discrepancies. Being married is presumed to be a less stressful and more satisfying experience for men than for women in western society where traditionally the women works for the husband, and does the housework, and looks after the children for him, while the man goes out to work, associates with colleagues, and earns money. Even if the married woman does work it is often in an intrinsically unsatisfying job. More recent workers have recognized that the experience of marriage may differ among groups of different educational attainments and social expectations, and have investigated the effects of such factors as social isolation, poverty, and the presence of children. These more searching studies have established that the relationship of marital status to psychiatric illness is complex, and differs

297

among groups of different educational attainments and social expectations, with social isolation, poverty, and the presence of children being important complicating factors (Meile *et al.* 1976; Pearlin and Johnson 1977; Cochrane and Stopes-Roe 1980).

Two opposing views are to be found in the literature. The first is that employment in women increases their role obligations (since they usually still retain their home-making tasks in addition to their paid employment), and that this may cause overload which predisposes the women to more ill-health than housewives. The other view is that employment increases affiliation and this extra social support is protective against morbidity. In addition, the extra role obligations make it less likely that such employed women will adopt a sick role.

Thus, while some studies find clear health advantages in employed women versus unemployed women (Cumming *et al.* 1975; Mostow and Newberry 1975; Nathanson 1980), such studies find that the relationship of employment status with psychiatric disorder is complicated by other factors such as duration of employment (Waldron 1976; Welch and Booth 1977), and the presence or absence of a confidante (Brown and Harris 1978).

Effect on reporting behaviour and diagnostic habits. This section examines the extent to which sex roles and sex stereotypes influence the illness behaviour of men and women, and the diagnostic habits of physicians. Four major hypotheses are examined. First, it has been suggested that women's traditional sex role as home-maker is more compatible with adoption of the sick role (visiting a doctor, taking medication, spending time in bed) than is men's traditional sex role as bread-winner (Mechanic 1965; Glaser 1970). There is vigorous opposition to this view. Parsons and Fox (1952) suggest that the nature of a woman's household and family responsibility make her illness more disturbing to family equilibrium than illness in her husband. Marcus and Seeman (1981) examined data from the Los Angeles Health Survey and demonstrated that role obligations do explain male/female differences in illness behaviour but not in illness *per se.*

Second, it has been suggested that differences in sex stereotypes result in men and women being socialized into different patterns of perception of illness and help-seeking behaviour based on those stereotypes (Mechanic 1964). There is speculation that women more readily translate diffuse feelings of psychological distress into conscious recognition of themselves as having emotional problems (Verbrugge 1979).

Several studies have suggested that it is culturally acceptable for women to be expressive about their difficulties while men are expected to bear their problems with greater self-control and to be reluctant to admit symptoms of distress (Komarovsky 1946; Phillip and Segal 1969; Cooperstock 1971). Psychological studies have indicated that women are more likely than men to disclose intimate information about themselves, especially unpleasant feelings such as anxieties and worries (Horowitz 1977; Briscoe 1982).

Jenkins, exploring several different aspects of illness behaviour in relation to minor psychiatric morbidity, reported that women without minor psychiatric morbidity have higher self-assessment of ill-health scores, a higher frequency of general practitioner consultations in the preceding twelve months, and take more sickness absence than do men without minor psychiatric morbidity (Jenkins 1985). There was no particular sex difference in prescribed medication or in 'over the counter' drug consumption in individuals without minor psychiatric morbidity. Increasing severity of psychiatric clinical state is associated with a greater increase in self-assessment of ill-health score, frequency of GP consultations, consumption of prescribed medication, and frequency and duration of sickness absence in men than in women. Thus it appears that women's illness behaviour may be less closely linked to the severity of their symptoms than is men's illness behaviour. It is as if men's illness behaviour is more 'realistic' than that of women. This may relate to the different socialization patterns of men and women and to their different tendencies to express their emotional difficulties (Briscoe 1982).

Third, it has been suggested that, because sex stereotypes exist, the social consequences of expression of symptoms differs between the sexes. Phillips (1964) presented subjects with descriptions of behaviour in which the disturbed individual was described as either a male or female. He found that men were rejected more than women for descriptions of the same behaviour. Phillips argues on the basis of his study that illness is stigmatizing for men but not so for women, and that, therefore, women are more willing to report symptoms in interview and are more likely to seek professional help for them. Unfortunately, although the majority of doctors are male, Phillips used only women as raters. These findings have received support from the studies of Broverman et al. (1970), Coie et al. (1974) and Hammen and Peters (1977), although Yamamoto and Disney (1967), using the same methods as Phillips (1964), failed to find differences in the rejection of disturbed individuals on the basis of their reported sex.

Fourth, it has been suggested that sex stereotypes affect the diagnostic habits of physicians. Broverman et al. (1970) have provided an empirical demonstration of a double standard of mental health among clinicians.

However, there is no evidence from recent studies that judges of either sex are partisan towards their own kind (Kosherak and Masling 1972; Lewittes et al. 1973; Schlosberg and Pietrofesa 1973; Werner and Block 1975; Zeldow 1975).

It may be concluded that, while evidence for the discrimination against women in the mental health field exists, the conditions for its occurrence are rather circumscribed and may be declining. There is some evidence that at least a part of the observed sex difference in the prevalence of depression in men and women may be attributed to women being more likely to recognize

299

problems in themselves and to seek help for them. It does, indeed, appear that illness is less stigmatizing for women than for men. The evidence that women are more likely to be diagnosed as ill than men remains conflicting. The fixed role obligations hypothesis explains sex differences in illness behaviour rather than in illness *per se*. However, the existence of these 'artefactual' mechanisms does not exclude the possibility that some of the observed sex difference is real, due to either inherited or acquired risks.

SUMMARY

Thus, a female excess in the prevalence of minor psychiatric morbidity is found in most of the treatment statistics, although not all, and in some community studies, with important and notable exceptions. Surveys of homogeneous populations, where care is taken to minimize occupational, social, and role differences between the sexes, do not reveal a female excess in the prevalence of minor psychiatric morbidity in schoolchildren, students, or young working adults aged 20–35. Any coherent theory of sex differences must, therefore, take these findings into account.

In view of the substantial genetic evidence that the excess of depression in women is environmental in origin rather than genetic; in view of the paucity of any direct endocrinological evidence linking mood change in men and women with gonadal hormones; in view of the evidence from homogeneous surveys that, when social variables are controlled and reduced, the sex difference disappears; and in the light of the nineteenth-century experience, all claims that the excess of depression in women is explained by their reproductive biology – or indeed by their constitution in general – should be treated with grave caution.

REFERENCES

Ananth, J. (1978) 'Psychopathology in Indian females', *Social Science and Medicine* 12: 177–8.

Ballinger, C.B. (1975) 'Psychiatric morbidity and the menopause: screening of a general population sample' *British Medical Journal* iii: 344–6.

Ballinger, C.B. (1976) 'Psychiatric morbidity and the menopause: clinical features', *British Medical Journal* i: 1183–5.

Ballinger, C.B., Buckley, D.E., Naylor, G.J.A., and Stansfield, DA. (1979) 'Emotional disturbance following childbirth: clinical findings and urinary excretion of cyclic AMP', *Psychological Medicine* 9: 293–300.

Bash, K.W. and Bash-Liechti, J. (1969) 'Studies of the epidemiology of neuro-psychiatric disorders among the rural population of the province of Khazestran, Iran', *Social Psychiatry* 4: 137–43.

Bash, K.W. and Bash-Liechti, J. (1974) 'Studies of the epidemiology of neuro-psychiatric disorders among the population of the city of Shiraz, Iran', *Social Psychiatry* 9: 163–71.

Bebbington, P., Hurry, J., Tennant, C., Sturt, E., and Wing, J.K. (1981) 'Epidemiology of mental disorders in Camberwell', *Psychological Medicine* 11: 561–79.

Briscoe, M. (1982) *Sex Differences in Psychological Well-Being* (Psychological Medicine Monograph Supplement 1), Cambridge: Cambridge University Press.

Broverman, L., Broverman, D., Clarkson, F., Rosenkranz, P., and Vogel, S. (1970) 'Sex role stereotype and clinical judgements of mental health', *Journal of Consulting and Clinical Psychology* 34: 1–7.

Brown, G.W. and Harris, T. (1978) *Social Origins of Depression: A Study of Psychiatric Disorder in Women*, London: Tavistock.

Carpenter, R.G. (1959) 'Statistical analysis of suicide and other mortality rates of students', *British Journal of Preventive and Social Medicine* 13: 163.

Chesler, P. (1971) 'Patient and patriarch: women in the psychotherapeutic relationship', in V. Gornick and B.K. Moran (eds) *Women in Sexist Society*, New York: Basic Books.

Chesler, P. (1972) *Women and Madness*, London: Allen Lane.

Chodorow, N. (1974) 'Family structure and feminine personality' in M.Z. Rosaldo and L. Larnphere (eds) *Woman, Culture and Society*, Stanford: Stanford University Press.

Clare, A.W. (1980) 'Psychological and social aspects of premenstrual complaint', MD thesis, National University of Ireland.

Cobb, S. (1976) 'Social support as a moderator of life stress', *Psychosomatic Medicine* 38: 300–14.

Cochrane, R. and Stopes-Roe, M. (1980) 'Factors affecting the distribution of psychological symptoms in urban areas of England', *Acta Psychiatrica Scandinavica* 61: 445–60.

Coie, J.D., Pennington, B.F., and Buckley, H.H. (1974) 'Effects of situational stress and sex roles on the attribution of psychological disorder', *Journal of Consulting and Clinical Psychology* 42: 559–68.

Comstock, G.W. and Helsing, K.J. (1976) 'Symptoms of depression in two communities', *Psychological Medicine* 6: 551–63.

Cooperstock, R. (1971) 'Sex differences in the use of mood modifying drugs: an explanatory model', *Journal of Health and Social Behaviour* 12: 238–344.

Cumming, E., Lazer, C., and Chisholm, L. (1975) 'Suicide as an index of role strain among employed and not employed married women in British Columbia', *Canadian Review of Sociology and Anthropology* 12 (4): 462–70.

Dekker, D.J. and Webb, J.T. (1974) 'Relationships of the social readjustment rating scale to psychiatric patient status, anxiety and social desirability', *Journal of Psychosomatic Research* 18: 125–30.

Dohrenwend, B.S. and Dohrenwend, B.P. (1974) *Stressful Life Events: Their Nature and Effects*, New York: Wiley.

Dohrenwend, B.P. and Dohrenwend, B.S. (1976) 'Sex differences and psychiatric disorders', *American Sociological review* 81: 1447–54.

Dube, K.C. and Kumar, N. (1973) 'An epidemiological study of manic depressive psychosis', *Acta Psychiatrica Scandinavica* 49: 691–7.

Farmer, R.D.J. and Harvey, P.G. (1975) 'Minor psychiatric disturbance in young adults', *Social Science and Medicine* 9: 461–74.

Finlay-Jones, R.A. and Burvill, P.W. (1977) 'The prevalence of minor psychiatric morbidity in the community', *Psychological Medicine* 7: 474–89.

Frankenhauser, M., Dunne, E., and Lundberg, U. (1976) 'Sex differences in sympathetic-adrenal medullary reactions induced by different stresses', *Psychopharmacology* 47: 1–5.

Frankenhauser, M., Rauste Von Wright, M., Collins, A., Van Wright, J., Sedvall, G., and Swahn, C.J. (1978) 'Sex differences in psychoneuroendocrine reactions to examination stress', *Psychosomatic Medicine* 40 (4): 334–43.

Gershon, E.S. and Bunney, W.E. (1976) 'The question of X-linkage in biopolar manic depressive illness', *Journal of Psychiatric Research* 13: 99–117.

Gershon, E.S., Bunney, D.L., and Goodwin, F.K. (1971) 'Towards a biology of affective disorders', *Archives of General Psychiatry* 25: 1–15.

Glaser, W.A. (1970) *Social Settings and Medical Organisation*, New York: Atherton Press.

Goldberg, D.P. and Huxley, P. (1980) *Mental Illness in the Community: The Pathway to Psychiatric Care*, London: Tavistock.

Golin, S. and Hartz, M.A. (1977) 'A factor analysis of the Beck Depression Inventory in a mildly depressed population', unpublished typescript from the University of Pittsburgh, quoted in Parker (1979).

Gore, S. (1978) 'The effect of social support in moderating the health consequences of unemployment', *Journal of Health and Social Behaviour* 19: 157–65.

Gove, W.R. (1972) 'The relationship between sex roles, mental illness and marital status', *Social Forces* 51: 34–44.

Graham, P. and Rutter, M. (1973) 'Psychiatric disorder in the young adolescent', *Proceedings of the Royal Society of Medicine* 66: 1226–9.

Graunt, J. (1667) *Natural and political observations mentioned in a following index, and made upon the bills of mortality*, quoted in Glass, D.V. (1963) 'John Graunt and His Natural and Political Observations', *Proceedings of the Royal Society* B159: 1–32.

Green, J.G. and Cook, D.J. (1980) 'Life stress and symptoms at the climacteric', *British Journal of Psychiatry* 136: 486–91.

Gurin, G., Veroff, J., and Feld, S. (1960) *Americans View Their Mental Health*, New York: Basic Books.

Haavio-Manilla, E. (1976) 'Ecological and sex differences in the hospitalisation of mental illness in Finland and Sweden', *Social Science and Medicine* 10: 77–82.

Hammen, C.L. and Padesky, C.A. (1977) 'Sex differences in the expression of depressive responses on the Beck Depression Inventory', *Journal of Abnormal Psychology* 86 (6): 609–14.

Hammen, C.L. and Peters, S.D. (1977) 'Differential response to male and female depressive reactions', *Journal of Consulting and Clinical Psychology* 45 (6): 974–1001.

Handley, S.L., Dunn, T.L., Waldron, G. and Baker, J.M. (1980) 'Tryptophan, cortisol and puerperal mood', *British Journal of Psychiatry* 136: 498–508.

Henderson, S., Duncan-Jones, P., Byrne, D.G., Adcock, S., and Scott, R. (1979) 'Neurosis and social bands in an urban population', *Australian and New Zealand Journal of Psychiatry* 13: 121–5.

Henderson, S., Byrne, D.G., Duncan-Jones, P., Scott, R.A., and Adcock, S. (1980) 'Social relationships, adversity and neurosis: a study of associations in a general population sample', *British Journal of Psychiatry* 136: 574–83.

Hinkle, L.E., Redmont, R., Plummer, N., and Wolff, H.G. (1960) 'An examination of the relationship between symptoms, disability and serious illness, in two homogeneous groups of men and women', *American Journal of Public Health* 50 (9): 1327–36.

Horner, M.S. (1972) 'Toward an understanding of achievement related conflicts in women', *Journal of Social Issues* 28: 157–75.

Horowitz, A. (1977) 'The pathways into psychiatric treatment: some differences between men and women', *Journal of Health and Social Behaviour* 18: 169–75.

Jenkins, R. (1983) 'Some epidemiological observations of minor psychiatric morbidity', MD thesis for Cambridge University.

Jenkins, R. (1985) 'Sex differences in minor psychiatric morbidity', *Psychological Medicine* (Monograph Supplement 7) Cambridge University Press.

Kendell, R.E., Rennie, D., Clarke, J.A., and Dean, C. (1981) 'The social and obstetric correlates of psychiatric admission in the puerperium', *Psychological Medicine* 11: 341–50.

Kidd, C.B., Caldbeck, J., and Meenan, J. (1966) 'A comparative study of psychiatric morbidity among students at two different universities', *British Journal of Psychiatry* 112: 57–64.

Komarovsky, M. (1946) 'Cultural contradictions and sex roles', *American Journal of Sociology* 52: 184–9.

Kosherak, S. and Masling, J. (1972) 'Noblesse oblige effect: the interpretation of Rorschach responses as a function of ascribed social class', *Journal of Consulting and Clinical Psychology* 39: 415–19.

Lewittes, D.J., Mosell, J.A., and Simmons, W.L. (1973) 'Sex role bias in clinical judgements based on Rorschach interpretations', in *Proceedings of the 81st Annual Convention of the American Psychological Association* 8: 495–6 referred to in Zelcher, P.B. (1978) 'Sex differences in psychiatric evaluation and treatment', *Archives of General Psychiatry* 35: 89–93.

Liem, R. and Liem, J. (1978) 'Social class and mental illness reconsidered: the role of economic stress and social support', *Journal of Health and Social Behaviour* 19: 139–56.

Linn, N.W., Hunter, K.L., and Perry, P.R. (1979) 'Differences by sex and ethnicity in the psychosocial adjustment of the elderly', *Journal of Health and Social Behaviour* 20: 273–81.

Lloyd, C. and Gartrell, N.K. (1981) 'Sex differences in medical student mental health', *American Journal of Psychiatry* 138 (10): 1346–51.

Marcus, A.C. and Seeman, T.E. (1981) 'Sex differences in health status: a re-examination of the nurturant role hypothesis', *American Sociological Review* 46: 119–23.

Mechanic, D. (1964) 'The influence of mothers on their children's health attitudes and behaviour', *Paediatrics* 33: 444–53.

Mechanic, D. (1965) 'Perceptions of parental responses to illness: a research note', *Journal of Health and Human Behaviour* 6: 253.

Meile, R.L., Johnson, D.R., and Peter, L. (1976) 'Marital role, education, and mental disorder among women: test of an interaction hypothesis', *Journal of Health and Social Behaviour* 17: 295–301.

Miller, P. Mc. and Ingham, J.G. (1976) 'Friends, confidantes and symptoms', *Social Psychiatry* 11: 51–8.

Mostow, E. and Newberry, P. (1975) 'Work role and depression in women: a comparison of workers and housewives in treatment', *American Journal of Ortho-psychiatry* 45: 538–48.

Murray, J., Dunn, G., Williams, P., and Tarnopolsky, A. (1981) 'Factors affecting the consumption of psychotropic drugs', *Psychological Medicine* 11: 551–60.

Myers, J.K., Lindenthal, J.J., and Pepper, M.P. (1971) 'Life events and psychiatric impairment', *Journal of Nervous and Mental Disease* 152: 149–57.

Myers, J.K., Lindenthal, J.J., and Pepper, M.P. (1975) 'Life stress, social integration and psychiatric symptomatology', *Journal of Health and Social Behaviour* 16: 421–7.

Nathanson, C.A. (1980) 'Social roles and health status among women: the significance of employment', *Social Science and Medicine* 14A: 463–71.

303

Newman, J.P. (1975) 'Sex differences in life problems and psychological distress', Master's Thesis, University of Wisconsin, Madison.

Nott, P.M., Franklin, M., Armitage, C., and Gelder, M.G. (1976) 'Hormonal changes and mood in the puerperium', *British Journal of Psychiatry* 128: 379–83.

Office of Population Censuses and Surveys (1980) *General Household Survey 1978* (Series GHS, No. 8) London: HMSO.

Office of Population Censuses and Surveys (1987) *General Household Survey (OPCS) 1985* (Series GHS, No. 14), London: HMSO.

O'Mahoney, P. and O'Brien, S. (1980) 'Demographic and social characteristics of university students attending a psychiatrist', *British Journal of Psychiatry* 137: 547–50.

Orley, J. and Wing, J.K. (1979) 'Psychiatric disorder in two African villages', *Archives of General Psychiatry* 36: 513–20.

Parker, G. (1979) 'Sex differences in non-clinical depression: review and assessment of previous studies', *Australian and New Zealand Journal of Psychiatry* 13: 127–32.

Parrish, P.A. (1971) 'The prescribing of psychotropic drugs in general practice', *Journal of the Royal College of General Practitioners* 21 (supplement 4): 1–71.

Parsons, R. and Fox, R. (1952) 'Illness, therapy and the modern urban American family', *Journal of Social Issues* 8 (4): 31–44.

Paykel, E.S., Prusoff, B.A., and Ulenluth, E.H. (1971) 'Scaling of life events', *Archives of General Psychiatry* 25: 340–7.

Pearlin, L.I. and Johnson, J.S. (1977) 'Marital status, life strains and depression', *American Sociological Review* 42: 704–15.

Personn, G. (1980) 'Life event ratings in relation to sex and marital status in a 70 year old urban population', *Acta Psychiatrica Scandinavica* 62: 112–18.

Phillips, D.L. (1964) 'Rejection of the mentally ill: the influence of behaviour and sex', *American Sociological Review* 29: 679–87.

Phillip, D.L. and Segal, B.E. (1969) 'Sexual status and psychiatric symptoms', *American Sociological Review* 34: 58–72.

Price, J. (1968) 'The genetics of depressive behaviour', in A. Coppen and A. Walk (eds) *Recent Developments in Affective Disorders* (British Journal of Psychiatry Special Publication No. 2) Ashford, Kent: Headley Brothers, 37–54.

Radloff, L.S., and Rae, D.S. (1979) 'Susceptibility and precipitating factors in depression: sex differences and similarities', *Journal of Abnormal Psychology* 88: 174–86.

Rheingold, H.L. and Cook, K.V. (1975) 'The contents of boys' and girls' rooms as an index of parents behaviour', *Child Development* 46: 459–63.

Rosenthal, D. (1971) *Genetics of Psychopathology*, New York: McGraw-Hill.

Rutter, M., Tizard, J., Yule, W., Graham, P., and Whitmore, K. (1976) 'Research report: Isle of Wight Studies 1964-1974', *Psychological Medicine* 6: 313–32.

Schepank, H. (1973) 'Erb-und Unweltfaktoren bei neurosen Ergebnisse der Zwilling Forschung und andere Methoden', *Nervenarzt* 44: 449–59, quoted in Katschnig, H. and Shepherd, M. (1976) 'Neurosis, the epidemiological perspective', in H.M. Van Praag (ed.) *Research in Neurosis*, Utrecht: Bohn, Schelerna and Holkena, pp. 5–21.

Schlosberg, N.K. and Pietrofesa, J.J. (1973) 'Perspectives on counselling bias: implications for counsellor education', *Counselling Psychology* 4: 44–54.

Seligman, M.E.P. (1975) *Helplessness: On Depression, Development and Death*, San Francisco: W.H. Freeman.

Shields, J. and Slater, E. (1971) 'Diagnostic similarity in twins with neuroses and personality disorders', in J. Shields and I.I. Gottesman (eds) *Man, Mind and Heredity: Selected Papers of Eliot Slater on Psychiatry and Genetics*, Baltimore: Johns Hopkins Press.

Slater, E. and Roth, M. (1969) *Clinical Psychiatry*, London: Balliere, Tindall & Cassell.

Sorenson, A. and Strömgren, E. (1961) 'Frequency of depressive states within geographically delineated population groups', *Acta Psychiatrica Scandinavica* supplement 162: 62–8.

Torgersen, S. (1983) 'Genetics of neuroses: the effects of sampling variation upon the twin concordance ratio', *British Journal of Psychiatry* 142: 126–32.

Verbrugge, L.M. (1979) 'Female illness rates and illness behaviour: testing hypotheses about sex differences in health', *Women and Health* 4: 61–79.

Veroff, J.B. (1981) 'The dynamics of help-seeking in men and women: a national survey study', *Psychiatry* 44: 189–200.

Waldron, I. (1976) 'Why do women live longer than men? Part I', *Journal of Human Stress* 2: 2–13.

Weeke, A.B., Videbeck, T.H., and Dupont, A. (1975) 'The incidence of depressive syndromes in a Danish county', *Acta Psychiatrica Scandinavica* 51: 28–41.

Weissman, M.M. and Klerman, G.L. (1979) 'Sex differences and the epidemiology of depression', in E.S. Gomberg and V. Franks (eds) *Gender and Disordered Behaviour: Sex Differences in Psychopathology*, New York: Brunner/Mazel.

Welch, S. and Booth, A. (1977) 'Employment and health among married women with children', *Sex Roles* 3: 385–97.

Werner, P.D. and Block, J. (1975) 'Sex differences in the eyes of expert personality assessor: unwarranted conclusions', *Journal of Personal Assessment* 39: 110–13.

Williams, J.E. and Best, D.L. (1982) *Measuring Sex Stereotypes: A Thirty Nation Study* London: Sage.

Yamamoto, K. and Disney, H. (1967) 'Rejection of the mentally ill: a study of attitudes of student teachers', *Journal of Counselling Psychology* 14: 254–68.

Zeldow, P.B. (1975) 'Clinical judgements: a search for sex differences', *Psychology Reports* 37: 1135–42.

Section Three

The Evaluation of Psychiatric Intervention

Introduction

Current resource constraints are increasingly focusing attention on the need to evaluate treatment modalities (Wilkinson and Williams 1985). This activity has not always been a priority in psychiatry, as Shepherd has noted:

> The relatively short history of modern psychiatry has witnessed the rise and fall of many different forms of treatment. At the present time few branches of medicine stand more in need of reliable methods for the assessment of their therapeutic claims. If this unsatisfactory state of affairs springs in some measure from an uncertainty about the causes and nature of most psychiatric illness it also reflects a failure on the part of many workers to have applied to psychiatry well recognised principles of clinical investigation. (Shepherd 1981: 99)

The three major treatment modalities in psychiatry are physical, psychosocial, and behavioural: chapters in the first subsection deal with each of the three. In the first, Malcolm Lader provides a 'state of the art' review of the methodology of clinical trials of psychotropic drugs. One of the most important of these was the trial of the treatment of depressive illness organized by a special subcommittee of the Medical Research Council (MRC 1965), of which Michael Shepherd was the secretary.

However, the conditions of a controlled clinical trial, in which drugs are prescribed for a carefully selected group of patients and their effects rigorously monitored, are clearly different from those that apply in routine clinical practice. Thus, in the comprehensive evaluation of psychotropic drugs, it is necessary to complement clinical trials with studies of utilization in a social context. This is the topic of the following chapter by Paul Williams and Jonathan Gabe.

While the introduction and development of psychotropic drugs is generally agreed to be a major advance, it is at the same time also acknowledged that social factors are a profound determinant of mental disorder and that psychosocial approaches constitute a necessary component of the management of psychiatric and emotional disturbance. The evaluation of such techniques are dealt with by Roslyn Corney and Joanna Murray. Their chapter and the one which follows, in which Ian Falloon describes behavioural approaches in the family management of schizophrenia, emphasize the importance of the multi-disciplinary team in this context. The concept of the multi-disciplinary team, and the nature and responsibilities of its members, are especially important at a time when, as at present, services are undergoing rapid change.

The second subsection is concerned with the evaluation of service provision. Traditionally, the focus of the psychiatric services has been the mental hospital, and David Watt appraises their current role. However, in many countries the provision of services is shifting from an institutional to a primary care and community base. Arguably the most radical change has taken place in Italy: it is appropriate, therefore, that the subsequent chapter, on the evaluation of community psychiatric services, is written by Michele Tansella. As he points out, the development of such services has provided plentiful opportunities for service evaluation; these have, regrettably, not been fully exploited.

It is now widely accepted that the primary care services play a pivotal role in providing mental health care to the community. This is exemplified in the conclusions of the WHO working party on psychiatry and primary medical care:

> the crucial question is not how the general practitioner can fit into the mental health services, but rather how the psychiatrist can collaborate most effectively with primary health services, and reinforce the effectiveness of the primary physician as a member of the mental health team.(WHO 1973: 27)

Here, the contribution of the general practitioner is discussed by Deborah Sharp and David Morrell, while Geraldine Strathdee and Michael King consider the interface between general and specialist psychiatric services.

Ultimately, the responsibility for the planning and provision of mental health services for populations rests with politicians, and hence policies and priorities are politically determined (even so, policy is often made *post hoc*: for example, Gronfein (1985) noted that in the USA closing mental hospital beds preceded the policy of deinstitutionalization by several years). The relationship between psychiatric research and public policy is ill-defined: Leon Eisenberg casts light on this topic in the final chapter in this section.

REFERENCES

Gronfein, W. (1985) 'Psychotropic drugs and the origins of deinstitutionalization', *Social Problems* 32: 437–54.

Medical Research Council (1965) 'Report by its clinical committee: clinical trial of the treatment of depressive illness', *British Medical Journal* i: 881–6.

Shepherd, M. (1981) *Psychotropic Drugs in Psychiatry*, New York: Jason Aaronson.

Wilkinson, G. and Williams, P. (1985) 'Priorities for research on mental health in primary care settings', *Psychological Medicine* 15: 515–20.

World Health Organization (1973) *Psychiatry and Primary Medical Care*, Copenhagen: WHO Regional Office for Europe.

Specific Treatment Approaches

20

Clinical Trials in Psychiatry

Malcolm Lader

Our inability upon all occasions to appreciate the efforts of Nature in the cure of disease, must always render our notions, with respect to the power of art, liable to numerous errors and multiplied deceptions.(Paris 1833:50)

Psychiatric disorders cover a range of conditions with a wide assortment of natural histories. Most are characterized by a fluctuating or relapsing/remitting course. Therefore, it is particularly important to assess the efficacy, and for that matter the apparent unwanted effects of psychiatric remedies in a manner which minimizes the influence of natural variations in severity and other biasses. This requirement applies to non-pharmacological as well as to drug treatments. For a variety of non-scientific reasons, such as the claimed difficulties in defining 'efficacy' in treatments involving dynamic psychotherapy, the assessment of treatments in psychiatry has been most systematic with respect to pharmacological agents (Johnson 1983).

But there are problems. Almost all psychotropic drugs used in psychiatry were discovered by accident, usually in the search for another class of drugs, sometimes after following a line of reasoning which turned out to be based on false premises (Ayd and Blackwell 1970). These remedies are established empirically not rationally and their efficacy has to be carefully established and not taken for granted because of an appealing theoretical rationale.

A second consequence of the serendipitous origins of many psychotropic agents relates to unwanted side effects. Because the drugs were stumbled on by chance, no prior attempts could be made to confine the range of activity of the compounds to wanted effects only. Both the antipsychotic and the antidepressant groups are notorious for their wide range and severity of side effects, often to the point of jeopardizing compliance. Thus, clinical trials must carefully assess the whole range of drug effects. Furthermore, practical field trials, such as post-marketing surveillance, are appropriate to assess the effectiveness in practice of any new drug and to complement the more formal clinical trials.

The area of psychopharmacology has not escaped the problem of serious adverse effects. The removal of zimeldine and nomifensine testifies to the powerful effects which psychotropic drugs can have outside the CNS. Because of the first such disaster, with thalidomide, regulatory agencies were set up to control the development and marketing of new compounds. These controls have been tightened inexorably with both commercial and scientific consequences. The former is that it now costs between fifty and a hundred million dollars to develop a new chemical entity to its launch on its market. The latter is that drug companies must design drug evaluation studies to accord with the requirements of the regulatory authorities whenever possible and appropriate.

In this article, I shall attempt to address some of the issues relating to the evaluation of psychiatric drugs. I shall sketch in the outlines rather than going into compendious detail and I shall concentrate on the principles rather than the practical minutiae. Some topics such as adverse effects and risk/benefit assessments are hardly touched upon (Walker and Asscher 1987).

AIMS OF TREATMENT

The aim of therapy is to restore 'health' or to prevent its breakdown. Doctors, including psychiatrists, seldom question this goal to which, indeed, most dedicate their working life. The WHO definition seems worthy but sententious: 'Health means more than freedom from disease, freedom from pain, freedom from untimely death. It means optimum physical, mental and social efficiency and well-being.' However, mental health is a complex concept which has been the subject of some fascinating essays (e.g. Lewis 1953). Perhaps more than with physical health, there is a positive aspect to mental health, the sense of well-being. This can, of course, become pathologically intense, as in mania.

By and large, drug treatments in psychiatry aim to rectify some behavioural or symptomatic abnormality. The behavioural abnormality may be phobic avoidance or a compulsive ritual or it may be a specific act such as suicide in the context of severe depression. Symptoms in psychiatry are psychological but physical symptoms may also be prominent, especially in anxiety and depression. In some instances the aims may appear quite modest and directed at the social consequences of a psychiatric disorder. For example, a patient suffering from chronic schizophrenia who is inert and unsociable may be 'activated' to the point where he is able to attend work punctually; this may seem a modest aim but may have immense consequences such as keeping the patient gainfully employed in the community.

Sometimes, the aims of treatment are difficult to define or different health professionals have different aims which may even be incompatible. For example, 'activating' a chronic schizophrenic in-patient may make him easier to rehabilitate but it may also make him truculent and aggressive. The social workers and nurses involved in his care would have very different views on the 'success' of the drug intervention. Drawing up a balance-sheet of the effectiveness of a drug requires input from several sources.

As well as different practical outcomes, there are ideological differences. The medically-trained psychiatrist is often primarily concerned with symptom reduction or the normalization of 'abnormal' or 'deviant' behaviour. The psychologically-trained behaviour therapist is concerned that drugs will facilitate rather than hinder his behaviour modification programmes. But the analytically-trained psychotherapist might eschew drugs altogether in the belief that any symptom reduction is more than outweighed by drug-induced interference with development of the personality and interpersonal relationships.

Finally, financial considerations obtrude. The costs of health care in all western countries continue to escalate, partly as a result of the changing demography, partly because medical technology has become much more sophisticated and expensive, and partly because health expectations have been raised. Psychiatry has taken part in these changes to a fairly modest extent. Nevertheless, the cost of drug treatments may become an important factor in the choice of therapy. For example, the discharge of a chronically institutionalized patient to the community may necessitate substitution of an expensive depot preparation for a cheap oral one. It is important to know the relative usefulness of the two forms of therapy, not just in terms of efficacies in a comparable clinical trial but also in day-to-day practice.

NATURE OF CLINICAL TRIALS

Pious platitudes abound concerning the usefulness of non-systematic clinical observations. Thus, it might appear that giving a drug to a patient and observing his or her response provides information concerning the efficacy of that drug in the treatment of the patient's disorder. Unfortunately, some inferences drawn from unsystematic observations may not merely be weak or unsubstantiated but actually wrong. The persistent use of venesection over a century or two despite the careful observations of thousands of practitioners testifies to the gullibility of the medical profession. Nor is our record since the mid-nineteenth century – the dawn of 'rational medicine' – unsullied by similar fads and fancies. In psychiatry this century, schizophrenic patients have undergone mutilating bowel excisions or dental extractions to expunge presumed foci of infection. The vigour with which these campaigns were conducted can only raise questions as to whether beliefs of delusional intensity were solely the prerogative of the patient. In psychopharmacology, a host of drug treatments was tried on no discernible rational basis and, worse, persisted in despite not one jot of evidence of any efficacy, but only of toxicity. The LSD episode provides a vivid example, Even now, some schizophrenic patients are exposed to exceedingly high doses of neuroleptic medication despite the lack of any evidence that such doses are needed routinely (Aubree and Lader 1980).

How has this come about? The roots of the problem lie in the difficulties of defining psychiatric syndromes, the chronicity and severity of many of these conditions, and the understandable wish on the part of the therapist to help his patient. The formal clinical trial is constituted in such a way as to minimize the biasses which bedevil apparently simple clinical observations.

The elements of the clinical trial have been thoroughly debated. The test treatment should be tested against a dummy treatment, the placebo, which contains all the attributes of the test treatment except for the active pharmacological principle, Patients meeting pre-set diagnostic and perhaps other criteria (e.g. demographic) should be allocated randomly to one or other of the treatments. Assessments of psychiatric state and symptom severity during treatment should be carried out 'double-blind', neither patient nor physician knowing which treatment has been given. Finally, appropriate statistics should be used to attempt to disprove the null hypothesis that the test and dummy treatments do not differ in efficacy.

Such an ideal trial is never attained in practice and each of the steps outlined above has its particular difficulties in clinical trials in psychiatry.

DEFINITION OF SAMPLES

The conclusions of a scientific experiment, clinical trials included, must be communicable to other scientists, otherwise the study is not worth doing. (Indeed, an unpublished study may raise ethical problems – a topic touched on later.) Essential to such communication is a well-defined clinical system of diagnoses. Unfortunately, psychiatric diagnosis is neither sufficiently standardized nor sufficiently reliable to provide more than an approximation to such precise definition of syndromes or disorders.

The clinician's solution to this problem is to use as his working standard, not a formal diagnosis, but an informal formulation. In this way he can communicate fairly succinctly the nub of a case without necessarily squeezing it into an ill-fitting diagnostic category. But this stratagem is too cumbersome for a research study. Furthermore, definitions and nosologies developed for the clinician or epidemiologist may not be entirely appropriate for the clinical researcher. For example, International Classification of Diseases (ICD–9) (1980) uses different types of criteria for different diagnostic categories and the DSM–III of the American Psychiatric Association (1980) also contains many inconsistencies although its operational definitions are often very useful. Perhaps the best categorical instrument for research purposes is the Research Diagnostic Criteria which is constructed in such a way as to ensure as few false positive inclusions as possible at the cost of some false negative

316

exclusions (Spitzer *et al.* 1978).

Of course, one can argue that such highly formalized criteria for patient definition run the risk of the trial ending up with such a spuriously homogeneous group as to be unrepresentative of the wider population in which the drug will actually be used. But this argument may lead to a worse outcome, namely that the indications for a medicine become so ill-defined as to be worthless scientifically and dangerous clinically. The widespread use of the benzodiazepines beyond definable anxiety disorders to any condition with any perceptible psychological component is a reminder of the dangers of this laissez-faire diagnostic policy. What is needed is a careful definition of a core group and establishment of the efficacy of a drug in that group. Then, other groups nosologically contiguous with the initial group are studied to provide a penumbra of indications.

But there is one other factor which is generally glossed over. This refers to the way in which patients come into the trial. In the UK, most patients are seen initially by a general practitioner who usually tries one or more treatments before admitting failure and referring the patient for specialist advice. If a patient is referred on without such trials-of-therapy, it generally means that he is untypical in terms of severity, chronicity, social or personality problems. The patient referred after treatments have failed is untypical by being refractory to those treatments. Thus, many out-patient trials of antidepressants are carried out on patients who have failed to respond to standard antidepressants such as prothiaden and amitriptyline favoured by UK general practitioners. Trials on depressed in-patients are subject to many other biasses, e.g. towards suicidal ideation and behaviour and social isolation. Sometimes, hospital-based doctors running clinical trials attempt to accelerate their recruitment rate by canvassing local general practitioners and asking them to send up newly-presenting patients of appropriate type, untreated, for prompt assessment and inception into the trial. This is perfectly legitimate provided this stratagem is clearly explained in the ensuing publication.

Differences between countries may be quite major. For example, in the USA many patients present directly to a psychiatrist who consequently sees a very different sample from his counterpart in the UK where general practitioner screening is the norm. Furthermore, some sick people in the USA may not seek help because of financial constraints. Some clinical trials recruit patients by publicity campaigns in the local media. Indeed, one enterprising researcher is supposed to have advertised for depressives on local radio at 5 a.m., thereby obtaining a sample characterized by early morning awakening. A further factor is that such subjects are motivated to enter and remain in the trial by the prospect of free treatment. For all these reasons, it is important to establish and document the provenance of patients studied in a clinical trial.

THE TYPE OF COMPARISON

Although the standard comparison should be between test medication and placebo, this is not always practicable, usually for ethical reasons. For example, it is generally accepted in the UK that tricyclic antidepressants are sufficiently effective in moderate-to-severe depressives to preclude the use of dummy medication. In the USA, placebo-controlled antidepressant trials are accepted, probably because the typical patient is mildly rather than moderately ill. However, because tranquillizers are viewed as only partially effective with appreciable side effects and are used in less important indications, placebos are generally accepted as comparators.

The solution to the antidepressant problem is to use a standard such as imipramine or amitriptyline. It is necessary, however, to establish the efficacy of the standard medication in the context in which it will be used. It cannot be taken for granted that, because an extensive literature attests to the efficacy, albeit not complete, of the standard, it will prove effective in that clinic in the particular type of patient seen. But this in itself poses a further problem in that the efficacy of the standard cannot be established against placebo because that study is regarded as unethical. The answer is to assess a cohort of patients in a manner as closely akin to that of a controlled trial as possible. For example, ratings are made, side effects sought, and compliance encouraged as if the patients were participating in a formal double-blind evaluation. The ratings are averaged and should follow those published in the literature. Without such a ploy, it is impossible to decide from the double-blind controlled comparison of test versus standard, which fails to refute the null hypothesis, whether the two drugs are equally effective or ineffective.

DESIGN CONSIDERATIONS

Clinical trials should be designed to answer one prime question, such as 'does this treatment lessen symptoms in this type of patient?' Other questions concerning onset of action, type of effect, side-effects, and so on must remain subordinate. Later, a fuller profile of the drug can be constructed. The experimental design must isolate and attempt to answer that main question.

The usual design is the parallel-groups design where patients are randomly allocated to one of two or more treatments. Cogent reasons are needed not to use this standard approach. The usual alternative is the cross-over design but this makes statistical assumptions that may be difficult to sustain. In particular, the cross-over design assumes that the state of the patient is the same at the start of each successive treatment, i.e., that the disorder is chronic and is not irreversibly affected in some way by any of the treatments.

Although many psychiatric disorders are distressingly chronic, most fluctuate and are influenced in subtle ways by treatments. Restoration of the status ante quo cannot be assumed. In favour of cross-over trials is the substantial reduction in the number of patients needed to show an effect when they are used as their own controls.

There are many other design strategies such as the sequential trial, incomplete block design, factorials, and so on, any of which may be appropriate for a specialized application. Expert statistical advice is needed to clarify the assumptions made.

BLINDEDNESS

Much ritual obeisance is paid to the principle of the double-blind procedure as the way to minimize bias in a comparative trial. The medications look, smell, and taste the same and neither the patient nor the rater know which treatment is being given. Such untainted assessments are especially needed in psychiatry where subjective evaluations are frequent and observational measures prone to error. Unfortunately, because of the fortuitous discovery of most psychotropic drugs, selectivity of action was not a property of the earlier compounds in each class – those which tend to be used as the standard. If a newer compound is more selective, with fewer side effects (and there is not much point introducing a less selective compound with more side effects), it may be quite apparent to the patient and in turn to the rater that major differences obtain between the two compounds. The rater inevitably becomes unblinded knowing, for example, that a complaint of dry mouth is attributable to amitriptyline rather than to a selective 5-HT uptake inhibitor or of restlessness to haloperidol rather than to a selective neuroleptic.

The extent of this problem can be assessed by asking the rater to guess which of the treatments the patient is receiving and seeing whether his accuracy is significantly greater than chance. It is also worth asking him why he made that guess. But this strategy cannot salvage a trial in which the blindedness has been significantly jeopardized. It is better to try and minimize bias by separating the rating of efficacy from that of side effects. This requires two raters, the first enquiring about general progress and side effects, and adjusting dosage if the regimen is a flexible one. The second rater confines his questioning to that needed for the formal assessments.

DOSAGE SCHEDULES

Too frequently, the dosage of psychotropic drugs is arrived at by a protracted sequence of trial-and-error and not by establishing a dose-effect curve. Regulatory authorities are becoming stricter in this respect and some such as

319

the Food and Drugs Administration in the USA recommend a four-group study: a) placebo; b) presumed subtherapeutic dose; c) presumed therapeutic dose; and d) presumed supratherapeutic dose. The risk-benefit ratio should be optimal with (c).

This can only establish the approximate mean effective dose. Biological variation will mean that the optimal dose will vary from patient to patient. Carrying out an efficacy trial at one single fixed dose, usually (c) above, may underestimate true efficacy and overestimate side effects. It is generally preferable to use a flexible dose regimen with pre-set decision points concerning raising or lowering the dose, which are adhered to closely. It may take a little time to establish the optimal dose for each patient but it is time well-spent. It also reflects clinical practice.

THE POWER OF THE TRIAL

Most trials are too small to yield worthwhile results (Freiman *et al.* 1978). Because of the modest improvements generally attained, expected differences between treatments are also narrow. For example, 70–80 per cent of depressed patients respond to a typical tricyclic antidepressant and about half that percentage to placebo. Consequently, it is difficult to show lesser effectiveness than the standard for a newer drug but also difficult to show differences from placebo. Even more of a problem would be posed by a test compound which helped 90 per cent of patients.

Power calculations result in some very high figures per group. For example, let us suppose that, in the case of a new antidepressant with a low incidence and severity of side effects, it is decided that it is only worth the expense of full development if it can be demonstrated with 95 per cent confidence (i.e, only a one in twenty chance of being wrong) that it is at worst 10 per cent less effective than amitriptyline. Let us assume the latter helps 70 per cent of patients, i.e., produces an adequate clinical response as measured by a standard rating scale. Even if we accept a 20 per cent risk that even if the drug is really equally effective one will fail to show it (a 20 per cent false negative risk), 332 patients are needed in each group. The typical study with thirty in each group will detect a standard response rate of 70 per cent and a test drug response rate of 40 per cent with the same degrees of confidence and error.

ORGANIZATION OF TRIALS

Increasing appreciation by regulatory authorities of the need for trials with large numbers of patients has led to major exercises involving several centres. Such multi-centre trials have been commonplace in, say, the area of cancer chemotherapy but are the exception in psychiatry. Those that have been conducted have generally been organized by official organizations such as the Medical Research Council or the National Institute of Medical Health. Recently, however, two large-scale studies have been mounted evaluating alprazolam in the control of panic attacks. The first trial involved hundreds of patients in several centres in the USA and Canada and compared alprazolam with placebo (Klerman *et al.* 1986). The second involved centres throughout the world, over a thousand patients, and compared alprazolam, imipramine, and placebo. Both required a great deal of preparation, organization, logistic support, quality control, and data handling. The major resources, human and financial, that were devoted to the task were beyond the bounds of most non-commercial funding agencies.

On a more modest scale are the co-ordinated general practitioner studies. These provide risk-benefit assessments in the milieu in which most psychotropic drugs are prescribed. The problem is that general practitioners do not accrue sufficient numbers of any but the most common psychiatric disorders. Multi-centre studies can too often threaten to degenerate into quasi-marketing exercises with each GP contributing less than ten patients. It is essential that the raters are properly trained and that they are 'calibrated' against more experienced researchers.

Epidemiological techniques can be used to evaluate the effectiveness of a medicine. for example, if lithium had had a major effect in preventing manic and hypomanic episodes, the rate of admission for these conditions should have fallen since the widespread introduction of lithium over the past two decades. A survey by Dickson and Kendall (1986) failed to show such an effect.

EXCLUSIONS AND DROP-OUTS

Clinical trial protocols include a section on inclusion and exclusion criteria. Some of the exclusion criteria relate to toxicological concerns, for example excluding pregnant women, others are more arbitrary and may reflect some pre-conceptions about the type of patient who should respond. Ethical considerations may be important: for example, severely disordered patients may be excluded from treatment with an untried remedy. It is, however, often illuminating to follow up patients excluded from a trial and presumably given standard treatment. For example, Leff and Wing (1971) attempted to follow up patients not included in a trial of maintenance therapy in schizophrenia and achieved a success rate of 95 per cent. Non-trial patients comprised those more ill and those less ill than trial patients.

The question of drop-outs is always a vexing one (May *et al.* 1981). But it is important to divide patients who fail to complete the study into those who terminate early because they recover, those whose treatment is changed because of failure to respond, and those whose side effects are too severe for them to continue. In addition, some patients drop out for administrative and operational reasons, e.g, moving away from the district. Analysing outcome data in terms of completers only may give a misleading estimate of the risk/benefit ratio of a compound (Sackett 1980). Including all patients who are entered into the trial – the 'intention-to-treat' approach – is better practice and is now usually required by regulatory authorities. In this strategy, the scores at the point of drop-out are carried forward to the end-point of analysis. Similarly, if the 'disposal' of the patient is being recorded, e.g, back to the GP or to continuing support, drop-outs should be included to render more valid comparisons between treatments.

Another instance where patients may be lost to a trial concerns placebo 'run-in' periods. Some trials incorporate a week or two of placebo treatment before allocation to the treatments proper. Spontaneous or placebo-related improvement may take place, lowering the patient's psychopathology score below that for inclusion. Placebo run-in periods may, however, distort the trial itself. Thus, if one group of patients is to receive placebo, the drug-placebo comparison will be vitiated because placebo responders have already been excluded and the active drug will appear more effective than it really is.

ASSESSMENT OF PSYCHOPATHOLOGY

Assessment in psychiatry usually refers to two features, the symptoms of the illness, if any, and behavioural abnormalities, if any. It has traditionally taken place in the course of an interview with the patient, together with interviews with friends, relatives, and nurses. Special observation of the patient's behaviour is instituted usually by nurse, doctor, or clinical psychologist (Burdock 1982). This informal approach has changed over the years with increasing sophistication and an emphasis on structured or semi-structured interviews, the results of which are recorded on specially constructed scales (Hamilton 1986).

The simplest form of assessment is an overall so-called Global Rating of Severity. Despite its apparent crudity, it is capable of yielding quite reliable data, sensitive to drug effects. Next, a simple check list of symptoms can be used, predicated on the principle that patients with a severe form of disorder will have more symptoms than those with a mild disorder. As long as the check list contains more than twelve or fifteen items, this holds good. However, no account is taken of the severity of each symptom.

On a more complex level, the development of item gradings is quite a sophisticated process. It is important that one dimension only is rated at a time; for example, frequency, severity, or subsequent handicap should not be mixed in one item. The next process, giving numbers to grades of frequency or severity, is recognized by psychometricians as a very arbitrary undertaking. It implies that the grades are equal in intervals when they are usually no more than ordinal. Nevertheless, the sum of items is generally regarded as a measure to which parametric statistics can be applied. By and large, no gross violations of statistical purity are perpetrated.

The types of scale available relate mostly to the user, the patient himself, or require an observer. The observer can be a psychiatrist, psychologist, nurse, or relative. Informal observations can be made or a structured or semi-structured interview undertaken.

It is most important to distinguish between instruments designed to measure change and those meant to establish a diagnostic or sometimes prognostic profile. The former contain items which are sensitive to change but which may not be pathognomonic of the condition. For example, the Hamilton Rating Scale for Anxiety contains items concerning depression, the Scale for Depression, anxiety items. This is justified as anxious patients are often depressed as well, and vice versa, and the symptoms resolve with treatment. It is important to recognize this 'cross-talk' in the evaluation of a therapeutic agent. Thus, an anxiolytic may show limited 'efficacy' in the treatment of depressed patients because the anxiety items such as initial insomnia alter, although true depressive ones do not.

The diagnostic profile instruments can be used as entry criteria to a study but not usually as measures of change. However, different instruments have different criteria and some may affect the responsiveness of a selected group to a particular medication.

Whatever scales are used, proper training in their use is essential. Raters should be skilled in the necessary assessments, especially when attempting to elicit psychotic phenomena. They should be 'calibrated' against experienced raters to avoid errors such as leniency, when they are reluctant to use an extreme score, and proximity, when similar scores are given to adjacent items.

Patients need careful instruction about self-rating. The purpose of the scale should be explained, together with the mechanics of rating. In particular, the time focus should be specified, i.e., whether the rating is here-and-now, for the past few days, or whatever. The first use of a scale by the patient should be carefully supervised and the patient corrected if all the ratings are extreme or absent. Computer-based assessments have become popular but, again, the patient must be familiarized with both the computer and the questions.

OBJECTIVE TESTING

The vagaries of rating scales are such, or at least are perceived as such, that many investigators have sought the Holy Grail of the objective test of the diagnosis of depression, or failing that the severity of depression. A host of measures from many disciplines have been tested, regarded as full of initial promise, intensively investigated, and then found to be insensitive, unreliable, nonspecific, or cumbersome, or any combination of these. Examples include the Sedation Threshold (Shagass 1954) and salivary flow rate (Palmai *et al.* 1967). Most recently, the Dexamethasone Suppression Test has been thoroughly studied on thousands of patients; little of clinical use has emerged (Gitlin and Gerner 1986). Nor do the biochemical tests of amine and neuroendocrine status seem any more promising.

More limited objectives are achieved by psychological tests. These include perceptual and cognitive tests such as the Cancellation and Digit Symbol Substitution Tests, memory tests, and psychomotor tests such as simple key-tapping speed. Many such functions are impaired in depressives and clinical recovery is attended by improvement (Lader *et al.* 1987).

Physiological, biochemical and psychological tests can all be used more effectively to quantify the side effects of psychotropic drugs. For example, antidepressants with anticholinergic properties lessen salivary flow and anti-psychotic drugs increase plasma prolactin concentrations. The elec-troencephalogram (EEG), usually quantified mathematically, provides a sensitive albeit empirical measure of dose-and time-effects as well as some qualitative impression of the type of psychotropic drug effect (Fink 1981).

All in all, however, such objective tests are of limited validity. Despite their high reliability, they remain research tools and have yet to establish themselves in the routine evaluation of new psychotropic chemical entities.

THE TYPE OF RESPONDER

In most comparative trials, attempts are made to identify the type of responder. First, the type of patient who responds to any treatment is sought. Some patients do well however they are treated. Others may respond to one but not another treatment and vice versa.

A good example of the former is provided by the multi-centre studies carried out by Rickels and his collaborators on responsiveness to antianxiety drugs. They found that older rather than younger, female rather than male, and higher than lower social classes responded better (Rickels *et al.* 1978). Patients who recognized that their symptoms were related to psychological problems and were prepared to try drug therapy did well. The closer the patient approximated to the text book description of Generalized Anxiety Disorder, the better the response, especially when more ill. Physicians could detect who would respond well, a finding with obvious implications for the design and conduct of clinical trials where doctors can exercise major influences on the selection of patients.

Differential responsivity has been sought repeatedly with respect to the two main groups of antidepressants, the tricyclic compounds and the monoamine oxidase inhibitors. Surprisingly few indicators have been found, the most robust being that depressed patients with phobic anxiety do well with MAOIs (Paykel *et al.* 1979).

COST-BENEFIT ANALYSIS

Escalating health costs have forced caring agencies, private and governmental, to evaluate treatments in economic terms (Hurst 1984). A large number of factors must be considered, especially as much psychiatric illness is chronic and results in social and occupational handicap (Rosser and Kind 1978). But non-economic values are also important. The benefits of relieving suffering are inestimable. And, family and friends also suffer seeing a loved one in anguished depression or in a truculent or inert phase of schizophrenia.

Thus, effective treatment for major mental disorders would have profound economic and humanitarian benefits. Drug therapy is relatively cheap compared, for example, with the total costs of an in-patient admission. But lesser conditions are common and mild symptomatic relief not to be undervalued. Against this, side effects are often frequent, severe, or chronic and must be entered into the equation.

ETHICS

This is a large topic which has been reviewed by doctors, moral philosophers, and theologians (e.g. Burkhardt and Kienzle 1978; Schafer 1982; Helmchen 1983). Particular problems relate to clinical trials in psychiatry, mainly with respect to informed consent and forcible detention of disturbed patients. Also, the doctor-patient relationship may be jeopardized.

However, provided the usual ethical guidelines are adhered to, psychiatric trials present the same dilemmas as psychiatric practice in general. As the treatment steps are detailed in the clinical trial protocol, the ethical problems are thrown into sharper relief. Flexibility is needed during the conduct of the trial, with the researcher remaining sensitive to the ethical issues involved. It is always helpful for the researcher's colleagues to be kept informed of the progress of the trial to constitute a sort of informal ethical peer review.

Then the study must be completed, analysed, written up, and published. It is unethical to expose patients to the hazards of research, however apparently minimal, and not to communicate the results of that research to the scientific community. Unfortunately, the bias in the traditional way of doing this – the refereed journal – is against publishing negative trials, those where the compound proves ineffective. It is to be hoped that the advent of the 'Information Revolution' will allow such data to be kept on file, but easily accessible by interested clinicians. Finally, the data must be communicated to clinicians in such a way as to influence their prescribing

(Avorn and Soumerai 1983). But that is another issue.

The clinician is compelled to hold the balance between the scales of laboratory data on the one hand and stochastic theory on the other. Though his experience and judgement are essential it will be necessary for him to adopt a more experimental role in the future if he is to cooperate fully with the pharmacologist and the statistician, whose techniques he should understand if full weight is to be given to observations made in the clinical setting. Shepherd (1959:S125)

REFERENCES

American Psychiatric Association (1980) *Diagnostic and Statistical Manual of Mental Disorders*: third edition, Washington, DC.

Aubrée, J.C. and Lader, M.H. (1980) 'High and very high dosage antipsychotics: a critical review', *Journal of Clinical Psychiatry* 41: 341–50.

Avorn, J. and Soumerai, S.B. (1983) 'Improving drug-therapy decisions through educational outreach: a randomized controlled trial of academically based "detailing"', *New England Journal of Medicine* 308: 1457–63.

Ayd, F.J. and Blackwell, B. (eds) (1970) *Discoveries in Biological Psychiatry*, Philadelphia: Lippincott.

Burdock, E.I. (1982) 'Problems and profits in quantitative evaluation', in E.I. Burdock, A. Sudilovsky and S. Gershon (eds) *The Behaviour of Psychiatric Patients*, New York: Marcel Dekker, 3–7.

Burkhardt, R. and Kienzle, G. (1978) 'Controlled clinical trials and medical ethics', *Lancet* 2: 1356–9.

Dickson, W.E. and Kendell, R.E. (1986) 'Does maintenance lithium therapy prevent recurrences of mania under ordinary clinical conditions?', *Psychological Medicine* 16: 521–30.

Fink, M. (1981) 'Classification of psychoactive drugs: quantitative EEG analysis of man' in H.M. van Praag *et al.* (eds) *Handbook of Biological Psychiatry, Part VI*, New York: Marcel Dekker, pp. 309–26.

Freiman, J.A., Chalmers, T.C., Smith, H., *et al.* (1978) 'The importance of beta, the type II error and sample size in the design and interpretation of the randomized control trial: survey of 71 "negative" trials', *New England Journal of Medicine* 299: 690–4.

Gitlin, M.J. and Gerner, R.H. (1986) 'The Dexamethasone Suppression Test and response to somatic treatment: a review', *Journal of Clinical Psychiatry* 47: 16–21.

Hamilton, M. (1986) *Assessment of Psychopathology* (Human Psychopharmacology Monographs, No. 1), Chichester: Wiley.

Helmchen, H. (1983) 'Ethical and practical problems in therapeutic research in psychiatry', in T. Helgason (ed.) *Methodology in Evaluation of Psychiatric Treatment*, Cambridge: Cambridge University Press, 251–64.

Hurst, J.W. (1984) 'Measuring the benefits and costs of medical care: the contribution of health status measurement', *Health Trends* 16: 16–19.

Johnson, A.L. (1983) 'Clinical trials in psychiatry', *Psychological Medicine* 13: 1–8.

Klerman, G.L., Coleman, J.H., and Purpura, R.P. (1986) 'The design and conduct of the Upjohn Cross-National Collaborative Panic Study', *Psychopharmacology Bulletin* 22: 59–64.

Lader, M.H., Lang, R.A., and Wilson, G.D. (1987) *Patterns of Improvement in Depressed In-patients*, Oxford: Oxford University Press.

Leff, J.P. and Wing, J.K. (1971) 'Trial of maintenance therapy in schizophrenia', *British Medical Journal* 3: 599–604.

Lewis, A.J. (1953) 'Health as a social concept', *British Journal of Sociology* 4: 109–24.

May, G.S., de Mets, D.L., Friedman, L.M., *et al.* (1981) 'The randomized clinical trial: bias in analysis, *Circulation* 64: 669–73.

Palmai, G., Blackwell, B., Maxwell, A.E., and Morgenstern, F. (1967) 'Patterns of salivary flow in depressive illness and during treatment', *British Journal of Psychiatry* 113: 1297–308.

Paris, J.A. (1833) *Pharmacologia* (eighth edition), London: Sherwood, Gilbert and Piper, p.50.

Paykel, E.S., Parker, R.R., Penrose, R.J.J., and Rassaby, E.R. (1979) 'Depressive classification and prediction of response to phenelzine, *British Journal of Psychiatry* 134: 572–81.

Rickels, K., Downing, R.W., and Winokur, A. (1978) 'Antianxiety drugs: clinical use in psychiatry' in L.L. Iversen, S.D. Iversen, and S.H. Snyder, (eds) *Handbook of Psychopharmacology, Volume 13*, New York: Plenum, 395–430.

Rosser, R. and Kind, P. (1978) 'A scale of valuations of states of illness: is there a social consensus? *International Journal of Epidemiology* 7: 347–58.

Sackett, D.L. (1980) 'The competing objectives of randomized trials', *New England Journal of Medicine* 303: 1059–60.

Schafer, A. (1982) 'The ethics of the randomized clinical trial', *New England Journal of Medicine* 307: 719–24.

Shagass, C. (1954) 'The sedation threshold: a method for estimating tension in psychiatric patients', *Electroencephalography and Clinical Neurophysiology* 6: 221–33.

Shepherd, M. (1959) 'Evaluation of drugs in the treatment of depression', *Canadian Psychiatric Association Journal* 4 (supplement): S120–8.

Spitzer, R.L., Endicott, J., and Robins, E. (1978) 'Research Diagnostic Criteria: rationale and reliability', *Archives of General Psychiatry* 35: 773–82.

Walker, S.R. and Asscher, A.W. (eds) (1987) *Medicines and Risk/Benefit Decisions*, Lancaster: MTP Press.

World Health Organization (1980) *International Classification of Diseases, 9th Revision, Clinical Modification: ICD*, Geneva: WHO.

21

Tranquillizer Use: Epidemiological and Sociological Aspects

Paul Williams and Jonathan Gabe

Although mood-altering drugs have been used for medicinal purposes throughout recorded history (Gabe and Williams 1986a), it is only recently that there has been a rapid development of a multiplicity of 'mood-altering' chemicals. This has in part resulted from the activities of the pharmaceutical industry, which, governed by market economics, sought to maximize profits (Rabin and Bush 1974). The bromides and chloral hydrate, which had replaced opium on the grounds that the latter was addictive (Berridge 1978), were themselves displaced in the 1930s by the barbiturates because they were considered 'safer'. By the 1950s the dependence-producing potential of barbiturates had also become clearly established, causing a great deal of concern (Hollister 1983). This encouraged the search for suitable non-barbiturate tranquillizers.

The first replacement was meprobamate, a drug which was received enthusiastically by physicians and much used in the late 1950s as an anti-anxiety agent until it too was found to cause dependence (Hollister 1983). The second was the benzodiazepine group of drugs which quickly made meprobamate obsolete, once it became clear that they were safer and more effective (Lader 1978). Chlordiazepoxide was the first benzodiazepine to be introduced in 1960, followed by diazepam in 1963. There are now eighteen generic benzodiazepine preparations available in Britain and their dominance of the field indicates that we are unquestionably living in the 'benzodiazepine era' (Hollister 1983: 13).

TRENDS IN PRESCRIBING

The large and regular increases in prescriptions for benzodiazepines and other tranquillizers that occurred during the late 1960s and early 1970s are well known. In 1960, some 28 million prescriptions for drugs classified as hypnotics or tranquillizers were dispensed at retail pharmacies in Great Britain: in 1974, the total was about 40 million, of which 25 million were

328

for benzodiazepines. The peak in benzodiazepine prescribing occurred in 1979 (31 million prescriptions): the estimated figure for 1985 is 26 million, a decrease of about 16 per cent in six years (Taylor 1987). This pattern – an increase until the mid- or late-1970s, and a subsequent levelling off and decrease – has been found in many countries (Marks 1983a).

Comparison of three population surveys of the consumption of tranquillizers and other psychotropic drugs suggest that in England at least, there was no comparable increase at that time in the proportion of the population who reported consuming such drugs. Williams (1983a) suggested that this disparity (between prescribing and consuming) could be explained by a decrease in compliance and an increase in long-term drug use. This interpretation is supported by Marks' demonstration of substantial increases, over the same time period, in the extent to which benzodiazepines are prescribed on a 'repeat' basis (Marks 1983b).

Conversely, the prime factor in the subsequent decrease in tranquillizer prescribing is most likely to have been a reduction in new prescribing rather than discontinuation of treatment by long-term consumers. This suggests that there is a cohort of long-term benzodiazepine users (created during the 'phase of enthusiasm' in the mid-1960s and early 1970s) from which members will slowly be lost (a small proportion will discontinue treatment, others will die) and to which few new members will be recruited, since a reduction in new prescribing will inevitably lead to fewer people becoming long-term users (however 'long-term' is defined).

THE GROWTH OF CONCERN ABOUT MINOR TRANQUILLIZERS

When benzodiazepines were first introduced they were accepted enthusiastically by the medical profession as highly effective and safe drugs which did not create dependence and which had few other side effects (Owen and Tyrer 1983). This impression was reinforced a few years later by favourable reports of clinical practice (Svenson and Hamilton 1966).

In the early 1970s, concern started to be expressed by physicians and social scientists (e.g. Dunlop 1970; Jefferys 1973) about the extent of benzodiazepine prescribing. Social scientists talked of an 'overmedicated society' (Muller 1972) and suggested that benzodiazepines, by providing symptomatic relief, discouraged the search for a social solution to problems with social origins (Lennard et al. 1971). Moreover, those social scientists influenced by feminist theory argued that tranquillizer prescribing represented a means of social control, because it encouraged women, the major recipient of these drugs, to deny or ignore the social concomitants of their distress, thereby minimizing pressure for social change (Waldron 1977).

Physicians questioned whether the increase in tranquillizer prescribing reflected an increase in the number of people suffering from anxiety, or a

too-ready recourse to a prescription (*Lancet* 1973a) by doctors who saw tranquillizers as a suitable way of modifying personal and interpersonal
processes: this was thought likely to fuel demand for tranquillizers among
patients (Trethowan 1975). Also questioned were the therapeutic (as opposed
to the commercial) value of increasing the number of benzodiazepines
available (Tyrer 1974), the cost of the drugs (Trethowan 1975), and the
possibility that tranquillizers were no more effective than placebos for those
suffering from minor mood changes (*Lancet* 1973b).

In the latter part of the 1970s the concern about prescribing levels abated,
to be replaced at the start of the 1980s by a new concern: that of physical
dependence on benzodiazepines. This possibility had been acknowledged as
far back as 1961 for those suddenly withdrawn from high dosages of
benzodiazepines (Hollister *et al.* 1961). Thereafter, the number of cases of
dependence reported did not increase above a trickle and these generally
referred to patients on high dosages (Tyrer 1980). Given the total number of
benzodiazepines consumed, what impressed during this period was the rarity
of benzodiazepine dependence: a view endorsed by Marks (1978) who
concluded, after a comprehensive review of published case histories of
dependence, that benzodiazepines had a negligible dependence risk if used in
therapeutic doses.

Two years later, the picture started to change. The Committee on the
Review of Medicines officially acknowledged for the first time a growing
concern about physical dependence, even though it concluded that: 'on
present available evidence the true addiction potential of benzodiazepines [is]
low' (Committee on the Review of Medicines 1980: 910). Soon afterwards
the evidence started to appear. Studies of relatively small numbers of people
(usually about forty) agreeing to or requesting withdrawal from long-term
benzodiazepine use at therapeutic dose found that a significant proportion
developed a withdrawal syndrome (Petursson and Lader 1981; Tyrer *et al.*
1983), and that these symptoms could last a year or more (Ashton 1984).
This was described as an 'epidemic in the making' (Lader 1981).

Current concern has not been limited to academics and clinicians. Recent
studies of patients have demonstrated a marked awareness of the side effects
of tranquillizers and, at best, an ambivalence about taking them (e.g. Gabe
and Lipshitz-Phillips 1982, 1984). This kind of concern suggests that tranquillizer use has become a public issue.

Why has this happened now, when the prescribing of tranquillizers is
actually declining? There are at least four reasons. *First* is the recent
coverage of tranquillizer dependence in the media. Once discovered, this
issue has featured regularly on television consumer programmes since at least
1981, in the up-market and popular press, and in women's magazines. Much
of this coverage has been sensationalizing in tone.

Furthermore, the impression has frequently been given that everyone on
tranquillizers is likely to be dependent on them and will automatically have

'terrible' withdrawal symptoms if they try and stop. Indeed, one recent television programme began with the statement that 'kicking the tranquillizer habit can be harder than coming off heroin'. As several commentators have remarked, this represents 'trial by media' (Lasagna 1980; Cohen 1983).

Second is the context of revived fears about *illegal* drug taking. The present climate in Britain is one of extreme concern if not outright panic over the use of illegal drugs (e.g. 'the greatest menace in peace time', Home Affairs Committee 1985). As the above quotation from a television programme illustrates, greater sensitivity to the deleterious effects of such drug taking is influencing responses to the use of tranquillizers.

Third, concern has also been fuelled by mental health campaigning bodies like MIND and RELEASE. These organizations have, with the help of one or two sympathetic academics, produced material on tranquillizer dependence for the general public (RELEASE 1982; MIND 1984), and have skilfully used and worked with the media in presenting their case.

Fourth, current concern has to be set against the backcloth of wider cultural changes. Over the last fifteen years or so there seems to have been a shift in attitudes away from a belief in the right to happiness and an unwillingness to tolerate 'normal' discomfort and malaise towards a more puritanical view of life based on abstinence, stoicism, and self-reliance (Hall 1983). The latter view has encouraged an attitude to drugs which Klerman (1971) has described as 'pharmacological calvinism'. Simply stated, this means 'if it makes you feel good it is wrong' (Blackwell 1977). The development of this 'anti-drug culture' (Gabe and Lipshitz-Phillips 1982) also coincides with increasing criticism of other forms of medical technology (Kennedy 1981) and the medical profession (Jefferys and Sachs 1983; Cartwright 1983), and an increasing enthusiasm for alternative medicines (Salmon 1985) and for self-help (Robinson 1978), at least among some social groups (Doyal 1983).

Not surprisingly, this concern about the danger of dependence is not shared to the same extent by all of those with an interest in tranquillizers. Some pharmaceutical companies, for example, have been fighting back by financing researchers who might provide ammunition to challenge the risks of benzodiazepine dependence. Other companies are developing alternatives to fill what they regard as a gap in the market (File 1987).

Also, some academics and clinicians have questioned the evidence about the extent of dependence (Rickels 1981), the adequacy of existing studies (Kraupl-Taylor 1984) and the availability of appropriate alternatives for chronic benzodiazepine users (Rickels *et al.* 1984). Even so, the future for benzodiazepines looks somewhat uncertain, given the level of current concern.

In Britain, this uncertainty is compounded by recent legislation concerning prescribing. As from 1 April 1985, the prescription under the NHS of seven categories of drug – including the benzodiazepines – has been limited in

331

range. That is, there is now a 'white list' of drugs which can be prescribed under the NHS and a 'black list' of drugs which cannot (although such drugs can still be prescribed privately).

The government's initial proposal was to limit the number of available benzodiazepines from eighteen to three, although, in the event, preparations of seven varieties were categorized as prescribable.

This legislation and the way in which it was introduced gives rise to a whole host of issues beyond the scope of this chapter (*British Medical Journal* 1984, 1985). However, from the point of view of tranquillizer use, there is some evidence that the regulations may have resulted in a sharp decline in NHS prescriptions. A recent press release from the DHSS (1987) claims that the NHS's financial outlay on benzodiazepines has been cut by £15.5m in a twelve-month period. Similarly, Taylor (1987) has asserted that the impact of the list has been to cut the NHS benzodiazepine drug bill by around 20 per cent in its first year of operation.

Even so, these figures only relate to prescriptions paid for under the NHS and not all prescriptions. No information is publicly available about trends in private prescribing, and it may well be that the fall in NHS prescriptions has been counterbalanced by a rise in private prescribing. There is certainly evidence that this happens in other countries. For example, in Italy, NHS prescriptions for benzodiazepines have decreased rapidly since their removal from the national formulary (Bellantuono *et al.* 1987), whereas sales have continued to increase (Williams *et al.* 1986). Thus, as Bellantuono *et al.* (1987) have observed, 'the exclusion of a drug or group of drugs from a national formulary, and their subsequent disappearance from official prescription audits, does not necessarily mean that the drugs will no longer be prescribed and (presumably) consumed'.

It is still too early to say what the long-term effect of the limited list will be on prescribing levels and on consumption patterns, especially among long-term users: close monitoring is essential.

LONG-TERM TRANQUILLIZER USE

The remainder of this chapter will be concerned with the long-term use of tranquillizers. Ideally, a prerequisite for research into such use is the development of a consensus about the interpretation of 'long-term'. One approach is to seek a common view as to 'how long is long'. Most researchers seem to regard the cut-off point as one year: using this criterion, the prevalence of long-term use in Britain is 1.5–3 per cent of the population (Rodrigo *et al.* 1988a).

An alternative, more realistic approach, is to regard the duration of use as a process rather than as a static criterion (Williams 1983b). Furthermore, more attention than is customary should be paid to distinguishing between intermittent and continuous use (Gabe and Thorogood 1986).

Clinical aspects of long-term use

Long-term users of tranquillizers report high levels of emotional distress. For example, half of the long-term users of anxiolytics studied in Mellinger *et al.*'s (1984) survey had high scores on a questionnaire measure of distress, as compared with 20 per cent of the non-users. They noted that 'the long-term users did not differ much from the other users in this respect', 45 per cent of whom were high scorers.

The study by Rodrigo *et al.* (1988a) is the first in which a standardized psychiatric assessment has been applied to long-term tranquillizer users in general practice. They found that twenty-four (38 per cent) of the sixty-four patients were rated as cases on the Standardised Psychiatric Interview (Goldberg *et al.* 1970). While in absolute terms this is a substantial level of psychiatric morbidity, it is not very different from that which would be found in an unselected series of general practice attenders (Marks *et al.* 1979). Rodrigo *et al.*'s study also found that three-quarters of the cases – i.e., just over a quarter of the long-term users – were classified under the rubric neurotic depression (ICD 300.4), and that none was assigned a diagnosis related to anxiety. This finding requires replication: if confirmed, it suggests that there exists a clearly-definable group of patients among whom a substantial proportion is suffering from unrecognized and untreated depression.

De novo prescription of benzodiazepines and other psychotropic drugs frequently occurs in response to physical rather than psychological disorder (Williams 1978). Similar findings apply to long-term users. For example, Murray and her colleagues (1982) interviewed twenty-two patients who had been prescribed psychotropic drugs continuously for six months or more. She found that 'chronic physical complaints were common in the sample (diverticulitis, arthritis, hypertension, migraine) and 13 people were long-term users of non-psychotropic prescribed drugs'. Furthermore, in a questionnaire of present and past long-term tranquillizer users (Murray 1981), only six out of 261 respondents scored as having no disability or physical symptoms on the Belloc scale (Belloc *et al.* 1971).

Mellinger *et al.* (1984) found that physical health distinguished between long-term users and other users more sharply than did any other factor. They noted that 'at least one-third of the long-term users reported four or more health problems – a rate twice that found among the other anxiolytic users and seven times that of the non users'. These differences persisted when age was controlled for, and much of the difference between the long-term users and the others was accounted for by cardiovascular disorders and arthritis.

The patients in Rodrigo *et al.*'s (1988a) study also reported substantial physical morbidity. For example, twenty-seven (42 per cent) had consulted their GP during the previous month for a physical illness (other than coughs, colds and influenza), and twenty-two (34 per cent) had attended medical or surgical out-patient clinics in the previous year.

Social factors in long-term use

There is general agreement that long-term tranquillizer users, as compared with all users, are older and predominantly women. These findings emerged from studies carried out in the late 1960s when barbiturates were still commonly used (Parish 1971). While the drugs may have changed in recent years, the relationship with age and sex has not (Cooperstock 1978, Mellinger *et al.* 1984, Rodrigo *et al.* 1988a).

The discussion here will focus on sex differences. Although most of the work in this area has been concerned with current, rather than with long-term, tranquillizer use, it can still throw light on the nature of long-term use.

One of the first social scientists to address this issue was the late Ruth Cooperstock (1971), who developed an explanatory model drawing on sex role theory. She hypothesized that women in western societies take more tranquillizers than men because (i) they are permitted greater freedom to explore their feelings than men, and are hence more likely to recognize emotional problems in themselves; (ii) they feel more able than men to bring their perceived emotional problems to the attention of a doctor; (iii) doctors – especially male doctors – expect women patients to be more expressive than men. They are therefore more likely to encourage such expressiveness among women patients and to prescribe tranquillizers.

Cooperstock's propositions were not tested empirically until the work of Mant *et al.* (1983) and Cafferata *et al.* (1983). Mant and her colleagues surveyed 1,300 adult patients attending fifteen randomly selected male general practitioners in Sydney, during a one-week period. They also collected information from these doctors on each of the patients in the sample.

They found clear support for a *consulting hypothesis* – i.e., that it is more socially acceptable for women than men to go to the doctor – and limited support for the *stereotyping hypothesis*, in that the doctors were much less likely to detect psychological ill-health among men. The findings did not support Cooperstock's *reporting hypothesis*, i.e., that it is more socially acceptable for women to admit to having symptoms, especially of emotional distress.

Cafferata and her colleagues (1983) broadened the debate by testing empirically not only the sex role theory but also *social support* and *social stress* theories. They conducted a secondary analysis of data on family circumstances and psychotropic drug use of adults in 11,000 households in the United States.

Evidence was found to support all three theories. For example, they reported that women in traditional families (in which the male is in paid work and the female fulfils the housewife role) were more likely than their spouses to be taking tranquillizers, suggesting that the traditional female role leads to more illness. They also found that women in non-intact families, and those caring for a spouse in poor health, were more likely to be using tranquillizers. This, they concluded, lent credence to social support and social stress theories, which suggest that women may be more sensitive than men to the effects of less supportive or more stressful family circumstances.

The views of long-term benzodiazepine users

The research on long-term use of benzodiazepines and other psychotropic drugs points to the importance of studying the point of view of the drug users themselves. While the term 'users' includes doctors as well as their patients (Cooperstock and Parnell 1982), relatively few studies have been concerned with doctors. For this reason, as well as constraints of space, we focus only on patients' views here.

It is only recently that researchers have begun to concern themselves, in a systematic way, with the views of the patients who use benzodiazepines and other tranquillizers on a long-term basis, and the impetus for such research has come primarily from social scientists rather than doctors. The methods used include postal surveys (Murray 1981), structured interviews and questionnaires (Rodrigo *et al.* 1988a), in-depth semi-structured interviews (Helman 1981; Gabe and Lipshitz-Phillips 1982, 1984; Gabe and Thorogood 1986) and group discussions (Cooperstock and Lennard 1979). Four issues arising out of this research will be discussed here: (i) long-term users' perceptions of the effects of the drugs; (ii) their views as to their continued need for their drugs; (iii) the way in which drug use is related to the availability of other resources for managing everyday life; and (iv) the meaning of long-term tranquillizer use.

Users' perceptions of the effects of tranquillizers. Do long-term users regard their drugs as helpful? It appears that, in a general sense, most do (Murray 1981, Rodrigo *et al.* 1988b). However, there is also evidence of considerable ambivalence: for example, 87 per cent of respondents in Murray's (1981) survey of women who were long-term psychotropic drug consumers agreed with the statement 'I don't like taking these tablets but I could not manage without them'. Furthermore, when Gabe and Thorogood (1986) asked women long-term users of benzodiazepines what they felt about taking the drugs, one-tenth of the sample emphasized the benefits, one-quarter the dangers, while the majority (about two-thirds) expressed mixed views. They also found that less ambivalence and fewer positive views were expressed by a sample of short-term users.

An important finding has been that when asked to specify the ways in which benzodiazepines and other tranquillizers are helpful, long-term users frequently mention social activities. For example, in Murray's (1981) questionnaire survey referred to above, travelling, shopping, mixing with people, and running the home were the four most frequently mentioned activities in this regard.

A similar finding emerged from Cooperstock and Lennard's (1979) series of group discussions with long-term benzodiazepine users. The women users in their study felt that taking the drug helped them to manage the strains they experienced in carrying out their traditional roles as wives, mothers, and homeworkers. Furthermore, over half of the long-term psychotropic drug users interviewed by Helman (1981) felt that withdrawal of the drugs would have a bad effect on their social relationships.

Users' views about their continued need for drugs. Fifty-eight per cent of the current long-term users surveyed by Murray (1981) said that they would find it 'very difficult' to manage without their drugs, and a further 33 per cent claimed that they would not be able to manage at all. A similar picture emerged from the long-term benzodiazepine consumers interviewed by Rodrigo *et al.* (1988b), most of whom were women. While only 17 per cent said that they could not 'do without', more than half (54 per cent) believed that they would need to take their drugs for 'years' or indefinitely.

An important aspect of the long-term use of prescribed drugs is the patients' perceptions of their doctor's attitude. Murray (1981) found a 'widespread belief in the general practitioner's acquiescence in continued drug taking' – 81 per cent of the respondents in her nationwide survey claimed that their doctors either wished them to continue or did not mind. Similarly, in Rodrigo *et al.*'s (1988b) study based in a two-doctor practice, thirty-three patients (52 per cent) had no idea as to their doctor's views, and a further twenty-four (38 per cent) believed that he encouraged their use. Fifty-two of the patients claimed that their GP had never suggested that they stop the drug. Conversely, the women interviewed by Gabe and Lipshitz-Phillips (1984), drawn from two practices with fourteen GPs, in general considered that their doctors were reluctant to prescribe benzodiazepines, and half of them said that their doctor had either restricted their supply or suggested that they cut down or stop taking the drug. A quarter of the users also believed that their doctors shared their doubts about benzodiazepines.

In Murray's (1981) and Rodrigo *et al.*'s (1988b) studies, users were asked to suggest alternative strategies that they would use if the drugs were not available. In both, the predominant strategy was the consumption of some alternative substance, other drugs, alcohol, and herbal remedies being the most frequently mentioned. Cigarette smoking was regarded as a resource by the women interviewed by Gabe and Thorogood (1986). In Rodrigo *et al.*'s study, 17 per cent of the patients interviewed could envisage no possible alternative to benzodiazepines and some expressed a fear of becoming mentally ill without their tablets.

The relationship between tranquillizer use and the availability of other resources. It is also important to consider how long-term users' tranquillizer use relates to the availability of other resources for the management of everyday life. As Gabe and Thorogood (1986) have argued, such resources are unequally distributed according to social group membership and can be variously experienced as enabling and/or constraining. In their study of working-class women, it was found that those who were long-term users of tranquillizers had access to fewer resources than other women in the study. Moreover, those resources that were available to them were rarely experienced in such a way as to enable them to manage their lives without recourse to tranquillizers.

Three resources in particular seemed to constrain the long-term users to maintain their pattern of drug use – paid work, children and partners, and leisure. Regarding paid work, Gabe and Thorogood found that the long-term users were not only markedly less likely to have a full-time job than other women, but that those who were so employed were more likely to express mixed feelings about their situation. It would thus seem that while the absence of paid work may deprive the long-term users of a resource which might make their lives easier, thereby reducing the need for tranquillizers, those users with access to this resource did not experience it in a sufficiently positive way to enable them to change the nature of their tranquillizer use.

The researchers also found that long-term use was related to being divorced and not having children living at home. Moreover, if these long-term users were living with partners and/or their children, they were less likely than the other women to find these kin supportive. It would thus appear that long-term users either lack access to potentially supportive social resources, or find that those that are available are unsupportive and a poor substitute for tranquillizers. In such circumstances, the existing pattern of drug use is likely to be maintained.

Gabe and Thorogood's study also revealed that long-term users were markedly more likely than other women to state either that they lacked all opportunities for leisure, or that they had few leisure options open to them. As this resource was only experienced as enabling and as a relaxant, these long-term users' limited access to it would seem to place them at a considerable disadvantage and further helps to explain why they continued to use tranquillizers to manage their daily lives.

Overall, then, it appears that three resources – paid work, children and partners, and leisure – had a particularly important influence upon the long-term drug users' behaviour. These women's access to and relationship with these resources combined with their views about tranquillizers to maintain their existing pattern of drug use.

The meaning of long-term use. Some of these various findings on users' perceptions and views can be integrated by using the concept of meaning, i.e., 'the interpretation a person gives to an object or event in his or her life' (Gabe and Williams 1986b). This approach has been taken by Helman (1981) and by Gabe and his colleagues (Gabe and Lipshitz-Phillips 1982, 1984;

337

Gabe and Thorogood 1986). Gabe has developed the concepts 'lifeline' and 'standby' to describe the meaning of benzodiazepines to consumers. Those who viewed their drugs as a lifeline felt them to be 'something which they needed to take regularly and depended on simply to keep going in the face of chronic, unresolved problems'. Others viewed their drugs as a standby, to be kept in reserve and used occasionally to meet some short-lived crisis, while a minority of their respondents characterized their drug-taking behaviour in terms of both these meanings.

Helman (1981) conducted in-depth interviews with fifty long-term (six months or more) benzodiazepine users. He found, on the basis of their beliefs, attitudes, and expectations concerning the drugs, that 'long-term users of psychotropics can be classified into three main groups – called "tonic", "food" and "fuel"'.

Patients classified as 'tonic' (about one-third of the sample) were those who expressed maximum control over the drug, its dosage, and when it was to be used, tending to use the drugs on an 'as required' (p.r.n.) basis rather than regularly. They placed the site of action of the drug on themselves rather than on their relationships, and tended to have more anti-drug views than the other groups. Patients classified as 'fuel' (some two-fifths of those interviewed) expressed a variable degree of control over their medication but nonetheless felt that the drug played an important and constant part in their daily lives. Its maximum effect was thought to be on their relationships with others: in some cases, the drug was seen as an essential constituent of the patients' relationships. Helman used the concept of 'fuel', since, as he observed, without the drug 'the patient would not disintegrate but would just not function in conformity with familial and social expectations'.

The third group of patients (about one-fifth of the sample), for whom benzodiazepines were conceptualized as a 'food', expressed least control over the drug, its ingestion, and over life generally. Helman noted that their psychological dependence was as much on the medical profession as on the drug. Furthermore, the drugs were seen by this group as acting both on the patient's emotional state and on social relationships: without it, both would disintegrate. Helman applied the concept of 'food' to these patients' drug use since, without it, they would not survive as an independent, sane person. There appears to be a parallel between Gabe's and Helman's categories. Helman's 'tonic' patients are similar to Gabe's 'standby' users, whereas his 'fuel' and 'food' patients are more like Gabe's 'lifeliners', being more dependent on their drugs.

CONCLUSION

It has long been recognized that the great majority of patients with a psychological problem are treated in primary medical care settings, rather than by specialists; the prescription of a psychotropic drug is one of the most commonly used methods of treatment for such problems in that setting (Shepherd *et al.* 1966).

While the previous chapter has dealt with the evaluation of psychotropic drugs in the context of the controlled clinical trial, this research strategy is, by its very nature, unable to throw light on the prescription and consumption of drugs in the real world. As we have demonstrated in this chapter, a purely medical approach is inadequate if a comprehensive understanding is to be obtained: indeed, it could be argued that a multi-disciplinary approach is mandatory rather than merely desirable (Gabe and Williams 1988).

Acknowledgement: The authors are supported by the Department of Health and Social Security.

REFERENCES

Ashton, H. (1984) 'Benzodiazepine withdrawal: an unfinished story', *British Medical Journal* 288: 1135–40.

Bellantuono, C., Fiorio, R., Williams, P., Martini, N. and Bozzini, L. (1987) 'Psychotropic drug monitoring in general practice in Italy: a two-year study', *Family Practice* 4: 41–9.

Belloc, N.B., Breslow, L., and Hochstim, J.R. (1971) 'Measurement of physical health in a general population survey', *American Journal of Epidemiology* 93: 328–36.

Berridge, V. (1978) 'Victorian opium eating: responses to opiate use in nineteenth century England', *Victorian Studies* 21: 437–61.

Blackwell, B. (1977) 'Medical, social and ethical issues in minor tranquilliser use', paper to the *World Congress in Mental Health*, Vancouver.

British Medical Journal (1984) 'Doctors, drugs and the DHSS: (editorial), *British Medical Journal* 289: 1397–8.

British Medical Journal (1985) 'Doctors, drugs and Government' (editorial), *British Medical Journal* 290: 880.

Cafferata, G.L., Kasper, J., and Bernstein, A. (1983) 'Family roles, structure and stressors in relation to sex differences in obtaining psychotropic drugs', *Journal of Health and Social behaviour* 24: 132–43.

Cartwright, A. (1983) 'Prescribing and the doctor-patient relationship', in D. Pendleton and J. Hasler (eds) *Doctor-Patient Communication*, London: Academic Press.

Cohen, S. (1983) 'Current attitudes about the benzodiazepines: trial by media', *Journal of Psychoactive Drugs* 15: 109–13.

Committee on the Review of Medicines (1980) 'Systematic review of the benzodiazepines', *British Medical Journal* 280: 910–12.

Cooperstock, R. (1971) 'Sex differences in the use of mood modifying drugs: an explanatory model', *Journal of Health and Social Behaviour* 12: 238–44.

Cooperstock, R. (1978) 'Sex differences in psychotropic drug use', *Social Science and Medicine* 12B: 179–86.

Cooperstock, R. and Lennard, H. (1979) 'Some social meanings of tranquilliser use', *Sociology of Health and Illness* 1: 331–47.

Cooperstock, R. and Parnell, P. (1982) 'Research on psychotropic drug use: a review of findings and methods', *Social Science and Medicine* 16: 1179–96.

Department of Health and Social Security (1987) 'Press release 87/127', 23 March.

Doyal, L. (1983) 'Women's health and the sexual division of labour', *Critical Social Policy* 7: 21–33.

Dunlop, D. (1970) 'The use and abuse of psychotropic drugs', *Proceedings of the Royal Society of Medicine* 63: 1279–82.

File, S. (1987) 'Beyond the benzodiazepines: the search for new anxiolytics', *Human Psychopharmacology* 2: 151–58.

Gabe, J. and Lipshitz-Phillips, S. (1982) 'Evil necessity? The meaning of benzodiazepine use for women patients from one general practice', *Sociology of Health and Illness* 4: 201–9.

Gabe, J. and Lipshitz-Phillips, S. (1984) 'Tranquillisers as social control?' *Sociological Review* 32: 524–46.

Gabe, J. and Thorogood, N. (1986) 'Prescribed drugs and the management of everyday life: the experiences of black and white working class women', *Sociological Review* 34: 737–72.

Gabe, J. and Williams, P. (1986a) 'Tranquilliser use: a historical perspective', in J. Gabe and P. Williams (eds) *Tranquillisers: Social, Psychological and Clinical Perspectives*, London: Tavistock.

Gabe, J. and Williams, P. (1986b) 'The meaning of tranquilliser use: introduction', in J. Gabe and P. Williams (eds) *Tranquillisers: Social, Psychological and Clinical Perspectives*, London: Tavistock.

Gabe, J. and Williams, P. (1988) 'A multidisciplinary approach to long-term tranquilliser use', unpublished paper, Institute of Psychiatry, London.

Goldberg, D., Cooper, B., Eastwood, M.R., Kedward, H.B., and Shepherd, M. (1970) 'A standardised psychiatric interview for use in community surveys', *Journal of Preventive and Social Medicine* 24: 18–23.

Hall, S. (1983) 'The great moving right show', in S. Hall and M. Jacques (eds) *The Politics of Thatcherism*, London: Lawrence & Wishart.

Helman, C. (1981) 'Tonic, fuel and food: social and symbolic aspects of the long-term use of psychotropic drugs', *Social Science and Medicine* 15B: 521–33.

Hollister, L. (1983) 'The pre-benzodiazepine era', *Journal of Psychoactive Drugs* 15: 9–13.

Hollister, L., Motzenbecker, F.P., and Degon, R.O. (1961) 'Withdrawal reactions from chlordiazepoxide (Librium)', *Psychopharmacologia* 2: 63–8.

Home Affairs Committee (1985) *Interim Report on Drug Misuse*, London: HMSO.

Jefferys, M. (1973) 'Medicine takers' *Journal of the Royal College of General Practitioners* 23 (supplement 2): 9–11.

Jefferys, M. and Sachs, H. (1983) *Rethinking General Practice*, London: Tavistock.

Kennedy, I. (1981) *The Unmasking of Modern Medicine*, London: Allen & Unwin.

Klerman, G. (1971) 'Drugs and social values', *International Journal of the Addictions* 5: 313–19.

Kraupl-Taylor, F. (1984) 'Benzodiazepines on trial', *British Medical Journal* 288: 1379.

Lader, M. (1978) 'Benzodiazepines: the opium of the masses?' *Neuroscience* 3: 159–65.

Lader, M. (1981) 'Epidemic in the making: benzodiazepine dependence', in G. Tognoni, C. Bellantuono, and M. Lader (eds) *The Epidemiological Impact of Psychotropic Drugs*, Amsterdam: Elsevier.

Lancet (1973a) 'Unreasonable profit' (editorial), *Lancet* i: 867.

Lancet (1973b) 'Benzodiazepines: use, overuse, misuse, abuse?' (editorial), *Lancet* i: 1101–2.

Lasagna, L. (1980)'The Halcion study: trial by media? *Lancet* i: 815–16.

Lennard, H.L., Epstein, L.J., Bernstein, A., and Ransom, D.C. (1971) *Mystification and Drug Misuse*, New York: Harper & Row.

Mant, A., Broom, D.H. and Duncan-Jones, P. (1983) 'The path to prescription: sex differences in psychotropic drug prescribing for general practice patients', *Social Psychiatry* 18: 185–92.

Marks, J. (1978) *The Benzodiazepines: Use, Overuse, Misuse and Abuse*, Lancaster: MTP Press.

Marks, J. (1983a) 'The benzodiazepines – for good or for evil?' *Neuropsychobiology* 10: 115–26.

Marks, J. (1983b) 'The benzodiazepines: an international perspective', *Journal of Psychoactive Drugs* 15: 137–49.

Marks, J., Goldberg, D., and Hillier, V.E. (1979) 'Determinants of the ability of general practitioners to detect psychiatric disorder', *Psychological Medicine* 9: 337–53.

Mellinger, G.D., Balter, M.B., and Uhlenhuth, E.H. (1984) 'Prevalence and correlates of long-term regular use of anxiolytics', *Journal of the American Medical Association* 251: 375–9.

MIND (1984) *Tranquillizers: Hard Facts, Hard Choices*, London, National Association for Mental Health.

Muller, C. (1972) 'The overmedicated society: forces in the marketplace for medical care', *Science* 176: 488–92.

Murray, J. (1981) 'Long-term psychotropic drug taking and the process of withdrawal', *Psychological Medicine* 11: 853–8.

Murray, J., Williams, P., and Clare, A.W. (1982) 'Health and social characteristics of long-term psychotropic drug takers', *Social Science and Medicine* 16: 1595–8.

Owen, R.T. and Tyrer, P. (1983) 'Benzodiazepine dependence: a review of the evidence', *Drugs* 25: 385–98.

Parish, P.A. (1971) 'The prescribing of psychotropic drugs in general practice', *Journal of the Royal College of General Practitioners* 21 (supplement 4): 1–77.

Petursson, H. and Lader, M. (1981) 'Benzodiazepine dependence', *British Journal of Addiction* 76: 133–45.

Rabin, D.L. and Bush, P.J. (1974) 'The use of medicines: historical trends and international comparisons', *International Journal of Health Services* 4: 61–87.

RELEASE (1982) *Trouble with Tranquillisers*, London: Release.

Rickels, K. (1981) 'Are benzodiazepines overused and abused?', *British Journal of Clinical Pharmacology* 11, (supplement 1): 71S–83S.

Rickels, K., Case, G.W., Winokur, A., and Svenson, C. (1984) 'Long-term benzodiazepine therapy: benefits and risks', *Psychopharmacology Bulletin* 20: 608–15.

Robinson, D. (1978) 'Self-help groups', *British Journal of Hospital Medicine*, September, 106–110.

Rodrigo, E., King, M., and Williams, P. (1988a) 'The health of long-term tranquilliser users', *British Medical Journal* 296: 603–6.

Rodrigo, E., King, M., and Williams, P. (1988b) 'Long-term tranquilliser use in a south London general practice', unpublished research report, Institute of Psychiatry.

Salmon, J.W. (1985) 'Introduction', in J.W. Salmon (ed.) *Alternative Medicines: Popular and Policy Perspectives*, London: Tavistock.

Shepherd, M., Cooper, B., Brown, A.C., and Kalton, G.W. (1966) *Psychiatric Illness in General Practice*, London: Oxford University Press.

Svenson, S.F. and Hamilton, R.G. (1966) 'A critique of over-emphasis of side effects with psychotropic drugs: an analysis of 18,000 chlordiazepoxide treated cases', *Current Therapeutic Research* 8: 455–64.

Taylor, D. (1987) 'Current usage of benzodiazepines in Britain', in H. Freeman and Y. Rue (eds) *The Benzodiazepines in Current Clinical Practice*, London: Royal Society of Medicine Services.

Trethowan, W.H. (1975) 'Pills for personal problems', *British Medical Journal* iii: 749–51.

Tyrer, P. (1974) 'The benzodiazepine bonanza', *Lancet* ii: 709–10.

Tyrer, P. (1980) 'Dependence on benzodiazepines', *British Journal of Psychiatry* 137: 576–7.

Tyrer, P., Owen, R., and Dawling, S. (1983) 'Gradual withdrawal of diazepam after long-term therapy', *Lancet* i: 1402–6.

Waldron, I. (1977) 'Increased prescribing of Valium, Librium and other drugs – an example of economic and social factors in the practice of medicine', *International Journal of Health Services* 7: 37–62.

Williams, P. (1978) 'Physical ill-health and psychotropic drug prescription: a review', *Psychological Medicine* 8: 683–93.

Williams, P. (1983a) 'Patterns of psychotropic drug use', *Social Science and Medicine* 17: 845–51.

Williams, P. (1983b) 'Factors influencing the duration of treatment with psychotropic drugs in general practice: a survival analysis approach', *Psychological Medicine* 13: 623–33.

Williams, P., Bellantuono, C., Fiorio, R., and Tansella, M. (1986) 'Psychotropic drug use in Italy: national trends and regional differences', *Psychological Medicine* 16: 841–50.

22

The Evaluation of Social Interventions

Roslyn Corney and Joanna Murray

Social interventions in the treatment of mental illness cover a broad spectrum of management techniques both of the individual's current symptoms and of the social circumstances with which they interplay. The focus of this chapter will be on social interventions directed at improving both the patient's symptoms and social functioning. We shall review studies of the effectiveness of various techniques employed primarily by trained social workers.

The crucial role of social factors in the causation of mental illness has been widely established and there exists a substantial literature documenting the positive associations between a number of socio-cultural factors (such as sex, socio-economic status and urban-rural location) and mental illness. The evidence has been reviewed by Dohrenwend and Dohrenwend (1969) and Dohrenwend (1975). The role of 'life events' and stress in the development of psychiatric morbidity has been investigated and discussed in a number of studies, although the theoretical difficulties in establishing the precise nature of the association remain to be resolved (Holmes and Rahe 1967; Brown and Birley 1968; Dohrenwend and Dohrenwend 1974; Paykel 1978). More recently there has been growing research activity in establishing the effects on illness of the presence or absence and the nature of personal relationships (Miller and Ingham 1976; Vaughn and Leff 1976; Brown and Harris 1978; Henderson *et al.* 1978).

In addition to the likely causative role in mental illness, social problems are found to exist with greater frequency in patients suffering from psychological disorders than in those unaffected. A higher degree of social impairment has been found in depressed patients than in normal subjects (Shepherd *et al.* 1966; Weissman and Paykel 1974; Brown and Harris 1978), and general practice patients with chronic neuroses have been shown to have a greater degree of social impairment than a matched group of non-psychiatric patients (Sylph *et al.* 1969; Cooper 1972). Although some of these problems may occur before the illness, the clinical symptoms themselves – such as irritability, anergia, and loss of libido – are likely to put extra strains on personal relationships and to have detrimental effects upon work performance and social activities.

Social factors play a major part in the prognosis of mental illness, chronicity being associated with long-term social difficulties. In a follow-up study of general practice patients, Kedward (1969) found that those who had chronic social problems were less likely to have improved after three years than patients without chronic problems. 'Situational' factors noted in these chronic patients were severe marital disharmony, housing problems, long-term physical illness, and bereavement. Kedward commented that a great deal of suffering might have been alleviated by interventions aimed at improving the patients' social conditions.

Two longitudinal studies have found that patients' social circumstances are the most powerful predictors of illness outcome. Huxley and Goldberg (1975) found that material and objective conditions predicted outcome at six months in a study of fifty non-psychotic patients. Stress and lack of support in patients' marital, family, and social life were found to predict continued illness at twelve months follow-up in a group of one hundred general practice patients initially diagnosed as having neurotic disorders (Jenkins et al. 1981). Further evidence of the key role of social supports and family tensions in determining outcome is to be found in the work of Bullock et al. (1972) and Vaughn and Leff (1976). The pioneering studies of the latter authors and their colleagues have isolated aspects of family interaction which are associated with episodes of schizophrenic illness. High levels of 'expressed emotion' and frequent criticism of the patient were found in those families in which readmissions to hospital occurred most often.

Given the evidence on the role of social factors, interventions aimed at ameliorating social problems should be considered along with psychological and physical treatments. However, the time available to general practitioners and psychiatrists to attempt to effect change in a patient's social condition is strictly limited (Shepherd et al. 1966; Royal College of General Practitioners 1973). Lack of knowledge of social agencies and their resources also limits the doctor's ability to intervene in this way (Jeffreys 1965). The changing nature of modern medicine, with greater emphasis on pharmacological and technological interventions, has also led to a change in the relation between doctor and patient to the point where counsel and support have become a much reduced aspect of medical practice (British Medical Association 1986). The lack of opportunity to vent the personal problems and social difficulties which they perceive to be associated with their illnesses, has led increasing numbers of patients to look to non-medical sources of help (BMA 1986). Recognition of the change in the doctor-patient relationship is demonstrated by the growing involvement of counsellors, clinical psychologists, and social workers in the management of psychological problems. This chapter will concentrate on social interventions in hospital and general practice settings, presenting the findings of clinical trials on social work treatment in the management of mental illness and its outcome. Trials of more analytic psychotherapies will be excluded and behavioural methods are discussed by Falloon in the following chapter.

METHODS OF EVALUATION: THE CLINICAL TRIAL

Although subjective impressions of social work involvement with the mentally disturbed indicate that social workers can offer a great deal of support and counsel, it is important to evaluate their therapeutic role in the management of mental disorder. The established method for the evaluation of any form of treatment is the controlled clinical trial. This technique has been used to measure the efficacy of psychotropic drugs both in hospital settings and in general practice (MRC 1965; Wheatley 1972), but it has been used infrequently to evaluate social treatments of psychiatric patients. The very nature of the intervention leads to a number of difficulties in conducting such trials. First, there are the problems of defining the disorders and assessing outcome. In addition, there are ethical and practical problems: many clinical trials are difficult to carry out because of the ethical issues arising from the withholding of treatment from the control group of patients. Practical difficulties arise when patients refuse the treatment offered, move from the district, or fail to attend for the follow-up interviews.

In double-blind drug trials, placebos can be given when medication is being tested and arrangements can be made for the patients, physicians, and assessors to remain unaware of who is receiving the active drug. Thus, the observations made are not biased by the attitudes of either the research worker or the client, and the physician's management of the patients is unaffected. In contrast, when social or psychological treatment is being tested there are no suitable placebos to allow double-blind procedures to be employed. Studies have to be planned so that the assessors, at least, are unaware of the treatment received by the patients. Trials of social work present extra difficulties because the treatment given is very difficult to standardize. Unlike drugs, for which a fixed dose can be prescribed, the practitioners, the clients, the relationship built up between them, and the content of the interventions all vary considerably (Truax and Carkhuff 1967; Bergin 1971). It is, therefore, important to record in detail and to attempt to codify the social work interventions that have occurred and the type of help given.

It is also difficult to decide by which criteria improvement will be assessed. Social treatment may, for example, fail to improve clinical symptoms (Weissman and Paykel 1974), but may alleviate social problems. Thus, the criteria used in the assessments must take into account the social worker's aims and treatment, and not rely on biomedical outcome measures. As we have said, social disadvantage and dysfunction are major components of much psychological illness, and their amelioration should be seen as a successful outcome of social therapy.

345

CLINICAL TRIALS OF SOCIAL WORK WITH PSYCHIATRIC PATIENTS

There have been very few studies on the effectiveness of social work with psychiatric patients, no doubt because of the many difficulties involved. This paper will focus on seven studies which have taken place in either out-patient or general practice settings and have included patients suffering from depression, chronic neurosis, and schizophrenia.

In hospital settings

The first of these studies was conducted in the United States and investigated the effects of psychiatric social work and drug treatment in depressed female out-patients (Klerman *et al.* 1974; Weissman and Paykel 1974). On entry to the study, the women were first given amitriptyline for four to six weeks. Those who responded to the drug were then accepted for maintenance treatment. They were randomly assigned to eight months of either the same antidepressant or a placebo or no tablet at all, with or without psychiatric social work, using a 2×3 factorial design. Women referred to the psychiatric social worker were seen once or twice a week with a minimum of one hour a week devoted to individual 'psychotherapy'. Their therapy was not so much psychodynamic as supportive, emphasizing their present state and circumstances and orientated towards the patients' descriptive accounts of their own problems. The results indicated that the psychotherapy did not prevent the recurrence of clinical symptoms but that it did affect social adjustment in those who remained well. After eight months, psychotherapy significantly reduced friction and anxious rumination, improved overall adjustment, work performance, and communication. The drug amitriptyline, on the other hand, reduced the possibility of relapse but had no effect on social adjustment. The authors concluded that combined drug treatment and psychotherapy was the most beneficial in alleviating clinical symptoms and improving social adjustment.

Another study in which social work was directed at improving patients' subjectively selected social problems involved patients who had been admitted to hospital after a drug overdose (Gibbons *et al.* 1978). It included 539 patients, 200 of whom were referred to the control group for 'routine' services and the same number to an experimental service employing a social worker. One hundred and thirty-nine patients were not referred to either group, as patients were excluded if they had a formal psychiatric illness requiring immediate psychiatric treatment, or if they were considered to constitute an immediate suicide risk, or if they were already in treatment with a psychiatrist or social worker. Ninety per cent of the experimental group received social work help limited to three months duration in which the social workers concentrated on specific tasks which had been identified by the patient as most needing to be changed (Butler *et al.* 1978).

The two groups were checked on repeated admissions for self-poisoning for a year after the index admission, and after four months a proportion completed the Beck self-rating depression inventory (Beck *et al.* 1961). There were no significant differences between the two groups in the repetition of self-poisoning or in scores on the Beck depression inventory. However, the patients differed in respect of their social scores and how they viewed the help given. This was measured by a semi-structured social questionnaire administered in hospital and repeated four months later. As in the study conducted by Weissman and Paykel (1974), the subjects receiving the social work service showed more improvement in their social scores than the control group. The patients in the experimental group also considered that they had received more help. One of the problems of this study was that the control group had more contact with the psychiatric services and also the social services department than the experimental group. This additional treatment might have had an effect on outcome, diminishing the difference between groups. Such problems are inherent in a study of this sort when it is impossible to restrict services given by other agencies or other departments.

The third study investigated outcome in 374 schizophrenics discharged from three Maryland state hospitals (Hogarty *et al.* 1974). Following discharge, patients were randomly assigned at clinic intake to 'major role therapy', defined as a combination of intensive social casework and vocational rehabilitation counselling. MRT was viewed as a problem-solving method designed to respond to the interpersonal, social, and rehabilitative needs of the study patients and their families. All patients were stabilized on chlorpromazine for two months and then randomly assigned identical-looking tablets of chlorpromazine or placebo. Relapse was defined as clinical deterioration of such magnitude that readmission to hospital was imminent. About 75 per cent of relapsed patients were actually readmitted.

At the end of the first year after discharge 68 per cent of placebo-treated patients and 31 per cent of drug-treated patients had relapsed. After two years, 80 per cent of the placebo group had relapsed in comparison with 48 per cent of the drug treated. 'Major role therapy' (MRT) had no effect on relapse rates in the first two years (46 per cent of the MRT group relapsed in comparison with 51 per cent of the non-MRT group in the first year) but did appear to lower relapse rates among those who survived in the community for six months after hospital discharge. Since the magnitude of the drug/placebo difference was the same for both sociotherapy (MRT) groups, the effects were judged to be additive rather than interactive.

In addition to relapse, patients were assessed at six, twelve, eighteen and twenty-four months on their personal and social adjustment and role performance. Among those patients who did not relapse, an interaction was found between drug treatment and MRT, suggesting that among drug-treated patients, those who received MRT adjusted better, and among placebo-treated patients those who did not receive MRT adjusted better. This effect was

347

observed on the ratings made by the social worker, physician, the patients themselves, and a relative. As with the study on female out-patients, the investigators concluded that maximum restorative benefits require both maintenance phenothiazine and psychological treatment continued beyond a single year following discharge.

A combination of maintenance medication and sociotherapy was found again to be a most effective combination in the final hospital-based study. Leff and his colleagues (1982) developed a 'package' of social interventions to counteract the risk factors found in earlier studies (Vaughn and Leff 1976) to be associated with schizophrenic breakdown. Provoking agents included high levels of 'expressed emotion' from the patients' immediate relatives and excessive amounts of close contact between the two. The social interventions included an education programme for relatives on the aetiology, symptoms, course, and management of schizophrenia; relatives' groups to provide support; and individual family sessions in their own homes which included the patient. Twenty-four patients at high risk of relapse were selected for the study, with half of the families allocated to an experimental group to receive social therapy and the other half assigned to routine out-patient care. All were maintained on neuroleptic drugs. The social interventions had a significant effect in reducing relapse rates to 9 per cent in the experimental group compared with 50 per cent in the control group. Operationally defined therapeutic aims had been set for each experimental family, and these were achieved in 73 per cent of cases; none of the patients in this group of families relapsed. The authors concluded that the combination of interventions was necessary to maintain the patients' stability.

In general practice settings

The first study conducted in this area investigated ninety-two patients who were considered by their general practitioners to have chronic neurosis and who had had symptoms continually for over a year (Cooper *et al.* 1975; Shepherd *et al.* 1979). The patients were suffering from depression, anxiety and phobias; they were all over 18 and of both sexes. Ninety-seven controls from practices in the same neighbourhood were selected for comparison.

The two groups were assessed by means of standardized psychiatric and social interviews. Patients in the experimental group were then referred to a special service operating in the practice, which included a psychiatrist and a social worker, while the controls were referred back to the doctor for routine treatment. After one year both groups were interviewed again using the same standardized instruments. Details were also collected from the medical notes on the psychotropic drugs prescribed, and the general practitioner was asked how much care and supervision had been necessary for each patient.

The special service included therapeutic intervention from both the research psychiatrist and the social worker, who met regularly with the general practitioners involved. The social worker was involved in the management of approximately two-thirds of the patients, working alone with three-quarters of them and jointly with the psychiatrist for the remainder. Her main role was in helping the patient and their family to deal with their practical problems. In most cases, the social worker was the key worker with the psychiatrist's main role limited to a reassessment interview. Some of the patients refused her help, while others were not regarded as suitable for referral, either because they had markedly improved or because the treatment they were receiving from the doctor was considered adequate. Many did not want any more specific help and were referred back to the general practitioner with recommendations.

Both groups showed a reduction in psychiatric symptoms at follow-up, but the fall was more pronounced in the experimental group, 38 per cent of whom had been taken off psychotropic drugs compared with 25 per cent of the controls. In addition, continued medical care and supervision were deemed necessary for only 60 per cent of the experimental patients compared with 77 per cent of the controls. The experimental patients also achieved much more improvement in their social functioning compared with the controls. Measurement of social adjustment included items on housing, finance, work, marriage, children, and other relationships.

Clinical outcome proved to be unrelated to the social worker's activities, much of which were devoted to solving practical problems. Those who received short-term intervention were more likely to improve than those receiving episodic or continuous social work support. This result cannot be taken to indicate that short-term social work intervention is more effective than a longer-term variety since the social worker was permitted to discontinue treatment as soon as her patient improved. By definition, therefore, clients who did not respond or who actually deteriorated were more likely to remain in longer contact.

The second study in general practice concerns the application of social work among women aged between 18 and 45 years attending with depression (Corney 1984). Such women place a great demand on GPs and also represent a high proportion of the referrals to social workers operating in GP attachment schemes. In this investigation eighty women were referred from a health centre and a single-handed practice to the study. They were assessed using the same psychiatric and social interviews as in the previous study. They were classified as either 'acutely depressed', having had symptoms for three months or less, or 'acute on chronic', having had symptoms for a longer period but with intensification in the past three months. The women were then randomly allocated either to the experimental group, where they were referred to one of four attached social workers, or to the control group, with referral back to their doctor. After six months, they were reinterviewed using the same instruments, and their medical notes were examined for one year after referral.

Both the experimental and control groups were initially similar in respect of psychiatric and physical health and demographic features. When reassessed at six months, approximately two-thirds of both groups had recovered from their depression and were no longer receiving psychotropic drugs. There was little difference in outcome between experimental and control groups on clinical and social scores, number of visits to the doctor in the previous six months, or length of time on psychotropic medication. These findings indicate that the additional involvement of a social worker had not helped these women in general on either clinical or social measures. However, analysis of covariance indicated that one subgroup of patients had benefited from the increased help. These patients were assessed initially as having major marital or boyfriend problems and were suffering from 'acute on chronic' depression. With this particular group of women, 80 per cent had improved at follow-up in comparison with 31 per cent of the controls. This difference persisted one year after referral when the medical notes were examined.

As the results suggested that social work intervention was more beneficial to certain patients than others, the social worker's records were analysed, taking into account these different groups. Women who benefited most from the social worker's help were considered by the social workers to be more highly motivated to receive help than the other groups. They also had more social problems and received more practical help from the social worker, including housing and financial help, day nursery placements, and liaison with other agencies.

The final study was also carried out with depressed patients referred from general practice (Ross and Scott 1985), although the social worker used cognitive therapy as opposed to casework or practical help as his main technique. Patients considered by their GP to be depressed were first assessed by a psychiatrist using the Present State Examination (Wing 1982), the Montgomery-Asberg depression scale (1979) and the Beck Depression Inventory (1981). Those whose scores met the criteria for inclusion were then randomly allocated to individual cognitive therapy, group cognitive therapy, or a waiting list control group. Patients in all three groups also received practical social work help so that any differences emerging between the groups would be attributable to cognitive therapy. After three months, cognitive therapy was found to have a statistically significant beneficial effect upon depression compared with 'normal treatment', as assessed by the Montgomery-Asberg scale and the Beck Depression Inventory. Group and individual cognitive therapy were found to be equally effective. In addition, comparison with the scores of those who were on the waiting list provided further evidence of the beneficial influence of cognitive therapy. These treatment gains were maintained at twelve months follow-up.

CONCLUSIONS

Studies in hospital settings

The results of the four studies on the outcome of more severe depressions and schizophrenias suggest that social interventions alone do not prevent relapse or reduce clinical symptomatology. However, all four studies showed evidence of treatment gains in terms of social adjustment, and in the study by Leff *et al.* (1982), in preventing relapse. All indicate the need for a combined approach of drug treatment and socio- or psychotherapy. In the social treatment of schizophrenia, the work of Vaughn and Leff (1976) suggests a number of interventions with an emphasis on changes in the family. The patient might be encouraged to move into a hostel rather than try to adjust to living with hostile or overbearing relatives; or the family might be better educated on the nature of the illness and their own role in preventing relapse.

The application of 'major role therapy' (Hogarty *et al.* 1974) appears to be disappointing; more specific operational definitions of social intervention might have led to greater consistency in treatment and consequent outcomes.

Studies in general practice

In this setting studies suggest that patients with more long-standing depressions and neuroses can be helped more than those with acute symptoms by a social worker's involvement. In the latter case, patients are more likely to recover spontaneously without outside help. Early intervention may be harmful, the social worker interfering with the client's own abilities to cope, or affecting the support received from informal sources, such as friends and relatives.

Depressed women with a poor relationship with their spouse or boyfriend may benefit more than other depressed women from the help of the social worker. Many of the women in the second study (Corney 1984) had inadequate social contact and no one in whom to confide, so that they more readily accepted the emotional support offered by a social worker. These findings are closely related to the theoretical work on the value of social supports and close confidants in protecting individuals from the development of mental disorder and in affecting the prognosis of an existing episode (e.g. Miller and Ingham 1976).

Practical help in managing social difficulties appears to be of most benefit to those with long-standing neurotic illness. In the general practice setting the effectiveness of social work with depressed and anxious patients depends on the duration of symptoms, the support received from others (including the spouse), the patient's motivation to accept help and the coexistence of chronic social problems. A more structured form of treatment, such as the cognitive therapy exemplified in the third study (Ross and Scott 1985), may bring advantages over and above the practical help of social work.

351

As we noted at the outset, social factors have an undoubted influence on the development, course, and outcome of mental illness. The limited number of studies available indicate a varying degree of effectiveness of social intervention under different conditions. There are intrinsic difficulties in establishing the optimum use of sociotherapy, in particular its content. The research to date sheds some light on the characteristics of patients who might benefit most from social intervention but, with the exception of the study by Leff *et al.* (1982), there has been little success in producing suitable detailed operational goals for social treatment.

A number of questions remain to be answered through detailed experimental studies, particularly on the role of trained social workers with the mentally ill:

(i) Are any aspects of social work unique? Apart from their statutory duties and abilities to liaise with other professionals and agencies, do social workers provide more than the befriending and supportive role of a sensitive volunteer?

(ii) Which elements of the social worker's skills (e.g. practical knowledge, counselling) are of most benefit and to what type of patient? Future studies of social therapy should develop operational goals and detailed treatment plans against which the effectiveness of interventions can be measured.

The current levels of demand for social work time are very high and there is little prospect of increased resources. The value of social intervention in psychiatric care will need to be fully justified by carefully designed research in order to make the case for the deployment of social workers in this area.

Acknowledgement: The authors are supported by the Department of Health and Social Security.

REFERENCES

Beck, A. (1981) *Cognitive Theory in Depression*, Chichester: Wiley.

Beck, A.T., Ward, C.H., and Mendelson, M. (1961) 'An Inventory for measuring depression', *Archives of General Psychiatry* 4: 561–71.

Bergin, A.E. (1971) 'The evaluation of therapeutic outcomes', in A.E. Bergin and S.L. Garfield (eds) *Handbook of Psychotherapy and Behaviour Change: An Empirical Analysis*, New York: Wiley.

Brown, G.W. and Birley, J.L.T. (1968) 'Crises and life changes and the onset of schizophrenia' *Journal of Health and Social Behaviour* 9: 203–14.

Brown, G.W. and Harris, T. (1978) *Social Origins of Depression: A Study of Psychiatric Disorder in Women*, London: Tavistock.

352

Bullock, R.C., Siegel, R., Weissman, M., and Paykel, E.S. (1972) 'The weeping wife: marital relations of depressed women', *Journal of Marriage and the Family* 34: 488–95.

Butler, J., Bow, I. and Gibbons, J. (1978) 'Task centred casework with marital problems', *British Journal of Social Work* 8: 393–409.

British Medical Association (1986) *Alternative Therapy*, London: BMA.

Cooper, B. (1979) 'Clinical and social aspects of chronic neurosis', in P. Williams and A. Clare (eds) *Psychosocial Disorders in General Practice*, London: Academic Press.

Cooper, B., Harwin, B.G., Depla, C., and Shepherd, M. (1975), 'Mental health care in the community: an evaluative study', *Psychological Medicine*, 5: 372–80.

Corney, R.H., (1984) 'The effectiveness of attached social workers in the management of depressed female patients in general practice', *Psychological Medicine*, Monograph supplement no. 6: 47.

Dohrenwend, B.P. (1975) 'Social, cultural and social psychological factors in the genesis of mental disorders', *Journal of Health and Social Behaviour* 16: 365–92.

Dohrenwend, B.S. and Dohrenwend, B.P. (1969) *Social Status and Psychological Disorder*, New York: Wiley.

Dohrenwend, B.S. and Dohrenwend, B.P. (1974) *Stressful Life Events: Their Nature and Effects*, New York: Wiley.

Gibbons, J.S., Butler, J., Unwin, P., and Gibbons, J.L. (1978) 'Evaluation of a social work service for self-poisoning patients', *British Journal of Psychiatry* 133: 111–18.

Henderson, S., Duncan-Jones, P., McAuley, H., and Ritchie, K. (1978) 'The patient's primary group', *British Journal of Psychiatry* 132: 74–86.

Hogarty, G.E., Goldberg, S.C., and Schooler, N.R. (1974) 'Drug and social therapy in the aftercare of schizophrenic patients', *Archives of General Psychiatry* 31: 603–18.

Holmes, T.H., and Rahe, R.H. (1967) 'The social readjustment rating scale' *Journal of Psychosomatic Medicine* 11: 213–18.

Huxley, P. and Goldberg, D.P. (1975) 'Social versus clinical prediction in minor psychiatric disorders', *Psychological Medicine* 5: 96–100.

Jeffreys, M. (1965) *An Anatomy of Social Welfare Services*, London: Michael Joseph.

Jenkins, R., Mann, A.H., and Belsey, E. (1981) 'The background, design and use of a short interview to assess social stress and support in clinical settings', *Social Science and Medicine* 15E(3): 195–203.

Kedward, H. (1969) 'The outcome of neurotic illness in the community', *Social Psychiatry* 4: 1–4.

Klerman, G.L., Di Mascio, A., Weissman, M., Prusoff, B., and Paykel, E.S. (1974) 'Treatment of depression by drugs and psychotherapy', *American Journal of Psychiatry* 131: 186–91.

Leff, J., Knupers, L., Berkowitz, R., Eberlein, Vries, R., and Sturgeon, D. (1982) 'A controlled trial of social intervention in the families of schizophrenic patients', *British Journal of Psychiatry* 141: 121–34.

Medical Research Council (1965) *Clinical Trial of the Treatment of Depressive Illness*, Report by Clinical Psychiatry Committee.

Miller, P. McC. and Ingham, J.G. (1976) 'Friends, confidants and symptoms', *Social Psychiatry* 11: 51–8.

Montgomery, S.A. and Asberg, M. (1979) 'A new depression scale designed to be sensitive to change', *British Journal of Psychiatry* 134: 382–9.

Paykel, E.S. (1978) 'Contribution of life events to causation of psychiatric illness' *Psychological Medicine* 8: 245–53.

Ross, M. and Scott, M. (1985) 'An evaluation of the effectiveness of individual and group cognitive therapy in the treatment of depressed patients in an inner city health centre', *Journal of the Royal College of General Practitioners* 35: 239–42.

Royal College of General Practitioners (1973) *Present State and Future Needs of General Practice* (third edition) (Reports from General Practice, No. 16) London: RCGP.

Shepherd, M., Cooper, B., Brown, A.C., and Kalton, G.W. (1966) *Psychiatric Illness in General Practice* London: Oxford University Press.

Shepherd, M., Harwin, B.G., Depla, C., and Cairns, V. (1979) 'Social work and primary care of mental disorder', *Psychological Medicine* 9: 661–69.

Sylph, J.A., Kedward, H.B., and Eastwood, M.R. (1969) 'Chronic neurotic patients in general practice', *Journal of the Royal College of General Practitioners* 17: 162–70.

Truax, C. and Carkhuff, R.R. (1967) *Towards Effective Counselling and Psychotherapy*, Chicago: Aldine.

Vaughn, C.E. and Leff, J.P. (1976) 'The influence of family and social factors on the course of psychiatric illness: a comparison of schizophrenic and depressed neurotic patients', *British Journal of Psychiatry* 129: 125–37.

Weissman, M.M. (1971) 'The social role performance of depressed women: comparison with a normal group', *American Journal of Orthopsychiatry* 41: 391–405.

Weissman, M.M. and Paykel, E.S. (1974) *The Depressed Woman: A study of Social Relationships*, Chicago: University of Chicago Press.

Wheatley, D. (1972) 'Evaluation of psychotropic drugs in general practice', *Proceedings of the Royal Society of Medicine* 65: 317–20.

Wing, J.K. (1982) 'The use of the Present State Examination in general population survey', *Acta Psychiatrica Scandinavica* (supplement), 285: 230–40.

23

Behavioural Approaches in the Family Management of Schizophrenia

Ian Falloon

A RATIONALE FOR FAMILY MANAGEMENT OF SCHIZOPHRENIA

The detrimental effects of environmental stress upon the course and outcome of schizophrenia have been investigated in a series of studies of patients living in the community. Much of this work has emanated from the Social Psychiatry Unit of the Institute of Psychiatry and has focused upon two stress factors a) ambient stress, chiefly household tension, and b) stressful life events.

High levels of ambient stress in the household in which the patient resides after partial or full recovery from an episode of schizophrenia are associated with more frequent exacerbations of florid symptomatology (Brown, Birley and Wing 1972; Vaughn and Leff 1976; Vaughn et al. 1984). The more discrete stress of life events appears to trigger episodes of schizophrenia (Brown and Birley 1970; Leff et al. 1973) even when ambient tension is low (Leff and Vaughn 1980). Other stress factors, such as the work environment, have not been studied in a systematic fashion (Wing et al. 1964).

It is apparent that optimal regimens of neuroleptic drugs provide a significant but incomplete buffer against these stressors (Vaughn and Leff 1976; Birley and Brown 1970). An alternative psychosocial strategy would involve the provision of a low-stress environment such as that offered by the old-style asylum (Dunham and Weinberg 1960). However, such an environment, while reducing florid symptoms, tends to enhance deficit or negative symptoms and their associated social morbidity (Wing 1978).

Community care of schizophrenia places a considerable stress on family caregivers (Creer and Wing 1974). Furthermore, high levels of family burden are associated with high levels of 'expressed emotion', a marker of high ambient stress in a household (Brown, Birley and Wing 1972). Family members make specific complaints about their lack of understanding about the nature of schizophrenia and its optimal management and their need for specific guidelines rather than non-specific social support (Creer and Wing 1974; Vaughn 1977).

Thus, an effective programme for family-based management of schizophrenia must encompass the following goals:

1. Educate patients and families about the nature of schizophrenia and its drug and psychosocial treatments;
2. Provide methods for the efficient resolution of environmental stressors, both ambient and life event stress;
3. Minimize the social morbidity of the disorder for both patient and family members;
4. Provide specific strategies for dealing with persisting behavioural disturbance associated with unremitting symptoms.

In order to provide a clear framework we chose to use a problem-solving model as the basis for family management. This involves teaching families to convene regular (at least weekly) meetings to discuss specific problems or goals within a clearly defined structure that facilitates creative solutions, careful planning, and review. As well as providing a means for resolution of all forms of stress, this model enables the family to work towards social goals for all members, and to develop strategies for coping with a wide range of behavioural problems.

ESTABLISHING CLINICAL EFFICACY

Assessment of the effectiveness of a management approach that combines drug and psychosocial treatment in a flexible manner is an extremely difficult problem. We chose to compare the family management approach with a carefully constructed version of the patient-oriented case management approach that was currently provided in most clinics for the long-term care of schizophrenia. This patient-oriented management combined optimal neuroleptic drug therapy, rehabilitation counselling, problem-solving psychotherapy, crisis intervention, and practical assistance with problems such as finances and housing. Efforts were made to ensure that the patient-oriented management was of similar intensity, and conducted over a similar time span, by therapists with similar skill and enthusiasm to the family management. The main distinction was that one approach was clearly family-based ánd conducted in the family home, whereas the comparative approach was focused on the individual patient and was conducted predominantly in the out-patient clinic.

We were aware that psychotherapy and pharmacotherapy researchers would both criticize our study on the grounds that we could not tease out the crucial ingredients that might account for any differential effectiveness. Essentially, we planned a trial of two contrasting management approaches. However, we included a wide range of process measures so that we could explore several potential mediators of outcome.

A further consideration was that effective management of schizophrenia entailed not merely controlling the florid symptoms of the disorder but necessitated the restoration of unrestricted social and family functioning. For this reason the assessment of outcome included a battery of social and family measures to supplement measures of clinical morbidity.

PATIENT SELECTION

The selection of patients was made on the basis of a high risk of recurrent or persistent florid symptoms of schizophrenia in cases, owing to continued daily involvement in a stressful parental household. An age range of 18 to 45 years was imposed and non-English speaking families were excluded.

Patients entered the study on recovery (partial or full remission) from an episode diagnosed as definite schizophrenia (Classes S and P) on PSE/CATEGO criteria. (Coincidently all patients also met DSM-III criteria for schizophrenic disorder.)

A stressful household was determined after Camberwell Family Interviews had been completed on all adult household members. High ratings of critical or over-involved attitudes expressed towards the patient (Vaughn and Leff 1976b) or evidence of high levels of persisting household stress not associated specifically with the patient's behavioural disturbance were employed as criteria predictive of a poor clinical prognosis independent of the previous history of the disorder (which in first episode cases could not be applied).

Consecutive admissions to Los Angeles County Hospital were screened soon after admission. A few cases were excluded on the basis of a lack of response to in-patient treatment with stabilization of florid symptoms. While substance abuse was not an exclusionary criterion, it is probable that some cases were excluded because the drug use obscured the diagnosis.

The thirty-nine cases selected for the study after application of these criteria included twice as many males as females; 42 per cent Caucasian, 36 per cent Afro-American and 17 per cent Hispanic-American; 86 per cent had completed high school. Most families were in the lower socio-economic classes and lived in the more deprived areas of Los Angeles. More than one-third were single-parent households. All but thirty-nine households were rated high on the expressed emotion index ('high EE').

Most patients (81 per cent) showed evidence of nuclear schizophrenia on CATEGO; one-quarter were experiencing their first episode; the average duration of illness was four years, with three hospital admissions.

Random assignment to the management approaches occurred once patients had left hospital and were stabilized on out-patient neuroleptic medication. This assignment procedure produced two clearly matched groups. Three cases dropped out in the early stages of the study, but did not affect the matching of the two groups. Chi-squared analyses revealed no differences

357

approaching statistical significance on any of the clinical or demographic variables.

THE THERAPEUTIC TEAM

Each patient and family received therapeutic interventions from a team of mental health professionals. The same team provided both forms of management according to strict protocol instructions. The psychosocial treatment of each case was co-ordinated by a primary therapist, who remained constant throughout the twenty-four month study period. A psychiatrist, social worker, and clinical psychologist, who had all been trained in behaviour therapy methods and psychiatric assessment, were the three primary therapists. They were all experienced in out-patient management of schizophrenia. They received specific training in behavioural family management prior to starting work in the study and continued to meet for weekly supervision sessions throughout the study.

Three pharmacotherapists with a minimum of five years experience in neuroleptic drug treatment of schizophrenia provided the drug treatment of schizophrenia and conducted serial assessment of mental status. A research nurse with considerable experience in the management of schizophrenia collected blood samples, administered intramuscular drugs, assisted in crisis intervention, and conducted regular blood pressure and heart rate assessments.

Two rehabilitation counsellors facilitated entry into vocational, day care, and residential rehabilitation services.

Team work was limited somewhat by the need to keep the pharmacotherapists blind to the psychosocial management approach employed for each patient. However, regular discussions between all clinicians occurred on all matters of clinical importance.

THE MANAGEMENT APPROACHES

The primary aim of the study was to examine the benefit of a family-based approach to the community management of schizophrenia when compared with a patient-based approach of similar intensity. These contrasting psychosocial components were applied to patients who were receiving optimal pharmacotherapy, twenty-four crisis management and rehabilitation counselling and services. Because each of the contrasting psychosocial modalities was only one part of the entire management programme, it was crucial that every component was carefully operationalized and applied in a standardized manner.

Neuroleptic drugs were prescribed in a manner designed to maximize their benefits and minimize unwanted effects. Chlorpromazine was the drug of first choice, with cases requiring more potent prophylaxis receiving fluphenazine hydrochloride. Where intramuscular preparations proved necessary, owing to irregular tablet taking or poor absorption of oral preparations, fluphenazine decanoate was given. Two cases received other neuroleptics (haloperidol and thiothixene) due to intolerance of the recommended preparations.

Patients were randomly assigned after regular adherence to maintenance medication had been established. Checks on tablet-taking behaviour were conducted at each medication appointment through interviews with patients and relatives and by tablet counts. This information was supplemented by serial assays of the plasma levels of the drugs and of serum prolactin. Any evidence of erratic compliance was considered a clinical crisis and was addressed urgently by the primary therapists and pharmacotherapists. On occasions this necessitated home visits by the pharmacotherapists, project nurse, and primary therapists.

Levels of drugs were reviewed monthly and were adjusted according to clinical ratings. Increased evidence of florid symptoms of schizophrenia led to increased drugs, a decrease in florid symptoms or severe side effects led to decreased drug levels. Drug and prolactin levels in blood samples supplemented clinical assessments. Additional anti-parkinsonian, anti-depressant, anxiolytic, and sedative drugs were used sparingly when indicated. At all times the pharmacotherapists aimed to minimize the levels of drugs prescribed to minimize psychopathology.

Behavioural family management was based on behavioural family therapy with the addition of education about the nature and management of schizophrenia and the use of a range of behaviour therapy strategies to deal with specific problems.

Weekly sessions of one hour duration with all adult members of the household, including the index patient, were conducted in the home for three months, decreasing in frequency to fortnightly until nine months, after which monthly sessions were provided, often in a multi-family group in a convenient community setting.

The first two or three sessions were devoted to comprehensive education about the nature of schizophrenia and the rationale for combined drug and psychosocial interventions. The value of efficient family management of stress in promoting a good outcome for schizophrenia was emphasized along with the need to maximize the efficacy of neuroleptic drugs.

The core component of the therapy was training the family to convene regular discussions that employed a structured problem-solving approach to develop clearly defined plans to resolve problem issues affecting any member of the family. These included the achievement of personal goals as well as stressful events and situations. Where major deficits in interpersonal communication precluded effective problem-solving discussions, training in communication skills such as expressing specific positive or negative feelings,

359

attentive listening, or making requests in a positive manner was implemented. Where specific problem issues such as parental conflict, aggressive behaviour, social skills deficits, persisting hallucinations, insomnia or depressive mood persisted in any family member, specific behaviour therapy strategies were employed within the problem solving framework. Details of this approach are available in a published manual (Falloon *et al*. 1984).

Patient-oriented management was based on a similar problem-oriented framework. It was of similar intensity and focus as the family-based approach, but directed primarily towards enhancing the community functioning of the index patient, while supporting his family in his care. Structured, goal-oriented sessions of one hour duration were conducted at the same frequency as the family sessions. Patients were educated about the nature of schizophrenia and the importance of drug and stress management in promoting adjustment. Specific behaviour therapy strategies, such as social skills training, anxiety management, or cognitive restructuring were employed where indicated.

Frequent contact was made with key family members to discuss treatment plans and to provide advice on patient care at home. These discussions were held in the absence of the patient in order to minimize problem-solving family discussions. Every effort was made to provide optimal community support.

Thus, the major differences between the two management approaches were a focus on enhancing family problem-solving efficiency; education of the entire family about schizophrenia and its management; home-based sessions; contrasted with a focus on solving the index patient's problems; education of the patient only; and clinic-based sessions. Identical drug therapy, crisis intervention, and rehabilitation services were provided to both management conditions.

STUDY DESIGN

Patients completed baseline assessments during a period of four to eight weeks of out-patient stabilization after an acute episode of schizophrenia. The final assessment included baseline measures of clinical, social, and family morbidity, as well as a series of family interaction measures. At the end of these assessments families were informed of their assignment and consent obtained to participate in the controlled study. The assignment to primary therapists was sequential with each therapist managing an equal number of cases in the two conditions. All index patients were scheduled to receive forty therapy sessions, twenty-four pharmacotherapy sessions, four vocational counselling sessions and four assessment sessions over twenty-four months. Additional sessions were scheduled when indicated according to clinical need.

ASSESSMENT PROCEDURES

Assessment of clinical, social, and family morbidity was conducted at baseline, nine and twenty-four months. Additional assessments of clinical morbidity were conducted monthly. Careful records were made of all contacts with medical and social agencies. Bi-weekly interviews with key family members were employed to assess family stress factors.

Clinical morbidity was assessed on several measures. These included:

a) *Clinical exacerbations:* The primary therapists assessed the mental status of each patient prior to therapy sessions using the Brief Psychiatric Rating Scale, BPRS (Overall and Goreham 1962) as a guideline. A time chart of all exacerbations of schizophrenia, affective disorders, anxiety disorders, emergent side effects, or other physical or mental disorders was maintained throughout the twenty-four months. Emergence of florid psychopathology that persisted for at least one week, or required a major management change was described as a 'major' exacerbation; less severe disturbance was described as a 'minor' exacerbation. These assessments were not standardized, not blind or independent although there was a high level of agreement among the three therapists concerning major exacerbations of schizophrenia.

b) *Community tenure:* All periods spent away from the family household were carefully recorded. These included hospital admissions, residential care and time spent in gaol. Decisions to admit patients to these institutions were made by personnel who were independent of the study.

c) *Target ratings of schizophrenia:* Two or three florid symptoms were selected that were most characteristic of the presentation of an acute episode of schizophrenia for each patient. These were rated monthly by blind assessors on a seven-point severity scale (1 = absent or trivial; 7 = severe). Inter-rater reliability was .95 (Pearson's product-moment coefficient).

d) *Brief Psychiatric Rating Scale, BPRS:* Blind ratings of the BPRS were made monthly. Four factors derived from this scale: assessed thought disorder, withdrawal ('negative' symptoms), hostile/suspiciousness, and depression/anxiety (Goldstein *et al.* 1978).

e) *Present State Examination, PSE:* At nought, nine, twenty-four months a blind assessment was made using the PSE to examine changes in the overall pattern of psychopathology.

f) *Hopkin's Symptom Checklist, HSCL:* The sixty-four item version of this self-report questionnaire was completed at nought, three and nine months to assess neurotic symptom patterns (Derogatis *et al.* 1974).

Social morbidity was assessed by therapists' observations, interviews with a key family member, and patients' self-reports. The measures included:

a) *Time spent in work and educational activity:* A careful record of all work and educational activity, both formal and informal, was made throughout the twenty-four months.

b) *Social Adjustment Scales, SAS-SR:* Patients completed a self-report measure of social functioning at nought, three and nine months (Weissman *et al.* 1978).

c) *Social Behaviour Assessment Schedule, SBAS:* Social morbidity was measured in an interview by a blind assessor with the family member most involved with the patient's care on an abbreviated version of the SBAS (Platt *et al.* 1980). This concerned impairment in social role functioning as well as the relatives' satisfaction with levels of functioning during three months before the interview.

Family morbidity was measured in terms of the social and clinical adjustment of each family member, the distress associated with living with the index patient, the problem-solving functions of the family unit, and the efficiency of coping with life stresses.

a) *Hopkin's Symptom Checklist, HSCL:* Each family member completed the HSCL at nought and nine months to assess patterns of clinical morbidity in the family.

b) *SBAS: distress and burden scales:* Scales measuring the distress and burden key family members experienced as a result of the index patient's morbidity were used from the SBAS interview conducted by the blind assessor.

c) *Family problem-solving functions:* At nought, three and twenty-four months the family unit participated in two ten-minute discussions about current problem issues in the households. These discussions were audiotaped, transcribed, and rated for the communication and problem-solving skills that were observed (Doane and Falloon 1985).

d) *Family stress and coping:* From nought to twelve months fortnightly interviews were conducted with a key member of each family to ascertain all potentially stressful events and situations that had occurred, and the manner in which the family unit had coped with these circumstances. The independent interviewers transcribed details of the events and associated behavioural and cognitive responses, which were subsequently reviewed by a blind rater for a) threatening life events (Brown and Harris 1978); b) effectiveness of coping responses.

THE RESULTS

Clinical morbidity: The multiple measures indicated that family management was associated with less clinical morbidity during the twenty-four-month study period than the patient-oriented approach. There were fewer exacerbations of schizophrenia (thirty-six vs. fifty-four); in particular, fewer major exacerbations (seven vs. forty-one). These differences were less marked when episodes of depression and anxiety were considered, with seven major episodes of affective symptoms in family management and sixteen in patient-oriented management. However, this difference remains noteworthy, particularly when one considers that affective episodes were not recorded during periods when florid schizophrenia was evident, thereby reducing the opportunity for affective episodes in the patient-oriented condition.

On average, patient-oriented cases spent almost seven of the twenty-four months in a state of clinical instability sufficient to warrant active acute management. Family managed patients averaged a little more than one month in a similar state. As a consequence, patient-oriented cases averaged twenty-three days in hospital over the two years and family cases a mere four days. Over twenty-four months 83 per cent of family cases had not experienced a major episode of schizophrenia, whereas only 17 per cent of patient-oriented cases had escaped a major exacerbation.

These clinicians' observations were supported by blind standardized ratings. A repeated measures analysis of covariance over the twenty-four monthly target symptom ratings, with the baseline ratings as covariates, indicated a significant trend favouring family management ($F = 16.73$, df 1,32; $p < .0003$). An overall tendency for improvement with time was noted ($F = 1.96$, df 23,816; $p < .005$). The management group $\times$ time interaction was not significant. This meant that, although all patients tended to improve over the twenty-four months, the family management tended to expedite that trend. PSE interviews at twenty-four months showed no continued evidence of any psychiatric abnormality in half the family managed cases, and two-thirds were in remission from schizophrenic or paranoid disorders. In contrast, fourteen (83 per cent) patient-oriented cases showed schizophrenic or paranoid symptoms and only one of the eighteen cases was free of psychiatric disorder.

The BPRS ratings showed similar patterns over the twenty-four months. Of particular interest was the near-significant trend on the withdrawal factor that suggested that family management was associated with greater reductions in negative symptoms than the patient-oriented approach ($F = 3.32$; df 1,34; $p < .09$).

It was evident that family management was associated with clear clinical benefits over a carefully applied patient-oriented approach, which itself appeared associated with beneficial trends. These benefits involved fewer episodes of serious psychopathology, less need for hospital care, fewer negative symptoms, and a trend towards restoration of mental health. However, it was evident that schizophrenic symptoms did emerge from time to time in most patients receiving family management. These episodes did not escalate into major crises and were readily contained in an out-patient setting. The value of a community-based service, in close contact with family caregivers, providing a twenty-four-hour service should not be underestimated in the achievement of such benefits. Furthermore, it is not sufficient merely to target emergent episodes of schizophrenic symptoms in the management of this disorder. In family managed cases depression and anxiety were prominent and specific therapeutic skills were essential to deal effectively with these episodes.

It could be argued that the clinical benefits associated with family management may have been achieved through more effective neuroleptic drug treatment for those cases. Our careful records of the pharmacotherapy enabled a detailed analysis to be conducted (Moss *et al.* 1985). We were able to establish that prior to 29 per cent of episodes of schizophrenia compliance with the prescribed dosage of medication was less than 75 per cent. These levels of reduced compliance remained the same before major and minor episodes, and prior to episodes experienced in both management conditions. Therefore, it seems unlikely that reduced intake of drugs could explain either the differential outcome of the two forms of management, or whether minor episodes escalated into major exacerbations.

Because the aim of pharmacotherapy was to reduce levels of drugs continually until symptom exacerbation appeared imminent, it was possible that the differential outcome was caused by excessively lower doses prescribed to the patient-oriented cases. This was not evident. The mean daily dosage of family cases was 245 mg of chlorpromazine, or its equivalent, compared with 338 mg for patient-oriented cases. Examination of the pattern of drug ingestion levels over the first nine months by comparing linear regression lines of the monthly dosage for each case revealed a near-significant trend indicating that lower dosages were ingested by family than patient-oriented cases (Mann-Whitney $U = 219.5$; df; $p < .07$).

On the basis of these data there seems little evidence to suggest that the benefits of family management could be explained on the grounds of more effective pharmacotherapy. On the other hand, it could be suggested that family management may facilitiate prophylaxis with lower doses of neuroleptic drugs, with the attendant benefits of few side effects.

Social morbidity: Although the clinical outcome of disorders tends to dominate our thinking, restoration of social functioning is a more important criterion of successful medical intervention. Family management showed clear benefits in enhancing the quality of life for patients. Over the twenty-four months, family cases spent an average of 12.6 months engaged in some form of work or educational pursuit, compared to 7.2 months for individual cases.

The self-reported assessment of social adjustment, SAS, showed significant advantages for the family management on scales of social and leisure activity ($F = 7.53$; dfl, 35; $p < .01$) and family relationships ($F = 4.58$; df 1,35; $p < .04$), as well as on the aggregate score ($F = 4.58$; df 1,35; $p < .04$).

The blind interviewer ratings of key relatives provided the strongest support for family management benefits. No evidence of significant social impairment was found at twenty-four months in 41 per cent of family cases, compared to 6 per cent (i.e., one case) who received patient-oriented management. A repeated measures analysis of covariance, using baseline scores as covariates, was performed on the seven social performance scales.

Family management was superior on households tasks (p < .001), decision-making (p < .05), and the aggregate score (p < .02), and approached significance on leisure activities (p < .10).

The key family members' dissatisfaction with the patient's social performance showed greater difference between the conditions, with significant differences between the groups on five of the seven scales. This suggested that family participation may have led to a greater acceptance of suboptimal social functioning in the cases where disability persisted. Such changes in attitude, combined with more efficient problem-solving by the family unit, appeared to contribute to the more effective rehabilitation associated with the family-based approach (Doane and Falloon 1985).

FAMILY MORBIDITY

At the start of the study half the fifty-four parents who completed the Hopkins' Symptom Checklist, HSCL, scored within the abnormal range on at least one of the five factors: somatization, obsessive-compulsive, interpersonal sensitivity, depression, anxiety. After nine months the proportion of family-based parents with abnormal scores had dropped, whereas the trend was for parents of patient-oriented cases to show an increased proportion of abnormal scores. However, the data were skewed, with more morbidity reported by family-based patients at the initial assessment. The changes observed at nine months could have resulted from regression toward the mean.

The SBAS scales of family distress and burden suggested that family-based management was associated with greater benefits to family members than the patient-oriented approach (Falloon and Pederson 1985). Only one family (i.e., 6 per cent) who received family-based management reported moderate or severe burden at the twenty-four-month assessment. A repeated measures analysis of covariance, with baseline scores as covariates, showed a significant between-group effect (F = 14.96; df 2,33; p < .0005).

Standardized assessment of family problem-solving behaviour revealed increases in the number of constructive problem-solving statements after three months of family therapy (mean of twelve statements at baseline versus thirty-six at three months). Families in the patient-oriented condition showed no increases. A Scheffé test of pre-post difference in the number of problem solving statements was significant (α = .05; df 1,30; p < .01). Significant differences between the two treatment conditions were also noted on non-constructive statements of criticism (F = 5.25; df 1,30; p < .05) and intrusiveness (F = 5.24; df 1,30; p < .05). These latter measures are behavioural correlates of the expressed emotion indices (Miklowitz et al. 1984). However, the reduction in non-constructive statements associated with the family approach was less striking than the *increase* in critical and

365

intrusive remarks made by family members in the patient-oriented condition.

These laboratory ratings of family problem-solving were reflected in measures of the effectiveness with which families coped with everyday problems and life events that impinged on all household members during the first twelve months of the study. The family-oriented approach was associated with an enhancement in the effectiveness with which families coped with stresses, whereas no change was noted in the patient-oriented families. A repeated measures analysis of variance showed a significant difference between the two management conditions (F = 26.5; df 3,30; p < .0001). A fine-grained analysis revealed that although families in both conditions encountered a similar number of life events, the better coping skills of those who received behavioural family therapy appeared to prevent stress escalating into major life events. Only 4 per cent of events experienced by family-oriented households were rated major, compared with 22 per cent of those experience in patient-oriented households (Hardesty *et al*. 1985).

ECONOMIC FACTORS

A detailed assessment of the comparative costs of the two management approaches was conducted (Cardin *et al*. 1985). The direct treatment costs for the family-oriented approach averaged US$5,952 per patient (1980/81 costs) for the first year of the study. This compared with US$5,514 for the patient-oriented approach. Nearly one-third of the cost of family management comprised the cost of travel time to conduct home visits, which proved substantial in Los Angeles County. However, the indirect treatment costs, that included hospital and residential care, emergency evaluation, and rehabilitation programmes, were substantially less for the family condition ($523 versus $2,760). Total costs to the community, which included all treatment costs as well as social security benefits and law enforcement services, averaged $8,880 for family-oriented cases, and $10,908 for patient-oriented cases – a 19 per cent saving for the family approach.

CONSUMER SATISFACTION

An important consideration in the development of new services is the level of satisfaction of the consumers. This is often assessed by the number of cases who discontinue attending the service. Over the two-year programme two patients dropped out of family management; one left during the first month of treatment, the other refused to complete the family assessment procedures and was excluded on this basis. Two patient-oriented cases withdrew from the study. No patients or families refused to be considered for the study during the recruitment and stabilization phases of the study. Thus, an overall attrition rate of 10 per cent was achieved. This contrasted with very high attrition from the usual services for schizophrenia in Los Angeles County.

A questionnaire survey of the satisfaction of patients and family members with the service provided was conducted at nine and twenty-four months. This indicated that consumer satisfaction was high in both management conditions (Falloon 1985). At twenty-four months, 89 per cent of patients and 100 per cent of family members considered the family-oriented approach either 'good' or 'very good'; 94 per cent of patients and 88 per cent of family members expressed similar levels of satisfaction with patient-oriented management.

THERAPIST SATISFACTION

The importance of maintaining therapists' enthusiasm is crucial to the development of new therapeutic approaches. Throughout the study the primary therapists completed ratings of their enthusiasm for the two management approaches at six-month intervals. Although the enthusiasm for family management remained higher than that for the patient-oriented approach, there was some reduction in therapist enthusiasm for this approach during the second half of the four-year research project. During this period therapists were conducting follow-up sessions and the family cases were either functioning well, needing little active therapy, or struggling with problems that could not be resolved by any therapeutic intervention.

Of greater significance to the differential outcome of the two contrasting management approaches was a series of assessments of the therapists' attitudes towards specific patients and their families conducted at one, six and nine months. No significant differences were noted between the management conditions in the therapists' levels of attraction for the patients, or enthusiasm, effort, and support for the patients. Nor did therapists differ in their perceptions of patients' needs for services in addition to those provided by the study approaches. They did believe that the family-oriented approach provided significantly greater contact and support for the families, and that it was a more effective approach (Falloon 1985).

It may be concluded that the therapists were biased in favour of the family-oriented management. However, this bias did not appear to affect the patients' and family members' perceptions which appeared highly positive towards both approaches.

CONCLUSIONS

This study provided evidence that a psychological intervention that aimed to reduce the impact of environmental stress on a person vulnerable to episodes of schizophrenia could add to the well-established benefits of long-term drug prophylaxis. A control group who received drug therapy alone was not considered feasible, because all drug therapy is supplemented by some psychosocial supportive interventions, albeit often merely to assist patients in coping with unwanted side effects and to maintain adherence to the drug regimen (Falloon 1984).

The patient-oriented comparison we employed was a clearly defined approach to provide continuous support to the patient and their family throughout the two-year study. Although this supportive approach did not appear to add to the clinical stabilizing effects of the drug therapy, there is little doubt that it provided benefits for many patients and their families in the overall management of their conditions. Only one-sixth of these patients and families were rated as experiencing no clinical, social, or family benefits over the two years. Mirror-image comparisons of the two years before and after entry to the study showed substantial reductions in the time spent in hospital during the study period.

Comprehensive crisis intervention that was available around the clock provided substantial support for patients and their families and probably contributed to the reduction in burden that many patient-oriented families reported, despite continued episodes of clinical instability.

Despite the apparent excellence of the community-based service provided in patient-oriented management, this approach did not appear to alter the course of the clinical morbidity of schizophrenia in a manner that would readily justify the extra costs involved. In contrast, the family-oriented approach appeared to provide substantial clinical, social, family and economic benefits. Similar benefits have been observed now in a series of studies that have compared family-based stress management methods with patient-based methods. There can be little doubt that these psychological interventions add to the prophylaxis of optimal drug therapy in a significant manner (Strachan 1986). The key question for future research is what are the clinical components of these interventions that are associated with these benefits.

It has been suggested that the benefits are achieved on the basis of improved adherence to drug therapy (Macmillan 1987). However, the clinical, social, and family morbidity associated with optimal pharmacotherapy for schizophrenia when adherence is assumed in trials of depot preparations is similar to that found in the patient-oriented management conditions (Falloon et al. 1978a, 1978b; Schooler et al. 1980; Hogarty et al. 1979). Although there was some evidence for inadequate adherence to drug regimens in this study, there was little evidence that this precipitated major exacerbations. Poor compliance with drugs appears to be a consequence of deteriorating cognitive function associated with florid episodes of schizophrenia, almost as often as it appears to precede such episodes.

However, it is extremely difficult to define the precise time that florid episodes begin. In clinic-based settings patients will avoid disclosing the earliest signs of cognitive dysfunction that presage a major exacerbation. A clear advantage of a family approach is the ability of family members to observe and report the earliest signs of behavioural disturbance and thereby alert the mental health team long before the patient may report symptoms. Furthermore, where patient and family have been alerted to links between environmental stressors and florid symptoms, they may begin looking for early signs after a stressful event, particularly where efforts to resolve the stress have proven unrewarding. The benefits of this collaboration between patient, family, and mental health professionals cannot be underestimated. But it is apparent that behavioural family therapy tended to facilitate its development. It is possible that this could have been achieved if the patient-oriented treatment sessions had also been conducted in the home.

One unexpected benefit of the family approach was the trend towards lower doses of medication (Moss *et al.* 1985). This may have contributed to the improved social functioning that was observed in this condition. Studies of low dosage pharmacotherapy have suggested that, despite a slightly higher frequency of minor exacerbation, improvements in social functioning, and a lower risk of side effects such as tardive dyskinesia, can be achieved (Kane 1983). If improved stability of florid symptoms can be promoted by combining low doses of neuroleptics with behavioural family interventions, this would seem to represent a major advance in the long-term management of schizophrenia. A multi-centred controlled trial is in progress to examine the interaction between behavioural family interventions and optimal, low (i.e., one-fifth the optimal dose), and targeted dose (i.e., drug given only when exacerbations begin to emerge) drug regimens. Two family approaches of differing intensity are compared: one similar to the method we have developed; the other a monthly family meeting that focuses on teaching families the practical skills of coping with the specific behavioural deficits that are associated with schizophrenia. The NIMH study should help advance our knowledge of the potential synergism between drug and psychosocial interventions.

It has been suggested that merely educating patients and their caregivers about schizophrenia and its management may enhance the clinical outcome. In a recently completed study Tarrier and Barrowclough and their colleagues (in press) demonstrated that education alone was insufficient to induce any major changes in the course of schizophrenia. However, a course that assisted families in resolving problems associated with the management of the disorder was effective in reducing clinical morbidity. However, benefits in terms of enhanced social functioning were not achieved by this essentially patient-focused approach.

The methodological difficulties of conducting research on multi-modal long-term management approaches are considerable. Despite this there is a substantial body of evidence that suggests that specific psychological interventions may enhance the outcome of schizophrenia and add to the benefits that can be achieved through drug therapy and psychosocial support. These methods are all effective in reducing the impact of environmental stress in the day-to-day lives of the patients. To date, lasting benefits and improvements in the quality of the lives of patients and caregivers have been limited to the behavioural family therapy method which has been shown to be highly cost-effective (Macmillan *et al.* 1987).

Several field trials of this method are being conducted in the US and Europe to examine its effectiveness in clinical settings. One such programme in Buckingham is examining the value of employing behavioural family management and low-dose neuroleptics to treat schizophrenia in its prodromal phase. Multi-disciplinary mental health teams have been integrated with primary care services in an effort to detect schizophrenia early in its development and to provide immediate intensive treatment. Early indications suggest new episodes of schizophrenia can be prevented by these interventions.

It would appear that the technology is now available that should enable persons who develop schizophrenia and their caregivers to enjoy lives relatively unrestricted by major clinical episodes or substantial functional disability. the introduction of such services is unlikely to prove costly, and may contribute to substantial savings in public expenditure, even in the initial phases of deployment. Continued research aimed at refining the components of drug and psychological interventions and the manner in which they are combined in the management of schizophrenia may prove as rewarding as the search for the causes of this disorder.

REFERENCES

Birley, J.L.T. and Brown, G.W. (1970) 'Crises and life changes preceding the onset or relapse of acute schizophrenia: clinical aspects', *British Journal of Psychiatry* 116: 327–33.

Brown, G.W., Birley, J.L.T., and Wing, J.K. (1972) 'Influence of family life on the course of schizophrenic disorders: a replication', *British Journal of Psychiatry* 121: 241–58.

Brown, G.W. and Harris, T.O. (1978) *Social Origins of Depression*, London: Tavistock.

Cardin, V.A., McGill, C.W., and Falloon, I.R.H. (1985) 'An economic analysis: costs, benefits and effectiveness', in I.R.H. Falloon (ed.) *Family Management of Schizophrenia*, Baltimore: Johns Hopkins University Press.

Creer, C. and Wing, J.K. (1974) *Schizophrenia at Home*, Surrey: National Schizophrenia Fellowship.

Derogatis, L.R., Lipman, R.S., Rickels, K., Uhlenhuth, E.H., and Cori, L. (1974) 'The Hopkins Symptom Checklist (HSCL)', in P. Pichot (ed.) *Modern Problems in Pharmacopsychiatry*, Basel: Karger.

Doane, J.A. and Falloon, I.R.H. (1985) 'Assessing change in family interaction: methodology and findings', in I.R.H. Falloon (ed.) *Family Management of Schizophrenia*, Baltimore: Johns Hopkins University Press.

Dunham, H.W. and Weinberg, S.K. (1960) *The Culture of the State Mental Hospital*, Detroit: Wayne State University Press.

Falloon, I.R.H. (1984) 'Developing and maintaining adherence to long-term drug-taking regimens: a behavioural analysis', *Schizophrenia Bulletin* 10: 412–17.

Falloon, I.R.H. (ed.) (1985) *Family Management of Schizophrenia: A Controlled Study of Clinical, Social, Family and Economic Benefits*, Baltimore: Johns Hopkins University Press.

Falloon, I.R.H., Boyd, J.L. and McGill, C.W. (1984) *Family Care of Schizophrenia*, New York: Guilford Publications.

Falloon, I.R.H. and Pederson, J. (1985) 'Family management in the prevention of morbidity of schizophrenia: The adjustment of the family unit', *British Journal of Psychiatry* 147: 156–63.

Falloon, I.R.H., Watt, D.C., and Shepherd, M. (1978a) 'A comparative controlled trial of pimozide and fluphenazine deconoate in the continuation therapy of schizophrenia', *Psychological Medicine* 8: 59–70.

Falloon, I.R.H., Watt, D.C., and Shepherd, M. (1978b) 'The social outcome of patients in a trial of long-term continuation therapy in schizophrenia: pimozide versus fluphenazine', *Psychological Medicine* 8: 265–74.

Goldstein, M.J., Rodnick, E.H., Evans, J.R., May, P.R., and Steinberg, M. (1978) 'Drug and family therapy in the aftercare treatment of acute schizophrenia', *Archives of General Psychiatry* 35: 1169–77.

Hardesty, J.P., Falloon, I.R.H., and Shirin, K. (1985) 'The impact of life events, stress and coping on the morbidity of schizophrenia', in I.R.H. Falloon (ed.) *Family Management of Schizophrenia: A Study of Clinical, Social, Family and Economic Benefits*, Baltimore: Johns Hopkins University Press.

Hogarty, G.E., Schooler, N.R., Ulrich, R.F. *et al.* (1979) 'Fluphenazine and social therapy in the aftercare of schizophrenic patients: Relapse analyses of a two-year controlled trial, *Archives of General Psychiatry* 36: 1283–94.

Kane, J.M. (1983) 'Low dose medication strategies in the maintenance treatment of schizophrenia', *Schizophrenia Bulletin* 9: 29–33.

Leff, J.P., Hirsch, S.R., Gaind, R., Rohde, P.D., and Stevens, B.C. (1973) 'Life-events and maintenance therapy in schizophrenic relapse', *British Journal of Psychiatry* 123: 659–60.

Leff, J. and Vaughn, C. (1980) 'The interaction of life events and relatives' expressed emotion in schizophrenia and depressive neurosis', *British Journal of Psychiatry* 136: 146–53.

Macmillan, J.F. (1987) 'Expressed emotion and relapse in first episodes of schizophrenia', *British Journal of Psychiatry* 151: 320–3.

Miklowitz, D., Goldstein, M.J., Falloon, I.R.H., and Doane, J.A. (1984) 'Inter-actional correlates of expressed emotion in the families of schizophrenics', *British Journal of Psychiatry* 144: 482–7.

Moss, H.B., MacDonald, N., Falloon, I.R.H., and Simpson, G.M. (1985) 'Biological factors affecting the outcome of schizophrenia', in I.R.H. Falloon (ed.) *Family Management of Schizophrenia: A Study of Clinical, Social, Family and Economic Benefits*, Baltimore: Johns Hopkins University Press.

Overall, J.E. and Gorham, D.R. (1962) 'The brief psychiatric rating scale', *Psychological Reports* 10: 799–812.

Platt, S., Weyman, A., Hirsch, S., and Hewett, S. (1980) 'The social behaviour assessment schedule (SBAS): rationale, contents, scoring and reliability of a new interview schedule', *Social Psychiatry* 15: 43–55.

Schooler, N.R., Levine, J., Severe, J.B. *et al.* (1980) 'Prevention of relapse in schizophrenia: an evaluation of fluphenazine decanoate', *Archives of General Psychiatry* 37: 16–24.

Strachan, A.M. (1986) 'Family intervention for the rehabilitation of schizophrenia: towards protection and coping', *Schizophrenia Bulletin* 12: 678–98.

Vaughn, C. (1977) 'Interaction characteristics in families of schizophrenic patients' in H. Katschnig (ed.) *Die andere Seite der Schizophrenie*, Vienna: Urban and Schwarzenberg.

Vaughn, E.E. and Leff, J.P. (1976a) 'The measurement of expressed emotion in the families of psychiatric patients', *British Journal of Social and Clinical Psychology* 15: 157–65.

Vaughn, C.E. and Leff, J.P. (1976b) 'The influence of family and social factors on the course of psychiatric illness: a comparison of schizophrenia and depressed neurotic patients', *British Journal of Psychiatry* 129: 125–37.

Vaughn, C.E., Snyder, K.S., Jones, S., Freeman, W.B., and Falloon, I.R.H. (1984) 'Family factors in schizophrenic relapse: a California replication of the British research on expressed emotion', *Archives of General Psychiatry* 41: 1169–77.

Weissman, M.M., Prusoff, B.A., Thompson, W.D., Harding, P.S., and Myers, J.K. (1978) 'Social adjustment by self-report in a community sample and in psychiatric outpatients', *Journal of Nervous and Mental Disease* 166: 317–26.

Wing, J.K. (1978) 'Social influences on the course of schizophrenia', in L.C. Wynne, R.L. Cromwell, and S. Matthysse (eds.) *The Nature of Schizophrenia*, New York: Wiley.

Wing, J.K., Bennett, D.H., and Denham, J. (1964) *The Industrial Rehabilitation of Long-Stay Schizophrenic Patients* (Medical Research Council Memo No. 42), London: HMSO.

Wing, J.K., Cooper, J.E., and Sartorius, N. (1974) *The Measurement and Classification of Psychiatric Symptoms*, London: Cambridge University Press.

Service Organization

24

Appraisal of Institutional Psychiatry

David Watt

A recent writer on the evaluation of psychiatric services observed that

> The evaluation of the psychiatric service of a community is a conceptually
> and technically difficult venture which calls for the exercise of a range of
> methods of epidemiological research and social enquiry . . . For the
> greater part of this enterprise, careful and comprehensive data collection
> is required. (Cawley 1983)

NATIONAL STATISTICS

National statistics clearly constitute 'comprehensive data collection' and are
typified in their most recent publication (DHSS 1980). This deals with
England only, a population of 46.4 million, and was the last of a series of
public productions from the National Mental Health Inquiry by which the
Ministry of Health collected information from all National Health Service
psychiatric hospitals on an individual patient basis. Returns were made for
each patient on admission and on discharge, or death, which recorded in standardized form comprehensive demographic information with some hospital
and social particulars. Diagnosis was the sole specifically clinical datum. This
information is arranged in the form of tables to show numbers of hospital
residents, admissions, discharges, and deaths which are divided according to
the type of hospital (psychiatric, general hospital unit, secure, and mental
handicap) and administrative Regions of the Health Service. They make a
separation of first admissions from readmissions because from readmission
tables the number of readmission events cannot be separated from the number
of persons involved, whereas for first admissions the number of events and
the number of persons is the same which, with knowledge of the size and
age-structure of the parent population, allows a calculation of the incidence
rate for mental disorder generally and for particular diagnoses. Variations in
incidence become manifest between Regions, and different types of service

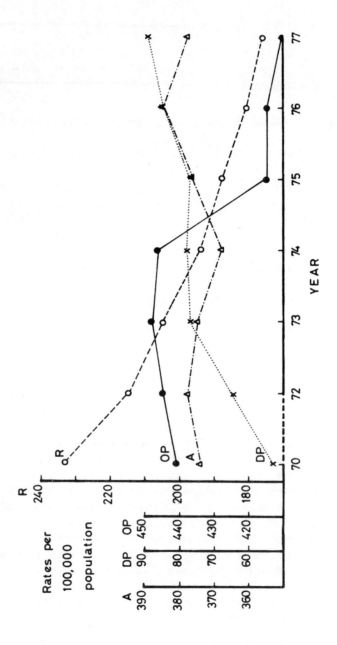

Figure 24.1 National statistics 1970–77 of psychiatric hospital residents (R, ○──────○), day patients (DP, ×-------×), out-patients (OP, ●──────●) and admissions (A, △------△).

Source Adapted from HMSO, 1980, p. 8.

(e.g. psychiatric hospitals and general hospital units) can be compared in this respect. Mortality rates and duration of stay can be used in a comparison of outcome. Tables are broken down by sex and age, showing, among other effects, the increase of mental disorder with increasing age and its excess in females.

The understanding afforded by national statistics is considerably increased by the examination of figures for consecutive years. These bring to light trends which may occur in association with social changes (e.g. in the incidence of alcoholism or drug addiction) or the introduction of new treatments. However, it is the effect of policy change that arouses most interest. Figure 24.1 shows data for psychiatric in-patients, against those for out-patients and day-patients for the years 1970–77. This shows an increase in day hospital attenders coincident with a decrease in hospital residents on which the commentary observes that 'The overall picture which emerges is of a shift away from in-patient care towards more prolonged or intensive out-patient and day care – this is, of course, the intention under the new pattern of services.' This interpretation, however, leaves out of account the simultaneous decrease in new out-patient attenders which the table also discloses, suggesting the equally probable explanation that the increase in day-patients accommodates a transfer of those who would formerly have been out-patients. Clearly interpretation of the aerial view which national statistics afford must be guided by detailed knowledge of the terrain.

A JOINT SURVEY OF THREE PSYCHIATRIC HOSPITALS

A sharper focus is brought to bear in a regional survey of psychiatric hospital performance undertaken by Norris (1959) in a London population of 1.7 million, which comprised the defined catchment population of three hospitals, each with over 2,000 beds. Particulars of all admissions to these hospitals during the triennium 1947–9 were extracted from case notes and administrative records. A follow-up from administrative records showing outcome of all admissions in terms of mortality and readmission to hospital was maintained until the end of 1951.

Data are presented for these mental hospitals as representative of London as a whole. The three hospitals are compared in respect of first admission rates, divided by sex, diagnosis, and age, totalling forty-two items of comparison. These, as would be expected, show many similarities, for instance, that in all three hospitals the rate for schizophrenia in persons below the age of thirty is substantially higher for men than for women. Less likely to be anticipated is the fact that in half of the comparisons there is a significant ($p < 0.01$) difference between hospitals in first admission rates. This is striking in the case of psychoses of old age where the difference in the male rates per million of the general population for hospitals 2 and 3 are 376 and 1,370 respectively and the female rates for hospitals 1 and 3 are 521 and 1,798. Such differences draw attention to what the author has designated 'nosocomial influences'; in the comparison just cited, the fact that psychogeriatric patients were more freely admitted to hospital 3, as a matter of policy, than to the other two hospitals.

To reduce the numerous, overlapping, and disputed diagnoses by which the multifarious conditions and behaviours encountered in persons admitted to a mental hospital are labelled to a manageable, reliable, and comprehensible form, the author adopts a broad classification under the four headings: schizophrenia, manic depressive psychosis, mental disorder of old age, other psychiatric disorder. The 'old age' category covers first admissions diagnosed as pre-senile, senile, and cerebrovascular psychoses, and confusional states in subjects of at least sixty years of age. The last category includes toxic, alcoholic, and epileptic conditions, organic psychoses (other than cerebrovascular), neuroses, mental deficiency, disorders of behaviour, and character, and ill-defined conditions in those under 60 years of age. Separate chapters show data obtained from the survey which are tabulated separately for each of these four groupings and for their constituent diagnostic categories. First admission rates (based on the general population) give the numerical expectation at which particular diseases will occur in populations of known composition in terms of age, sex, and civil state. Outcome is similarly quantified for each category of disease in terms of discharge rates (by age, sex, and civil state) according to time since admission, mortality, duration of stay in hospital, frequency and duration of readmissions in the two years following discharge, and the proportion of patients remaining in hospital according to time since admission. Besides allowing a comparison in both expectation and outcome between the diagnostic categories adopted, these data, using information routinely and uniformly collected by hospitals and administrative bodies, provide a baseline for comparison between hospitals and between regions, and for the appraisal of varying types of service. The large numbers here (e.g. 2,279 schizophrenics of whom more than half were first admissions), the definition of catchment areas and their populations, the detailed local knowledge (e.g. of population structure, of diagnostic conventions; of preferential admission of specific diagnostic categories to particular hospitals), together with the author's combined medical, statistical, and epidemiological expertise, gave the findings of this survey and the authors' reservations particular authority and value for comparative purposes.

COMPARATIVE SURVEY AT SEPARATE PERIODS IN A SINGLE HOSPITAL

A different design is adopted in a study (Shepherd 1957) in which, instead of an interhospital comparison, a single hospital is compared at two periods of time (1931–3, 1945–7) between which social influences and the direction of policy changed considerably. A notable feature of this study was the considered choice of the hospital selected for study because of uncommon features in its situation favourable to precise definition and representativeness of the population served. The catchment area (about 400,000) was limited by the boundaries of an administrative county and had remained so for eighty years and was characterized by a fairly even balance of urban and rural character. The hospital had a central position within the catchment area for which the staff formed virtually the only source of psychiatric service. The choice of periods for study ensured that upheavals of the war years were avoided. The choice of the starting year of the study to coincide with the year of national census secured the most accurate denominator available for the calculation of rates. The maximum statutory bed provision during the periods of study was 600 (1.5 per 1,000, acute and long-stay) but occupation reached 800.

The aims of the study were to produce estimates of minimal incidence of illness, demand on hospital resources, outcome and variation of these features with time. Outcome was judged by duration of stay in hospital, readmissions, and mortality during the period of index admission and during a five-year follow-up period. For each triennium of the study first admission and readmission rates are given by sex, age, diagnosis, marital status, and legal status (voluntary or detained). Outcome is reported in the same categories in terms of discharge, transfer, continued residence or death in hospital, readmissions in the five years following discharge, and the time spent in and out of hospital during the five-year follow-up.

A substantially improved outcome is demonstrated for patients admitted during later triennium, in that less time was spent in hospital during the index admission and follow-up; continuous residence and mortality were reduced. At the same time, more frequent readmission during follow-up of patients admitted with a history of previous admission and greater numbers of female patients admitted in the later period adumbrated national trends prominent during subsequent decades, while the increased mean age of admissions was premonitory of the overwhelming surge in elderly psychiatric admissions, consequent upon the life-prolonging advances made in medicine, which have since required large administrative and policy adjustments.

The single hospital, relatively encapsulated population, and unitary psychiatric service studied here provide a reliable basis for estimating incidence and outcome. Detailed knowledge of social pressures on the service and the response in terms of policy make possible a firm quantitative indication of the predominant influences, among which nosocomial factors are prominent, on indices of performance and outcome. The hospital had, for instance, 800 beds for a population of 500,000, which is sparse compared with the London hospitals in Norris's survey (1959), each of which had approximately the same catchment population as the Buckinghamshire hospital and around 2,000 beds. This discrepancy is reflected in overall first admission rates (per million per annum) which for the three London hospitals in 1949 were 791, 599 and 1,079 respectively (average 823) while for the Aylesbury hospital for 1931–3 and 1945–7 they were 434 and 395; that is, the average rate for the London hospitals was double that of the hospital in Buckinghamshire.

In the London and Buckinghamshire surveys performance and outcome of the institutional psychiatric service are evaluated entirely in terms of socio-demographic features of the general population, of the population admitted to hospital and the statistics of hospital events (admission, discharge, and death). These data sources have the advantages of being recorded routinely, precise, and suitable for statistical manipulation. They can be appraised in the perspective of national figures. Interpretation, however, which requires circumspection and illumination from local knowledge, is often tentative and inconclusive, demanding softer data to flesh out the skeletal framework such studies provide.

HOSPITAL EVALUATION USING CLINICAL AND BEHAVIOURAL OBSERVATIONS INCLUDING THE EFFECT ON FAMILY

In a prospective comparative evaluation of three hospitals, Brown and his colleagues (1966) extended their enquiry to include clinical progress and social functioning of patients. The hospitals surveyed had catchment populations ranging from 400,000 (hospital 3) to 650,000 (hospital 1) each with roughly 3,000 beds per million population. The areas they served were mainly: Hospital 1, the periphery of South London; Hospital 2, the compact industrial city of Nottingham and its surroundings; Hospital 3, a scattered rural area of Essex including three small towns and also a section of east London periphery. The feature of these hospitals most pertinent to the investigation, however, lay in the differing philosophy which informed and moulded the organization of their services: 1 emphasized an active rehabilitation programme within the hospital and aimed not to discharge patients before employment was available or, preferably, had been tried before departure; 2 had the poorest facilities both within the hospital and extramurally; 3 concentrated on early discharge of patients, mobilization of extramural services, and support for relatives undertaking care. The authors' purpose was to measure the effect of these differences in organization of service on the five-year outcome of schizophrenia.

380

For this purpose, during 1956, all patients admitted aged 15–59 whose address lay in the catchment area and where schizophrenia was exclusively diagnosed from hospital case records (independently by two psychiatrists applying prescribed criteria) formed a cohort for each of the three hospitals. Negligible numbers of patients from the catchment areas were found to have been admitted to other hospitals or to have been treated (in the case of hospital 3) without admission. Comparability of the three cohorts was checked in respect of socio-demographic data and no significant initial differences were apparent.

Information during follow-up, besides being provided from hospital, out-patient and after-care agencies, and employment records, was obtained by interview at home visit with the patient and separately with a relative. The interview was free in form but covered prescribed topics. To ensure uniformity the senior interviewer attended every tenth interview and the interviewers compared their procedures regularly. In this way clinical state, duration and competence in employment (including house-keeping and care of children), decline in occupational status, time unoccupied, leisure activity and recreation were assessed and given numerical value or ordinated.

Symptomatology which issued as decline or disruption in patients' social behaviour during a six-month period was recorded. Threats, violence, and destructiveness; slowness and withdrawal; inappropriate and embarrassing behaviour; moods and invalidism were recorded and each item rated minimal, moderate, or marked according to the degree of social disturbance each caused.

The restrictions and other disadvantages experienced by relatives were recorded and included limitation of employment, leisure, and social life; distress and ill-health; adverse effect on children; financial and accommodation difficulties. Both the patients' behaviour and the effect on relatives were quantified in terms of frequency, duration, and severity. The association of domestic living group (parents, wives, dependent children, supporting children) with outcome of patient's illness was assessed.

Table 24.1 shows how these indices of outcome were distributed in the three hospitals which are labelled 1. high standard hospital care; 2. community care; and 3. low standard hospital care, as a crude shorthand indication of their main difference in character. The distinction between hospital 2 (community care) and hospitals 1 and 3 is highlighted in the markedly shorter duration of admissions in hospital 2, the longer time spent in community care, the greater use of out-patient consultation, day hospital, and visits by mental welfare officers (MWO). There were no statistically significant differences between the three hospitals on the measures of outcome but certain tendencies appear; notably, the greater time spent employed in the community by patients in hospital 2, their higher proportion of disturbed behaviour, and the higher proportion of their children adversely affected. The trends are most prominent when the community care hospital

Table 24.1 Comparison of three hospitals, in terms of various criteria employed, during five-year follow-up

	Hospital 1: High hospital care	Hospital 2: Community care	Hospital 3: Low hospital care
Hospital criteria			
% time spent in hospital	30	20	31
% subjects readmitted	55	70	62
Community care criteria			
Average OP attendances per patient	1.4	2.1	1.1
% time in day hospital (final year)	0.3	14.0	–
MWO routine visits in final year	1.5	48.0	1.5
Duration under community care	8 times more in hospital 2 than in 1 and 3		
Patient criteria			
Employment			
% time employed for first admissions	62	60	47
% time employed for readmissions	31	20	26
% time in community unemployed for 1st admissions	9	28	26
% time in community unemployed for readmissions	20	48	28
Clinical			
% chronic course of illess (first and previous admissions combined)	41	41	40
Behavioural			
% disturbed behaviour for first admissions	65	63	66
% disturbed behaviour for readmissions	58	74	73
% danger to self or others for first admissions	25	39	19
% danger to self or others for readmissions	30	44	41
Effect on relatives			
% having three or more problems	18	41	28
% health affected	36	43	37
% children adversely affected	15	59	41
% relatives expressing welcoming attitude	86	63	74

Source: Brown *et al.* 1980.
MWO = mental welfare officer; OP = outpatient

(2) is compared with hospital 1 (high standard of in-patient care). An overall index of severe disability during the final six months of follow-up was constructed from the three most valid indices of outcome (hospitalization, severe disturbance, unemployment). By this meaure 35–45 per cent of first admissions and 59–66 per cent of readmissions suffered serious handicap in follow-up and there were no statistically significant differences between the hospitals.

In discussing their results, the authors refer to 'the reservations that must be attached to any conclusions drawn from the comparative data' and are restrained by a number of these reservations in expressing their own judgements. However, even allowing for their provisos, it can be firmly concluded that no superiority was demonstrated for community care over an accomplished high standard of hospital care as judged by the patients' clinical and social outcome, employment, the extent of disturbed or dangerous behaviour in the community, the adverse effects and disadvantages for relatives and children.

THE RELATION BETWEEN ENVIRONMENT AND INSTITUTIONALISM

In a subsequent study using the same three hospitals, the authors (Wing and Brown 1970) narrowed the field of examination, bringing into sharper focus the syndrome of 'institutionalism' which, although not confined to psychiatric hospitals, was first identified in these institutions, and has become a major charge in their blanket indictment. 'Institutionalism' appears in chronic schizophrenia as clusters of characteristic clinical features (Liddle 1987), comprising withdrawal, flatness of affect, poverty or incoherence of speech, coherent delusions, socially inappropriate behaviour, and hospital dependence. By the use of standardized scales these items were scored for a cohort of long-stay female schizophrenics at each of the three hospitals. Similarly, the social milieu of the hospitals was assessed in terms of patients' personal possessions, time spent unoccupied, occupation, contacts with the outside world, and restriction of spontaneous activity, to give indices of environmental poverty.

Over a period of four years a programme of improvement was undertaken at the hospitals. The measures of social milieu were repeated at the end of this time and all showed a substantial reduction of environmental poverty. Similarly, assessment of the clinical items characterizing institutionalism was repeated and showed an overall amelioration of this condition in a third of patients, which was most marked in hospital 3 which had originally shown the most severe degree of environmental poverty and of 'institutionalism' in patients.

A further refinement of the method used in this comparison of hospitals was the demonstration of associations between specific items of hospital

383

environmental poverty and particular features of institutionalism in patients. For instance, those patients who showed greatest increase in the proportion of time for which they were employed and decrease in time for which they were unoccupied showed greatest improvement in clinical features of institutionalism.

INTERNATIONAL COMPARISON OF HOSPITALS

It could not be assumed that the measures employed in the appraisal of hospitals in these studies would be applicable to all psychiatric hospitals in Britain and still less to those in other countries. In the case of indices derived from administrative records (e.g. duration of hospital stay), discrepancies in computing (e.g. through the method of recording patients' leave) will probably be discovered in preliminary scrutiny and taken into account. However, discrepancies in less standard, culture-bound features which are not routinely recorded (e.g. measures of hospital social milieu) are less likely to be readily evident. To test the feasibility of generalization Wing and Brown (1970) undertook a comparison of a British and an American hospital in respect of hospital environmental standards and the level of institutional syndrome in patients. The British hospital was number 2 in the study already described, a standard county mental hospital responsible for the care of all types of psychiatric illness, which had developed community care services to a degree exceptional at the time of this study. The American hospital was a relatively small unit (325 inmates) specializing in the care of long-stay patients with psychiatrically unqualified staff. Forty-five residents similar to the sample from the British hospital were selected for comparison. Assessments of social withdrawal, socially embarrassing behaviour, and patient attitude to discharge were made as had been done for the British hospital cohort, giving a measure of 'institutionalism'. Similarly, the measures of hospital social milieu that had been made in the comparison of British hospitals were applied in the American hospital. These two hospitals could thus be compared for significant features. The American hospital, for instance, adopted a more protective policy towards women patients which resulted in a notably higher average ward restrictiveness score for the American women (22.9) than for the British women (11.9) and there was a significant excess in average social withdrawal scores in the American (3.9) over British patients (2.3). The experience and results of this preliminary study enabled the authors to conclude that 'a full-scale comparative survey of the kind outlined here is feasible', provided that modifications are made to take account of sampling problems and socio-demographic differences and that 'under these conditions tentative hypothesis testing might be possible even using international comparisons'.

384

EVALUATION OF PSYCHIATRIC SERVICE AS CONTROLLED TRIAL

The appraisal of a psychiatric service involves comparison of the service to be evaluated with the measured outcome of an evaluated alternative. It shares its essential principle with that of the controlled trial; here two populations, identical in all respects except for the item to be evaluated, are compared as to the effect of the item for evaluation. Criteria for detecting and measuring the effect(s) of the item(s) for evaluation must be standardized and applied impartially to both populations. The widespread application and analysis of the controlled clinical trial during the last forty years has secured considerable refinement in the adaptations required in rigorously applying the principle in varying practical circumstances. Although the studies in the evaluation of institutional psychiatry examined here demonstrate the practical feasibility of the principle, application has been dilatory and little progress has been made. This is particularly true of 'community care' service which, as front-runner in the race to replace psychiatric hospitals, needs to know the direction in which it is heading and whether it can stand the pace or last the distance.

REFERENCES

Brown, G.W., Bone, M., Dalison, B., and Wing, J.K. (1966) *Schizophrenia and Social Care*, London: Oxford University Press.

Cawley, R.H. (1983) in M. Shepherd and O.L. Zangwill (eds) *Handbook of Psychiatry, Volume 1*, Cambridge: Cambridge University Press, 242.

Department of Health and Social Security (1980) *In-patient Statistics from the Mental Health Enquiry for England, 1977* (Statistical and research report series no. 23), London: HMSO.

Liddle, P.F. (1987) 'The symptoms of chronic schizophrenia: a re-examination of the positive-negative dichotomy', *British Journal of Psychiatry* 151: 145–51.

Norris, V. (1959) *Mental Illness in London*, London: Chapman and Hall.

Shepherd, M. (1957) *A Study of the Major Psychoses in an English County*, London: Chapman and Hall.

Wing, J.K. and Brown, G.W. (1970) *Institutionalism and Schizophrenia*, Cambridge: Cambridge University Press.

25

Evaluating Community Psychiatric Services

Michele Tansella

In the past twenty years there has been an increasing interest in the evaluation of health care delivery systems. This has been mainly due to the need for a more efficient utilization of resources in an era of steadily increasing costs. In mental health care a gradual move from hospital to community care, with substantial changes in the organization and use of mental health services, occurred in the same period, and this has also emphasized the importance of descriptive and evaluative studies.

In the report of a WHO symposium on *Trends in Psychiatric Care* it is stated: 'All participants accepted the need for evaluation of new services. It is no longer advisable to set up a new service alone. Its objectives must be stated and ways and means devised for assessing how far its aims are achieved' (WHO 1971: 14). The same point was made some fifteen years later by Professor John Wing, who underlined the importance of ensuring that 'planning and evaluation go hand in hand' (Wing 1986: 36) and pointed out the differences between policy makers and evaluators in their approach to the process of evaluation, as well as the utility of creative collaboration.

Similar statements on the importance of evaluating psychiatric services have often been made in the last two decades. In spite of this long history of suggestions and good advice for a wider evaluative approach to the delivery of mental health care, in recent years there has been much more planning and implementation than services evaluation. Moreover, there are no good reasons to be optimistic about creative collaboration between planners and researchers so far (Sartorius 1982; Kreitman 1984; Tansella 1985) and this possibility remains an interesting challenge for the future.

Several volumes on the evaluation of psychiatric services have appeared to date (Gruenberg 1966; Williams and Ozarin 1968; Wing and Hailey 1972; Wing and Häfner 1973; Feldman and Windle 1973; Struening and Guttentag 1975; Guttentag and Struening 1975; Coursey *et al.* 1977; EEC 1981; Wing 1982; Stahler and Tash 1982). However, the literature on evaluation research which goes beyond the descriptive stage is relatively scanty and the evidence on one particular aspect of evaluation, namely cost-benefit analysis, is inconclusive (Glass and Goldberg 1977; Frank 1981; McGuire and Weisbrod 1981; Weisbrod 1982; Wilkinson and Pelosi 1987).

In spite of recent progress on data gathering and processing and of the increasing availability of indicators of service use as well as standardized instruments for psychological and psychiatric assessment, there is still a long way to go to make the cycle of planning and evaluation of mental health care a productive one.

The aims of this chapter are, first, to focus on the aspects of evaluation which are particularly relevant for community psychiatric services and, second, to describe the first steps in the evaluation of the South-Verona Community Psychiatric Service (CPS), a new service set up in 1978 according to the provision of the Italian psychiatric reform.

DEFINITIONS

The title of this chapter contains two key concepts which need to be defined: evaluation and community psychiatric services. According to Sartorius (1983: 59): 'Evaluation at its best is a systematic way of learning from experience and using the lessons learned to improve both current and future action. At its worst, it is an activity used to justify the selection of a scapegoat for past failures.' Twenty years ago Suchman (1967) used the term 'evaluative research', stating that it is appropriate when scientific methods and techniques are used in making an evaluation. On the other hand, Roemer (1972) pointed out that, at its highest level, the evaluation of health services measures the extent to which the ultimate objective of a programme – an improvement in the health of the people serviced – has been attained. But, he observed, if this is the best type of evaluation to undertake, doubtless it is also the most difficult. One could argue that, of course, a clear outcome measure may be obtained only when the objectives to be achieved have been clearly identified and made explicit in advance, in the planning phase of the programme. In other words the evaluative process must start in the planning phase. Schulberg (1977) called the function of assessing the degree to which the objectives are being accomplished as the 'assessment of performance', to be differentiated from the 'assessment of adequacy' which refers to re-evaluating the validity of objectives and providing feedback, through the recycling of information, to systems change. The latter approach, which views programme outcomes from a more global perspective, has been referred to by Bachrach (1980, 1982) as 'impact evaluation'.

As may be seen from these definitions, the process of evaluating mental health services should be a timely, long-term, and complex process, and different approaches and strategies as well as various techniques need to be used. I will come back to this issue later.

As far as the terms 'community psychiatric services' and 'community care'

387

are concerned, I have discussed in a previous paper several definitions and their implications (Tansella 1986). It is worthwhile to recall here the risk that 'that over used word community' (Acheson 1985: 3) degenerates into a slogan and loses its actual meaning, becoming a generic expression to label different, not homogeneous functions and institutions. In this context, community care, as applied to mental health, is intended as:

> A system of care devoted to a defined population and based on a comprehensive and integrated mental health service, which includes out-patient facilities, day and residential training centres, residential accom-modation in hostels, sheltered workshops and inpatient units in general hospital and which ensures [with multidisciplinary team work], early diagnosis, prompt treatment, continuity of care, social support and a close liaison with other medical and social community services and, in particular, with general practitioners. (Tansella 1986: 664)

HISTORICAL BACKGROUND

Historical perspectives in evaluating mental health care have been outlined by Cooper and Morgan (1973), by Sartorius and Harding (1984) as well as by Coursey (1977), who made particular reference to the American scene. It is sufficient to mention here that some evaluative-type activity took place as early as the mid-1800s in mental hospitals, in the form of tabulating admissions, discharges, and deaths. This record system, usually independent of individual case notes, 'monitored the demography and economy of a closed institution' (Sartorius and Harding 1984: 228). Afterwards hospital statistics became more patient-oriented and included information on diagnosis, treatment, and natural evolution of psychiatric disorders. The implementation of new extramural mental health services, often consisting of various independent agencies, together with the change of focus of treatment from the mental hospital to this more dispersed community-based system of care, demanded more sophisticated and integrated approaches in the description and evaluation of care provided. It became necessary, wherever possible for evaluation to be a continuing process rather than an isolated, occasional activity. Instruments for the assessments of specific conditions were developed (Sartorius and Harding 1984) while psychiatric case registers covering defined population areas proved to be, in many parts of the world, valuable and potent tools for monitoring and evaluating mental health services (Wing and Fryers 1976; Gibbons et al. 1984). The methodology derived from the work of social scientists and the availability of computers and of advanced databases recently made possible a wide range of other approaches, such as goal attainment, management by objectives, and systems analysis (Coursey 1977). However, until now evaluators have not gone very far along these new roads.

DESCRIPTIVE AND EVALUATIVE RESEARCH. FROM MONITORING SERVICE ACTIVITIES TO EVALUATING THEIR EFFICACY AND OUTCOME

Although 'it is never possible to be purely descriptive' (Wing 1972: 27), a distinction should be made between research which is mainly descriptive (the monitoring of services, which describes how many patients are in contact and what pattern of contacts they make over time) and that which goes beyond the descriptive stage to measure the extent to which the stated objectives have been attained. The former 'is an essential first step in an evaluation research, usually provides much important information regarding the operation of the service, and is frequently all that is required to answer the questions being posed' (Burvill 1978: 189). Indeed Wing *et al.* (1970: 3–4) some years ago stated that, if the need for services is defined in terms of reduction or containment of morbidity, evaluative studies may be elaborated in the form of six questions:

1. How many and what kinds of individuals are in contact with existing services?
2. What are their needs and those of their relatives?
3. Are the services at present provided meeting these needs effectively and economically?
4. How many others, not in touch with existing services, also have needs, and are they different from the needs of patients who do not see psychiatrists?
5. What new services, or modifications to existing services, are likely to cater for unmet needs?
6. When innovations are introduced, do they in fact meet these needs?

It is clear that only the first question may be answered by the use of descriptive statistics, particularly those provided by case registers. Other approaches and techniques, including surveys of the population not in touch with existing services as well as the planning and evaluation of *new* services, are required to answer the remaining questions.

EVALUATING COMPREHENSIVE, COMMUNITY-BASED PSYCHIATRIC SERVICES

The rationale for a shift from mental hospitals to a community-based system of care as well as the main critical views on this move and the distinctive features of 'alternative' community services have been reported elsewhere (Tansella and Zimmermann-Tansella 1988). It has been recently stated that several randomized controlled studies (Weisbrod *et al.* 1980; Fenton *et al.*

389

1982; Hoult *et al.* 1983; Cardin *et al.* 1985) show that 'care provided around the clock, seven days a week in the community has clinical, social and economic advantages over hospital care' (Wilkinson and Pelosi 1987: 140). A similar view was expressed by Tantam (1985), who, however, stated that 'the essential elements of the alternatives to hospital remain to be determined' (Tantam 1985: 3).

It is generally recognized that evaluation of community services is more difficult than the evaluation of a mental hospital. Examples of evaluative studies of comprehensive community services for patients from a defined catchment area are the evaluations of the 'Worthing Experiment' (Carse *et al.* 1958), of the Dutchess County Project in New York State (Hunt *et al.* 1961), of the Chichester service (Grad and Sainsbury 1966), of the Southwest Denver Program (Polak 1978), of the Madison experience (Stein and Test 1980), of the Swedish Nacka Project (Cullberg and Stefansson 1981; Cullberg *et al.* 1981), of the community service in Mannheim (Häfner and Klug 1982), of the Samsø project in Denmark (Munk-Jørgensen 1985) and the New South Wales (Australia) experience (Hoult 1983; Hoult *et al.* 1986). Classic studies are those conducted in England, in Camberwell (Wing and Hailey 1972; Wing 1982, 1986) and in Salford (Fryers and Wooff 1985). Other important studies are actually in progress, such as the Worcester Development Project (Tombs 1987). Studies on services for particular groups of patients, for example, the elderly or the mentally retarded have not been mentioned here.

Specific issues arising in the evaluation of comprehensive, community-based psychiatric services are:

1) The evaluation should become part of a longitudinal, long-term programme, 'with defined mechanisms to carry it out in an "integrated" manner (i.e., planning and implementing it together with service development)' (Sartorius and Harding 1984: 234).
2) Contacts with the psychiatric services, as well as data about type and amount of mental health care provided at the primary care level, particularly by GPs, have to be collected. Information about filters as well as about levels of the Goldberg and Huxley model (Goldberg and Huxley 1980) are essential for effective planning. It is well known that a *minor* increase in the permeability of the filter number 3 (general practice vs. psychiatric services) may well require a *substantial* increase in service provision at the specialist levels (Shepherd *et al.* 1966).
3) Information is needed on the socio-cultural context (characteristics of the area and of the resident population), and on the political and legal context (legislation regulating the delivery of mental health care, social assistance, provisions of pensions and subsidies, etc.).
4) Indicators need to be developed of the extent to which various agencies

and services providing care to the resident population are integrated. It may be expected that the same amount of resources may well have different outcomes in areas with well-integrated or unintegrated services, and this appears to be an interesting topic for future research.

STEPS IN THE EVALUATION OF THE SOUTH-VERONA COMMUNITY PSYCHIATRIC SERVICE (CPS)

The legal context

In the 1960s in Italy the existing gap between the principle and the practice of psychiatry began to be subjected to stringent criticism by professionals as well as by lay people. In those years rapid political, social, and cultural changes occurred, while the practice of psychiatry (which was taking place almost exclusively in old-fashioned, large mental hospitals) was still governed by statutes and regulations dating from 1904 and 1909 respectively. This contradictory situation provided a fertile background for the development of a movement for psychiatric reform which finally resulted in new psychiatric legislation, passed by the Italian parliament in 1978. The features of this movement and those of its final outcome (Law 180) have been described in detail elsewhere (De Plato and Minguzzi 1981; Tansella and Williams 1987).

The main proposal of the Italian reform was to develop comprehensive and integrated community services while blocking admissions to mental hospitals without inducing rapid and massive deinstitutionalization. For many years the pressure of policy and the call for action were allowed to overshadow the crucial need for evaluation, so there are now many community-based services, providing a high standard of care, but which do not produce quantitative data and have no evaluative studies in progress to support the quality of their practice. Although quantitative national and regional data have been analysed (Williams et al. 1986, 1987b; Tansella et al. 1987), the main issue remains whether or not the new pattern of psychiatric care delivery is effective where it is fully applied.

The South-Verona area and the psychiatric case register

South-Verona is a mainly urban area of 75,000 inhabitants in northern Italy where a Community Psychiatric Service (CPS) was set up in 1978, according to the principles of the Italian reform (Zimmermann-Tansella et al. 1985). Its care delivery is comprehensive and is based on staff intensive domiciliary visits, and on out-patient care and day care, designed to avoid hospitalization as much as possible (Jablensky and Henderson 1983; Burti et al. 1986). The style of intervention is psychosocial and special emphasis is given to integrating different interventions such as medication, family support, and social work. To ensure continuity of care all staff members (except for a group of hospital nurses) work both in hospital and in the community. The

391

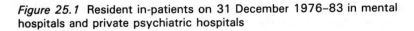

Figure 25.1 Resident in-patients on 31 December 1976–83 in mental hospitals and private psychiatric hospitals

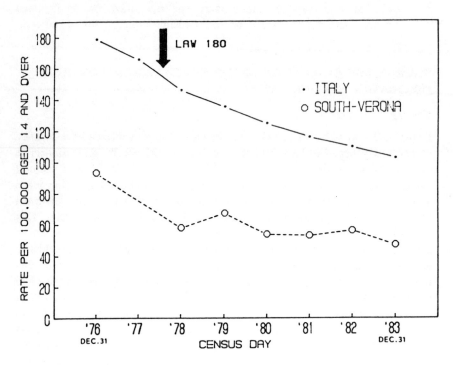

South-Verona CPS is run by the Institute of Psychiatry, University of Verona, which also provides training for undergraduate and post-graduate students (Burti and Mosher 1986). The area has been monitored since January 1979 by a Psychiatric Case Register (PCR) (Tansella *et al.* 1985) and by an epidemiological/evaluative research team.

Descriptive statistics

Figure 25.1 shows the trend in the rates for bed occupancy in mental hospitals and private psychiatric hospitals, in Italy (ISTAT, Roma) and in South-Verona (South-Verona PCR, unpublished annual reports) from December 1976 (more than one year before the psychiatric reform) to December 1983 (five years after).

It may be seen that South-Verona has lower rates than Italy (a gradual process of deinstitutionalization started before 1976) and that, after 1978, the decreasing trend in the in-patient population is more evident at the national than at the local level. In most recent years this decline is mainly due to death rather than discharge. Since the front doors of public mental hospitals have been closed since 1982, admissions are only possible to fifteen-bed

Figure 25.2 South-Verona. Build-up of 'new' long-stay patients (non-resident in mental hospitals, private psychiatric hospitals and general hospitals' psychiatric units for one year or more on triennial census days, but long-stay on subsequent annual census days)

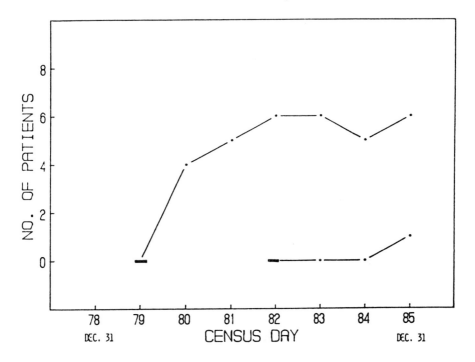

general hospital psychiatric units (with a length of stay that in most cases does not exceed two months – one such a unit is part of the South-Verona CPS) or to private psychiatric hospitals (where patients may remain a long time – there are two such hospitals in Verona and their total bed complement is 220). It is interesting to note that, under these circumstances, there was a negligible build-up of *new long-stay patients* in South-Verona.

The two curves in figure 25.2 indicate the number of people who have become long-stay since the two given starting dates and are still in hospital at the end of each subsequent year. This pattern, which is unusual as compared with international standards (Häfner and Klug 1982; Gibbons *et al.* 1984), is mainly due to the ban on new admissions (from 1978) and on all admissions (from 1982) to mental hospitals, the main places where long-stays are produced. It is also due to the change in psychiatric practice and to the development, since 1978, of an expanding community service. The South-Verona CPS is now taking care of most psychiatric patients who before the

393

Figure 25.3 South-Verona. Build-up of 'new' long-term patients (not in 'continuous care' in the community for one year or more on triennal census days, but long-term community patients on subsequent annual census days)

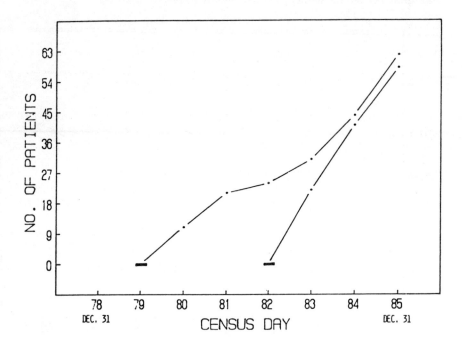

reform would have been admitted to the mental hospital, becoming long-stay. They receive intensive and continuous care in the community (out-patient care, including home visits and crisis intervention, and day care) and have spells of admission to hospital (the psychiatric unit in general hospital or private psychiatric hospitals) when necessary. In all settings but the private hospital they are under the care of the same team. The patients under continuous care (without a break between contacts of ninety-one days or more) for 365 days or longer may be defined as long-term patients. Figure 25.3 shows the build-up of 'new' long-term patients since 31 December 1980.

The curves show that the number in both cohorts are consistently rising. The clinical and social implications of the build-up of long-term patients *instead* of long-stay in-patients need to be considered. In fact, the outcome, in terms of service use, seems to be different in the two groups. In a follow-up study we showed that while 88 per cent of patients of the long-stay cohort were still long-stay after two years, only 45 per cent of the long-term patients remained long-term over the same period (Balestrieri *et al.* 1987). Further

394

Figure 25.4 South-Verona. Total number of days in hospital (long-stay in mental hospital included), total number of days in day hospital and centre (day care started in 1982) and all out-patient contacts (out-patient visits, home visits, attendances at the casualty departments, ward referrals, attendances at the Community Mental Health Centre). Drug addicts not included.
NB From 1982 onward admissions to neurological wards of general hospitals with psychiatric diagnosis, are also included

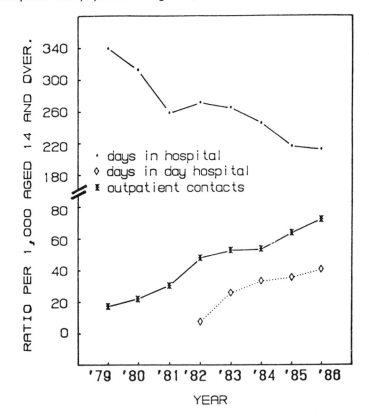

studies, using appropriate outcome measures, are necessary before concluding that long-term community care by the South-Verona CPS is inducing to a lesser extent dependence on the services and chronicity of their use, as compared with the old hospital-centred system of care.

One important aspect of the Italian model of community psychiatry is that hospital psychiatry is considered complementary to community care and not vice versa. The 1978 Italian reform prescribes that, as a rule, treatment would be made available to psychiatric patients in their own environment and that hospitalization, both voluntary and compulsory, would be regarded as an extraordinary intervention. We wanted to check if this is actually taking place in our area.

395

Several case-register studies showed that in South-Verona the great majority of patients (more than 70 per cent) are treated outside the hospital *only*, confirming the community orientation of our programme (see Burti *et al*. 1986; Tansella *et al*. 1987), and that compulsory admissions were much lower after the psychiatric reform (in 1979–86, mean number of 11 admissions/100,000 adult population per year) than before (in 1977, 55 admissions/100,000) (South-Verona PCR, unpublished annual reports).

Figure 25.4 confirms that, over the years, in South-Verona, out-patient care and day care are consistently increasing, while the extent of in-patient care is decreasing. This shows that, as expected, community care requires adequate time for implementation, even in places such as Italy where a radical policy has been adopted.

Monitoring patterns of care

The utilization of mental health services is a topic of special interest in areas where a major change in the organization of care provision has occurred. The South-Verona PCR has been used in several studies designed to describe patterns of care. For example, we studied high users and long-term users of the mental health services and showed that, after excluding long-stay in-patients and single consulters, 9.4 per cent of the patients seeking care in one year were high users and 12.1 per cent were long-term users. A log-linear analysis demonstrated a strong association between the pattern of service use and diagnosis, occupational status, and previous psychiatric contacts (Tansella *et al*. 1986a).

To study the relationship between the amount of care provided by specialist and by primary care services, the extent of patient contact for affective disorders at the extramural psychiatric service level (number of contacts) and its monthly fluctuations were compared with those at the in-patient level (number of admissions) and at the GP level (number of antidepressant prescriptions), in 1983 and 1984. Patients with a diagnosis of affective disorder accounted for about 20 per cent of the total number of patients contacting the specialized services in one year. The extent of patient contact was approximately ten times greater at the GP level (in one year about 150 antidepressant prescriptions per 1,000 adult inhabitants) than at the out-patient/community psychiatric service level. Similarly, the extent of patient contact at the latter level was approximately ten times greater than at the in-patient level. There was a clear correspondence between monthly fluctuations in the extent of care for affective disorders provided at the two community levels in 1984, but not in 1983 (Tansella *et al*. 1986b). The implications of these findings for service planning and evaluation have been discussed in the above quoted papers.

The study of seasonal variation in the expression of morbidity of several psychiatric disorders may be relevant not only to the investigation of the causes, but also to the organization, planning, and evaluation of psychiatric services. Seasonal variation in new episodes of affective disorders was investigated using the South-Verona PCR. Case-register data have considerable advantages over hospital admission statistics for this type of study, especially in case-register areas where community psychiatric care is well developed, as in South-Verona. We found evidence for a cyclical pattern in the occurrence of affective psychosis, but this was statistically significant only for the males; there was no cyclical variation in depressive neurosis (Williams *et al.* 1987a).

Monthly variation in the demand for extramural psychiatric care was also studied. Using harmonic analysis, a complex pattern of seasonal variation emerged, but the first harmonic (1 cycle/per year) was consistently the most important (in both sexes and in all diagnostic groups, except schizophrenic psychosis). The seasonal variation in extramural contacts could not be accounted for by variation in the number of patients in contact, but was found to be partly due to variation in the availability and supply of psychiatric care. After examining the amplitude of the cyclical fluctuation we concluded that it has trivial implications for service organization, thus supporting previous findings from the primary care setting (Balestrieri *et al.* 1987).

Descriptive surveys

In order to understand the decision to hospitalize at the first contact, rather than utilize the other services of a community-based system of care, forty-six consecutive patients who were admitted on first-contact with the South-Verona CPS were compared with all other in-patients over a two-year period with respect to socio-demographic characteristics, ICD-9 diagnosis and symptoms (on the PSE Syndrome Check List). Results suggested that first-contact hospitalized patients have significantly more neurotic depressive features than other in-patients and that alternatives to immediate admission were considered more often for patients with psychoses (except those with organic psychoses) than for those with depressive neurosis (Faccincani *et al.* 1987).

A survey of all sixty-one schizophrenia patients from the South-Verona area who contacted the psychiatric services in 1979 was conducted seven years later. Fifty-seven patients (93 per cent) were traced and all those still alive (N = 46) interviewed using PSE-9, DAS-2, PIRS, and other standardized instruments. The results are currently being analysed.

The risk of mortality over five to eight years for a total one-year prevalence cohort of schizophrenic patients, extracted by means of the South-Verona PCR, was assessed using three methods: case control with both non-psychotic patients and general population (matched for sex and age), indirect standardization using mortality tables, and indirect standardization with survival tables, according to the method described by Sturt (1983). All methods yielded an excess mortality: that is, around the two-fold increase described in other studies. Moreover, the findings do *not* support the view that excess mortality in South-Verona is linked to suicide, but to natural causes (Lesage *et al.* 1988).

It is well recognized that another index of the efficacy of a community service is its ability to help patients to maintain themselves in their community, without migration. Although the circumstances of migration, the quality of life, symptoms, and social disability of patients who migrate and those who do not need to be taken into account, the simple quantitative findings on migration are the first necessary step for evaluating this aspect of the practice of new services. Migration of the 1982 cohort of all South-Verona schizophrenic patients over a five-year period was compared to non-psychotic and general population control groups. The migration outside the catchment area was highest in the general population sample, but no significant difference was found between the groups. On the other hand, schizophrenic patients tended to migrate less than neurotics within South-Verona. These findings suggest that, following the application of the Italian psychiatric reform in South-Verona, schizophrenic patients do not drift from this small northern city of 270,000 into big cities. Moreover, except for mental hospital long-stay in-patients, the schizophrenic cohort shares the potential mobility of the general population (Lesage and Tansella 1988).

One of the limitations of the register method is related to the geographical mobility of the population outside the area covered by the case register. It is obvious that high mobility limits the value of longitudinal analyses conducted using register data. It is important, therefore, to have, from each register area, quantitative information on this demographic variable in order to evaluate the stability over time of the denominators of case-register analyses and to calculate the expected number of patients, among those in contact with the psychiatric services in one day and/or in one year, who may lose contact with the register simply because of migration and may therefore be excluded from any case-register follow-up.

For example, in the study quoted above, we showed that, over a five-year period (1982–86), 13.8 per cent of a South-Verona population sample moved outside the register area. The corresponding figures for the schizophrenic and the non-psychotic groups were 7.3 per cent and 11.8 per cent respectively (Lesage and Tansella 1988). If we use the highest figure and consider that one-day and one-year treated prevalence rates (mean values for the years 1982–86) in South-Verona were 257/100,000 and 1,184/100,000 respectively, we can assume that in a five-year case-register follow-up of cohorts of patients in contact with services in one day and in one year, the risk of being considered out of care due to migration out of the case-register area applies to 35 and 163 patients/100,000 residents respectively. In areas with higher geographical mobility and/or with higher treated prevalence rates this bias may have a substantially greater effect on longitudinal case-register analyses.

CONCLUSIONS

It was stated that 'The scope, extent and impact of community care are difficult to estimate. Official figures provide a starting point, but they may hide as much as they purport to disclose' (Wilkinson 1985: 1371). A number of properly designed studies, intensively conducted over a sufficiently long period of time, are therefore necessary. Case registers are invaluable tools for service use descriptions, and may well provide the sampling frame for *ad hoc* surveys and outcome evaluations. The work done until now in South-Verona shows that the Italian reform is effective and that our community-based system of care is able to cope with all the problems presented by the patients living in our area, without 'back up' from the psychiatric hospital, where only a small group of old long-stay in-patients (N = 18 on 31 December 1986) continues to reside. The efficacy of the system needs to be further evaluated and a cost-benefit analysis needs to be undertaken.

To conclude, I would like to refer to Pascal's dictum, recently quoted by Professor Michael Shepherd (1987), that words differently arranged have a different meaning and meanings differently arranged have a different effect. What is important in community care is not only the number and characteristics of various services, but the way in which they are actually arranged and integrated. Different arrangements of similar services may have a very different effect. The outcome due to the type of arrangement and collaboration among services in a particular area, in other words the outcome due to the existing *model of coordination and integration*, has been subjected to little assessment and evaluation until now. Reliable measures of process and outcome, as well as of the costs and benefits, need to be developed for this particular purpose. The effects due to the particular organization of psychiatric services which is operating in South-Verona and qualititative as well as quantitative aspects of the offered care deserve further studies.

Acknowledgements: This study has been supported by the Consiglio Nazionale della Richerche (CNR, Roma), Progetto Finalizzato Medicina Preventiva e Riabilitativa 1982–1987, Contract No. 86.01962.56, and by the Regione Veneto, Ricerca Sanitaria Finalizzata, Contract No. 134.03.86.

I am indebted to Dr M. Balestrieri and Mr R. Fianco, as well as to the staff of the South-Verona Psychiatric Case Register and especially to Mr G. Meneghelli, for their valuable help. Many thanks are also due to Dr D. De Salvia for the collection of national data reported in figure 25.1.

REFERENCES

Acheson, E.D. (1985) 'That over-used word community', *Health Trends* 17: 3.
Bachrach, L.L. (1980) 'Overview: model programs for chronic mental patients', *American Journal of Psychiatry* 137: 1023–31.

399

Bachrach, L.L. (1982) 'Assessment of outcomes in community support systems: results, problems, and limitations', *Schizophrenia Bulletin* 8: 39–61.

Balestrieri, M., Micciolo, R., and Tansella, M. (1987) 'Long-stay and long-term psychiatric patients in an area with a community-based system of care: a case-register follow-up study', *International Journal of Social Psychiatry*, 33, 251–62.

Balestrieri, M., Williams, P., Micciolo, R., and Tansella, M. (1987) 'Monthly variation in the pattern of extramural psychiatric care', *Social Psychiatry* 22: 160–6.

Burti, L. and Mosher, L.R. (1986) 'Training psychiatrists in the community: a report of the Italian experience', *American Journal of Psychiatry* 143: 1580–4.

Burti, L., Garzotto, N., Siciliani, O., Zimmermann-Tansella, Ch., and Tansella, M. (1986) 'South-Verona's psychiatric service: an integrated system of community care', *Hospital and Community Psychiatry* 37: 809–13.

Burvill, P.W. (1978) 'Evaluation of psychiatric services', *Australian and New Zealand Journal of Psychiatry* 12: 189–95.

Cardin, V.A., McGill, C.W., and Falloon, I.R.H. (1985) 'Economic analysis: costs, benefits and effectiveness', in I.R.H. Falloon, C.W. McGill and J.L. Boyd (eds) *Family Management of Schizophrenia. A Study of Clinical Social, Family, and Economic Benefits*, Baltimore: Johns Hopkins University Press.

Carse, J., Panton, N.E., and Watt, A. (1958) 'A district mental health service: the Worthing experiment', *Lancet* 1: 39–41.

Cooper, B. and Morgan, H.G. (1973) *Epidemiological Psychiatry*, Springfield: Thomas.

Coursey, R.D. (1977) 'Introduction: the need, history, definition, and limits of program evaluation', in R.D. Coursey, G.A. Specter, S.A. Murrell, and B. Hunt (eds) *Program Evaluation for Mental Health: Methods, Strategies, and Participants*, New York: Grune & Stratton.

Coursey, R.D., Specter, G.A., Murrell, S.A., and Hunt, B. (eds) (1977) *Program Evaluation for Mental Health: Methods, Strategies, and Participants*, New York: Grune & Stratton.

Cullberg, J. and Stefansson, C.G. (1981) *An Evaluation of the Nacka Project*, Stockholm: Spri Publications.

Cullberg, J., Stefansson, C.G., and Wennersten, E. (1981) 'Psychiatry in young low status dwelling areas', *Psychiatry and Social Science* 1: 117–23.

De Plato, G. and Minguzzi, G. (1981) 'A short history of psychiatric renewal in Italy', *Psychiatry and Social Science* 1: 71–7.

European Economic Community (1981) *Evaluation and Mental Health Care: Third European Seminar on Health Policy*, Brussels: Report EUR 7172.

Faccincani, C., Mignolli, G. and Munk-Jørgensen, P. (1987) 'Hospital admission as first contact with a community-based psychiatric service: a two-year study in South-Verona', *European Archives of Psychiatry and Neurological Sciences* 236: 247–50.

Feldman, S. and Windle, W. (1973) 'The N.I.M.H. approach to evaluating the community mental health centers program', *Health Services Report* 88: 174–99.

Fenton, F.R., Tessier, L., Contradiopoulos, A., Nguyen, H., and Struening, E.L. (1972) 'A comparative trial of home and hospital psychiatric treatment: financial costs', *Canadian Journal of Psychiatry* 27: 177–87.

Frank, R. (1981) 'Cost-benefit analysis in mental health services: a review of the literature', *Administration in Mental Health* 8: 161–76.

Fryers, T. and Wooff, K. (1985) 'Il controllo di servizi di salute mentale in una citta inglese', in M. Tansella (ed.) *L'Approccio Epidemiologico in Psichiatria*, Torino: Boringhieri.

Gibbons, J., Jennings, C., and Wing, J.K. (1984) *Psychiatric Care in Eight Register Areas*, copies obtainable from Southampton Case Register, Knowle Hospital, Fareham, PO17 5NA.

Glass, N.J. and Goldberg, D. (1977) 'Cost benefit analysis and the evaluation of psychiatric services', *Psychological Medicine* 7: 701–7.

Grad, J. and Sainsbury, P. (1966) 'Evaluating the community psychiatric service in Chichester: results', in E.M. Gruenberg (ed.) *Evaluating the Effectiveness of Mental Health Services*, New York: Milbank Memorial Fund.

Gruenberg, E.M. (ed.) (1966) *Evaluating the Effectiveness of Mental Health Services*, New York: Milbank Memorial Fund.

Guttentag, M. and Struening, E.P. (eds) (1975) *Handbook of Evaluation Research: Volume 2*, Beverley Hills: Sage.

Häfner, H. and Klug, J. (1982) 'The impact of an expanding community mental health service on patterns of bed usage: evaluation of a four-year period of implementation', *Psychological Medicine* 12, 177–90.

Hoult, J. (1986) 'Community care of the acutely mentally ill', *British Journal of Psychiatry* 149: 137–44.

Hoult, J., Reynolds, I., Charbonneau-Powis, M., Weekes, P., and Briggs, J. (1983) 'Psychiatric hospital versus community treatment: the results of a randomised trial', *Australian and New Zealand Journal of Medicine* 17: 160–7.

Hunt, R.C., Gruenberg, E.M., Hacken, E., and Huxley, M. (1961) 'A comprehensive hospital-community service in a state hospital', *American Journal of Psychiatry* 117: 817–21.

Istituto Centrale di Statistica (ISTAT) *Annuario Statistico Italiano*, 1979–1986 editions, Roma: ISTAT.

Jablensky, A. and Henderson, J. (1983) 'Report on a visit to the South-Verona community psychiatric service', WHO Assignment Report, Geneva and Copenhagen, WHO.

Kreitman, N. (1984) 'Operational research in a faltering economy', *Social Psychiatry* 19: 1–2.

Lesage, A.D. and Tansella, M. (1988) 'Migration of schizophrenic patients, non-psychotic patients and general population in a case register area', submitted for publication.

Lesage, A.D., Trapani, V., and Tansella, M. (1988) 'Excess mortality measured according to 3 methods: a study on a cohort of schizophrenic patients in the years following the Italian psychiatric reform', submitted for publication.

McGuire, T.G. and Weisbrod, B.A. (eds) (1981) *Economics and Mental Health*, Washington: US Government Printing Office.

Munk-Jørgensen, P. (1985) 'Cumulated need for psychiatric service as shown in a community psychiatric project', *Psychological Medicine* 15: 629–35.

Polak, P.R. (1978) 'A comprehensive system of alternatives to psychiatric hospitalization', in L.I. Stein and M.A. Test (eds) *Alternatives to Mental Hospital Treatment*, New York: Plenum Press.

Roemer, M.I. (1972) *Evaluation of Community Health Centres* (Public Health Papers, No. 48), Geneva: WHO.

Sartorius, N. (1982) 'Epidemiology and mental health policy', in M.O. Wagenfeld, P.V. Lemkan and B. Justice (eds) *Public Mental Health*, Beverly Hills: Sage.

Sartorius, N. and Harding, T.W. (1984) 'Issues in the evaluation of mental health care', in W.W. Holland (ed.) *Evaluation of Health Care*, Oxford: Oxford University Press.

Schulberg, H.C. (1977) 'Issues in the evaluation of community mental health programs', *Professional Psychology* 560–72.

Shepherd, M. (1987) 'Jean Starobinski', *Lancet* 6 April: 798.

Shepherd, M., Cooper, B., Brown, A.C., and Kalton, G.W. (1966) *Psychiatric Illness in General Practice*, London: Oxford University Press.

Stahler, G.J. and Tash, W.R. (eds) (1982) *Innovative Approaches in Mental Health Evaluation*, New York: Academic Press.

Stein, L.I. and Test, M.A. (1980) 'Alternative to mental hospital treatment: 1. Conceptual model, treatment program and clinical evaluation', *Archives of General Psychiatry* 37: 392–7.

Struening, E.L. and Guttentag, M. (1975) *Handbook of Evaluation Research*, California: Sage.

Sturt, E. (1983) 'Mortality in a cohort of long-term users of community psychiatric services', *Psychological Medicine* 13, 441–6.

Suchman, E.A. (1967) *Evaluation Research: Principles and Practice in Public Service and Social Action Programs*, New York: Russel Sage Foundation.

Tansella, M. (1985) 'Approccio epidemiologico e psichiatria italiana del dopo-riforma', in M. Tansella (ed.) *L'Approccio Epidemiologico in Psichiatria*, Torino: Boringhieri.

Tansella, M. (1986) 'Community psychiatry without mental hospitals: the Italian experience: a review', *Journal of the Royal Society of Medicine* 79: 664–9.

Tansella, M. and Williams, P. (1987) 'The Italian experience and its implications', *Psychological Medicine* 17: 283–9.

Tansella, M. and Zimmermann-Tansella, Ch. (1988) 'From mental hospitals to alternative community services', in J.G. Howells (ed.) *Modern Perspectives in Clinical Psychiatry*, New York: Brunner-Mazel (in press).

Tansella, M., Faccincani, C., Mignolli, G., Balestrieri, M., and Zimmermann-Tansella, Ch. (1985) 'Il registro psichiatrico di Verona-Sud: epidemiologia per la valutazione dei nuovi servizi territoriali', in M. Tansella (ed.) *L'Approccio Epidemiologico in Psichiatria*, Torino: Boringhieri.

Tansella, M., Micciolo, R., Balestrieri, M., and Gavioli, I. (1986a) 'High and long-term users of the mental health services: a case-register study in Italy', *Social Psychiatry* 21: 96–103.

Tansella, M., Williams, P., Balestrieri, M., Bellantuono, C., and Martini, N. (1986b) 'The management of affective disorders in the community', *Journal of Affective Disorders* 11: 73–9.

Tansella, M., De Salvia, D., and Williams, P. (1987) 'The Italian psychiatric reform: some quantitative evidence', *Social Psychiatry* 22: 37–48.

Tantam, D. (1985) 'Alternatives to psychiatric hospitalisation', *British Journal of Psychiatry* 146: 1–4.

Tombs, D.A. (1987) personal communication.

Weisbrod, B.A. (1982) 'A guide to benefit-cost analysis, as seen through a controlled experiment in treating the mentally ill', *Journal of Health Political Policy Law* 7: 808–45.

Weisbrod, B.A., Test, M.A., and Stein, L.I. (1980) 'Alternative to mental hospital treatment: II Economic benefit-cost analysis', *Archives of General Psychiatry* 37: 400–5.

Wilkinson, G. (1985) 'Community care: planning mental health services', *British Medical Journal* 290: 1371–3.

Wilkinson, G. and Pelosi, A.J. (1987) 'The economics of mental health services', *British Medical Journal* 294: 139–40.

Williams, P., De Salvia, D., and Tansella, M. (1986) 'Suicide, psychiatric reform, and the provision of psychiatric services in Italy', *Social Psychiatry* 21: 89–95.

Williams, P., Balestrieri, M., and Tansella, M. (1987a) 'Seasonal variation in affective disorders: a case register study', *Journal of Affective Disorders* 12: 145–52.

Williams, P., De Salvia, D., and Tansella, M. (1987b) 'Suicide and the Italian psychiatric reform: an appraisal of two data collection systems', *European Archives of Psychiatry and Neurological Sciences* 236: 237–40.

Williams, R.D. and Ozarin, L.D. (eds) (1968) *Community Mental Health*, San Francisco: Jossey-Bass.

Wing, J.K. (1972) 'Principles of evaluation', in J.K. Wing and A.M. Hailey (eds) *Evaluating a Community Psychiatric Service*, London: Oxford University Press.

Wing, J.K. (ed.) (1982) 'Long-term community care experience in a London borough', *Psychological Medicine*, Monograph supplement no. 2.

Wing, J.K. (1986) 'The cycle of planning and evaluation', in G. Wilkinson and H. Freeman (eds) *The Provision of Mental Health Services in Britain: The Way Ahead*, London: Gaskell.

Wing, J.K. and Fryers, T. (1976) *Psychiatric Services in Camberwell and Salford, 1964–1974*, Manchester: University Department of Community Medicine.

Wing, J.K. and Häfner, H. (eds) (1973) *Roots of Evaluation*, London: Oxford University Press.

Wing, J.K. and Hailey, A.M. (1972) *Evaluating a Community Psychiatric Service: The Camberwell Register 1964–71*, London: Oxford University Press.

Wing, J.K., Wing, L., and Hailey, A. (1970) 'The use of case registers for evaluating and planning psychiatric services', in J.K. Wing and E.R. Bransby (eds) *Psychiatric Case Registers*, London: HMSO.

World Health Organization (1971) *Trends in Psychiatric Care: Day Hospitals and Units in General Hospitals*, Copenhagen: WHO Regional Office for Europe.

Zimmermann-Tansella, Ch., Burti, L., Faccincani, C., Garzotto, N., Siciliani, O., and Tansella, M. (1985) 'Bringing into action the psychiatric reform in South-Verona: a five year experience', in C. Perris and D. Kemali (eds) *Focus on the Italian Psychiatric Reform* (Supplement of *Acta Psychiatrica Scandinavica*, No. 316), 71: 71–86, Copenhagen: Munksgaard.

26

The Psychiatry of General Practice

Deborah Sharp and David Morrell

In Great Britain, health care is organized in a two-tier system. Primary care is provided by National Health Service general practitioners who are effectively responsible for most of the referrals into the second tier – the hospitals, where the service is provided by consultants in the different specialities. Ninety-eight per cent of the population is registered with a general practitioner; 60–70 per cent of whom consult at least once each year and only about 10 per cent will not consult at all in any three-year period. Thus, the general practitioner can be regarded as a personal physician who has access to the medical history and social background of his patients and who, by virtue of the continuity of care he provides, not only for the patient but often for the whole family, is in an unique position to monitor psychosocial disorder in the community.

It is commonly believed that between one-quarter and one-third of all illnesses treated by general practitioners comprise some form of psychological disorder (Goldberg and Blackwell 1970; Goldberg and Bridges 1987). On average each patient consults his or her general practitioner between three and four times a year. Thus, with an average list size of 2,000, most general practitioners will be confronted with a large amount of psychiatric morbidity.

Table 26.1 compares general practitioner consultation rates for diagnosed psychiatric disorders with those for out-patient and day-patient attendances and rates of admissions to psychiatric institutions. Despite the shortcomings of the data available for general practice from the Third National Morbidity Study (1986), mainly on account of problems in the classification of mental illness and inter-practice variation, it can be seen that consultations for psychiatric disorder in general practice outnumber psychiatric out-patient attendances by nearly 7:1.

In 1973 a WHO working party on psychiatry in general practice (WHO 1973) identified the general practitioner as playing a major role in mental health care. They argued that: 1) patients with psychosocial problems are high users of medical care and thus are well known to primary care physicians who may utilize this relationship for psychotherapeutic intervention;

404

Table 26.1 Comparative rates of attendance for different levels of psychiatric care (rates per 100,000 general population, all ages and sexes combined, in 1981)

	General practitioner consultations*	Out-patients attendances +	Day hospital attendances +	Psychiatric admissions +
ICD-9 290–315 Mental Disorders	22,980	3,532	4,943	397

* Obtained from *Morbidity Statistics from General Practice* 1981–1982, Third National Study, RCGP, OPCS, DHSS.
+ Obtained from *Mental Health Enquiry for England*, 1981

2) patients with emotional disorders experience less stigma when treated by a primary care physician than by a psychiatrist; 3) physical and psychiatric complaints tend to co-occur and are often difficult to separate in diagnosis and treatment, which makes the non-psychiatrist, who is more able to treat the 'whole' person, the first choice as physician; 4) primary care physicians are best placed to provide long-term follow up and be available for successive episodes of illness.

IDENTIFICATION OF PSYCHIATRIC DISORDER IN GENERAL PRACTICE

The study of psychiatric disorder in general practice has received increasing interest in the last two decades (Clare and Lader 1982; Shepherd *et al.* 1986). The starting point for much of this work was the study by Shepherd and his colleagues at the Institute of Psychiatry over twenty years ago (Shepherd *et al.* 1966). They studied a one in eight sample of patients attending forty-six general practices in London for a period of one year. Of the 15,000 patients at risk, approximately 14 per cent consulted their doctor at least once for a condition diagnosed as entirely or largely psychiatric in nature. More than half of these conditions had been present for at least one year. However, less than one in twenty of these patients were known to have received specialist psychiatric care during the survey year. Doctors varied greatly in their estimates of psychiatric morbidity, reporting rates between 3.7 per cent and 65 per cent.

The arrival of psychiatric screening questionnaires linked to standardized psychiatric interviews has meant that it is now possible to make estimates of the prevalence of psychiatric illness in general practice that are independent of the varying abilities of general practitioners in making such assessments. The General Health Questionnaire (GHQ) (Goldberg 1972) has been used in

405

several studies which aimed to estimate the prevalence of psychiatric morbidity in general practice. This instrument is designed to identify non-psychotic psychiatric ill health in the community and was originally constructed to function as a first-stage screening tool in studies where the Clinical Interview Schedule (CIS) (Goldberg et al. 1970) was to be used to provide a standardized approach to confirming or denying the presence of psychiatric morbidity.

In order to try and quantify the disparity between the true prevalence of psychiatric morbidity in general practice and that identified by the general practitioner, Goldberg and Blackwell (1970) used the GHQ to screen for probable 'caseness' in 200 patients who were also assessed by psychiatrist, using the CIS. The 'conspicuous psychiatric morbidity', as assessed by the general practitioner and validated by the psychiatrist, was calculated to be 20 per cent and 'hidden psychiatric morbidity' accounted for one-third of all disturbed patients. They found that those patients with 'hidden psychiatric morbidity' were more likely to present their illness in somatic terms but that their illnesses were no less severe in terms of prognosis. Similar findings were reported by Skuse and Williams (1984) where the general practitioner regarded 24 per cent of a sample of consecutive attenders as 'psychiatric cases' and the true prevalence as assessed by the CIS was found to be 34 per cent.

The detection of psychiatric morbidity by primary care physicians has an important influence on the amount and type of disorder that is subsequently cared for in the mental health sector. Goldberg and Huxley (1980) have constructed a hierarchical model of levels and filters to describe the nature of psychiatric disorder in the community and how this is reflected in the organization of care (see figure 26.1). Level 1 refers to all psychological disorders in the community, a large proportion of which pass through filter 1 into level 2 when the patient decides to consult the general practitioner. However, a great deal of this psychological morbidity is not recognized by general practitioners, so these people do not pass through filter 2. Level 3 is therefore the 'conspicuous psychological morbidity' most of which will be treated by the general practitioner. A proportion will however be referred to the specialist mental health services, i.e., pass through filter 3 into level 4. An even smaller proportion will require admission to hospital, i.e., pass through filter 4 into level 5.

The large between-general practitioner variation in detecting psychiatric morbidity has already been mentioned. Filter 2, that separating the hidden and conspicuous psychiatric morbidity, allows about 60 per cent of morbidity through into level 3, and represents the doctor's ability to detect psychiatric disorder. Passage through this filter is affected by characteristics of both the patient and the doctor. Two particular aspects of the doctor's ability to detect these disorders are thought to be important. The first is bias – the tendency of a general practitioner to over- or under-identify psychiatric disorder. This

Figure 26.1 Goldberg and Huxley's model

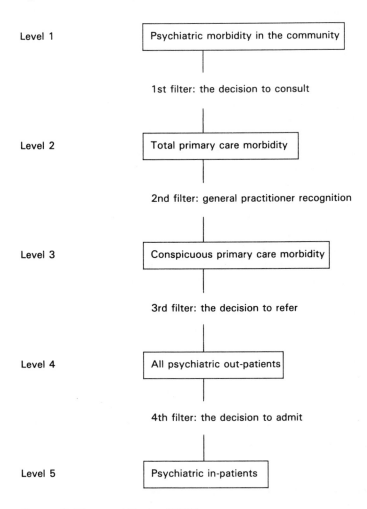

Level 1 — Psychiatric morbidity in the community

1st filter: the decision to consult

Level 2 — Total primary care morbidity

2nd filter: general practitioner recognition

Level 3 — Conspicuous primary care morbidity

3rd filter: the decision to refer

Level 4 — All psychiatric out-patients

4th filter: the decision to admit

Level 5 — Psychiatric in-patients

Source: Goldberg and Huxley (1980).

is thought to be determined by factors such as personality, attitudes, training, and experience. The second is accuracy, which is the degree to which the general practitioner is correct in his assessment.

Marks *et al.* (1979) studied in detail some of the factors associated with general practitioners' ability to detect psychiatric morbidity. They suggested that the most important factor is the ability of the general practitioner to conduct a simple mental state examination in an empathic manner, together with an understanding of the association of psychiatric morbidity with social dysfunctioning. It appears that some aspects of the doctors' behaviour in the consultation can be modified so as to increase their accuracy. Replicating this British study with a study of family practice residents in the USA, Goldberg *et al.* (1980) showed that videotape feedback training can improve the accuracy with which they rated psychiatric disturbance (using an agreement coefficient, kappa, between their ratings and patients' symptom levels as reported on the GHQ). He also found that doctors who were self-confident and outgoing with high academic ability in general made more accurate assessments. More recently a further replication study has been undertaken in South London (Boardman 1987). While the GHQ results were similar in both studies, the general practice estimates of morbidity were much lower in this latest study, reinforcing the need for further training of general practitioners in psychiatric case detection.

The self-report questionnaires constructed originally for screening purposes may also have a role in improving the recognition of psychiatric morbidity by general practitioners. In a study to assess the efficacy of the GHQ in the secondary prevention of minor psychiatric illness in general practice (Johnstone and Goldberg 1976), patients with hidden psychiatric morbidity were randomly assigned to treated and control groups. The effects of case detection and treatment were beneficial – patients were more likely to get better quickly and have fewer symptoms at follow-up. In addition, identification of psychiatric disorder altered consulting behaviour, with patients in the treated group increasing their consultations for emotional complaints at the expense of consultations for physical symptoms during the follow-up year.

Wright and Perini (1987) suggested that the GHQ may be a useful clinical tool if the cut-off point is raised above that recommended for epidemiological research, i.e., increasing specificity at the expense of sensitivity. They found it particularly useful in patients with physical symptoms not conforming to any recognizable clinical pattern and in patients who had chronic physical illness or were frequent attenders. More recently, studies in the USA using the GHQ (Rand *et al.* 1987) and the Zung Self-rating Depression Scale (Zung and Magruder-Habib 1987) have also shown that feedback of screening results to general practitioners improves recognition of psychiatric morbidity.

It has been proposed that there are two types of clinical decision: the 'diagnostic decision' and the 'management decision' (Howie 1972). The relationship between diagnosis and treatment in psychiatry is not necessarily a strong one and this is particularly true in the general practice setting. Furthermore, while a psychiatric diagnosis may be only relatively infrequently recorded by a general practitioner, the record of the 'reason for visit', the prescribing of psychotropic drugs or the provision of psychotherapy suggest that recognition of 'distress' may be much more common but is not diagnosable in current terminology.

What are the characteristics of these patients with neurotic disorders, mainly anxiety and depression, that will enable a general practitioner to make a psychiatric diagnosis and is it necessary to make such a diagnosis before management can be considered? Indeed, does making a diagnosis really determine what is to be done and by whom?

As described by Eastwood elsewhere in this volume, many studies have found that psychiatric morbidity is often associated with physical complaints. It is widely believed by patients that doctors expect to hear about physical symptoms. In addition, it is still more socially acceptable to have a physical illness than a psychiatric one. Thus, depressed patients may well present a physical symptom to their general practitioner rather than their psychological symptoms. But this may also occur because a depressed patient is often more introspective than usual and will be more aware of their general bodily functions. Thus, a physical symptom which has been present for some time may appear worse in a period of emotional distress and thus will be presented as their main complaint to the doctor. On the other hand, depression may occur as a consequence of a physical illness or symptom and, while it is appropriate to offer the physical illness to the general practitioner, the onus is on the general practitioner to be aware of the likely psychological consequences of a serious or chronic physical illness. In addition, there appears to be a real association of physical illness with psychiatric illness. This was noted by Shepherd *et al.* (1966) and investigated further by Eastwood and Trevelyan (1972), and is discussed by Eastwood elsewhere in this volume.

Another group of patients in general practice who frequently suffer from psychological disorders are those who are subject to acute life events or chronic social stresses. Although there are individual and biological differences in the extent to which people are vulnerable to mental illness, many studies support the notion that adverse social circumstances are also aetiologically important (Cooper 1972). These social factors may, in addition, determine what sort of symptoms a patient develops and what 'treatment' he seeks. Social factors may also be relevant in the development or relapse of illnesses such as schizophrenia.

Stressful life events, often masquerading as an acute minor physical ailment or the exacerbation of a chronic symptom, are frequently the cause of depression in general practice patients (Cooper and Sylph 1973). Brown and Harris (1978), in a study of women in the community, found that working-class women were more prone to depression, in part due to an increased incidence of adverse life events.

Chronic social difficulties such as financial hardship, social isolation, and lower social class have also been shown to be associated with an increased prevalence of mental illness. When consultation rates are examined, those patients who consult their general practitioners and are found to have minor psychiatric morbidity more frequently tend to be women, often separated or divorced, of lower social class, who are unemployed with consequent housing and financial difficulties. The question as to whether women do actually experience more psychiatric ill health than men or whether they are just more likely to consult their general practitioner (Shepherd *et al.* 1966), and whether the general practitioner is more likely to detect psychiatric illness in women (Marks *et al.* 1979), has not been definitively answered. It would seem that women, especially if separated or divorced, with a family to bring up and without employment, are likely to be socially isolated and, thus lacking social support, are vulnerable to psychiatric illness (Henderson 1981). However, a recent study of a relatively homogeneous sample of British civil servants showed that there was no sex difference in the prevalence of minor psychiatric morbidity between these men and women of similar age, education, occupation, and social environment. The women did, however, report more somatic symptoms of psychogenic origin (Jenkins 1985). A survey of general practice attenders in Dundee (Ballinger *et al.* 1985; Hobbs *et al.* 1985) showed that psychiatric disturbance as assessed by GHQ score was more likely in men in association with ill health, unemployment, lower social class, poverty, being divorced or having a poor marital relationship, or having a wife who was ill or had a psychiatric history. Women were more likely to have a high GHQ score in the presence of poor personal relationships, having three or more children, low social class, and gynaecological symptoms. It is now generally accepted that depression and anxiety brought on by social stress are just as real and legitimate as those not so associated and as such merit attention and possibly treatment by general practitioners.

The conclusion from most of these studies is that a patient's 'life situation' is very likely to affect both their physical and their psychological functioning. A plethora of self-report questionnaires and interview schedules are now available to help the general practitioner assess social stresses – the Social Assessment Schedule (Clare and Cairns 1978), the Interview Schedule for Social Interaction (Henderson 1981) and the Social Support and Stress Interview (Jenkins *et al.* 1981) are all well validated instruments which could be used in the primary care setting to improve information gathering with a view to increasing the recognition of psychiatric disorder. Certain illnesses such as post-natal depression may be more specifically enquired for. The Edinburgh Postnatal Depression Scale (Cox *et al.* 1987) is a validated, ten-item self-report questionnaire which reliably predicts depression in post-partum women. Quick and simple to use, such questionnaires may help general practitioners, who are often short of time, in getting to the root of the problem more quickly.

DIAGNOSIS OF PSYCHIATRIC ILLNESS IN GENERAL PRACTICE

Psychiatric disorder, like most illness, behaves as a continuously distributed variable and a valid question from the general practitioner might therefore be 'how much of it is present?' In psychiatry there is an even more fundamental

410

question – deciding what 'it', the disorder – actually is. The general practice setting further compounds the problem of psychiatric case definition – there is a high incidence of transient morbidity and the illness is often seen in its very early stages, before the full clinical picture has developed. For these reasons, in particular, the classifications of psychiatric disorder in current use are quite inappropriate for primary care, i.e., the Diagnostic and Statistical Manual of Mental Disorders, Third Edition (DSM-III), the International Classification of Disease, Ninth Edition (ICD-9), as well as the International Classification of Health Problems in Primary Care, Second Edition (ICHPPC-2). This latter system was in fact devised by and for general practitioners who recognized that the ICD did not provide satisfactory diagnostic labels for many of the problems seen in primary care.

For example, in ICD-9, the emotional disorders which occur at the level of primary care are classified not only in chapter V, 'Mental Illness', but also in chapter XVI, 'Symptoms, signs and ill defined conditions', and chapter XVIII, 'Supplementary classification of factors influencing health status and contact with health services' – known as the 'V' code. That there is an 'a priori' need to change from the ICD system, which is based on a mixture of symptomatology and aetiology, to a multi-axial system which would take into account a patient's personality and social status as well as symptom state was the conclusion of a study of outcome of neurotic illness in general practice (Mann et al. 1981). They found that apart from the initial severity of psychiatric morbidity, the quality of social life at the time of follow-up was the only other factor to predict psychiatric state after one year. A study of the classification of mental ill health in general practice was undertaken in order to underline the need for a new system of classification appropriate to primary care (Jenkins et al. 1985). They invited twenty-seven experienced general practitioners to watch videotaped real-life consultations and to record their diagnoses, using both ICD-9 and ICHPPC-2. They found a very high degree of inter-observer variation, with ICHPPC-2 performing no better than ICD-9.

When rates of diagnosis for general practice from the Third National Morbidity Survey are compared with in-patient statistics from the Mental Health Enquiry for England (1981/2), the rates for neuroses and psychoses are reversed. Thus it appears that not only are general practitioners seeing the majority of psychiatric morbidity in the population, but what they see, the psychoneuroses, is quite different from what the psychiatrist, who deals mainly with the psychoses, dementia, personality disorders, mental retardation, alcoholism, and drug addiction, sees. But at what point does a set of complaints become serious enough to be considered epidemiologically, sociologically, or clinically significant? The criterion of 'caseness' has been greatly enhanced by the availability of structured psychiatric interviews and diagnostic instruments such as the Present State Examination (PSE) (Wing et al. 1974) and the Research Diagnostic Criteria (RDC) (Spitzer et al. 1978).

However, there is evidence to suggest that such diagnostic criteria derived from and for patients seen in specialist psychiatric practice may incorporate threshold levels which are inappropriate for non-specialist settings.

There will of course always be a 'hard core' of patients who have a definable mental illness classifiable by any diagnostic schema and for whom medical treatment is of proven value. At the other end of the spectrum are those patients who do not really have a psychiatric illness as such at all, although they may well exhibit illness behaviour or be complaining of psychological symptoms. These patients either have too few symptoms for a formal 'syndrome' diagnosis to be made or their symptoms are transient and self-limiting, perhaps temporarily related to some external happening such as an 'anniversary'. Also in this group are patients whose symptoms are long standing, related to a 'life situation' and whose distress is understood by the doctor but not considered by either to require 'treatment'.

Patients with minor affective disorders, mainly depression with or without anxiety, form the largest group requiring treatment in primary care, although most of these cases would only be identified at the minimum threshold level on instruments such as the PSE.

Studies of diagnosis of psychiatric disorder in primary care have concentrated largely on depressive disorders. One by general practitioners in South West London (Sireling et al. 1985; Freeling et al. 1985) reported on three groups of depressed patients – those prescribed antidepressants, those given other treatment, and those missed by the general practitioner. The majority of patients qualified as psychiatric cases on the PSE Index of Definition, with those given other treatment most often failing to meet diagnostic criteria. The patients with unrecognized depression were less obviously depressed, more likely to have a concurrent physical illness, and their illness had lasted longer.

A review by Blacker and Clare (1987) addresses the issue in some detail. They conclude that the traditional notion that general practice depression is mild, self-limiting, and clinically unimportant is mistaken, and that, apart from the consequences of non-diagnosis for the patient, untreated patients also impose an increased burden on the primary care service.

MANAGEMENT OF PSYCHIATRIC DISORDER IN GENERAL PRACTICE

When faced with a patient in whom he identifies psychological symptoms, the general practitioner has a variety of treatment options open to him. The first decision to make may well be whether the patient requires any treatment at all. Sharing and understanding a transient situational disturbance or acknowledgement of a chronic life stress may be all that is required or the general practitioner may decide that he can treat the patient himself with drugs and/or some form of 'listening treatment'. This may be supplemented by simple guidance and advice, supportive non-directive counselling or psychotherapy. The doctor as the 'drug' is a concept developed by Michael Balint in the 1950s who adapted psychoanalytically based psychotherapy to meet the needs and realities of general practice (Balint 1957). Balint's views have wielded considerable influence, particularly among those doctors who have been able to attend training seminars based on his methods. These 'entail a limited, though considerable change in the doctor's personality' (Balint 1957). They have, however, also been criticized for not being appropriate in the primary care setting (Sowerby 1977; Madden 1979), particularly on the grounds of the time it requires both in the consultation and in supervision. An adaptation of the Balint technique to the 'six minute' consultation is the flash technique (Balint and Morrell 1973), whereby the doctor helps the patient develop insight into the meaning of his symptoms within the constraints of normal practice. Balint never intended to convert general practitioners into psychoanalysts, but all general practitioners should be able to provide supportive intervention for their patients when required. One of the most commonly employed treatments for psychiatric disorder in general practice is the prescription of a psychotropic drug. Trends in psychotropic drug prescription and factors which relate to the prescription and consumption of psychotropic drugs are described in the chapter by Williams and Gabe.

Attempts have also been made to identify the characteristics of general practitioners which might account for their prescribing behaviour. A study by Raynes (1979) aimed to test some of Howie's hypotheses on decision-making (Howie 1972). She compared the consultation process leading to the prescription of a psychotropic or an antibiotic and found that the focus of both patient and doctor on physical, social, and emotional issues was the commonest characteristic in consultations where a psychotropic was prescribed. To encourage an alternative approach to the treatment of minor affective disorder, patients selected by their general practitioners as suitable for anxiolytic medication were randomly divided into a drug group and a counselling group (Catalan et al. 1984). Similar improvements were found in both groups on measures of psychiatric symptoms and social functioning at follow-up one month and seven months later. This study has, in conjunction with the government restrictions on the prescribing of benzodiazepines, been instrumental in dissuading general practitioners from relying solely on pharmacotherapy in the treatment of minor affective disorders.

A second option open to the general practitioner is to involve other members of the 'multi-disciplinary primary health care team' in management – this may include social workers, counsellors, psychologists, or community psychiatric nurses.

These different professionals bring with them a variety of skills with which to approach the patient suffering from a psychiatric illness. Social workers and general practitioners have historically tended to work quite

413

separately, although both are the responsibility of the same government department. The Seebohm Committee (1968) recommended greater liaison between the two professions and accordingly a social work attachment scheme was set up in South London and was the subject of several observational and experimental studies. Corney and Briscoe (1977) showed that general practitioners referred different patients to attached social workers when they became aware of the social workers' skill in dealing with social and emotional problems. Furthermore, it appears that clients referred to attached social workers, rather than an area team, present more emotional problems and spend more time with the social worker (Corney and Bowen 1980). Referral to social workers also seems to have beneficial effects in that patients with depression improve more when they have help from a social worker compared with only seeing their general practitioner (Cooper 1972; Corney 1981). The advantages and disadvantages of closer collaboration between general practitioner and social workers have been extensively reviewed (Clare and Corney 1982).

Recently, an increasing number of clinical psychologists have developed links with general practice and, instead of receiving referrals in the hospital, are beginning to see patients in the community and developing attachment schemes similar to those of social workers. The advantages of a primary-care-based clinical psychology service are reviewed by Johnston (1978) and include access to psychological help for patients who would not otherwise receive it owing to problems associated with travel, work, stigma, and the type of presenting complaint, such as agoraphobia. Increased communication between general practitioner and therapist, more flexible and relevant therapy, and seeing the patient in their own setting are also advantageous. Two studies (Ives 1979; Koch 1979) have reported that patients seeing a psychologist in the general practice make fewer visits to the surgery and are prescribed fewer psychotropic drugs in the months after treatment and that those changes are maintained one year later. About 27 per cent of psychology posts in England now include some involvement with general practice (Hall et al. 1986). The sorts of problems most often referred are phobias, anxiety states, panic attacks, habit disorders, and interpersonal, social, and marital problems. The methods used by psychologists are predominantly those of behaviour therapy, cognitive therapy (Teasdale et al. 1984), and supportive psychotherapy. There is currently some discussion about the types of assessment which have been used in determining the benefits of psychological treatment to patients (Trepka and Griffiths 1987). They suggest that rather than assessing the global effects of treatment, a more differentiated approach to evaluation is required to fully assess the effectiveness of clinical psychologists in primary care.

Some of these treatment options are equally well carried out with nurse therapists. A study by Marks (1985) showed that patients who had phobic or obsessive/compulsive symptoms and received behavioural psychotherapy from a community psychiatric nurse reported significantly greater benefit compared with patients who had routine treatment from a general practitioner. The patients seemed to prefer treatment in the primary care setting rather than in the hospital and the placing of nurse therapists in this setting may also save on health care resources. A study reporting a similar role for psychiatric nurses in the community found that neurotic patients who had been attending the psychiatric hospital were cared for equally well when nurses provided supportive home visits (Paykel *et al.* 1982). Social workers, psychologists, and community psychiatric nurses, despite having somewhat different backgrounds, all have certain therapeutic skills which make them the ideal people to treat the neurotic disorders so common in primary care, many of which respond to behaviour therapy (Gelder 1979).

Counsellors are not quite so specialized in their role. Their attachment to primary care teams is also on the increase and their value lies mainly in providing supportive 'psychotherapy' for those patients who are distressed by social, marital, and interpersonal problems. The effectiveness of some of these specialist mental health treatments in general practice is reviewed in a meta-analysis by Balestrieri *et al.* (1988). The third option open to the general practitioner is to refer the patient for a specialist psychiatric opinion. As was pointed out earlier, the number of new patients seen each year in psychiatric out-patient clinics represents somewhat less than 10 per cent of the total psychiatric morbidity recognized by general practitioners. Referred patients are not a random sample of the conspicuous psychiatric morbidity. Filter 3 (figure 26.1) is 'selectively permeable' to younger people, men, the more severely ill, and the psychotic.

Brook (1978) suggested four main motives behind general practitioners' referrals:

1) to obtain an expert opinion so that he can then continue treatment himself;
2) to arrange specialist treatment that he cannot provide himself;
3) to share the burden of a patient for whom little can be done;
4) to be relieved of the patient for a while.

An important move in the last few years has been the delivery of psychiatric care by psychiatrists consulting in general practices. A recent survey showed that one in five consultant psychiatrists now spend some time in general practice settings (Strathdee and Williams 1984). They describe three different models of working – the consultation model, the shifted out-patient model, and the liaison attachment team model. Although there are some logistic problems in getting both sides together, with increasing acceptance of the psychiatrist by the primary care team, the benefits of liaison psychiatry appear to outweigh the costs (Mitchell 1985; Tyrer 1986).

CONCLUSION

Much of the research on psychiatric disorders in the primary care setting has, over the last two decades, been carried out by psychiatrists rather than by general practitioners themselves. This is not surprising in that this has been a period in which investigative methods have been slowly evolving, resulting in a variety of questionnaires and scales which have been validated and are now accessible to those without specialist training who wish to work in this field. In addition, the enormous problems described in this chapter are concerned with effective labelling of psychiatric disorders and have deterred all but the most reckless or the very brave. Finally, the level of basic training in psychology and psychiatry which has characterized undergraduate medical training until recent years has not ensured the production of a cadre of general practitioners with the necessary interest or skills to develop research.

Hopefully, the situation is changing with improvements in medical education and with the closer communication between general practitioners and psychiatrists inherent in many of the experimental situations in which psychiatrists are now conducting clinical work in general practice. Imaginative training fellowships for general practitioners wishing to develop research skills in psychiatry, and introduced three years ago by the Mental Health Foundation, have pointed the way to developments in this field. They will hopefully be copied by the Department of Health whose financial concerns with mental illness must surely make them cognizant of the need for research in this field.

Much of the early work has been concerned with identifying and quantifying mental ill health in the community. There is now a growing need for the evaluation of the outcome of different modes of management and for what will undoubtedly be the most challenging task, the prevention of mental illness.

Acknowledgement: Deborah Sharp is supported by the Mental Health Foundation.

REFERENCES

American Psychiatric Association (1980) *Diagnostic and Statistical Manual of Mental Disorders*, third edition (DSM-III), Washington, DC: AMA.
Balestrieri, M., Williams, P. and Wilkinson, G. (1988) 'How effective is specialist mental health treatment in general practice?', *Psychological Medicine* (in press).
Balint, M. (1957) *The Doctor, his Patient and the Illness*, London: Pitman Medical.
Balint, E. and Norrell, J.S. (1973) *Six Minutes for the Patient: Interactions in General Practice Consultation*, London: Tavistock.

Ballinger, C.B., Smith, A.H.W. and Hobbs, P.R. (1985) 'Factors associated with psychiatric morbidity in women – a general practice survey', *Acta Psychiatrica Scandinavica* 71: 272–80.

Boardman, A.P. (1987) 'The General Health Questionnaire and the Detection of Emotional Disorder by General Practitioners: A replicated study', *British Journal of Psychiatry* 165: 373–81.

Blacker, C.V.R. and Clare, A.W. (1987) 'Depressive disorder in primary care', *British Journal of Psychiatry* 150: 737–51.

Brook, A. (1978) 'An aspect of community mental health – consultative work with general practice teams', *Health Trends*, 10: 37–9.

Brown, G.W. and Harris, T. (1978) *Social Origins of Depression: a Study of Psychiatric Disorder in Women*, London: Tavistock.

Catalan, J., Gath, D., Edmonds, G. and Ennis, J. (1984) 'The effects of non-prescribing of Anxiolytics in General Practice I. Controlled evaluation of psychiatric and social outcome', *British Journal of Psychiatry* 144: 593–602.

Clare, A.W. and Cairns, V.E. (1978) 'Design, development and use of a standardized interview to assess social maladjustment and dysfunction in community studies', *Psychological Medicine* 8: 589–605.

Clare, A.W. and Corney, R.H. (1982) *Social Work and Primary Health Care*, London: Academic Press.

Clare, A.W. and Lader, M. (eds) (1982) *Psychiatry and General Practice*, London: Academic Press.

Cooper, B. (1972) 'Clinical and social aspects of chronic neurosis', *Proceedings of Royal Society of Medicine* 65: 509–12.

Cooper, B. and Sylph, J. (1973) 'Life events and the onset of neurotic illness: an investigation in general practice', *Psychological Medicine* 3: 421–35.

Corney, R.H. (1981) 'Social work effectiveness in the management of depressed Women', *Psychological Medicine* 11: 417–23.

Corney, R.H. and Bowen, B.A. (1980) Referrals to social workers: a comparative study of a local authority intake team with a general practice attachment team. *Journal of the Royal College of General Practitioners* 30: 139–47.

Corney, R.H. and Briscoe, M.E. (1977) 'Social workers and their clients: a comparison between primary health care and local authority settings', *Journal of the Royal College of General Practitioners* 27: 295–301.

Cox, J.L., Holden, J.M. and Sagovsky, R. (1987) 'Detection of postnatal depression. Development of 10–item postnatal depression scale', *British Journal of Psychiatry* 150: 782–6.

Eastwood, M.R. and Trevelyan, M.H. (1972) 'Relationship between physical and psychiatric disorder', *Psychological Medicine* 2: 363–72.

Freeling, P., Rao, B.M., Paykel, E.S., Sireling, L.I. and Burton, R.H. (1985) 'Unrecognised depression in general practice', *British Medical Journal* 290: 1880–3.

Gelder, M.G. (1979) 'Behavioural treatment for psychiatric disorders in general practice: preliminary communication', *Journal of the Royal Society of Medicine* 72: 421–4.

Goldberg, D.P. (1972) *The Detection of Psychiatric Illness by Questionnaire*, (Maudsley Monograph No. 21), London: Oxford University Press.

Goldberg, D.P. and Blackwell, B. (1970) 'Psychiatric illness in general practice: a detailed study using a new method of case identification', *British Medical Journal* ii: 439–43.

Goldberg, D.P. and Bridges, K. (1987) 'Screening for psychiatric illness in general practice: the general practitioner versus the screening questionnaire', *Journal of the Royal College of General Practitioners* 37: 15–18.

417

Goldberg, D.P., Cooper, B., Eastwood, M.R., Kedward, H.B. and Shepherd, M. (1970) 'A standardised psychiatric interview for use in community surveys', *British Journal of Social and Preventative Medicine* 24: 18–23.

Goldberg, D.P. and Huxley, P. (1980) *Mental Illness in the Community: the Pathway to Psychiatric Care*, London: Tavistock.

Goldberg, D.P., Steele, J.J., Smith, C. and Spivey, L. (1980) 'Training family doctors to recognise psychiatric illness with increased accuracy', *Lancet* ii: 521–3.

Hall, J., Koch, H., Pilling, S. and Winter, K. (1986) 'Health Services information and clinical psychology', *Bulletin of British Psychological Society* 39: 126–30.

Henderson, S. (1981) 'Social relationships, adversity and neurosis: an analysis of prospective observations', *British Journal of Psychiatry* 138: 391–8.

Hobbs, P.R., Ballinger, C.B., McClure, A., Martin, B. and Greenwood, C. (1985) 'Factors associated with psychiatric morbidity in men – a general practice survey', *Acta Psychiatra Scandinavica* 71: 281–6.

Howie, J.G.R. (1972) 'Diagnosis – The Achilles Heel?' *Journal of the Royal College of General Practitioners* 22: 310–15.

Ives, G. (1979) 'Psychological treatment in general practice', *Journal of the Royal College of General Practitioners* 29: 343–51.

Jenkins, R. (1985) 'Sex differences in minor psychiatric morbidity: a survey of a homogeneous population', *Social Science and Medicine* 20: 887–9.

Jenkins, R., Mann, A.H. and Belsey, M. (1981) 'Design and use of a short interview to assess social stress and support in research and clinical settings', *Social Science and Medicine* 3: 195–203.

Jenkins, R., Smeeton, N., Marinker, M. and Shepherd, M. (1985) 'A study of the classification of mental ill health in general practice', *Psychological Medicine* 15: 403–9.

Johnston, M. (1978) 'The work of a clinical psychologist in primary care', *Journal of the Royal College of General Practitioners* 28: 661–7.

Johnstone, A. and Goldberg, D. (1976) 'Psychiatric screening in general practice: a controlled trial', *Lancet* i: 605–8.

Koch, H.C.H. (1979) 'Evaluation of behaviour therapy intervention in general practice', *Journal of the Royal College of General Practitioners* 29: 337–40.

Madden, T.A. (1979) 'The doctors, their patients and their care: Balint reassessed', *Psychological Medicine* 9: 5–8.

Mann, A.H., Jenkins, R. and Belsey, E. (1981) 'The twelve month outcome of patients with neurotic illness in general practice', *Psychological Medicine* 11: 535–50.

Marks, I. (1985) 'Controlled trial of psychiatric nurse therapists in primary care', *British Medical Journal* 290: 1181–4.

Marks, J.N., Goldberg, D.P. and Hillier, V.F. (1979) 'Determinants of the ability of general practitioners to detect psychiatric illness', *Psychological Medicine* 9: 337–53.

Mitchell, A.R.K. (1985) 'Psychiatrists in primary health care settings', *British Journal of Psychiatry* 147: 371–9.

Paykel, E.S., Mangen, S.P., Griffith, J.H. and Burns, T.P. (1982) 'Community psychiatric nursing for neurotic patients: a controlled trial', *British Journal of Psychiatry* 140: 573–81.

Rand, E.H., Badger, L.W. and Coggins, D.R. (1987) 'Recognition of mental disorders by family practice residents: the effect of GHQ feedback', paper given at 'Mental Disorder in General Health Care Settings: A Research Conference', Seattle, USA.

Raynes, N.V. (1979) 'Factors affecting the prescribing of psychotropic drugs in general practice consultations', *Psychological Medicine* 9: 671–9.

Royal College of General Practitioners, Office of Population Censuses and Surveys, Department of Health and Social Security (1986) *Morbidity Statistics from General Practice* (Third National Study 1981–2).

Shepherd, M., Cooper, B., Brown, A.C. and Kalton, G.W. (1986) *Psychiatric Illness in General Practice*, London: Oxford University Press.

Shepherd, M., Wilkinson, G. and Williams, P. (eds) (1986) *Mental Illness in a Primary Health Care Setting*, London: Tavistock.

Sireling, L.I., Paykel, E.S., Freeling, P., Rao, B.M. and Patel, S.P. (1985) 'Depression in general practice: case thresholds and diagnoses', *British Journal of Psychiatry* 147: 113–19.

Skuse, D. and Williams, P. (1984) 'Screening for psychiatric disorders in general practice', *Psychological Medicine* 14: 365–77.

Sowerby, P. (1977) 'The doctor, his patient and the illness: a reappraisal', *Journal of the Royal College of General Practitioners* 27: 583–9.

Spitzer, R.L., Endicott, J. and Robins, E. (1978) 'Research diagnostic criteria: rationale and reliability', *Archives of General Psychiatry* 35: 773–82.

Strathdee, G. and Williams, P. (1984) 'A survey of psychiatrists in primary care: the silent growth of a new service', *Journal of the Royal College of General Practitioners* 34: 615–18.

Teasdale, J.D., Fennell, M.J.V., Hibbert, G.A. and Amies, P.L. (1984) 'Cognitive therapy for major depressive disorder in primary care', *British Journal of Psychiatry* 144: 400–6.

Trepka, C. and Griffiths, T. (1987) 'Evaluation of psychological treatment in primary care', *Journal of the Royal College of General Practitioners* 37: 215–17.

Tyrer, P. (1986) 'What is the role of the psychiatrist in primary care?', *Journal of the Royal College of General Practitioners* 36: 373–5.

Wing, J.K., Cooper, J.E. and Sartorius, N. (1974) *The Measurement and Classification of Psychiatric Symptoms*, Cambridge: Cambridge University Press.

World Health Organization (1973) *Psychiatry and Primary Medical Care*, Copenhagen: WHO, Regional Office for Europe.

World Health Organization (1980) *International Classification of Diseases, 9th revision, Clinical Modification: ICD*, Geneva: WHO.

Wright, A.F. and Perini, A.F. (1987) 'Hidden psychiatric illness: use of the General Health Questionnaire in general practice', *Journal of the Royal College of General Practitioners* 37: 164–7.

Zung, W.W.K. and Magruder-Habib, K. (1987) 'Depressed patients in general medical care', paper given at 'Mental Disorder in General Health Care Settings: A Research Conference', Seattle, USA.

27

The Interface Between Primary and Secondary Psychiatric Care

Geraldine Strathdee and Michael King

In Britain there has long been a sharp division between the primary and secondary levels of medical care, with hospital out-patient clinics forming the main focus of interaction between the two. Inevitably, training and research have been similarly separated, resulting in two distinctive ideologies in the provision of patient care.

This chapter traces the nature of the interface between the two levels of service beginning with an historical perspective, subsequent developments in the last two to three decades, and finishing with a view of the future.

HISTORICAL PERSPECTIVE

Service

The strength of primary medicine in Britain is unique among western countries in that 98 per cent of the population are registered with a general practitioner from whom they receive all their primary medical care. Access to the secondary services is largely at the discretion of the general practitioner with little room for patient-initiated approaches to specialists. It is only in the past twenty years that it has been recognized that psychological disorders comprise a significant part of the workload of these primary care physicians (Shepherd et al. 1966).

As Goldberg and Huxley (1980) have demonstrated, the filter between those patients identified by the GP and those referred to secondary care is relatively impermeable in that only one in twenty are referred on to specialists. In the vast majority of cases this is to hospital out-patient clinics. Psychiatric out-patient departments arose from an uncritical replication of the general medical model. The function of this expedient development has never been officially defined and even attempts to delineate the referred patient population on an empirical basis have raised more questions than they have answered (Kessel 1963).

Little has been done to evaluate either the nature or quality of service delivered by the clinics from the perspective of either primary or secondary care. However, the two substantive studies in this area have shown deficiencies in the clinical and referral outcomes and considerable dissatisfaction among patients and doctors alike (Kaeser and Cooper 1971, Johnson 1973a, 1973b). In addition, a careful examination of communication patterns between primary and secondary care doctors revealed a significant lack of understanding of each other's needs (Williams and Wallace 1974). As both areas of enquiry have shown, the result for patients was a variable level of care in both short and long term. Thus, it would seem that a rigid hospital-based out-patient service precluded effective dialogue or consensus management between GP and specialist.

Training

The training relationship in psychiatry and primary care has likewise followed the traditional medical model. Very few psychiatric trainees have had any exposure to post-graduate general practice and those GP trainees on vocational training schemes which included a psychiatric placement received an almost exclusively hospital-based training. Both the appropriateness and adequacy of this training, often sited as it is in large mental hospitals for the severely mentally ill, has been questioned as an adequate preparation for dealing with the broad spectrum of psychosocial morbidity encountered in primary care (Lesser 1983).

For GPs established in practice the only in-service training available was either in Balint groups with a psychotherapeutic emphasis, in the occasional hospital-based study day which often focused on theoretical rather than practical management issues, or the infrequent clinical associate attachment. The only other training mechanism has been through scientific and educational journals.

Research

The foundations of psychiatric research in primary care were laid by Shepherd and his colleagues in the 1960s (Shepherd *et al.* 1966). These early studies have been described in the chapter by Sharp and Morrell. As they also noted, important fields of enquiry stemming from this work have included the development of questionnaires and interviews for the identification of psychiatric morbidity and social dysfunction, and the performance of the general practitioner as a case detector.

Considerable work has also been directed at the GPs themselves with regard to their attitudes to psychiatry, their training, their referral patterns, and their ability to recognize psychological disorder (Shepherd *et al.* 1966; Rawnsley *et al.* 1962; Gardiner *et al.* 1974).

THE INTERFACE OF THE 1980S

Service

The past decade has seen the development of a unique service innovation which is altering the whole nature of the interaction between psychiatry and primary care. In a survey reported from the General Practice Research Unit, it was established that a growing number of psychiatrists (almost one in five) in England and Wales had moved their out-patient service from their hospital bases and established liaison-consultation clinics in primary care (Strathdee and Williams 1984). This service was unique in the sense that it arose *de novo*, undirected by any official policy, that there were no monetary incentives, and that its proponents were largely rurally based, front-line, clinical psychiatrists.

In contrast to the traditional 'referred away' approach of hospital out-patient departments, these liaison-consultation clinics facilitated GP and specialist working together. Three integrated methods of working were described. First, there was the consultation method in which the psychiatrist undertook assessment of the patients with an agreed treatment plan being carried out by the referring GP. Second and more common, in the shifted out-patient model, the psychiatrist both assessed and treated the patient in a series of short-term therapeutic interventions, with the GP remaining involved and informed of the management. In the third pattern, which evolved in long-standing attachments, the psychiatrist, after developing working and training links with the primary care team, adopted a predominantly supervisory or consultative role.

The context of this innovative service has recently been identified (Strathdee 1987) and correlated with major changes in primary care, psychiatry, and the relationship between the two. Within general practice the old dissatisfactions with long waiting lists and unsatisfactory clinical outcome associated with hospital clinics (Morgan and Strathdee 1987) have been voiced yet again. Moreover, GPs had increasingly begun to question the role of out-patient clinics in all specialities. There had also been a growing criticism of the propensity of hospital specialists to assume long-term clinical responsibility and exclude the referrer from the therapeutic process (Todd 1984; Marsh 1982). In particular the proclivity of hospital clinics to create 'chronic careers' for patients has been decried. One critic has gone so far as to suggest that their *only* function was as training fodder for an ever-changing series of junior doctors (Todd 1984). Research in the 1980s into the communication process reflected similar findings (Pullen and Yellowlees 1985) to that of the 1970s (Williams and Wallace 1974) in that specialists and generalists continued to be unaware of each other's requirements.

The 1980s have seen an acceleration of changes in the structure and organization of primary care, which had begun some years earlier, and which were to have profound effects on its role within medicine. The rapid expansion of vocational training schemes and the growth of academic departments of general practice has improved the status of the discipline within the medical establishment. In addition, the majority of GPs now work in partnership with other doctors and increasingly are based in health centres, facilitating the development of multi-disciplinary teams which have included health visitors, practice nurses, practice managers, and occasionally social workers and psychologists (Jeffreys and Sachs 1983). To many GPs the logical extension of the primary care team is the involvement of specialists and, in addition to the psychiatric attachments already described, reports indicate that similar trends are occurring in obstetrics, paediatrics, dermatology, and ENT.

Psychiatry itself has also undergone radical reorientation in the impetus to establish a more community-based service. Hospital closures and the need to establish community initiatives have forced psychiatrists to break the 'short umbilical cord syndrome' and recognize that working in the community behoves them to learn new skills beyond the purely clinical (Sturt and Waters 1985). In particular, the importance of developing management, communication, and administrative expertise has been underlined by the Royal College of Psychiatrists (1984). The ability to recognize and mobilize resources is fundamental to this approach. Specialists have generally failed to take account of what in Great Britain can be seen as a unique resource – the strength of the primary care network. Jones (1982) has reminded psychiatrists to recognize the consequent opportunity cost of failing to take advantage of this resource. In countries without a primary infrastructure such as the USA it may seem logical to create a first contact mental health service in the form of community health centres, but in Great Britain it could be argued that the World Health Organization view that the GP must form the 'cornerstone' of community psychiatry should be upheld. A working party cited six reasons why the GP and not the psychiatrist should remain the doctor of first contact for patients with psychiatric disorder (WHO 1973). These included the frequent presentation of psychiatric disorder in physical terms, the close relationship between psychiatric and social problems, and the lesser stigma associated with the primary care setting.

Psychiatry has begun to address itself to two important issues, the first being how can it assist GPs in providing better care to the bulk of those with psychiatric disorder who remain within primary care. Secondly, how might it best interact with GPs in this era of community psychiatry. One suggested model is that of the hive system (Tyrer 1985) which has, at the centre of a well-defined catchment area, a hospital base co-ordinating peripherally sited sub-units of care such as day hospitals, day centres, and health centre outpatient clinics located in areas of greater psychiatric morbidity. Others have emphasized a more mobile team approach concentrating on personnel rather than buildings. Falloon (personal communication) in an English rural setting has established a core multi-disciplinary team which responds quickly to referrals initially processed by community psychiatric nurses based in each general practice within a catchment area. In this system treatment takes place almost exclusively in the home setting thereby greatly reducing the need for in-patient care.

The hierarchical nature of the specialist-generalist relationship has come under increasing scrutiny. As in the changing face of doctor-patient relationships, the paternalistic model whereby the consultation is perceived as all-powerful is being replaced by a system whereby authority is based on expertise. This may be a difficult step for many GPs whose attitudes are a legacy from their training as junior doctors where consultants were regarded as omnipotent in carrying ultimate responsibility. Earlier commentators have pointed out that the optimal balance in this relationship can only effectively be achieved by an decrease in the power and authority of the specialist accompanied by a greater sharing in the burden of work and responsibility by all concerned (Horder 1986, Editorial 1978).

Training

More recently both the Royal College of Psychiatrists (Working Party report in progress) and the Royal College of General Practitioners (1980) have outlined the need for a reorientation in training to take account of the greater community emphasis in the provision of psychiatric care. There have been a number of innovations in this direction in the 1980s. First, GP trainees have been increasingly involved in the primary-care-based out-patient clinics already described. Among advantages cited are that they encounter psychiatrically ill patients in a setting akin to their future working environment and they acquire the practical skills of assessment and treatment adapted to the primary care setting. In addition, experience of the team approach common to community psychiatry will give them an understanding of how, in their future role as general practitioners, they might best liaise and communicate with the specialist services.

Second, for trainee psychiatrists, experience in liaison to general practice has introduced them to the need to develop more than purely clinical skills. It is envisaged that they will be able to identify and utilize resources not found in the hospital, as well as learn administrative, management, and communication skills essential for specialists working in the community. Working in a non-hospital setting may give the trainee a better understanding of the psychosocial components of psychiatric disorder and a recognition that psychiatric care involves much more than the period of hospital contact either as an in-patient or out-patient. More recently, a London teaching school has introduced a scheme whereby trainee psychiatrists work as general practitioners themselves for a limited period in order that they might gain a better understanding of the limitations and resources available within the primary care setting. This is in keeping with the General Medical Council's Education Committee's recommendation that all post-graduate education should include a mandatory six-month attachment in general practice (Turner 1987).

Third, established general practitioners have also reported substantial training benefits from close interaction with visiting specialists (Strathdee 1987). This has included increased theoretical knowledge about the nature of psychiatric disorders and treatments, as well as the mastery of practical skills of mental state assessment and management. These were acquired from face-to-face discussions and formal case presentations as well as directly from the joint management of patients.

Finally, psychiatric specialists gain a greater understanding of the limitations of time, interest, and skills of GPs and of the difficulties encountered in primary care psychiatry (Strathdee and Williams 1986). These include the assessment of earlier, less differentiated presentations of psychological disorder. Their GP colleagues often face patients whose behaviour and mental state seems clearly to separate them from the norm, but for whom, at the time of initial consultation, psychiatric diagnosis is unclear. Diagnosis is reached by a process of exploration by the doctor which inevitably leads to organization of the symptoms by the patient. Often this process only culminates on arrival at hospital when specialists, unaware of this resolution process, may be critical of GPs' diagnostic acumen, because of what is (by then) a classical clinical entity. While this is a problem in medicine or surgery, for example the vague abdominal pain referred by the GP which becomes an unquestionable appendicitis on arrival at casualty, it is even more compounded in psychiatry by the dimension of patient insight and the difficulties inherent for patients describing their own psychic phenomena. An example in psychiatry might be the 'disturbed' adolescent who isolates himself from peers, plays loud music, and loses interest in school work and his family. Even though the GP may feel that this patient is *qualitatively* distinct from other difficult adolescents, it may take some time for the patient himself to be able to divulge and discuss his bewildering array of psychotic experiences.

Research

Following on from the early work concentrating on the attitude and training attributes of GPs and their ability to recognize psychiatric disorders has been a generation of studies aimed at ways of improving identification and treatment skills (Goldberg *et al.* 1987).

Principal among these areas of development have been studies of depression among primary care populations, with a focus on recognition (Freeling *et al.* 1985; McDonald 1986; Blacker and Clare; 1987), intervention (Blackburn *et al.* 1981), Teasdale *et al.* 1984), and outcome (Blacker *et al.* 1987). The direction of work on minor psychiatric disorder has concentrated on treatment and outcome studies (Catalan *et al.* 1984: Corney 1984: Mann *et al.* 1981; Rodrigo *et al.* 1988, Johnstone and Shepley 1986), although the exact phenomenology of this syndrome remains rather vague. Other specific disorders which have received attention include problem drinking (Clements 1986: King 1986a; Wallace *et al.* 1987; Heather *et al.* 1987), eating disorders (Meadows *et al.* 1986; King 1987), and phobic disorders (Marks 1985).

Out of this research several training texts and manuals have been developed specifically to assist family doctors undertake psychological intervention in primary care (Williams 1984; France and Robson 1986).

In the 1980s research has expanded on the earlier evaluations of the service provided by psychiatric out-patient clinics. New impetus has come from the development of psychiatric clinics based in primary care. Conclusions from three studies have identified that moving the location of the clinics into the primary care setting results in an alteration of the spectrum of referrals to psychiatrists. This patient population more closely reflects the composition of patients with psychiatric morbidity in the community, i.e., more women, more chronically ill, and a wider representation of ethnic minorities (Tyrer 1984; Browning *et al.* 1987; Brown *et al.* 1988; Strathdee *et al.* 1988).

INTERFACE IN THE FUTURE

Services

One of the most crucial questions for the future structure of mental health services has been posed by the World Health Organization. In its First Contact Mental Health Care document (WHO 1983) it asks:

> in what ways should mental health specialist services interact with primary health services? Should the model be one of supervision and of direction, or one of collaboration and working directly with families in the community? Are all members of the mental health team equally relevant to the work in primary care? . . . These questions raise issues of integration, teamwork, collaboration and co-ordination.

Within the development of community services in Great Britain the role of primary care within these parameters remains largely unexplored. To reiterate, we believe that the GP will continue to remain the point of first contact for the mentally disturbed in the community. He or she is involved in acute and emergency care, continuing care, and the follow-up of the chronically mentally ill discharged from hospital units. Although there has been little quantitative evaluation of this role, services need to be set up so as to maximize the potential of this important resource.

The development of medical services has historically proceeded in a largely ad hoc, unevaluated fashion. We would emphasize that the expansion of community psychiatry should be accompanied by systematic evaluation going beyond mere description of the process. Initiatives requiring this approach include the provision of crisis intervention teams; community psychiatric nurses based in primary care; the further expansion of general practice out-patient clinics; working links with community day hospitals and centres; and the co-ordination of the care of the long-term mentally ill. In addition, contacts between GPs and psychiatric units in district general hospitals, particularly the communication aspects and continuity of care, need to be evaluated. Only such a careful clinical and economic assessment will allow new services to respond to changing needs.

Much more emphasis needs to be placed on the importance of prevention. The Royal College of General Practitioners (1981) has already led the way with a thoughtful report on the possibilities for prevention of psychiatric morbidity in primary care. GPs and other members of the primary care team are particularly well placed to provide education on such areas as stress reduction, alcohol and drug use, eating habits, and the psychological health of mothers and babies. In particular, they have an important role in crisis pre-emption and would benefit from increased education on crisis prevention.

Training

It is uncertain what degree of extra work load new community services will place on GPs. Equally, it appears that with the move into the community the work of psychiatrists and other mental health workers will alter. The success of these changes will rest on innovative changes in training of all staff concerned.

Clear-cut lines of responsibility and a formalized support system need to be established. Psychiatrists need to become more responsive to the needs of GPs by being prepared to offer supervision and training for a whole range of psychotherapeutic interventions, such as elements of cognitive and behavioural therapies, marital and family therapy. There is fruitful ground for study of how these techniques can best be adapted to the primary care field. However, the success of this training can only come about given that psychiatrists themselves become more aware of the constraints of general practice. It would seem logical that this can be achieved only by continuing integration of vocational schemes for both trainee psychiatrists and GPs in the community setting itself.

In centres where the traditional hospital model continues, the training potential of existing contacts between the two specialities should be maximized. For example, information in the assessment letters of psychiatrists might serve a more practical function by paying more attention to management techniques and their rationale, and less to lengthy historical accounts and diagnostic debate. The educational potential of shared care cards such as exist in obstetrics has never been explored, nor has their role in improving continuity of care, particularly for the chronically mentally ill.

The need for established GPs to become more involved in post-graduate education has been stressed in a recent government green paper 'Primary Health Care, An Agenda for Discussion' (DHSS 1986). Courses for these doctors should have an emphasis on the development of practical clinical skills. There is much scope for the development of a multi-disciplinary-based diploma course in psychosocial medicine on the same lines as for geriatric medicine and paediatrics. Already in England there are moves afoot to set up such a diploma (Higgs 1988).

Similar considerations must likewise apply to other professionals, such as social workers, community psychiatric nurses, psychologists, and counsellors. While the exact role of each group remains unclear they, too, will have to adapt to the new patterns of care both within their own work and in their relationship to the other disciplines.

Research

With the current economic constraints, patterns of research may change. At one level it could be argued that all practitioners should critically evaluate their services. This process of service audit is best undertaken by collaborative research between specialist and generalist. In the future therefore, it might be hoped that the current haphazard developments be replaced by a more planned approach which takes account of and adapts to joint efforts at evaluation.

At the other level there remain many areas where the possibilities for research are limitless. There has been a recent emphasis on the importance of establishing the natural history of psychiatric disorder. This can only be effectively delineated by studies which include the population at large rather than the narrow spectrum of disorders that present to hospital. Primary care, at least in the UK, represents an important community resource for this type of work. The importance of intervention and outcome studies has received increasing attention and it is a prerequisite for all such studies that we have a firm understanding of the natural history of the conditions in question. The work on intervention by GPs in the areas such as alcohol abuse (Heather *et al.* 1987) needs to be replicated and extended to other conditions with a psychiatric component.

It will be necessary to establish guidelines for collaborative management of psychiatric conditions, particularly the chronically ill. There are many models of integration between health professionals, staff of other agencies, and informal carers including the family, few of which have been systematically evaluated.

Little of the research into psychiatry in primary care has been undertaken by GPs themselves in contrast to areas such as family planning and medicine. Of course, it has been only in the last two decades that academic general practice has been widely established. Although the funding of primary care research remains problematical, the future is not so bleak. New developments in the primary care field, such as more universal use of age-sex and disease registers, computerization, together with recognition of the importance of research (Royal College of General Practitioners 1985) is likely to facilitate an expansion of research initiatives.

Economic appraisal of health care is a necessary component of all the above research considerations, but implicit in such an approach is a greater awareness and training in basic methods of economic evaluation. This is discussed elsewhere in this volume by Wilkinson and Pelosi.

The question of whether research leads or merely documents service developments has never been fully addressed. However, in the area of referral to specialists, research findings can inform clinical practice. It has been well established that the clinical reasons form only one part of the overall rationale for referral to psychiatrists. The other administrative and social reasons are seldom confronted in the standard out-patient consultation, resulting in the high level of dissatisfaction on the part of both consumers and doctors. Future research needs to establish if greater attention to these factors facilitates improved clinical outcome.

Finally, but of crucial importance for the direction of future research, is a consideration of how patients move in and out of treatment. Little attempt has been made to establish what influences movement of patients *back* into the community. Specialists need to accept that the time spent in contact with the hospital service represents only a small fraction of the total episode of illness. Goldberg and Huxley (1980) identified that the nature of the patient, his or her social environment, and the attitudes and training of the family doctor were the deciding factors in the referral of patients to psychiatric services. Although in their model little emphasis was placed on the nature of the service at each level, research has shown that there are considerable differences in the pattern of referral and outcome depending on whether the service is community or hospital-based (Grad and Sainsbury 1966, Brown *et al.* 1988). Moreover, as yet we know little about the effects of joint management by specialists and GPs.

The factors which determine the re-entry of patients back from hospital to out-patients to primary care and finally to the community, for even a single episode of illness, have not been identified. We would postulate that important among these might be the nature of the psychiatric and primary care services, the form and chronicity of the illness, treatment employed and patient compliance, social support, and the involvement of other community agencies. Delineation of the factors determining movement in either direction along this pathway might provide useful information for innovative changes in community services.

CONCLUSIONS

The specialist-generalist relationship forms the nidus of effective patient care.

429

Throughout the last three decades this interface has been subjected to increasing scrutiny with the result that the sharp division that characterized the early years is beginning to give way to closer collaboration. This has come about because of the growing strength of primary care as a speciality and new innovations in training in both specialities. Further impetus has arisen from the growing dissatisfaction with the traditional out-patient clinic, a new emphasis on evaluation which informs clinical practice and the increasing community orientation in psychiatry

In the future the interaction between psychiatrist and family doctor needs to be seen in the broader context, emphasizing that the interface between the two disciplines is only one component of the full circle of care. This will form a fruitful basis for future service, training and research initiatives.

Acknowledgement: The authors are supported by the Department of Health and Social Security.

REFERENCES

Blackburn, I.M., Bishops, S., Glen, A.I.M., Whalley, L.J. and Christie, J.E. (1981) 'The efficacy of cognitive therapy in depression: a treatment combination', *British Journal of Psychiatry* 139: 181–9.

Blacker, C.V.R., Clare, A.W. and Thomas, J. (1987) 'Depression in primary care', paper presented to 'Mental Disorders in General Health Care Settings', Seattle, USA.

Blacker, C.V.R. and Clare, A.W. (1987) 'Depressive disorder in primary care', *British Journal of Psychiatry* 150: 737–51.

Brown, R.M.A., Strathdee, G., Christie-Brown, J.R.W. and Robinson, P.H. (1988) 'A comparison of referrals to primary care and hospital outpatients clinics', *British Journal of Psychiatry*, in press.

Browning, S.M., Ford, M.F., Goddard, C.A. and Brown, A.C. (1987) 'A psychiatric clinic, in general practice: a description and comparison with an out-patient clinic', *Bulletin of the Royal College of Psychiatrists* 11, (4): 114–17.

Catalan, J., Gath, G., Edmonds, G., Bond, A., Mertin, P. and Ennis, J. (1984) 'Effects of non-prescribing of anxiolytics in general practice, 1. controlled evaluation of psychiatric and social outcome; 2. factors associated with outcome', *British Journal of Psychiatry*, 144: 593–610.

Clements, S. (1986) 'The identification of alcohol-related problems by general practitioners', *British Journal of Addiction* 81: 257–64.

Cooper, B., Harwin, B.G., Depla, G. and Shepherd, M. (1975) 'Mental health care in the community: an evaluative study', *Psychological Medicine* 5 (4): 372–80.

Corney, R.H. (1984) *The Effectiveness of Attached Social Workers in the Management of Depressed Female Patients in General Practice* (Monograph supplement 6) Cambridge: Cambridge University Press.

Department of Health and Social Security (1986) *Primary Health Care: An Agenda for Discussion*, London: HMSO.

Editorial (1978) 'General Practitioners and Psychiatrists – a new relationship', *Journal of the Royal College of General Practitioners* 28: 643–5.

France, R. and Robson, M. (1986) *Behaviour Therapy in Primary Care*, London: Croom Helm.

Freeling, P., Rao, B.M., Paykel, E.S., Sireling, L.I. and Burton, R.H. (1985) 'Unrecognised depression in general practice', *British Medical Journal* 290: 1880–82.

Gardiner, A., Petersen, J., and Hall, D. (1974) 'A survey of general practitioners' referrals to a psychiatric outpatient service', *British Journal of Psychiatry* 124: 536–41.

Goldberg, D.P., Bridges, K., Duncan-Jones, P. and Grayson, D. (1987) 'Dimensions of neurosis seen in primary care settings', *Psychological Medicine* 17: 461–70.

Goldberg, D. and Huxley, P. (1980) *Mental Illness in the Community: The Pathway to Psychiatric Care*, London: Tavistock.

Grad, J. and Sainsbury, P. (1966) 'Evaluating the community psychiatric service in Chichester: results', in E.M. Gruenberg (ed.) *Evaluating the Effectiveness of Mental Health Services*, New York: Milbank Memorial Fund.

Heather, N.M., Campion, P.D., Neville, R.G. and Maccabe, D. (1987) 'Evaluation of a controlled drinking minimal intervention for problem drinkers in general practice (the DRAMS scheme)', *Journal of the Royal College of General Practitioners* 37: 358–63.

Higgs, R., Strathdee, G., Corney, R. and Dammers, J. (1988) Personal communication.

Horder, J.P. (1986) 'The balance between primary and secondary care: a personal view', *Health Trends* 17: 64–8.

Jeffreys, M. and Sachs, H. (1983) *Rethinking General Practice*, London: Tavistock.

Johnson, D.A. (1973a) 'An analysis of out-patient services', *British Journal of Psychiatry* 122: 301–6.

Johnson, D.A. (1973b) 'A further study of psychiatric outpatient services in Manchester', *British Journal of Psychiatry* 123: 185–91.

Johnstone, A. and Shepley, M. (1986) 'The outcome of hidden neurotic illness treated in general practice', *Journal of the Royal College of General Practitioners* 36: 413–15.

Jones, K. (1982) 'Scull's dilemma', *British Journal of Psychiatry* 141: 221–6.

Journal of the Royal College of General Practitioners (1978) 'General practitioners and psychiatrists – a new relationship', editorial, *Journal of the Royal College of General Practitioners* 28: 643–5.

Kaeser, A.C. and Cooper, B. (1971) 'The psychiatric out-patient, the general practitioner and the out-patient clinic; an operational study: a review', *Psychological Medicine* 1: 312–25.

Kessel, N. (1963) 'Who ought to see a psychiatrist?' *Lancet* 1: 1092–5.

King, M. (1986) 'At risk drinking among general practice attenders: prevalence, characteristics and alcohol related problems', *British Journal of Psychiatry* 148: 533–50.

King, M. (1987) 'Eating disorders in general practice', *British Medical Journal* 293: 1412–14.

Lesser, A.L. (1983) 'Is training in psychiatry relevant for general practice?', *Journal of the Royal College of General Practitioners*, 39: 617–18.

Liaison Committee of the Royal College of Psychiatrists and the Royal College of General Practitioners (1980) 'Experience desirable for the general practice trainee occupying a senior house officer post in psychiatry', *Journal of the Royal College of General Practitioners* 30: 625–8.

MacDonald, A.J.D. (1986) 'Do general practitioners "miss" depression in elderly patients?', *British Medical Journal* 292: 1365–7.

Mann, A.H., Jenkins, R. and Belsey, E. (1981) 'The twelve month outcome of patients with neurotic illness in general practice', *Psychological Medicine* 11: 535–50.

Marks, I. (1985) 'Controlled trial of psychiatric nurse therapists in primary care', *British Medical Journal* 240: 1181–4.

Marsh, G.N. (1982) 'Are follow-up consultations in medical outpatient departments futile?', *British Medicine Journal* 284: 1176–7.

Meadows, G.N., Palmer, R.L., Newball, E.V.M. and Skentick, J.M.T. (1986) 'Eating attitudes and disorder in young women: a general practice based survey', *Psychological Medicine* 16: 351–7.

Morgan, D. and Strathdee, G. (1987) 'An ethnography of psychiatric referrals', unpublished research report.

Pullen, I. and Yellowlees, A.J. (1985) 'Is communication improving between general practitioners and psychiatrists?', *British Medical Journal* 290: 31–3.

Rawnsley, K., Loudon, J. and Miles, M. (1962) 'Factors influencing the reference of patients by general practitioners', *British Journal of Preventive and Social Medicine* 16: 174.

Rodrigo, E., King, M.B. and Williams, P. (1988) 'The health of long-term benzodiazepine consumers', *British Medical Journal*, in press.

Royal College of General Practitioners (1981) *Prevention of Psychiatric Disorders in General Practice* (Report of a Sub-Committee of the Royal College of General Practitioners' Working Party on Prevention).

Royal College of General Practitioners (1985) 'Quality of General Practice', *Policy Statement* 2: RCGPs.

Royal College of Psychiatrists (1984) 'Management Training', *Bulletin of the Royal College of Psychiatrists* 9: 84.

Royal College of Psychiatrists (1987) 'The front line of the health service'.

Shepherd, M., Cooper, B., Brown, A.C. and Kalton, G.W. (1966) *Psychiatric Illness in General Practice*, London: Oxford University Press.

Strathdee, G. (1987) 'Primary care – psychiatry interaction: a British perspective', *General Hospital Psychiatry* 9: 102–10.

Strathdee, G., King, M., Araya, R. and Lewis, S. (1988) 'The clinical and social status of patients referred to hospital and primary care outpatient clinics', unpublished research report.

Strathdee, G. and Williams, P. (1984) 'A survey of psychiatrists in primary care: the silent growth of a new service', *Journal of the Royal College of General Practitioners* 34: 615–18.

Strathdee, G. and Williams, P. (1986) 'Patterns of collaboration', in M. Shepherd, G. Wilkinson and P. Williams (eds) *Mental Illness in Primary Care Settings*, London: Tavistock.

Sturt, J. and Waters, H. (1985) 'Role of the psychiatrist in community-based mental health care', *Lancet* i: 507–8.

Teasdale, J.D., Fennell, M.J.V., Hibbert, G.A.R. and Amies, P.L. (1984) 'Cognitive therapy for major depressive disorder in primary care', *British Journal of Psychiatry* 144: 400–6.

Todd, J.W. (1984) 'Wasted resources: referral to hospital', *Lancet* 2: p. 1089.

Turner, T. (1987) 'GPs may soon train other specialists', *General Practitioner*, November 13: 4.

Tyrer, P. (1984) 'Psychiatric clinics in general practice: an extension of community care', *British Journal of Psychiatry* 145: 9–14.

Tyrer, P. (1985) 'The hive system: a model for a psychiatric service', *British Journal of Psychiatry* 146: 571–5.

Tyrer, P., Seivewright, N. and Wollerton, S. (1984) 'General practice psychiatric clinics: impact on psychiatric services', *British Journal of Psychiatry* 145: 15–19.

Wallace, P.G., Brennan, P.J. and Haines, A.P. (1987) 'Drinking patterns in general practice patients', *Journal of the Royal College of General Practitioners* 37: 354–7.

Williams, J.M.G. (1984) *The Psychological Treatment of Depression. A Guide to the Theory and Practice of Cognitive-Behaviour Therapy*, London: Croom Helm.

Williams, P. and Wallace, B.B. (1974) 'General practitioners and psychiatrists – do they communicate?' *British Medical Journal* 1: 505.

World Health Organization (1973) *Psychiatry and Primary Medical Care*, Copenhagen: WHO Regional Office for Europe.

World Health Organization (1983) *First Contact Mental Health Care* (report on a working group), Copenhagen: WHO Regional Office for Europe.

28

The Relationship Between Psychiatric Research and Public Policy

Leon Eisenberg

The relationship between psychiatric research and public policy embraces two separate but interrelated issues: how public policy for the support and regulation of research is, or should be, formulated, on the one hand; and the ways in which research findings are, or should be, utilized in formulating public policy, on the other. The two are obviously closely connected: the extent to which the public in a democratic society is persuaded that research can lead to more effective policy for the control of disease and the promotion of health will obviously influence the funds allocated to, and the latitude afforded for, health research. Drawing primarily on examples from the United States, I will first consider national policy for the support of research and then examine the extent to which research findings inform the debate on public policy.

POLICY GOVERNING RESEARCH SUPPORT

Although a National Institute of Health (NIH) was first created in 1930 (as successor to the Hygienic Laboratory established at the US Marine Hospital on Staten Island in 1887), its funding was quite modest. Not until the years following the Second World War did support for medical research in the federal budget begin to become substantial. The visible success of the wartime Office of Scientific Research and Development had persuaded the US Congress that investment in basic and applied research would lead to tangible results for public health. Between 1956, when federal appropriations for NIH were $98 million, and 1959, they tripled in response to a new health science coalition (Shannon 1987); by the late 1960s, funding passed the unprecedented $1 billion mark. Year after year, Senator Lester Hill and Representative John Fogarty, chairing the relevant Congressional committees, provided the leadership for an almost exponential increase in the commitment of public funds to health research; the Congress has authorized larger sums than successive Presidents have proposed in all but eight of the annual budgets between 1933 and 1987 (Marshall 1987)!

Obviously such a rate of increase could not continue for long (or, as one wag proclaimed, half of the US population would soon be employed doing health research on the other half). The rate began to slow in the late 1960s and appropriations actually fell (in dollars corrected for inflation) during some budget years in the 1970s and again in the early 1980s. Allocations for health research and development from all sources in the US remained about level in constant dollars between 1975 and 1983 (Office of Program Planning and Evaluation 1986: 4). Fortunately, over the last five years, NIH funding has once again attained sustained growth amounting to 70 per cent in dollars appropriated and 28 per cent in real terms; it reached $6.2 billion for fiscal year 1987 (Wyngaarden 1987).

The National Institute of Mental Health (NIMH), a component of NIH from its founding in 1946 until it was split off in 1974 together with the National Institutes for Alcoholism and Alcohol Abuse (NIAAA) and for Drug Addiction (NIDA) to form a separate Alcohol, Drug Abuse and Mental Health Administration (ADAMHA), began more modestly and its research budget did not reach $100 million until 1966. Had the NIMH research budget kept pace with inflation or had it paralleled the growth at NIH during the 1970s and 1980s, it would have exceeded $300 million by 1983 (Institute of Medicine 1984); however, because of the lower priority assigned to mental health by the Congress, the actual allocation was $158 million, one-sixth of the amount awarded to the National Cancer Institute and one-quarter of that awarded to the National Heart, Lung and Blood Institute in that year.

I have thus far merely outlined the history of what has been a remarkable national commitment to the support of health research, unparalleled elsewhere, although it has not fully satisfied the scientific community and has at times proceeded by fits and starts. As the President's Biomedical Research Panel noted:

> The scientific enterprise needs stability and predictability. It does not require growth and expansion at the rate achieved in the 1950's and 1960's, but it cannot survive being turned on and off, nor will it succeed if held at a standstill without any opportunity for growth.
>
> (Murphy and Ebert 1976:3).

Concerns about stability, costs, and cost effectiveness in health research led Joseph Califano, the then Secretary of the Department of Health, Education and Welfare, to convene a National Conference on Health Research Principles in January of 1979 to help develop 'a multi-year research strategy to guide the allocation of limited government health research dollars' (Office of the Director, NIH 1979: 99). Many in the academic community were concerned that the conference was convened with a greater emphasis on 'limited government health research dollars' than on a 'multi-year research strategy'; yet it was clear that 'public funds . . . will be made available to us only insofar as we are able to make a persuasive case for their utility' (Eisenberg 1979: 97).

What are the grounds that justify government support of health research? Are there guidelines for the total amount that should be committed? And how should priorities be set for allocating monies to particular health problems within the total?

Justifying a national commitment to health research

To many in the academy, the justification for basic science is the pursuit of knowledge for its own sake. Although this intellectual position does not carry much cachet in political debates, it remains the case that science enriches human understanding; science is a way of knowing. In the words of Adam Smith, it 'introduces order into the chaos of jarring and discordant appearances . . . and [restores the imagination], when it surveys the grand revolutions of the universe, to that tone of tranquillity and composure, which is most agreeable in itself, and most suitable to its nature' (Smith 1790: 45). The gratification of man's aesthetic sensibilities is not often persuasive to the public as a rationale for expending tax funds; the body politic is much more likely to respond to the substantial practical benefits scientific discovery brings with it. As Francis Bacon put the matter in his Third Aphorism 'concerning the interpretation of nature and the kingdom of man' in the *Novum Organum*, 'Human knowledge and human power meet in one; for where the cause is not known the effect cannot be produced. Nature to be commanded must be obeyed' (Bacon 1620: 259).

Bacon's proposition that knowledge is power was borne out in the late Julius Comroe's (1976) analysis of the scientific patrimony of ideas which proved ultimately of great benefit to patient care; 41 per cent of the work essential for later clinical advance was not clinically oriented at the time it was undertaken (Comroe and Dripps 1976). Although the chemist von Baeyer synthesized barbituric acid as early as 1864, it was not until Fischer and von Mering produced barbital in 1903 that barbiturates were employed as sedatives. Even when scientists pursue health-related ends, the applicability of their findings may not be apparent. Michael Heidelberger and Walter Jacobs synthesized sulfanilamide in the laboratory in 1915; yet twenty years were to pass before sulfonamides were first used against infectious diseases; the concept that inhibiting the uptake of metabolites would produce bacteriostasis had not been conceived. In 1970, David Baltimore and Howard Temin independently found evidence for an enzyme in RNA viruses capable of constructing double-stranded DNA from single-stranded RNA templates. The discovery of reverse transcriptase was acknowledged as a scientific landmark by the award of a Nobel Prize five years later. That work was to provide the foundation for understanding the pathophysiology of the Acquired Immune Deficiency Syndrome, a disease not identified until 1981 (Centers for Disease Control 1981a, 1981b); its cause, the HIV retrovirus employing reverse transcriptase to integrate itself into the host cell genome, was not identified until 1983 (Barre-Sinoussi *et al.* 1983; Gallo *et al.* 1983). The pursuit of basic knowledge in the laboratory yielded a concept and a methodology essential for the understanding of an unprecedented epidemic (Eisenberg 1986a); it provides major insights into the evolutionary origins of genetic information (Varmus 1987).

The most common rationale for research support is its direct benefit for health. The goals of health research have been epitomized as: advancing the fundamental knowledge base; translating that knowledge into improved diagnostic, treatment, and preventive interventions in order to alleviate suffering, improve the quality of life, and enhance survival; providing the basis for regulatory actions to promote safety and health; and providing the basis for informed decision making on health policy (Institute of Medicine 1979: 11). The Presidential Panel Report heralded the promise of biomedical and behavioural science in these terms:

> Human beings have within reach the capacity to control or prevent human disease. Although this may seem an overly optimistic forecast, it is, in fact, a realistic, practical appraisal of the long term future . . . There do not appear to be any impenetrable, incomprehensible diseases.
>
> (Murphy and Ebert 1976: 2).

A decade later, it is not likely that the promise of biomedical science for creating a disease-free society would be stated in such self-confident terms. It is not that the capabilities of the scientific enterprise have diminished in the interim; indeed, they have increased. But so has our awareness of the complexity of disease virulence, the multiple determinants of host resistance and the ecologic consequences that follow technological fixes (Eisenberg 1986b). As this decade ends, we have reason to recall the words of Rene Dubos:

> There is no reason to doubt . . . the ability of the scientific method to solve each of the specific problems of disease by discovering causes and remedial procedures . . . But solving problems of disease is not the same thing as creating health . . . In the world of reality, places change and man also changes . . . Health and happiness cannot be absolute and permanent values . . . Biological success in all its manifestations is a measure of fitness, and fitness requires never-ending efforts of adaptation to the total environment, which is ever changing. (Dubos 1959: 22–5)

The goal of interdisciplinary research in the health sciences must become a more complete understanding of the interactions between human populations and their salient physical, biological, and social environments.

The final – and least credible – argument for supporting research is a promise of reduction in health care costs. Advocates cite as a prototype the spectacular success of the WHO campaign against smallpox, which, by eliminating the virus, even removed the need for continuing vaccination costs. But that example has limited relevance. The biology of smallpox is unique: no animal reservoir, virtual life-long immunity after infection or vaccination, visible evidence of the immune state through scarification, transmissibility only while the vesicular eruption lasts, and no carrier state (Breman and Arita 1980). Other disease prevention measures are much less efficient and none has yet sufficed to eliminate the causal agent. Vaccinating those sixty-five and over against influenza costs an additional $2,000 for each year of life gained, even though the vaccine is cheap and hospitalization for the complications of influenza dear, because the economic calculus takes into account the additional costs for medical care from other causes among those who survive (Office of Technology Assessment 1981).

None of this argues against research in disease prevention in order to diminish morbidity and mortality; to the contrary, prevention must be in the forefront of our endeavours (Eisenberg 1987a). But the claims for cost reduction are illusory. They are likely to discredit the research enterprise when it does not yield the vaunted benefits. As Gori and Richter (1979) and Russell (1986) have pointed out, prevention delays death but does not eliminate cumulative morbidity. Increased survivorship into later years inexorably foretells higher costs (unless one clings to the fantasy of eliminating all chronic diseases). Americans 65 and over, some 11 per cent of the population in 1980, 'consumed' 29 per cent of personal health care expenditures; by 2020, when they will constitute 26 per cent of the population, the figure for expenditures will rise to 40 per cent (Rice and Feldman 1983). Success in prolonging meaningful life is a cause for celebration, but it does not come cheap. To claim that health research will lower overall health costs is to issue an unredeemable promissory note.

How much is enough?

Are there guidelines governments might usefully employ to determine appropriate resource allocations for medical research? In the heady years of the 1950s and early 1960s in the United States, with the GNP increasing each year, little thought was given to the sustainable limits to expansion in the research enterprise. In the late 1970s and 1980s, at a time of budget deficits, a slow-down in growth of the GNP, and an unfavourable trade balance, the question of limits has become prominent in policy debates. In 1976, the President's Panel had stated:

> In other fields of technological endeavor . . . it is customary to invest between 5 and 10 per cent of the total budget on research and development . . . At the present time the health industry as a whole invests a

considerably smaller percentage in research . . . While 5 per cent would represent an abruptly large increase if committed overnight, it seems to us a rational percentage to head toward as a long-range goal.

(Murphy and Ebert 1976: A22)

In 1976, total health research and development costs were 3.6 per cent of total health costs; the estimate for 1985 was 3.1 per cent (Office of Program Planning and Evaluation 1986: 2).

US health care expenditures for 1987 can be expected to total more than $500 billion. If the Panel's recommendation for a 5 per cent set aside for health research had been in effect, that would have justified an allocation of some $25 billion. What are the actual figures likely to be be? Over the past decade, the NIH budget has provided from 35 per cent to 40 per cent of all national support for health research and development, with other federal sources providing 15 per cent to 20 per cent and industry about 30 per cent to 39 per cent (Office of Program Planning and Evaluation 1986: 4). *If* similar ratios obtain in 1987 (an uncertain assumption) with an NIH budget of $6.2 billion, total support will equal some $16 billion, about 3.2 per cent rather than 5 per cent of 'industry' costs. Moreover, what is listed under 'research and development' in the national total is likely to reflect expenditures for development far more than basic research.

The relative generosity of research funding in the US stands in stark contrast to the situation in the UK, which invests only 1.5 per cent of the NHS budget in medical research, according to Sir Walter Bodmer, Director of the Imperial Cancer Fund. The most recent commentary in *Nature* remarked bitterly:

For want of sufficient renewal over 15 years, the research community is aging. The depth and variety of its pattern of work, already constrained by the lack of funds, will be further restricted by the reorganizations now in the cards. There are good reasons to fear that the permanent loss of able people is potentially another undermining influence. The flight of able young people into fields other than science, made possible and even necessary by the British educational system, is a greater if more distant worry. Bankruptcy tomorrow is a threat. (*Nature*, editorial, 1987: 745)

From this side of the Atlantic, the state of affairs in the UK can only be described as appalling. Lacking detailed knowledge of the British scene, I have no insights to offer into the reason for the meanness of government policy toward scientific research. I am, however, acutely aware of the loss for us when British scientists are handcuffed. Science is an international enterprise; its fruits are shared by all. When its future is in jeopardy in any country, that must be a matter of concern to scientists and citizens everywhere.

Setting priorities within the research budget

Within the health research budget, how are priorities to be assigned for allocations to particular disease problems? A rationalist might argue that decisions should be based on a close analysis (a) of the scientific opportunity for discovery in a given area (the existence of exciting new concepts and the availability of reliable methods) and (b) of the health burden produced by the diseases under consideration. For example, a cogent argument can be made on both grounds for a much increased investment in research on Alzheimer's disease. Localization of the gene controlling the production of amyloid on chromosome 21 (Goldgaber et al. 1987; St George-Hyslop et al. 1987: Tanzi et al. 1987) in familial Alzheimer's disease offers a powerful weapon to dissect the molecular biology of the disease. Aggregate net social costs over their remaining lifetimes for all cases of Alzheimer's disease diagnosed in a single year have been estimated at some $30 billion (Hay and Ernst 1987). Further, a substantial increase in incidence and prevalence of Alzheimer's disease is inevitable because of the gains in longevity among those over 75, the most striking demographic phenomenon in our era.

The Board on Mental Health and Behavioral Medicine of the Institute of Medicine (1984) has argued that psychiatric research is grossly underfunded in relation both to progress in neuroscience and to the health burden produced by mental disorders. In 1980, mental disorders entailed direct health care costs of $20 billion (without taking into account their contributions to morbidity from cirrhosis, drunk driving accidents, chronic pain syndromes, etc.), exceeded in aggregate expense only by costs resulting from circulatory and digestive diseases. A five per cent set aside rule would have warranted $1 billion for ADAMHA research; the actual figure did not reach half that amount for all three institutes under its aegis until 1987. When indirect costs secondary to lost productivity, restricted activity, welfare transfer payments, and other social liabilities (i.e., losses from crime and the costs of law enforcement because of opiate addiction) are added, the overall fiscal impact of major mental disorders and addictive states was estimated by the Board to total $185 billion a year (Institute of Medicine 1984: 7). The Board called for annual expenditures of $300 million for NIMH and $100 million for each of the other two Institutes (in 1983 dollars). In 1987, ADAMHA research budgets, which I have converted into 1983 dollars by means of the NIH Biomedical Research and Development Price Index, were the equivalent in 1983 dollars of $198 million for NIMH, $107 million for NIDA and $57 million for NIAAA, not quite three-quarters of the total recommended four years earlier.

The fact is that the politics of the budgetary process reflect the power of constituencies extending well beyond the scientific establishment. The National Institute of Health became the National Institutes with the proliferation of disease-oriented Institutes at the insistence of patient groups and their lobbyists, the most recent being the splitting of the National Institute for

Arthritis, Diabetes, and Digestive and Kidney Disease into new Institutes for Arthritis and Musculoskeletal and Skin Disease and for Diabetes and Digestive and Kidney Diseases because of legislative lobbying for sports medicine (Booth 1987). The National Cancer Institute (NCI), founded in 1944, became the best endowed component of the entire complex with the passage of the National Cancer Act in 1971 for a 'war against cancer'. Although academic purists opposed each of the new Institutes in turn (at the same time that academics who foresaw greater funding for their own research lobbied for the change), it is probable that the overall research budget grew as rapidly as it did because more citizens had a tangible reason to support budgets targeted against diseases with a personal meaning for them.

THE USES OF RESEARCH IN THE FORMULATION OF PUBLIC POLICY

At a time when Thatcherism and Reaganism reign supreme in our two countries, laissez-faire has become the ideal public policy. Conservative politicians call for a return to Adam Smith's 'invisible hand' which ensures that individuals, motivated solely by self-interest, 'without intending it, without knowing it, advance the interests of the society, and afford means to the multiplication of the species' (Smith 1759: 304). In this view, the discipline of the market leads to self-regulating order; *sans* conscious plan, regulation, or enforcement, the market place co-ordinates the individual behaviours of the multitude of vendors and buyers for the common good. In the debate between those who believe that government to be best which governs least and those who opt for the planned use of the taxing and regulatory powers of the state, conviction rests on philosophical rather than empirical grounds. There are no 'controlled clinical trials' on such questions (think for a moment about the meaning of 'informed consent' for such trials!).

Whatever the virtues of the market for the exchange of material goods, 'the invisible hand' clearly does not suffice for the provision of services unaffordable to those in the greatest need of them. Psychiatric services for the chronically impaired stand as a compelling instance. Curiously enough, the most convinced advocates of laissez-faire are quite prepared to support laws to enforce monogamy, to ban abortion, or to uphold the sovereignty of private property. Moreover, every modern state since the time of Bismarck's Prussia transfers funds from those who work to those who are retired rather than leaving it to individuals to provide for their security in old age. Every western state, save the US, entitles its citizens to health care by insurance or a national system; the Thatcher government, though it is progressively depleting the NHS of resources, continues to profess allegiance to it.

Highlighting the follies which he supposed to result from interference with the marketplace, Adam Smith had this to say about planners:

The man of system . . . is apt to be very wise in his own conceit, and is often so enamoured with the supposed beauty of his own ideal plan of government, that he cannot suffer the smallest deviation from any part of it. He goes on to establish it completely and in all its parts, without any regard either to the great interests or to the strong prejudices which may oppose it: he seems to imagine that he can arrange the different members of a great society with as much ease as the hand arranges the different pieces upon a chess-board; he does not consider that the pieces on the chess board have no other principle of motion besides that which the hand imposes on them; but that, in the great chess-board of human society, every single piece has a principle of motion of its own, altogether different from that which the legislature might choose to impress upon it.

(Smith 1759: 380–1)

The notion that the 'man of system . . . wise in his own conceit' is able to establish his 'ideal plan of government . . . completely and in all its parts' corresponds as little with the reality of the planning process as does his free market with today's international market. Rudolf Klein (1972), in a fascinating essay, has contrasted the 'optimizing, rationalizing' model of the decision-making process with the 'satisficing' model. The latter is based on a course of action that is good enough: cautious, incremental, and based on compromises dictated by the conflicting claims of competing constituencies. In the case of the NHS, those constituencies include the DHSS and the Treasury, civil servants in the bureaucracy, physicians (themselves divided among competing speciality groups), regional health authorities and public opinion (or what is judged to be public opinion). Klein concluded his article with these words:

The problem for policy makers – and those who try to assess the outcome of the process – is to know whether the right balance has been struck between overestimating the frictional costs, and thus missing an opportunity for improvement, and underestimating the frictional costs, and thus creating a situation of opposition to evolving change. (Klein 1972: 420)

These prefatory remarks may help to clarify some of the reasons for the divergence between the views of the planning process held by government officials, on the one hand, and physicians and scientists, on the other. The political agenda is such that decisions must be made in the face of limited (and sometimes absent) data. The policy-maker wants answers now and is impatient with the scientist's reiteration of the need for more research. Moreover, politicians operate within a time frame set by the next election; yet the impact of policy changes (or failures to change) should be assessed over much longer periods. Scientists complain that research findings are ignored, that debates proceed without data, and that politicians are unwilling

442

to submit proposals to empirical trial; i.e., comparing alternative policies in separate geographic areas. All too often, they feel that research findings are cited when they seem to support politically palatable alternatives and ignored when they don't (a phenomenon not unknown in medical debates).

Research findings are indeed often ignored, in part because they are themselves debatable, in part because larger political considerations come into play. An example may be informative. In 1965, as part of the War on Poverty, a national Head Start Program was established to provide pre-school education for economically disadvantaged children in order to improve their chances for successful performance when they enter elementary school. As programme costs mounted, the Westinghouse Learning Corporation (1969) was given a contract to evaluate effectiveness. Its report concluded that the increases in IQ for disadvantaged children observed early in the programme were not sustained after the children entered primary grades. The report diminished enthusiasm for the programme in the Nixon White House and reinforced efforts to reduce funding. Yet, despite the negative Westinghouse evaluation, funding has continued to grow in the years up to the present.

Head Start had, and continues to have, a large political constituency in local communities. Its emphasis on the children of the poor draws support even from those who oppose other welfare transfer payments. The Westinghouse study was heavily criticized because it lumped together data from programmes of very different quality and used IQ as the proxy for outcome rather than school progress. If its results were grist to the mill of Head Start opponents, they were roundly criticized as flawed by Head Start proponents. It was not until the 1970s and 1980s (Lazar et al. 1982; Berrueta-Clement et al. 1984) that longitudinal studies provided persuasive evidence of programme effectiveness: better school progress, fewer drop-outs, less delinquency, and an improved record of employment after high school. In the event, such research 'findings' as were available had little impact on a political process set in motion as part of a much larger national agenda.

Even when clinical and research data are solid, they may be unwelcome if they lead to social policy implications that contravene deeply held beliefs defined as 'moral'. Consider the prevalence of teenage pregnancy and of low birthweight infants, two strongly interconnected public health problems with high risk for maternal and neo-natal mortality and neuropsychiatric morbidity in both mothers and infants (Eisenberg 1987b). Among industrialized countries, the US has the highest teenage pregnancy, abortion, and birth rates because US teenagers have the lowest rate of contraceptive use (Jones et al. 1985). Although the percentage of unmarried adolescent women having had intercourse is higher by half in Sweden than in the US, pregnancy rates are only half as high because Sweden provides a compulsory sex education curriculum in its schools, closely linked to contraceptive clinic services. Evidence from US studies that school clinics lead to lower birth rates among secondary school students (Kenney 1986) and that they are associated with a *delay* in the age at which coitus is initiated (Zabin *et al*. 1986) has not deterred the Reagan Administration, and the 'moral majority' it speaks for, from opposing public health measures of demonstrated effectiveness.

Low birthweight is a major determinant of neo-natal mortality, total infant mortality and developmental retardation among the infants who survive (McCormick 1985). The Institute of Medicine (1985) has estimated that current rates of low birthweight in the US could be reduced by 15 per cent among whites and 12 per cent among blacks if all women began pre-natal care in the first trimester of pregnancy and continued to receive care through delivery. Yet, since 1978 the proportion of women in the US not receiving care until the third trimester or receiving no care at all has remained unchanged. What has been missing is a national commitment to abolishing the barriers to care. The problem persists, not because of a lack of knowledge, but because of a lack of social will. The issue is not further research, though much more remains to be done to improve on present performance, but the creation of a political coalition to press for universal access to the medical and social measures already available.

An impediment of a different kind arises when research yields strong, replicated, and important findings but the policy measures to change current practices are not readily implemented. Twenty years ago, Michael Shepherd and his colleagues demonstrated the crucial role of general practitioners in the provision of mental health care. They concluded that 'The cardinal requirement for improvement of the mental health services in this country [the UK] is not a large expansion and proliferation of psychiatric agencies, but rather a strengthening of the family doctor in his therapeutic role' (Shepherd *et al*. 1966: 176). Goldberg *et al*. (1978) and Regier *et al*. (1978) obtained comparable data for the United States and came to similar conclusions. Moreover, there is solid evidence from a number of studies, of which those by Hankin *et al*. (1982) and Williams *et al*. (1986) are representative, that patients with mental disorder use general medical services at a disproportionate rate. Yet, there has been little progress in upgrading psychiatric training for family doctors and less in creating the conditions necessary in the US for changing practice patterns (i.e., providing adequate reimbursement for time spent in delivering mental health care). In his most recent commentary on the problem, Shepherd (1987) suggests that psychiatric protectionism may be an additional major obstruction.

What are the policy implications of these findings? Medical curricula are controlled locally rather than nationally; they are constructed by faculty committees on which psychiatrists have little representation. Proposals to increase funding for mental health services in primary care will be coldly received in a climate of cost control unless they include mechanisms to reduce payments in other sectors of the health service. As rational as that would be for improving primary care, it faces bitter opposition from procedure-based specialities whose incomes would fall. Nonetheless, I am persuaded that a more rational redistribution of health care funds is inevitable; that change, when it occurs, will provide a more powerful stimulus to needed curriculum reform than purely internal educational forces are able to muster (Eisenberg 1987c).

The failure of research to inform policy for the care of psychotic patients is clearly evident in the number of homeless mentally ill persons in the US, estimated in the hundreds of thousands. Massive release of formerly hospitalized patients followed upon policy decisions undertaken without systematic evaluation of the consequences. Wyatt and DeRenzo (1986) contrast the stringent demands established by the Food and Drug Administration before drugs are allowed on the market with the absence of any requirement for trials of efficacy and toxicity for social policy innovations. Thoughtful scholars had indeed warned against the danger of substituting good intention for evidence. Freedman had cautioned that a tradition in America of:

> veneration for change leads some to envision abandonment of all state hospitals immediately without thought to feasibility or consequences . . . [There is a danger that] in paying increased attention to the socially deviant and the neurotic in the community, the traditional responsibility of psychiatry for caring for the severely disturbed or psychotic will be minimized or abandoned. (Freedman 1967)

When short-term studies seemed to demonstrate the feasibility of caring for acutely psychotic patients in the community with psychotropic drugs *and* appropriate social support, the second part of the message (the costly part) was lost in the stampede to deinstitutionalization in hope of transferring costs from state to federal budgets. Moreover, no provision was made for care over the long run for patients whose disorders are chronic and marked by periodic exacerbations. The fate of the research by Pasamanick and his colleagues (1967) provides a distressing instance of the way in which good results can be transformed into tragedy when the long-term needs of patients are not met.

The study was designed to determine whether actively psychotic patients could be treated more effectively at home than in hospital. Patients eligible for entry into the trial were those diagnosed as schizophrenic, between 18 and 60 years of age, neither homicidal nor suicidal, resident within a defined geographic area, and with a family able and willing to provide supervision in the home. Note the age limitations, the exclusion of violent patients, and the requirement for a supportive family. Those eligible were randomized to conventional state hospital care or to home care on drug or placebo. The outcome was unequivocal. Those cared for at home with psychotropic drugs (but not placebos), visiting public health nurses, and psychiatric and social work back-up available as needed did better on all of the outcome measures than the hospital control cases. Even after an initial hospitalization averaging three months and remission of gross symptoms, the hospitalized patients were judged as treatment failures more often than were the home care patients at the termination of the study.

Despite its clear success, funding for the home care programme was not continued by state authorities after the NIMH supported research ended. What was the fate of the patients over the next five years? The investigators set out to determine the facts. To their distress, though not to their surprise, they found no significant differences between groups on any of the indicia of outcome; worst of all, the majority of patients, whatever their initial treatment assignment, showed evidence of major psychiatric and social impairment. They conclude bitterly:

> We must raise questions about the social implications of science, the expenditure of funds and personnel on research whose results are not utilized, and all the personal frustrations of investigators who must feel the tremendous anger of what are, fundamentally, wasted professional lives.
> (Davis *et al*. 1974: xii)

The situation is not quite so grim as it was when those words were written. Public policy is beginning to move toward a recognition of responsibility for chronic mental patients. There is great promise in the current joint effort by the Robert Wood Johnson Foundation and the US Department of Housing and Urban Development to establish model urban programmes for the care of chronic mental patients, with equal emphasis on the provision of social services and clinical care. The lesson still to be learned is that the effectiveness of the best designed model must be measured, not only when it is new and is under carefully chosen leadership, but also when it becomes the basis for routine and inevitably bureaucratized services. What is needed is the equivalent of post-marketing surveillance after the introduction of new drugs. Only by setting up a system sensitive to toxicity and ensuring the feedback and use of data obtained can we be confident that what works in a demonstration project in fact continues to perform as expected when it becomes the basis of routine care.

CONCLUSION

Public policy for the support of psychiatric research takes its primary justification from evidence that the results of research improve the health of the population. When discoveries come in the form of more effective new drugs and procedures, they are readily introduced into practice. When they come in the form of remedies which counter deeply held beliefs or are costly and manpower-intensive, they compete in the political arena with other social values.

Though I have limited this account to issues internal to the health policy sector, the fight for medical research and the application of its funding demand attention to broader questions of resource distribution. What is spent for 'defence' is not available for the improvement of health care. Advocates of public health must be prepared to challenge the disproportionate allocations of tax monies to military expenditures, themselves the greatest threat to the health of populations.

REFERENCES

Bacon, F. (1620) *Novum Organum*, in J.M. Robertson (ed.) (1905) *The Philosophical Works of Francis Bacon*, London: George Routledge and Sons, Ltd.

Barre-Sinoussi, F., Chermann, J.C., Rey, F., *et al.* (1983) 'Isolation of a T-lymphotrophic virus from a patient at risk for Acquired Immune Deficiency Syndrome', *Science* 220: 868-71.

Berrueta-Clement, J.R., Schweinhart, L.J., Barnett, W.S., *et al.* (1984) *Changed Lives: The Effects of the Perry Preschool Program on Youths Through Age 19*, Ypsilanti, Michigan: The High/Scope Press.

Booth, W. (1987) 'Arthritis Institute tackles sports', *Science* 237: 846-7.

Breman, J.G. and Arita, I. (1980) 'The confirmation and maintenance of smallpox eradication', *Science* 164: 262-70.

Centers for Disease Control (1981a) 'Pneumocystis pneumonia – Los Angeles', *Morbidity and Morality Weekly Report* 30: 250-2.

Centers for Disease Control (1981b) 'Kaposi's sarcoma and pneumocystis pneumonia among homosexual men – New York City and California', *Morbidity and Mortality Weekly Report* 30: 305-8.

Comroe, J.H. (1976) 'Lags between initial discovery and clinical application to cardiovascular and pulmonary surgery', in F.D. Murphy and R.H. Ebert, *Report of the President's Biomedical Research Panel*, Appendix B, 1-33.

Comroe, J.H. and Dripps, R.D. (1976) 'Scientific basis for the support of biomedical science', *Science* 192: 105-11.

Davis, A.E., Dinitz, S. and Pasamanick, B. 1974 *Schizophrenics in the New Custodial Community: Five Years After the Experiment*, Columbus, Ohio: Ohio State University Press.

Dubos, R. (1959) *Mirage of Health: Utopias, Progress and Biological Change*, New York: Harper and Brothers.

Eisenberg, L. (1979) 'The National Conference on Health Research Principles: bread and circuses or the great debate?' *Clinical Research* 27: 95-7.

Eisenberg, L. (1986a) 'The genesis of fear: AIDS and the public's response to science', *Law, Medicine and Health Care* 14: 243-9.

Eisenberg, L. (1986b) 'Human ecology and health: disease prevention and control', presented at a World Health Organization Meeting on Human Ecology and Health, Delphi, Greece, 30 September-3 October.

Eisenberg, L. (1987a) 'Preventing mental, neurological and psychosocial disorders', *World Health Forum* 8: 245-53.

Eisenberg, L. (1987b) 'Preventive pediatrics: the promise and the peril', *Pediatrics* 80: 415-22.

Eisenberg, L. (1987c) 'Science in medicine: too much or too little and too limited in scope:' presented at the Kaiser Family Foundation Conference on Biopsychosocial Medicine, Wickenburg, Arizona, 13 May 1987.

Freedman, A.M. (1967) 'Historical and political roots of the Community Mental Health Centers Act', *American Journal of Orthopsychiatry* 37: 487–94.

Gallo, R.C., Sarin, P.S., Gelmann, E.P., *et al.* (1983) 'Isolation of a human T-cell leukemia virus in Acquired Immune Deficiency Syndrome', *Science* 220: 865–7.

Goldberg, I.D., Babigian, H.M., Locke, B.A., *et al.* (1978) 'Role of non-psychiatrist physicians in the delivery of mental health services: implications from three studies', *Public Health Reports* 93: 240–5.

Goldgaber, D., Lerman, M.I., McBride, O.W., *et al.* (1987) 'Characterization and chromosomal localization of a cDNA encoding amyloid of Alzheimer's disease', *Science* 235: 877–80.

Gori, G.B. and Richter, B.J. (1979) 'Macroeconomics of disease prevention in the United States', *Science* 200: 1124–30.

Hankin, J.R., Steinwachs, D.M., Regier, D.A., *et al.* (1982) 'Use of general medical care by persons with mental disorders', *Archives of General Psychiatry* 39: 225–31.

Hay, J.W. and Ernst, R.L. (1987) 'The economic costs of Alzheimer's disease', *American Journal of Public Health* 77: 1169–75.

Institute of Medicine (1979) *DHEW's Research Planning Principles*, Washington, DC: National Academy of Sciences.

Institute of Medicine (1984) *Research on Mental Illness and Addictive Disorder: Progress and Prospects*, Washington, DC: National Academy Press.

Institute of Medicine (1985) *Preventing Low Birth Weight*, Washington, DC: National Academy Press.

Jones, E.F., Forrest, J.D., Goldman, N. *et al.* (1985) 'Teenage pregnancy in developed countries: determinants and policy implications', *Family Planning Perspectives* 17: 53–63.

Kenney, A.M. (1986) 'School-based clinics: a national conference', *Family Planning Perspectives* 18: 44–6.

Klein, R. (1972) 'NHS reorganization: the politics of the second best', *Lancet* ii: 418–20.

Lazar, I., Darlington, R., Murray, H., *et al.* (1982) *Lasting Effects of Early Education* (Monographs of the Society for Research in Child Development 47 (1–2, Serial No. 194).

McCormick, M.C. (1985) 'The contribution of low birth weight to infant mortality and childhood morbidity', *New England Journal of Medicine* 312: 82–90.

Marshall, E. (1987) 'OMB stalks the "burgeoning growth of biomedicine"', *Science* 237: 847–8.

Murphy, F.D. and Ebert, R.H. (1976) *Report of the President's Biomedical Research Panel*, Washington, DC: DHEW Publication No. (OS) 76–500.

Nature (1987) 'Formative turbulent months ahead', editorial in *Nature* 328: 745–6.

Office of the Director, NIH (1979) *DHEW Health Research Principles, Volume 1*, Washington, DC: DHEW(NIH).

Office of Program Planning and Evaluation (1986) *NIH Data Book*, Washington, DC: US Department of Health and Human Services.

Office of Technology Assessment (1981) *Cost Effectiveness of Influenza Vaccination*, Washington, DC: US Government Printing Office.

Pasamanick, B., Scarpitti, F. and Dinitz, S. (1967) *Schizophrenics in the Community: An Experimental Study in the Prevention of Hospitalization*, New York: Appleton-Century-Crofts.

Regier, D.A., Goldberg, I.D., and Taube, C.A. (1978) 'The de facto U.S. mental health services system: a public health perspective', *Archives of General Psychiatry* 35: 685–93.

Rice, D.P. and Feldman, J.J. (1983) 'Living longer in the United States: demographic changes and health needs of the elderly', *Milbank Memorial Fund Quarterly/Health and Society*, 61: 362–96.

Russell, L.B. (1986) *Is Prevention Better than Cure?* Washington, DC: The Brookings Institution.

St George-Hyslop, P.H., Tanzi, R.E., Polinsky, R.J., *et al.* (1987) 'The genetic defect causing familial Alzheimer's disease maps on chromosome 21', *Science* 235: 885–90.

Shannon, J.A. (1987) 'The National Institutes of Health: some critical years, 1955–1957', *Science* 237: 865–8.

Shepherd, M. (1957) 'An English view of American psychiatry', *American Journal of Psychiatry* 114: 417–20.

Shepherd, M. (1987) 'Mental illness and primary care', *American Journal of Public Health* 77: 12–13.

Shepherd, M. and Blackwell, B. (1968) 'Prophylactic lithium: another therapeutic myth', *Lancet* ii: 968–71.

Shepherd, M., Cooper, B., Brown, A.C. and Kalton, G.W. (1966) *Psychiatric Illness in General Practice*, London: Oxford University Press.

Smith, A. (1759) *The Theory of Moral Sentiments*, republished 1976, Indianapolis: Liberty Classics.

Smith, A. (1790) *The History of Astronomy*, reprinted (1980) in W.P.D. Wightman and J.C. Bryce (eds) *Essays on Philosophical Subjects*, Oxford: Clarendon Press.

Tanzi, R.E., Gusella, J.F., Watkins, P.C., *et al.* (1987) 'Amyloid beta-protein gene: cDNA, mRNA distribution, and genetic linkage near the Alzheimer locus', *Science* 235: 880–4.

Varmus, H. (1987) 'Reverse transcription', *Scientific American* 257: 56–64.

Westinghouse Learning Corporation (1969) *The Impact of Head Start: An Evaluation of Head Start on Children's Affective and Cognitive Development, (Volumes I and II)*, Athens, Ohio: Ohio University.

Williams, P., Tarnopolsky, A., Hand, D., and Shepherd, M. (1986) 'Minor psychiatric morbidity and general practice consultations: the West London Survey', *Psychological Medicine* (Monograph Supplement 9).

Wyatt, R.J. and DeRenzo, E.G. (1986) 'Scienceless to homeless', *Science* 234: 1309.

Wyngaarden, J.B. (1987) 'The National Institutes of Health in its Centennial year', *Science* 237: 869–74.

Zabin, L.S., Hirsch, M.B., Smith, E.A., *et al.* (1986) 'Evaluation of a pregnancy prevention program for urban teenagers', *Family Planning Perspectives* 18: 119–26.

Section Four

The International Perspective

Introduction

Social and epidemiological psychiatry are, by their very nature, not confined within national boundaries: the requirement for a global perspective is thus self-evident. This helps to orientate the international research community to prevalent and socially relevant problems; to enhance local research potential, particularly in developing countries; to generate and disseminate appropriate research methods and techniques; and to facilitate international collaboration (Sartorius 1980).

In appraising these issues, it is useful to consider the five headings which characterize the research component of the WHO mental health programme (Sartorius 1980): (i) the development of a common language; (ii) characteristics of mental and neurological disorders and of psychosocial problems of major public health importance; (iii) development and improvement of treatment methods; (iv) organization of mental health services – assessment and development of new models; and (v) psychosocial aspects of general health care and high risk group research.

As well as reflecting these topics, the papers included in this section are concerned with three levels – international, national, and local. These distinct but related levels apply not only to the nature of the enquiry but also to the organization and implementation of the research.

In the first paper, Assen Jablensky gives an overview of the WHO multi-centre studies of schizophrenia: these underline the heuristic importance of a global view. One of the most interesting results to emerge has been that, while the incidence of schizophrenia is relatively constant across cultures, the outcome is not, a finding which raises many important questions for further research.

While these WHO studies exemplify all three levels – international, national and local – the focus of the second paper in this section is national. Darrel Regier describes the psychiatric epidemiology research programme being undertaken at the National Institute of Mental Health (NIMH) in the USA. He draws particular attention to the Epidemiologic Catchment Area (ECA) Program, one of the largest and most ambitious studies of its kind. While a national programme of research is addressed to national priorities and many of the detailed findings are specially pertinent to the catchment areas involved, the experience gained and the broader implications of the findings are of international significance.

Both WHO and NIMH research activities have been directly influenced by Michael Shepherd's contributions. Moreover, his research unit at the Institute of Psychiatry in London has played an important role in training research workers from America, Asia, Europe, and the Third World, three of whom have written the third chapter in this section. Jair Mari, Biswajit Sen, and

Tai-Ann Cheng draw upon their experiences in studying psychiatric disorder in the community and in primary care settings in Brazil, India, and Taiwan respectively, and use them to make some observations on the problems which arise in the cross-cultural measurement of psychiatric morbidity.

The location of much of this research – the primary medical care setting – serves as a reminder that, as has been discussed previously, it has become widely accepted that the focus of the provision of mental health care should shift from specialist to general medical settings. This policy is endorsed by, among others, WHO (1973) and NIMH (1980): Michael Shepherd's work has played a seminal part in its formulation.

REFERENCES

National Institute of Mental Health (1980) *Mental Health Services in Primary Care Settings: Report of a Conference* Series DN: Health/Mental Health Research, DHHS publication no. (ADM)80-995), Washington, DC: US Government Printing Office.

Sartorius, N. (1980) 'The research component of the WHO mental health programme', *Psychological Medicine* 10: pp. 175–85.

World Health Organisation (1973) *Psychiatry and Primary Care*, Copenhagen: WHO Regional Office for Europe.

29

An Overview of the World Health Organization Multi-centre Studies of Schizophrenia

Assen Jablensky

Comparative psychiatry is to the study of the nature of mental disorders what comparative anatomy once was to the construction of a scientific taxonomy of the living organisms: a systematic search for the right building blocks of a nosology that could accommodate and reduce the outwardly bewildering variation of the phenomena of mental illness. While modern biological taxonomy is reaching beyond phenotypical variations and is now capable of classifying many living things on the basis of similarities in strings of DNA, psychiatry has yet to resolve the question whether its elementary units of observation, the psychopathological symptoms and syndromes, represent a universal code of abnormal mental life.

COMPARATIVE PSYCHIATRY: SOURCES AND BACKGROUND

With characteristic foresight, the need for comparative 'observation of mental disorders in different groups of people' was advocated more than eighty years ago by Kraepelin (1904), who suggested at least two ways in which cross-cultural studies could advance knowledge: by 'throwing light on the causes of mental disorders' and by providing 'means of determining the influence which the patient's personality exerts on the particular form his illness assumes'.

Kraepelin was himself wary of the methodological obstacles:

Reliable comparison is, of course, only possible if we are able to draw clear distinctions between identifiable illnesses, as well as between clinical states; moreover, our clinical concepts vary so widely that for the foreseeable future such comparison is possible only if the observations are made by one and the same observer.

His own explorations of psychoses in Java were one of the few attempts at the time to pursue the strategy of comparative research in a field which soon after became increasingly dominated by a psychoanalytically-oriented cultural anthropology. The latter was practically divorced from psychiatric epidemiology which in the 1920s and 1930s attained a level of sophistication marked by such milestones as Goldberger's discovery of the dietary aetiology of pellagra (Goldberger 1927), Brugger's census surveys (Brugger 1933), Faris and Dunham's studies on the social ecology of psychosis (Faris and Dunham 1938), and Strömgren's genetic epidemiological investigation of an entire insular population (Strömgren 1938).

However, the application of the epidemiological method remained restricted mainly to European and North American populations; it was not until the Taiwan studies (Rin and Lin 1962), the Mauritius survey (Murphy and Raman 1971), and the WHO International Pilot Study of Schizophrenia (WHO 1973), that comparative psychiatric epidemiology ventured into cultural settings different from the one in which its own concepts and methods originated.

At an early stage of WHO's involvement in cross-cultural mental health issues, the methodological problems facing psychiatric epidemiological research were reviewed by a WHO Expert Committee (WHO 1960) which, in a seminal report, pointed to: (a) the existence of 'individual factors in the causes and manifestations of many psychiatric diseases which . . . because they belong to the sphere of values, cannot be fully quantified'; (b) the 'essentially multifactorial' nature of the aetiology of mental disorders, complicated by the fact that 'in few branches of medicine are genetic, physiological and psychological factors as evenly distributed in the origin and distribution of disease as in psychiatry'; (c) the 'incongruities in the diagnostic appraisal in different countries and schools' and a 'tendency to use technical terms in different senses according to the theory favoured'; (d) the presence of 'considerable social and cultural differences in what is considered psychically abnormal in different surroundings, and the way such abnormality is treated'; and (e) the problem of 'infinite variations' in human character and behaviour deviations 'ranging from severe psychosis to mild personality disorders which many would not consider to be the concern of psychiatry'. The Committee concluded that 'these problems may make it difficult to advance the study of epidemiology of mental disorders as quickly and consistently as might be hoped'.

For all the thoroughness of its diagnosis of the problems, the Committee was overly guarded in its prognosis. The resolving of the difficulties barring the progress of comparative psychiatric research (and of mental health action consequent upon such research) became the chief objective of the mental health programme of WHO in the 1960s and 1970s. As an inter-governmental organization of a practically universal membership, WHO was in a unique position to set up a framework for cross-national mental health research which ensured access to: (a) populations representing a wide variation in socio-economic development, ecology, and culture; (b) individual experts and teams of investigators willing to apply their knowledge and skills to collaborative research.

One of the first steps resulted from the realization of the lack of a 'common language' in mental health research. In 1959 WHO requested Professor E. Stengel to review critically the field of psychiatric classification and to make recommendations about the future work of the Organization in this respect. In his comprehensive report, Stengel concluded that:

The lack of a common classification of mental disorders has defeated attempts at comparing psychiatric observations and the results of treatments undertaken in various countries or even in various centres in the same countries . . . Diagnoses can rarely be verified objectively and the same, or similar conditions, are described under a confusing variety of names. This situation militates against the ready exchange of ideas and experiences, and hampers progress.   (Stengel 1959)

THE WHO MENTAL HEALTH PROGRAMME

Stengel's findings provided a stepping-stone for the first major component of the WHO mental health programme: the so-called 'Programme A' which envisaged the development of common rules of usage of psychiatric concepts and terms; the standardization of methods and instruments; and the training of investigators in different parts of the world in using such a technology in a manner that is both congruent with their own culture and enabling them to generate comparable data. This was the prerequisite to the subsequent extension of the WHO programme into substantive areas such as:

(i) Research to explore the existence of culturally invariant reference points in mental morbidity, e.g. the occurrence of comparable forms of schizophrenia or depression and the applicability of diagnostic concepts in different cultures;

(ii) Investigation of the extent of culture-related variation in areas such as the phenomenology of mental disorders or their 'natural history';

(iii) The comparative incidence and disease expectancy of the major mental disorders in different populations;

(iv) Delineation of new syndromes or enrichment of the description of established clinical entities with data on their manifestation in different cultures;

(v) Identification of predictors of course and outcome and search for significant associated, and possibly causal, factors.

The WHO mental health programme has been consistent in pursuing the above objectives in spite of variable political winds and recurrent financial

457

uncertainties. It should be noted that epidemiological and social psychiatry is only one of the several major areas of concern of the WHO mental health programme which includes, among other things, work on the psychosocial aspects of general health, service-orientated activities (including the designing and implementation of training programmes for mental health workers), research in alcohol- and drug-related problems, support to international legislative action concerning the control of psychoactive substances, studies on neurological disorders, and promotion of research in biological psychiatry. The mental health programme is an integral component of the WHO General Programme of Work which is renewed every six years (the seventh programme cycle ends in 1989) and contains three objectives in the area of protection and promotion of mental health: (i) psychosocial and behavioural factors in the promotion of health and human development; (ii) prevention and control of alcohol and drug abuse; and (iii) prevention and treatment of mental and neurological disorders.

WHO is a less monolithic body than most United Nations organizations; in fact, it consists of six regional organizations (Africa, the Americas, Eastern Mediterranean, Europe, South-East Asia, and the Western Pacific), each governed by a Regional Committee and managed by a Regional Office. The WHO Headquarters in Geneva is the strategic centre which is entrusted with global policy development and co-ordination (mandated by the World Health Assembly and the Executive Board) and with many of the research initiatives, especially those concerning global or inter-regional problems. In the past fifteen years, the ethos of WHO has been permeated by concerns about social issues, the predicament of the Third World, and the role of health in socio-economic development, a philosophy strongly espoused by its Director-General, Dr Halfdan Mahler. Since 1977, WHO has adopted a militant policy platform, epitomized in the idea of Health for All by the Year 2000, which (against all odds) is gradually acquiring the operational features of a structured and technically supported approach to health planning.

A glimpse of the background is indispensable for an understanding of the operation of the WHO mental health programme, because, in contrast to academic and research centres engaged in the pursuit of pure knowledge, the former is essentially a public health enterprise, in service of a constituency including over 165 member countries of extremely varied perception of needs and priorities. The *raison d'être* of epidemiological and social psychiatry within the WHO mental health programme has been expressed in a position paper entitled 'Social Dimensions of Mental Health' in the following terms:

There is a mass of neglected mental and neurological disorders, and associated social malfunctions, which specialized mental health services can never reach. Many of them can be managed by community health and other social sector workers, trained, supervised and supported by mental health professionals, in a primary health care setting. Although much improvement can be achieved if available knowledge were to be applied there are significant gaps in our understanding of mental and neurological functioning and disease. (WHO 1981)

It is precisely these 'significant gaps' that the research programme in epidemiological and social psychiatry set itself to cover, to the extent that is made possible by the opportunities provided by WHO's position *vis-à-vis* very different countries and cultures. The overall development of the research component of the WHO programme has been described by Sartorius (1980). What follows below is a summary of several activities, spanning over nearly two decades of research, and illustrating the way in which WHO has launched its 'attack on the lacunae in knowledge relating to the clinical epidemiology of mental disorders' (Shepherd 1983) with the example of schizophrenia, a condition of great public health importance and of inexhaustible scientific interest.

THE WHO MULTI-CENTRE STUDIES ON SCHIZOPHRENIA

The programme of collaborative clinical and epidemiological research into schizophrenia and related disorders, which began in the late 1960s, aimed to develop a methodology that would clear the way for reliable comparative investigations in different populations. It involved psychiatrists and other investigators in over twenty research centres in seventeen countries. The strategy of the programme was characterized by three principal features: (i) use of standardized instruments for case-finding, history-taking, and mental state assessment, translated into equivalent versions of the local languages of the study area population; (ii) data collection by highly qualified psychiatrists trained to use reliably the research instruments (the comparability of assessment was monitored through regular reliability exercises and tests); (iii) a two-tier diagnostic classification of the clinical data, including a clinical diagnosis made by the local team and a reference classification of the standardized mental state data, produced centrally at the study headquarters, using the CATEGO computer program (Wing *et al.* 1974); (iv) multiple assessments of the cases, with periodic follow-up examinations.

The schizophrenia programme included three major studies. The first (1969–77) was the International Pilot Study of Schizophrenia (IPSS) (WHO 1973–79), which involved nine centres in Africa, Asia, Europe, and North America, with a total of 1,202 patients aged 15–44. The patients were selected for presence of psychotic symptoms and for absence of gross organic brain pathology, chronicity, alcohol- or drug-dependence, sensory defects, and mental retardation. The majority of the patients (811) had a clinical diagnosis of schizophrenia; the remaining 391 were classified as affective disorders, reactive psychoses, neuroses, and personality disorders. Each

patient had a detailed standardized clinical examination at the point of inclusion into the study and full reassessments two years and five years later. The
principal research instruments used in the IPSS were the Present State
Examination (PSE) (Wing et al. 1974), a psychiatric history schedule, and a
social description form.

The second WHO study aimed to explore the behavioural impairments and
social disabilities in schizophrenic patients of recent onset. It included 520
patients in seven countries who were examined initially and also at one-year
and two-year follow-up investigations. In addition to the PSE and a history
schedule, two new instruments, the Psychological Impairments Rating
Schedule (PIRS) and the WHO Disability Assessment Schedule (WHO-DAS),
were developed for this study (Jablensky et al. 1980). The PIRS was
designed to describe and quantify negative symptoms, such as deficits in
social and communication skills, while the purpose of the WHO-DAS was to
elicit and rate data on social role performance and the environmental factors
influencing such performance.

The third study (1978–1984), bearing the title 'Determinants of Outcome
of Severe Mental Disorders' (Sartorius et al. 1986; Jablensky et al. 1988),
had a more complex design and included 1,379 patients assessed at twelve
research centres in ten countries. The core of the project was an
epidemiological case-finding and clinical study in which data were collected
on the incidence of schizophrenic disorders in defined geographical areas in
different cultures, the frequency of particular syndromes, the distribution of
various patterns of course, and the dependence of incidence estimates on
alternative schemes of diagnostic classification of the cases (a clinical ICD-9
diagnosis and a reference classification by the CATEGO computer program).
The case-finding method involved an active search for people contacting any
community facilities (medical services, social agencies, traditional or
religious healers) for the first time in their lives because of symptoms that
on screening could be considered psychotic. Each person with a suspected
psychotic illness was given a full examination using standardized instruments
(PSE, a psychiatric and personal history schedule, and a diagnostic and
prognostic form). Follow-up re-examinations took place one year and two
years after the initial evaluation. The series of incident cases collected in this
manner were of particular interest from the point of view of psychiatric
epidemiology because the great majority of them (over 85 per cent) had been
identified within twelve months of the onset of the disorder, i.e., early
enough to rule out any significant pathoplastic effects of treatment or of the
social response to the symptoms. Apart from the standard clinical, social, and
diagnostic assessment of all the cases, subgroups of the patients participated
in special investigations. e.g. a study on the incidence of stressful life events
prior to the acute onset of psychosis (Day et al. 1987), on the relationship
between an index of expressed emotion in the family and the course of the
disorder (Wig et al. 1987; Leff et al. 1987), on the perception of the

patient's behaviour by the social environment, and on the rate of development of behavioural and social role dysfunctions.

CONTRIBUTIONS OF THE WHO STUDIES TO THE KNOWLEDGE BASE ON SCHIZOPHRENIA

The three studies referred to above have produced results which contribute to: (i) the completion of the spectrum of clinical manifestations of schizophrenia; (ii) the assessment of morbid risk; (iii) the establishment of outcome; (iv) the evaluation of the efficacy of treatment; and (v) the conceptual construction of the diagnosis and classification of the group of schizophrenic disorders – five categories which, according to Shepherd (1984), sum up the principal contributions of epidemiology to clinical psychiatry.

Spectrum of clinical manifestations

The major psychopathological syndromes defining the clinical entity of schizophrenia since its delimitation by Kraepelin (1896) and Bleuler (1911) were found to occur in all the populations and geographical areas covered by the WHO studies. Although the clinical picture of schizophrenia was shown to be highly variable (no single symptom being invariably present in every patient and in every setting), the overall profiles of psychopathology associated with a clinical diagnosis of schizophrenia were remarkably similar in the different cultures (figure 29.1).

Schizophrenic patients everywhere tended to have high PSE scores on lack of insight, suspiciousness, delusional mood, delusions or ideas of reference and persecution, flatness of affect, auditory hallucinations, and the delusion of being controlled by an external agency (table 29.1). Furthermore, there was a high degree of concordance between the clinical diagnosis made in the local research centre and the computer reference diagnosis made at the study headquarters (between 63 per cent and 95 per cent of the cases assessed in the different centres as schizophrenic were assigned to a CATEGO class selecting schizophrenic disorders on the basis of formalized classification rules). An average of 56 per cent of the patients with a clinical diagnosis of schizophrenia in the different centres also exhibited one or more of the 'first-rank' symptoms proposed by Schneider (1957) to serve as reliable demarcating features from other non-organic psychotic illnesses. The 'first-rank' symptoms defined a sub-population of schizophrenic patients characterized by generally elevated scores on 'positive' psychotic symptoms. These patients manifested an even greater similarity across the cultures than the total study population.

The spectrum of psychopathology of schizophrenia also includes variations in the presentation of the disorder in the different cultures. The principal

461

Figure 29.1 Profiles on 44 selected PSE items of 586 patients in developing countries and 746 patients in developed countries all meeting 'broad' diagnostic criteria for schizophrenia and related disorders

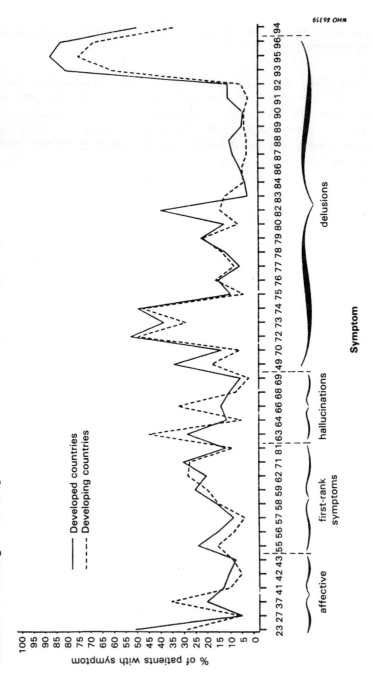

Source WHO Study on Determinants of Outcome of Severe Mental Disorders

Key to figure 29.1 *44 PSE symptoms used to construct psychopathology profiles of subgroups of patients*

AFFECT
23. Depressed mood
27. Morning depression (rating 2 only)
37. Early waking
41. Expansive mood
42. Ideomotor pressure
43. Grandiose ideas and actions

SUBJECTIVE THOUGHT
DISORDER
55. Thought insertion
56. Thought broadcast
57. Thought echo
58. Thought withdrawal
59. Thoughts being read
49. Delusional mood

HALLUCINATIONS
62. Voices in third person

63. Voices speaking to subject
64. Dissociative hallucinations
66. Visual hallucinations
68. Olfactory hallucinations
69. Delusion of smell
70. Other hallucinations

DELUSIONS
71. Control
72. Reference
73. Delusional misinterpretation
74. Persecution
75. Assistance
76. Grandiose abilities
77. Grandiose identity
78. Religious
79. Paranormal
80. Physical forces

81. Alien forces
82. Primary delusions
83. Subcultural
84. Morbid jealousy
86. Sexual
87. Fantastic
88. Guilt
89. Appearance
90. Depersonalization
91. Hypochondriacal
92. Catastrophe
93. Systematization of delusions
94. Evasiveness
95. Preoccupation with delusions or
    hallucinations
96. Acting out of delusions

Table 29.1 International Pilot Study of Schizophrenia (IPSS). Ten most frequently positive 'units of analysis' in patients with diagnosis of paranoid schizophrenia in Aarhus, Agra, Cali, Ibadan, London, Moscow, Prague, Taipei, and Washington

1) Lack of insight	55% (Was) – 100% (Agr, Mos)
2) Suspiciousness	67% (Pra) – 93% (Agr)
3) Delusions of persecution	60% (Cal) – 93% (Agr)
4) Delusions of reference	54% (Mos) – 73% (Agr)
5) Ideas of reference	46% (Aar) – 86% (Tai)
6) Uncooperativeness	28% (Lon) – 82% (Aar)
7) Inadequate description	32% (Lon) – 83% (Was)
8) Delusional mood	36% (Pra) – 75% (Cal)
9) Flatness of affect	41% (Iba) – 68% (Lon)
10) Auditory hallucinations	31% (Was) – 64% (Pra)

differences observed in the WHO studies were those between patients in the Third World and patients in the industrialized countries, and they are likely to reflect a pathoplastic effect of culture. For example, a significantly greater proportion of patients in the developing countries had an acute onset of the disorder, exhibited fewer affective symptoms (such as depression) in the initial phase of the disorder, and had higher scores on auditory and visual hallucinations. On the other hand, a higher percentage of the patients in the developed countries had Schneiderian 'first-rank' symptoms and systematized delusions. However, these were differences of degree rather than of kind, and the symptoms concerned did not cluster together in a way that would suggest separate culture-specific syndromes, different from the central schizophrenic syndrome which was present in all study areas.

Incidence and morbid risk

The WHO study on 'Determinants of Outcome of Severe Mental Disorders' was the first cross-cultural investigation in which the incidence of a major psychiatric disorder, such as schizophrenia, was assessed simultaneously in several different cultural settings, using a uniform methodology (a prospective monitoring of the first contacts with services over two years and an in-depth evaluation of each individual case including a special inquiry about the time and mode of onset of psychotic manifestations.). The incidence of schizophrenic illnesses diagnosed according to ICD-9 was found to be quite comparable in populations which are culturally distant from one another. It varied by no more than a factor of three between areas with high rates (such as the rural area of Raipur Rani near Chandigarh, India) and areas with low rates (such as the county of Aarhus, Denmark). Although the differences observed among those six centres which throughout the study maintained an effective coverage of all first contacts were statistically significant ($p < 0.05$), the size of these differences was not of an order that would suggest major

Figure 29.2 Annual incidence rates per hundred thousand population age 15–54 (both sexes); for the 'broad' and for the 'restrictive' definition of schizophrenia

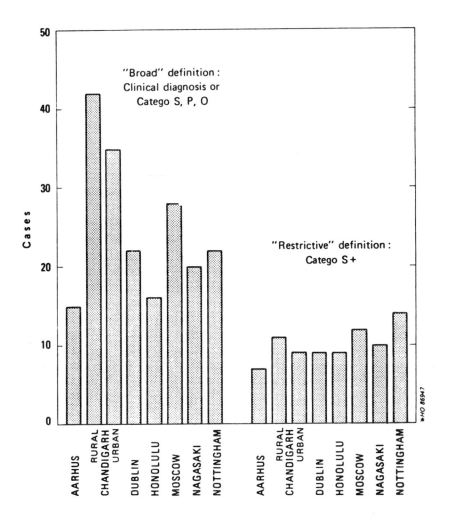

contrasts in the incidence of schizophrenia in different cultures (figure 29.2). Furthermore, a statistical comparison of the rates of the 'nuclear' schizophrenic syndrome (as defined by the CATEGO diagnostic class S+) failed to detect significant differences among the areas and resulted in a reduction of the inter-area variation of the incidence rates. This was contrary to the expectation that, as the mean rates of occurrence of a disease in several

Table 29.2 Morbid risk (percentage) for age 15–54 for a 'broad' and for a 'restrictive' case definition of schizophrenia

Centre	Clinical diagnosis or Catego S,P,O			Catego S+		
	M	F	M+F	M	F	M+F
Aarhus	0.66	0.49	0.52	0.33	0.20	0.27
Chandigarh (rural)	1.48	2.03	1.72	0.54	0.40	0.48
Chandigarh (urban)	1.04	1.21	1.10	0.22	0.42	0.30
Dublin	0.85	0.80	0.83	0.31	0.32	0.32
Honolulu	0.55	0.47	0.50	0.27	0.26	0.26
Moscow	1.08	1.17	1.13	0.39	0.54	0.47
Nagasaki	0.79	0.65	0.72	0.39	0.34	0.37
Nottingham	0.98	0.62	0.80	0.60	0.47	0.54

locations are lowered, the inter-area variation would increase as a result of a susceptibility of the low rates to random variation. The absence of this effect supported the tentative, potentially weighty conclusion that a 'core' schizophrenic syndrome occurs at a similar rate in very different populations.

Since different pathological processes may underlie the same phenotypical expression of a syndrome, it was essential to find supportive evidence, other than the pattern of psychopathology, that the schizophrenic illnesses observed in the different settings belong to the same genus of morbidity. Such evidence was provided by the highly characteristic and consistent age and sex distribution of onsets (a clustering of onsets in the age groups younger than 24 in males and a higher mean age at onset in females) which showed the same pattern in the different study areas. In the 'core' group of CATEGO S+ patients the age- and sex-related patterns of onset were even more sharply delineated than in the entire series of clinical schizophrenia. The age- and sex-specific incidence rates obtained in the WHO study made it possible to establish estimates of disease expectancy (morbid risk) which are shown in table 29.2.

Establishment of outcome

Against this background of important similarities in the incidence and presentation of schizophrenic illnesses in different parts of the world, there were also some striking differences, most pronounced in the longitudinal aspects of the disorder. In both the IPSS and the 'Determinants of Outcome' follow-up studies, there was a marked contrast between the symptomatological similarity of the initial picture of schizophrenia, both within and across the study areas, and the variation in course and outcome which was observed within a period of up to five years after the first examination. Schizophrenia presenting with reliably established symptoms that would meet the current operational criteria of the disorder did not exhibit a single pattern of course.

466

Figure 29.3 Distribution of 233 followed-up schizophrenic patients in developing countries and 295 followed-up schizophrenic patients in developed countries over 5 categories of 2-year overall outcome

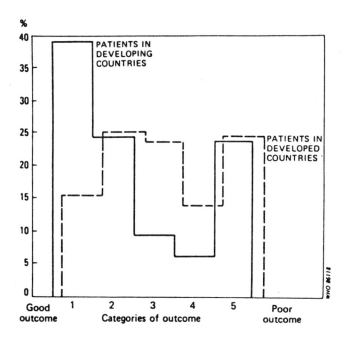

Source WHO International Pilot Study of Schizophrenia

In a proportion of the cases the initial psychotic episode was of a limited duration and resulted in a clinical and social recovery which remained stable throughout the follow-up. At the other extreme, there were cases of a similar initial symptom profile which, however, remained continuously ill and became severely incapacitated in the course of follow-up. There was also an intermediate group of patients with several psychotic attacks and interposed remissions of varying quality. This tripartite distribution of the temporal patterns of schizophrenic illnesses appeared in varying proportions in the different areas, the most marked differences being those between the series of patients in the developing countries and the series of patients in the developed countries. On most course and outcome dimensions (such as the cumulative percentage of the follow-up period during which psychotic symptoms were present, the quality of remissions, the degree of social impairment, and the overall pattern of course) the patients diagnosed as

467

schizophrenic in the developing countries scored significantly better than the patients in the developed countries (figure 29.3).

A number of statistical predictors of the course and outcome of schizophrenic illnesses were identified by stepwise multiple regression and log-linear types of analyses. In summary, the remitting type of schizophrenia was best predicted by an acute onset, absence of previous episode of psychiatric illness, and a stable family background. The chronic pattern represented usually the extension of an illness which had started insidiously in the past, in a socially withdrawn person with other manifestations of abnormal behaviour who was also likely to be single, divorced, or separated from spouse. The recurrent pattern was more frequent in females and the initial episodes of the illness were characterized by an admixture of schizophrenic, affective, and neurotic symptoms. Notably, neither the clinical ICD-9 subtypes of schizophrenia, nor the CATEGO classes predicted course and outcome as effectively as the fairly general characteristics of person and process referred to above. This underscores the difficulty of integrating within a single diagnostic schema the two dimensions of schizophrenia, one providing a symptomatological profile and the other describing course and outcome.

SIGNIFICANCE AND IMPLICATIONS OF THE FINDINGS

First and foremost, the WHO findings on schizophrenia provide a firm epidemiological foundation for further comparative research on the clinical, biological, and psychosocial aspects of a major mental disorder which, in spite of seven decades of research, remains the *Ding an sich* of psychiatry. By demonstrating that a characteristic profile of symptoms, and an age- and sex-related pattern in their occurrence, can be identified reliably in widely varying populations and cultural settings, these studies add significantly to the plausibility of a disease theory of schizophrenia. The tables of comparative age- and sex-specific incidence rates in different populations contain material of critical value to genetic epidemiology, while the standardized psychopathological and 'natural history' data provide ample opportunities for the testing of new clinical and diagnostic hypotheses. It is essential, therefore, that the unique WHO databases on schizophrenia, built up in the course of two decades, and containing over 3,000 patient records, be maintained in a manner that would make it accessible for secondary analysis.

Regardless of any future uses of the WHO data, certain research questions can be asked now, leading to conjectures about the nature of the disorder. For example, the similarity of the form in which the characteristic manifestations of schizophrenia appear in different cultures is a puzzling finding. Considering the variety of social norms, beliefs, attitudes, and stress coping techniques which exist in different cultures, the similarities in the subjective

468

experience of schizophrenic symptoms reported by patients as distant from each other in background and culture as a Yoruba farmer in Nigeria and a Danish fisherman are striking. Why should they experience hallucinatory voices discussing their thoughts and actions precisely in the third person, or perceive their innermost feelings as being bared to others? Unless this observation is shown to be an artefact of the interviewing technique (which is unlikely), it can only suggest that certain basic forms of schizophrenic experience, i.e., the specific disorders of perception, thought, self-image, and ideation, have common pathophysiological mechanisms at a level of function which is relatively untouched by cultural learning. If this is the case, then at least some of the 'first rank' symptoms which index highly specific intra-psychic phenomena might serve as quasi-markers of those schizophrenic syndromes that merit a systematic investigation for underlying commonalties at a neurophysiological and biochemical level.

However, even if certain schizophrenic symptoms are shown to have a common pathophysiological basis in different cultures, the causation of the disorder need not be exclusively construed in 'biological' terms. The finding of similar incidence rates in different populations raises more questions than can be answered at present. Taking into account the genetic, constitutional, nutritional, and other biological differences among the populations studied, the ascertainment of similar incidence rates would hardly be expected. Schizophrenia appears to behave differently from other multifactorial diseases like diabetes or ischaemic heart disease, which show much greater variation in incidence both across and within populations. If schizophrenia is not a single disease of uniform aetiology and pathophysiology, but rather a 'final common pathway' for a variety of pathological processes and developmental anomalies – some with strong genetic contribution and some resulting primarily from environmental factors – then the relatively invariant rate of its occurrence could be the expression of a similarly distributed liability for a schizophrenic type of response to different causes rather than a reflection of a similar distribution of an identical primary cause. Analogies are provided by two other disorders which are known to be aetiologically heterogeneous and to occur with comparable rate of incidence in different populations: epilepsy and mental retardation. Both can be understood as a phenotypical expression of a liability anchored in the general structural and neuro-physiological organization of the brain which can be actuated by a variety of lesions, stresses, or developmental events.

In the instance of schizophrenia, there is also the possibility that some environmental contribution may be provided by psychosocial or cultural conditions modulating the probability of a 'schizophrenic' response to a genetic or developmental lesion. The WHO finding of a more favourable outcome of schizophrenia in the developing countries may be interpreted as an indication that in technologically less complex cultures schizophrenia is less likely to develop into a chronic, deteriorating condition than in societies imposing upon their members more complex, conflicting, and potentially disorienting cognitive requirements. This hypothesis is in need of further exploration, especially in societies which are more contrasting among each other than those already covered by the WHO research programme, e.g. in pre-literate cultures or hunter–gatherer groups in comparison with societies in transition to modernity and 'post-industrial' societies.

In a discussion of possible future strategies of schizophrenia research, Shepherd wrote:

It is now clear that the design of a study aiming to elucidate the natural history of schizophrenia must take account of at least four factors: (1) the identification of all cases in a defined population during a fixed period of time; (2) the application of standardized diagnostic procedures with criteria of known reliability; (3) prospective follow-up procedures, preferably from the onset of first attachment for at least five years, with interim as well as end-point assessments and, preferably, uniform treatment regimes throughout the follow-up period; (4) standardized and independent clinical and social measures of outcome. (Shepherd 1987)

The WHO programme on comparative cross-cultural research in schizophrenia has succeeded in meeting most of these methodological requirements. The real pay-off of the enterprise will be seen in the extent to which its results focus future investigations on those aspects of the disorder which point to its roots in basic and universal characteristics of human nature.

REFERENCES

Bleuler, E. (1911) *Dementia Praecox oder die Gruppe der Schizophrenien*, Leipzig, Wien: Deuticke.

Brugger, C. (1933) 'Psychiatrische Ergebnisse einer medizinischen, anthropologischen und soziologischen Bevölkerungsuntersuchung', *Zeitschrift für Neurologie und Psychiatrie* 146: 489–524.

Day, R., Nielsen, J.A., Korten, A., *et al.* (1987) 'Stressful life events preceding the acute onset of schizophrenia: a cross-national study from the World Health Organization', *Culture, Medicine and Psychiatry* 11: 123–205.

Faris, R.E.L. and Dunham, H.W. (1939) *Mental Disorders in Urban Areas*, Chicago: University of Chicago Press.

Goldberg, J. (1927) *DeLamar Lectures*, Baltimore: Williams & Wilkins.

Jablensky, A., Schwarz, R., and Tomov, T. (1980) 'WHO collaborative study on impairments and disabilities associated with schizophrenic disorders', *Acta Psychiatrica Scandinavica* 62 (supplement 285): 152–63.

Jablensky, A., Sartorius, N., Ernberg, G., *et al.* (1988) *Schizophrenia: Manifestations, Incidence and Course in Different Cultures: A World Health Organization Ten-Country Study* (Psychological Medicine Monograph), to be published.

Kraepelin, E. (1896) *Psychiatrie*, V Auflage, Leipzig: Barth.

Kraepelin, E. (1904) 'Comparative psychology', in S.R. Hirsch and M. Shepherd (eds) *Themes and Variations in European Psychiatry*, Bristol: Wright.

Leff, J., Wig, N.N., Ghosh, H., *et al.* (1987) 'Expressed emotion and schizophrenia in North India; III: Influence of relatives' expressed emotion on the course of schizophrenia in Chandigarh', *British Journal of Psychiatry* 151: 166–73.

Murphy, H.B.M. and Raman, A.C. (1971) 'The chronicity of schizophrenia in indigenous tropical peoples: results of a twelve-year follow-up survey in Mauritius', *British Journal of Psychiatry* 118: 489–97.

Rin, H. and Lin, T.Y. (1962) 'Mental illness among Formosan aborigines as compared with the Chinese in Taiwan', *Journal of Mental Science* 108: 134–46.

Sartorius, N. (1980) 'The research component of the WHO mental health programme', *Psychological Medicine* 10: 175–85.

Sartorius, N., Jablensky, A., Korten, A., *et al.* (1986) 'Early manifestations and first-contact incidence of schizophrenia in different cultures', *Psychological Medicine* 16: 909–28.

Schneider, K. (1957) 'Primäre und sekundäre Symptome bei der Schizophrenie', *Fortschrifte der Neurologie und Psychiatrie* 25: 487–90.

Shepherd, M. (1978) 'Epidemiology and clinical psychiatry', *British Journal of Psychiatry* 133: 289–98.

Shepherd, M. (1983) *The Psychosocial Matrix of Psychiatry: Collected Papers*, London, New York: Tavistock, 277.

Shepherd, M. (1984) 'The contribution of epidemiology to clinical psychiatry', *American Journal of Psychiatry* 141: 1574–5.

Shepherd, M. (1987) 'Formulation of new research strategies on schizophrenia', in H. Häfner, W.F. Gattaz and W. Janzarik (eds) *Search for the Causes of Schizophrenia*, Berlin, Heidelberg, New York, London, Paris, Tokyo: Springer, 29–38.

Stengel, E. (1959) 'Classification of mental disorders', *WHO Bulletin* 21: 601–3.

Strömgren, E. (1938) 'Beiträge zur psychiatrischen Erblehre, auf Grund von Untersuchungen an einer Inselbevolkerung', *Acta Psychiatrica et Neurologica*, supplement 19.

WHO (1960) *Epidemiology of Mental Disorders: Eighth Report of the Expert Committee of Mental Health* (Technical Report Series No. 185), Geneva: WHO.

WHO (1973) *Report of the International Pilot Study of Schizophrenia, Volume I*, Geneva: WHO.

WHO (1979) *Schizophrenia: An International Follow-Up Study*, Chichester: Wiley.

WHO (1981) *Social Dimensions of Mental Health*, Geneva: WHO.

Wig, N.N., Menon, D.K., Bedi, H., *et al.* (1987) 'Expressed emotion and schizophrenia in North India: I. Cross-cultural transfer of ratings of relatives' expressed emotion', *British Journal of Psychiatry* 151: 156–60.

Wing, J.K., Cooper, J.E., and Sartorius, N. (1974) *Measurement and Classification of Psychiatric Symptoms*, Cambridge: Cambridge University Press.

30

The NIMH Epidemiological Research Program: Past, Present, and Future

Darrel Regier

An overview will be provided of significant epidemiologic research conducted within the National Institute of Mental Health (NIMH). Admittedly selective in its emphasis, the paper will review a range of studies conducted since the initiation of the NIMH research programmes in 1949. Epidemiological research areas included are defined in textbooks as descriptive, analytic, or experimental studies (Morris 1964: Regier and Burke 1984) – areas which form the bases for much of clinical research in medicine (Feinstein 1985). The role of the NIMH in these studies is multifaceted and includes co-ordinating peer review of research applications, financial support judgements, 'state-of-the-art' analyses of scientific fields, stimulation of research fields to overcome barriers to further progress, administrative co-ordination and collaborative research in multi-centre studies, and the conduct of certain types of research – some of which cannot be accomplished by investigators outside a federal research setting.

NIMH was developed at the end of the Second World War during a period of widespread public concern about the extent of mental disorders in military recruits and in the general population. A basic laboratory research programme was established in the intramural programme under Seymour Kety and extramural research studies were supported for university-based investigators. Early intramural basic research studies included fundamental neuroscience work on brain physiology which led to a Nobel Prize for Julius Axelrod's work in identifying the metabolism of chemical neurotransmitters, their uptake at the presynaptic neurone, and the effect of psychoactive drugs in inhibiting such uptake (Axelrod 1970). A major advance in basic neuroscience techniques was accomplished by Sokoloff's Lasker Award winning development of the deoxyglucose method for determining brain metabolic activity – a method critical for the development of positron emission tomography (PET) scanning of the brain (Sokoloff et al. 1977). Among some of the earliest extramural research studies supported were descriptive epidemiological studies in Sterling County (Nova Scotia), mid-town Manhattan, and New Haven, Connecticut, to determine prevalence rates of mental

472

disorders in the civilian population and their possible stress-related aetiology.

A major implicit objective of the Institute has been to integrate research findings about basic biological mechanisms with studies of clinical psychopathology and the behavioural expression of physiological mechanisms. Shepherd (1978) has described epidemiology as a useful integrating framework for bridging the gap which remains between basic and clinical research. Such a framework incorporates epidemiologically focused studies as an essential part of clinical research and a means of testing the strength of biological as well as psychosocial correlates of clinical disorders. This presentation uses the framework suggested by Shepherd to illustrate how epidemiological research has developed within the National Institute of Mental Health and how it has begun to bridge the gap between basic physiology and more descriptive clinical research. It will focus most specifically on the areas of affective disorders (depression), with illustrations of findings from a range of these studies, and will outline future opportunities now in the planning stage at the NIMH.

The basic framework of descriptive, experimental, and analytic epidemiological research will include selected examples of individual research studies in these areas and related developments in research methods. NIMH staff functions will also be emphasized in the previously described roles of carrying out research support judgements, 'state-of-the-art analyses' of scientific field opportunities and needs, collaborative research and co-ordination, and other direct participation of NIMH scientists in the conduct of research.

DESCRIPTIVE EPIDEMIOLOGY – COMMUNITY STUDIES

Shortly after the founding of the NIMH, there were three major community studies in the US and Canada that received NIMH support. These included the Stirling County (Leighton *et al.* 1963), Midtown-Manhattan (Srole *et al.* 1962), and Baltimore Morbidity (Commission on Chronic Illness 1957) studies. The first two studies used a range of case-identification methods which relied heavily on symptom scales to determine rates of mental disorder in the community whereas the Baltimore study relied on diagnoses by general medical physicians – diagnostic judgements were reviewed by psychiatrists in all three studies. Because of the absence of explicit research diagnostic criteria in these studies, it is difficult to interpret the prevalence rates of specific disorders. High symptom levels consistent with mental disorder diagnoses with 'significant impairment' were found at rates ranging from 10 per cent to 24 per cent of the population.

After these major community prevalence studies in the 1950s, additional smaller studies were conducted to disentangle the reasons for finding higher rates of severe psychiatric disorders in lower socio-economic classes (Dohrenwend and Dohrenwend 1969). There was continued reliance on dimensional scales, including a new one developed by the NIMH to identify rates of depressive symptomatology – the Center for Epidemiological Studies Depression (CES-D) Scale (Radloff and Locke 1986: Comstock and Helsing 1976). Additional studies were supported to examine the role of stress in the aetiology of mental disorders and a vigorous effort focused on stress related to major life events (Dohrenwend and Dohrenwend 1981).

In the mid-1970s, Weissman was able to conduct a community follow-up study by using the Schedule for Schizophrenia and Affective Disorders (SADS-L) (Endicott and Spitzer 1978) in a newly adapted lifetime form for use in community epidemiological surveys (Weissman and Myers 1978). The major significance of this NIMH-supported study was that it represented the first application of a structured diagnostic interview, based on the explicit Research Diagnostic Criteria (RDC) (Spitzer *et al.* 1978) ever performed in a community survey. The demonstration that such a survey could be carried out with non-psychiatrist interviewers was of major importance in paving the way for the later Epidemiological Catchment Area (ECA) studies in the US.

DESCRIPTIVE EPIDEMIOLOGY – SPECIALIZED TREATMENT SETTINGS

In addition to general population studies to determine prevalence rates of mental disorders and their correlation with domestic psychosocial stresses (in contrast to war-related stress), other descriptive studies focused on the correlates of disorders in treatment settings. A major study in this category was the Hollingshead and Redlich study of *Social Class and Mental Illness* in New Haven (Hollingshead and Redlich 1958). This landmark study graphically illustrated the higher rates of severe mental disorders and of institutionalization for those in lower social classes. Social concerns stimulated by this study included the inadequacy of community treatment for mental disorders which, in turn, helped launch the US Community Mental Health Centers legislation in the mid-1960s.

Two of the most significant and productive NIMH staff contributions to descriptive epidemiology were provided by Morton Kramer during his thirty-year tenure as Director of the NIMH Biometry Branch, a unit which later evolved into the Division of Biometry and Epidemiology and more recently reorganized with components in a Division of Clinical Research and a Division of Biometry and Applied Sciences. During his NIMH tenure, Dr Kramer, along with Drs Pollock and Taube, developed the NIMH National Reporting Program (Redick *et al.* 1983). This mental health statistical programme monitors psychiatric admissions and discharges, along with associated diagnoses, to in-patient and out-patient mental health facilities in the US. It has successfully traced variations in treated prevalence rates through the early 1950s period of increasing hospitalization for mental illness, and the period from the mid-1950s to the late 1970s covering deinstitutionalization and the expansion of community psychiatric services.

Kramer's second contribution was made possible by the availability of comparable mental health statistics from England and from the US National Reporting Program. Kramer noted that US mental hospitals were reporting rates of schizophrenia several times higher, and rates of affective disorder several times lower, than some facilities in the United Kingdom (Kramer 1961). This 'state-of-the art' analysis rapidly led to a US/UK study, supported by the NIMH, to determine the reason for these different treated prevalence rates. The findings of the study demonstrated that differences in observed treated prevalence rates for schizophrenia and affective disorders reflected differences in the application of relatively vague diagnostic criteria instead of any real differences in mental disorder rates (Kramer 1969: Cooper *et al*. 1972).

Under the auspice of the World Health Organization, the NIMH subsequently supported the International Pilot Study of Schizophrenia (IPSS) in nine countries to determine if any differences could be found in the characteristics of schizophrenia associated with widely varying cultures (WHO 1973). This landmark study also involved intramural and extramural NIMH scientific participation, including Wynn, Strauss, Carpenter, Kramer, and Bartko, and demonstrated the existence of a similar type of schizophrenic disorder in every culture studied (Sartorius *et al*. 1974). A longitudinal follow-up study of patients with schizophrenia was subsequently supported through WHO to assess the differential course of schizophrenia in different cultures and the 'determinants' of any differences in outcomes (Sartorius *et al*. 1986).

DESCRIPTIVE EPIDEMIOLOGY – PRIMARY CARE TREATMENT SETTINGS

Since large-scale community studies up to the mid-1970s were generally unable to assess prevalence rates of specific disorders, and specialized mental health treatment settings tended to include only the more seriously ill, prevalence studies in general medical practice settings offered several advantages. Such practices enable coverage of at least 70 per cent of the population in any one year who visit a general medical physician, they permit cross-sectional diagnoses based on a longitudinal relationship with a patient, and the general medical practitioner is a highly trained interviewer with the potential for making valid diagnostic assessments.

During the 1960s and 70s, there was a particular interest among NIMH investigators to follow a British tradition of examining prevalence rates of mental disorders in general medical practice settings. In England, these studies took on a more rigorous form under the direction of Michael Shepherd and the General Practice Research Unit (Shepherd *et al.* 1966). Stimulated in part by this interest, NIMH investigators Locke, Goldberg, and Rosen conducted a series of collaborative studies identifying rates of psychiatric disorder in primary care settings (Locke and Gardner 1969: Rosen *et al.* 1972). Goldberg, in particular, linked studies of prevalence with service use to determine the relative effect in decreasing use of general medical services when referrals to psychiatric specialists were made (Goldberg *et al.* 1970).

In the late 1970s, a Primary Care Research Section was established by Regier and Goldberg in the NIMH Division of Biometry and Epidemiology (Burns *et al.* 1979). This section was modelled in large part after the General Practice Research Unit of Shepherd and was developed to study systematically the prevalence rates of mental disorders (Goldberg *et al.* 1979: Goldberg *et al.* 1980; Hoeper *et al.* 1980), the level of service utilization by patients with these disorders (Hankin *et al.* 1982), the most appropriate division of responsibility between generalists and specialists in the care of these disorders (Regier *et al.* 1982), and the role of primary care physicians in caring for the chronic mentally ill (Regier *et al.* 1985). This research programme has continued with significant contributions from Burns, Burke, Kessler, Kamerow *et al.* (1986) and a wide range of investigators supported in extramural academic institutions.

DESCRIPTIVE EPIDEMIOLOGY – LINKAGE OF COMMUNITY, SPECIALIZED TREATMENT SETTING, PRIMARY CARE SETTING, AND SERVICE RESEARCH

The President's Commission on Mental Health

In the late 1970s, the President's Commission on Mental Health (1978) was established immediately after President Carter entered office. This Commission was a special concern of the First Lady, Rosalyn Carter, who personally guided its development. In the White House Executive Order establishing the Commission, the first priority given was to describe how the mentally ill were being served, determine the extent of underservice, and determine who was affected by such underservice (The White House 1977). An NIMH staff group of Regier, Goldberg, and Taube conducted a 'state-of-the-art' secondary analysis of prevalence data, and compared these data with service use or treated prevalence data obtained from the NIMH National Reporting Program and from the primary care sector research. The resulting synthesis of the most conservative estimate of prevalence, incidence, and service use rates in the US was published in the final report of the Commission and as a freestanding paper entitled, 'The *De Facto* U.S. Mental Health Services System'. The findings included an estimated 15 per cent annual prevalence of mental disorders with only 3 per cent (one-fifth of those affected) using specialist mental health services in one year (Regier *et al.* 1978). Of special note was the estimate that 54 per cent of individuals with these disorders were seen exclusively in the primary care sector although the level of specific mental health services could not be determined.

Despite a considerable effort to document the data sources in support of prevalence and service use estimates, this undertaking highlighted the major gaps in our knowledge of prevalence rates of specific mental disorders and how these related to service utilization in general medical, specialized mental health, and other human service settings. The ADAMHA Administrator, at that time Dr Gerald Klerman, requested an agency-wide review of epidemiological, service system, and statistical reporting programmes (Regier and Rosenfeld 1979). Following this review, research programmes were announced in mental health service systems research and there was expansion of the Primary Care Research Section established in 1977. In addition, a framework for developing a clinical services research programme that would assess the effectiveness of primary care mental health services was conceptualized and developed by Burke.

A mental health economics research programme was established under Taube to address the health insurance and other financing issues affecting the delivery of mental health services (Taube *et al.* 1985). Finally, support was obtained to launch a new generation of psychiatric epidemiology studies that would use the new diagnostic criteria of DSM-III (American Psychiatric Association 1980) to identify prevalence rates, incidence rates, and service use rates that would more directly address a major need, identified by the President's Commission, to link epidemiology and services research findings.

The Epidemiological Catchment Area (ECA) study

Analyses for the President's Commission, reported on earlier, led the NIMH staff to conceptualize a comprehensive epidemiological and health services research study that would fill several of the major gaps identified. The Epidemiological Catchment Area (ECA) study was designed to start with a sample survey to determine the prevalence and incidence of mental disorder in a total (community and institutionalized) population. Individuals so identified would subsequently be followed longitudinally to determine their utilization of mental health services in all general medical, specialized mental health, or other human service facilities. Both prevalence and utilization data would then allow analysis of the population groups most affected by mental disorder and by an under-utilization of services (Regier *et al.* 1984).

Before any study could be conducted, it was necessary to develop a diagnostic instrument for use in a large enough population survey to obtain a sufficient number of subjects with low prevalence disorders, such as schizophrenia, to do meaningful analyses. The NIMH staff reviewed all available instruments and decided to develop a new one that was modelled on the St Louis, Renard Diagnostic Interview (Helzer *et al.* 1981) and would use the soon-to-be-published DSM-III criteria. Lee Robins was provided a contract to develop the interview along with Robert Spitzer who received a separate contract to assure its coverage of the DSM-III criteria. The NIMH Diagnostic Interview Schedule (DIS) was the instrument developed for this study and it has subsequently been used in many additional national and international investigations (NIMH 1981: Robins *et al.* 1981). It is useful to note that several major diagnostic interviews now in active research use – the Present State Examination (PSE) (Wing *et al.* 1974), the SADS, the SADS-L, and the DIS – were all developed (or significantly refined) for specific NIMH-related collaborative research studies.

The ECA was a major collaborative study between the NIMH and academic investigators in five university sites including Yale, Johns Hopkins, Washington University – St Louis, Duke, and UCLA. The study would also never have been conducted without the active support of Mrs Carter who was called upon during the Office of Management and Budget (OMB) clearance process to certify that this study, and all of the sensitive data to be collected, were supported by the President's Commission recommendations.

Since the study design has been adequately described elsewhere (Eaton *et al.* 1984: Eaton and Kessler 1985), only a few of the major findings relating to affective disorders will be described. Data on the six-month prevalence (Myers *et al.* 1984: Blazer *et al.* 1985; Burnam *et al.* 1987), six-month service utilization (Shapiro *et al.* 1984; Hough *et al.* 1987), and life-time prevalence (Robins *et al.* 1984: Karno *et al.* 1987) have now been published for all five sites. One-month, six-month, and life-time prevalence rates, combined and standardized to the US population by age, sex, and race are also in press (Regier *et al.* 1988). The data to be presented here are drawn from the US standardized six-month prevalence data and service utilization analyses. They will be used to illustrate the linkage between community prevalence, specialized mental health treatment setting, primary care setting, and general service utilization studies.

ECA affective disorder results

In the first wave of interviews in the study, it was possible to determine that 19.1 per cent of the adult population could be identified as having at least one alcohol, drug abuse, or mental disorder. Affective disorders were found in 5.8 per cent of the population including 0.5 per cent with bipolar disorder, 3.0 per cent with major depressive episode, and 3.3 per cent with dysthymia. Overall, female rates (7.5 per cent) were found to be about twice those found for men (3.9 per cent) although rates for bipolar disorder were not significantly different by gender groups. Among age groups, the rates were highest in the 25–44 year age group with non-significant differences in the next highest age group of 45–64. When all other variables are controlled, there are no significant differences between white, or black, or Hispanic race/ethnicity groups or between socioeconomic status groups. Significantly higher rates were found for separated/divorced and widowed persons in comparison with the married group.

Given the substantial number of people affected by depressive disorders, an immediate analytic issue was to determine the extent to which they receive some type of care in the mental health, general health, or other human service settings. Our analyses show that during a six-month period, slightly less than one in five (19 per cent) are seen by mental health specialists, three-quarters (74 per cent) are seen by general medical physicians, less than one in ten (9 per cent) are seen by other human service agencies (e.g. social service or clergy), and 21 per cent are not seen by any professional. Although there is significant overlap in service between mental health specialists and general medical physicians, 54 per cent of individuals with depressive disorders are seen exclusively by primary care physicians.

From a treatment perspective, a major issue is to determine the number identified as having a disorder and receiving treatment specifically for mental disorders in general medical and other human service settings. Despite the fact that three-quarters visit general medical physicians for some reason, only 17 per cent of individuals with these disorders receive some mental health treatment in these general medical settings. About 5 per cent receive mental health services in other human service settings. There is minimal overlap in services provided in general medical and other human service settings with the 19 per cent seen in specialized mental health settings. Fully 63 per cent receive no mental health treatment during a six-month time period. Individuals with major depression have the highest rate of treatment in specialized or general medical settings at 38 per cent, followed by 33 per cent with bipolar disorder and 24 per cent with dysthymia.

An additional question relates to the level of treatment intensity for individuals with these disorders. The average number of visits to any of the three service settings for all individuals, regardless of diagnosis, is three visits per person/six-months of which one in three is for a mental health reason. About one-half (48 per cent) of these visits are to mental health specialists, only 13 per cent are to general medical providers, and 38 per cent are to other human service professionals. For individuals with affective disorders, the average number of visits is three times as high (nine visits per six-months), of which five out of nine are for mental health reasons and slightly more than half (54 per cent) of these are to mental health specialists. If only the health sector is considered, 84 per cent of the mental health visits are to specialists.

A final question, which has yet to be addressed in a systematic way, is how effective are the mental health services provided in any of these treatment settings? The translation of research on treatment efficacy in controlled clinical trials, addressed in the next section, into treatment effectiveness in routine clinical practice is a major challenge in clinical medicine. The application of epidemiological methods to answer these questions is the field of clinical services research now under development at the NIMH (Regier and Burke 1984).

479

Conclusions from this analysis of depressive disorders include the following:

1. Affective disorders are widespread (about 6 per cent in six-months) and 80 per cent of affected persons are seen in professional settings in six-months where they could be screened, diagnosed, and treated.
2. The major location for early recognition and treatment is in the general medical sector where 74 per cent are seen in six-months.
3. Individuals with depression are heavy users of medical services, visiting for non-mental health reasons twice as frequently as the average and three times more frequently overall.
4. Of those with a depressive disorder who visited a general medical setting, only 23 per cent (17 per cent of the 74 per cent visiting) acknowledged receiving a mental health service in that setting. Overall about two-thirds of individuals with these disorders receive no mental health services.
5. In the absence of a robust method of primary prevention, the greatest potential for decreasing prevalence lies in the early identification and treatment of these disorders to reduce their duration and associated morbidity, and to prevent relapse. A new NIMH prevention programme, entitled the Depression Awareness, Recognition, and Treatment (D/ART) Program, has recently been launched. This programme is aimed at improving the recognition of affective disorders among the general public and general medical practitioners as well as increasing knowledge about the latest treatment advances.

EXPERIMENTAL EPIDEMIOLOGY – CONTROLLED CLINICAL TRIALS

The introduction of controlled clinical trials of psychotropic drugs received major support from the NIMH in the past twenty-five years. Clinical trials of phenothiazines (May 1968), antidepressants (Klerman and Cole 1965: Klein *et al*. 1980), and lithium (Baastrup *et al*. 1970; Prien *et al*.1973) have introduced prospective cohort intervention designs into the mainstream of psychiatric research. The same experimental epidemiology designs have more recently been applied to the study of psychosocial interventions for the treatment of depressive disorders (Elkin *et al*. 1985).

The need for methodological rigour in interpreting the results of controlled clinical trials was a recurrent theme for Shepherd (Blackwell and Shepherd 1968). Such an emphasis, although associated with considerable controversy in the case of lithium trials, ultimately contributed to clear methodological principles for clinical trials more generally (Grof *et al*. 1970; Medical Research Council Drug Trials Subcommittee 1981: Meinert 1986).

ANALYTIC EPIDEMIOLOGY – CASE CONTROL STUDIES

Collaborative depression studies

During the 1960s and early 1970s, NIMH staff developed a major interest in identifying biological and psychosocial correlates of affective disorders. The psychobiology of depression collaborative research studies, initiated by NIMH staff (Katz *et al.* 1979) and senior extramural research investigators, provided a major contribution to refining diagnostic criteria and developing standardized interviews. This study was responsible for development of the RDC and the SADS diagnostic interview. It also used a prospective cohort for examining multiple potential biological (Koslow *et al.* 1983) and psychosocial correlates of affective disorders. Longitudinal follow-up studies to examine naturalistic treatment of these disorders (Keller *et al.* 1986), clinical course, and familial aggregation (Klerman *et al.* 1985) have made significant contributions to this field.

Population genetic studies

Addressing the issue of schizophrenia from a more aetiological framework, Seymour Kety and David Rosenthal of NIMH and their Danish collaborators recognized an opportunity to separate environmental and genetic influences in the development of schizophrenia through the Danish Adoption Study. This classic case-control study identified higher rates of 'exposure' of adoptees with schizophrenia to a genetic history of schizophrenia in their biological relatives than was found in the genetic history of adoptees without the disorder (Kety and Rosenthal 1968).

It is ironic that one of the most significant studies to establish a biological predisposition to development of schizophrenia, was conducted by a biological psychiatrist (Kety) with no formal epidemiological training or disciplinary identification. The fact that an epidemiological research design was used to carry out such a study gives added credence to Shepherd's contention that epidemiology can serve the bridging function of integrating biological and clinical research.

Population and molecular genetic studies

Of all the epidemiological studies supported by the NIMH in the past forty years, none comes closer to the ideal of integrating basic and clinical research than the recent NIMH-supported study by Egeland *et al.* (1987). This study of affective disorders in an Amish population began as a population genetics epidemiological study and was supported for over a decade under the careful stewardship of the NIMH project officer Ben Locke. Despite several less-than-enthusiastic peer reviews of the study and modest priority scores, Locke facilitated expert technical assistance and exercised funding judgements to assure payment out of priority score order. He saw the excellent potential of this study and encouraged the linkage of molecular genetics experts with the population genetics originators of the study. The ultimate outcome of the study was identification of a specific gene fragment that was transmitted on chromosome 11 between three generations in one family, and was associated with transmission of bipolar affective disorder.

The linkage of clinicians, descriptive epidemiologists, population geneticists, and molecular genetics staff again supported Shepherd's contention that epidemiology can serve as the bridge between clinical and basic research. Future research studies should benefit from a greatly expanded thrust to develop other biological correlates which may in turn be studied for their naturally occurring rates in larger populations representative of the community and of the specific disorders.

RESEARCH METHODS

A distinguishing characteristic of epidemiology research, in contrast to clinical practice, is that such research focuses on a group as the unit of study rather than on individual patients. The ability to conduct studies in groups, large or small, is dependent upon a reliable case identification or diagnostic method which incorporates clinically relevant diagnostic criteria. The individual clinician may develop his or her own interviewing and physical examination procedure to apply to the group of patients in an individual practice. Although consistency in diagnosis may be relatively good for all patients in one clinician's practice, the US/UK study and others have shown the discrepancies that may be introduced in diagnoses involving large numbers of patients.

Since research studies require comparable diagnoses in all members of a group, there is considerable concern for development of good statistical reporting systems, clear diagnostic criteria, and the reliable application of these criteria. Statistical measures, such as Cohen's 'kappa' have been developed to assess reliability or the degree to which diagnostic agreement is obtained over that expected by chance alone. Increasingly explicit diagnostic criteria and structured diagnostic instruments, which facilitate consistent and thorough reviews of psychopathological symptoms, have become essential for advances in all clinical and epidemiological research.

Because of the centrality of diagnostic criteria and assessment instruments to the advancement of epidemiological research, NIMH staff have been actively involved in these activities since the beginning of the NIMH. Kramer was a key consultant to the committees developing ICD-8 and ICD-9 as well as the first and second editions of the American Psychiatric Association (APA) Diagnostic and Statistical Manuals (DSM-I and DSM-II). The NIMH also supported research studies that developed the Research Diagnostic Criteria (RDC) and then supported many of the subsequent diagnostic workgroups and field trials of DSM-III and DSM-IIIR – a set of diagnostic criteria that followed closely in the tradition of the RDC. NIMH staff have continued to serve as active participants in the evaluation of this major advance in psychiatric nosology (Regier 1987). With regard to diagnostic instruments, the previously described developments in the PSE, SADS, CES-D, and DIS instruments have all received substantial support from NIMH.

In 1978, the US Alcohol, Drug Abuse and Mental Health Administration (ADAMHA) Administrator, Gerald Klerman, and the World Health Organization (WHO) Mental Health Director, Norman Sartorius, initiated a joint programme to review diagnostic criteria on a world-wide basis (WHO/ADAMHA 1985). The formal co-operative agreement supporting this endeavour has advanced through the first two phases of multiple diagnostic workgroups (1979–82) and a major international conference (Copenhagen 1982) to the third phase focused on development of diagnostic instruments for use in epidemiological and clinical research studies. Field trials are now being conducted for several of these instruments including the Composite International Diagnostic Interview (CIDI), which combines elements of the DIS and PSE; the schedule for Clinical Assessment in Neuropsychiatry (SCAN), which is based on a tenth revision of the PSE; and the Personality Disorder Examination (PDE). All of these instruments are being constructed in conjunction with the new ICD-10 and DSM criteria developments. Although not covered under the co-operative agreement, ADAMHA staff are co-ordinating the North American field trial of the ICD-10 to assure a throrough review of these new international diagnostic criteria.

Within the US, NIMH has been involved in supporting Spitzer and Williams' development of the Structured Clinical Interview for DSM-III (SCID) through contracts and grants. This interview has been used in several international pharmacotherapy trials of anxiety disorders and in a multi-site NIMH collaborative study on treatment strategies for schizophrenia. A final diagnostic interview that has been under development by NIMH for the past several years is a Diagnostic Interview Schedule for Children (DISC) which will be used for future epidemiological studies of children and adolescents.

FUTURE DIRECTIONS

Epidemiological research studies supported by the NIMH have begun to bridge the gaps between clinical practice and research on basic mechanisms underlying psychopathology. Work on diagnostic criteria and assessment instruments required for epidemiological studies has greatly advanced the precision of clinical and research communication. It is now possible for clinicians around the world to specify both the explicit criteria used in describing a patient, and the operational application of those criteria in a diagnostic instrument. The potential for comparing more homogeneous patient populations in controlled clinical trials or in risk factor (biological or psychosocial

483

correlate) studies is greatly enhanced by these developments.

Of particular importance in future studies involving biological correlates, such as the Egeland *et al.* (1987) genetic studies, is the possibility of developing a reciprocal interaction between the initial descriptive diagnostic criteria and a more refined biologically-based diagnostic criterion which emerges from genetically similar subtypes of a disorder. In order to prevent spurious correlations, epidemiological studies will be necessary to assess the frequency of putative biological correlates of mental disorders in representative samples of individuals with those disorders. Past difficulties in replicating biological markers, such as Dexamethasone Suppression Test (DST) correlates with affective disorders, may be attributed in part to an insufficient attention to patient sampling.

We look forward to an increasingly synergistic relationship between clinical practice, clinical research, and basic research that will build on the existing scientific base briefly reviewed in this paper. Two new research programmes have just been launched within the NIMH including a 'National Plan for Research on Schizophrenia' and a programme directed toward 'Opportunities for NIMH Neuroscience Research – the Decade of the Brain'. Investments in these enterprises will clearly provide returns of higher quality if the epidemiological framework recommended by Shepherd finally enters the mainstream of psychiatric research. Such a framework will no longer confuse descriptive epidemiological studies, concerned only with mental disorder prevalence or incidence rates, with the whole of epidemiological research. Rather, such research will be seen as part of the research fabric that will eventually unlock us from our continuing ignorance of the basic mechanisms underlying some of humanity's most disabling disorders.

REFERENCES

American Psychiatric Association, Committee on Nomenclature and Statistics (1988) *Diagnostic and Statistical Manual of Mental Disorders*, third edition, Washington, DC: APA.

Axelrod, J. (1970) *Noradrenaline: Fate and Control of its Biosynthesis*, The Nobel Foundation.

Baastrup, P.C., Poulson, J.C., Schou, M., Thomsen, K. and Amdisen, A. (1970) 'Prophylactic lithium: double-blind discontinuation in manic-depressive and recurrent disorders', *Lancet* 2: 326–30.

Blackwell, B. and Shepherd, M. (1968) 'Prophylactic lithium: another therapeutic myth? An examination of the evidence to date', *Lancet*, i: 968–71.

Blazer, D., George, L.K., Landerman, R., Pennybacker, M., Melville, M.L., Woodbury, M., Manton, K.G., Jordan, K. and Locke, B.A. (1985) 'Psychiatric disorders: rural/urban comparison', *Archives of General Psychiatry* 42: 651–6.

Burnam, M.A., Hough, R.L., Escobar, J.I., Karno, M., Timbers, D.M., Telles, C.A. and Locke, B.Z. (1987) 'Six-month prevalence of specific psychiatric disorders among Mexican Americans and non-Hispanic whites in Los Angeles', *Archives of General Psychiatry* 44: (8): 687–94.

Burns, B.J., Regier, D.A., Goldberg, I.D. and Kessler, L.G. (1979) 'Future directions in primary care/mental health research', *International Journal of Mental Health* 8: 130–40.

Commission on Chronic Illness (1957) *Chronic Illness in the United States, IV: Chronic Illness in a Large city: The Baltimore Study*, Cambridge, Mass: Harvard University Press.

Comstock, G.W. and Helsing, K. (1976) 'Symptoms of depression in two communities', *Psychological Medicine* 6: 551–63.

Cooper, J.E., Kendell, R.E., Gurland, G.J., Sharpe, L., Copeland, J.R.M. and Simon, R. (1972) *Psychiatric Diagnosis in New York and London*, London: Oxford University Press.

Dohrenwend, B.P. and Dohrenwend, B.S. (1969) *Social Status and Psychological Disorder: A Causal Inquiry*, New York: Wiley.

Dohrenwend, B.S., And Dohrenwend, B.P. (1981) *Stressful Life Events and Their Contents*, New York: Prodist.

Eaton, W.W., Holzer, C.E., Von Korff, M., Anthony, J.C., Helzer, J.E., George, L., Burnam, M.A., Boyd, J.H., Kessler, L.G. and Locke, B.Z. (1984) 'The design of the Epidemiologic Catchment Area Surveys', *Archives of General Psychiatry* 41 (10): 942–8.

Eaton, W.W. and Kessler, L.G. (eds) (1985) *Epidemiologic Field Methods in Psychiatry: The NIMH Epidemiologic Catchment Area Program*, New York: Academic Press.

Egeland, J.A., Gerhard, D.S., Pauls, D.L., Sussex, J.N., Kidd, K.K., Allen, C.R., Hosterrer, A.M. and Housman, E.D. (1987) 'Bipolar affective disorders linked to DNA markers on chromosome 11', *Nature* 325: 783–7.

Elkin, I., Parloff, M.B., Hadley, S.W. and Autry, J.H. (1985) 'NIMH treatment of depression collaborative research program', *Archives of General Psychiatry* 42: 305–16.

Endicott, J. and Spitzer, R.L. (1978) 'A diagnostic interview: the schedule for affective disorders and schizophrenia', *Archives of General Psychiatry* 35: 837–44.

Feinstein, A. (1985) *Clinical Epidemiology: The Architecture of Clinical research*, Philadelphia: W.B. Saunders.

Goldberg, I.D., Krantz, G. and Locke, B.Z. (1970) 'Effect of a short-term outpatient psychiatric therapy benefit on the utilization of medical services in a prepaid group practice medical program', *Medical Care* 8: 419–28.

Goldberg, I.D., Regier, D.A., McInerny, T.K., Pless, I.B. and Roghmann, K.J. (1979) 'The role of the pediatrician in the delivery of mental health services to children', *Pediatrics* 63 (6): 898–909.

Goldberg, I.D., Regier, D.A. and Burns, B.J. (eds) (1980) *Use of Health and Mental Health Outpatient Services in Four Organized Health Care Settings*, National Institute of Mental Health, Series DN, No. 1, DHHS Publication No. (ADM) 80–859.

Graf, P., Schou, M., Angst, J., Baastrup, P.C. and Weis, P. (1970) 'Methodological problems of prophylactic trials in recurrent affective disorders', *British Journal of Psychiatry* 116: 599–619.

Hankin, J.R., Steinwachs, D.M., Regier, D.A., Burns, B.J., Goldberg, I.D. and Hoeper, E.W. (1982) 'Use of general medical care services by persons with mental disorders', *Archives of General Psychiatry* 39: 225–31.

Helzer, J.E., Robins, L.N., Croughan, J.L. and Weiner, A. (1981) 'Renard Diagnostic Interview', *Archives of General Psychiatry* 38: 393–8.

Hoeper, E.W., Nycz, G.R., Cleary, P.D., Regier, D.A. and Goldberg, I.D. (1980) 'Estimated prevalence of RDC mental disorder in primary medical care', *International Journal of Mental Health* 8 (2): 6–15.

485

Hollingshead, A.B. and Redlich, F.C. (1958) *Social Class and Mental Illness*, New York: Wiley.

Hough, R.L., Landsverk, J.A., Karno, M., Burnam, M.A., Timbers, D.M., Escobar, J.I. and Regier, D.A. (1987) 'Utilization of health and mental health services by Los Angeles Mexican Americans and non-Hispanic whites', *Archives of General Psychiatry* 44 (8): 702–9.

Kamerow, D.B., Pincus, H.A. and Macdonald, D.I. (1986) 'Alcohol abuse, other drug abuse, and mental disorders in medical practice: prevalence, costs, recognition and treatment', *Journal of the American Medical Association* 255 (15): 2054–7.

Karno, M., Hough, R.L., Burnam, M.A., Escobar, J.I., Timbers, D.M., Santana, F. and Boyd, J.H. (1987) 'Lifetime prevalence of specific psychiatric disorders among Mexican Americans and non-Hispanic whites in Los Angeles', *Archives of General Psychiatry* 44 (8): 695–701.

Katz, M.M., Secunda. S., Hirschfeld, R.M.A. and Koslow, S.H. (1979) 'NIMH Clinical Research Branch Collaborative Program on the Psychobiology of Depression', *Archives of General Psychiatry* 36: 765–71.

Keller, M.B., Lavori, P.W., Klerman, G.L., Andreasen, N.C., Endicott, J., Coryell, W., Fawcett, J., Rice, J.P. and Hirschfeld, R.M.A. (1986) 'Low levels and lack of predictors of somatotherapy and psychotherapy received by depressed patients', *Archives of General Psychiatry* 43: 458–66.

Kety, S.S., Rosenthal, D., Wender, P.H. and Schulsinger, F. (1968) 'The types and prevalence of mental illness in the biological and adoptive families of adopted schizophrenics', in D. Rosenthal, and S.S. Kety (eds) *Transmission of Schizophrenia*, London: Pergamon Press.

Klein, D., Gittelman, R., Quitkin, F. and Rifkin, A. (eds) (1980) *Diagnosis and Drug Treatment of Psychiatric Disorders in Adults and Children*, second edition, Baltimore: Williams and Wilkins.

Klerman, G.L. and Cole, J. (1965) 'Clinical pharmacology of imipramine and related antidepressant compounds', *Pharmacological Reviews* 17: 101–41.

Klerman, G.L., Lavori, P.W., Rice, J.., Reich, T., Endicott, J., Andreasen, N.C., Keller, M.B. and Hirschfeld, R.M.A. (1985) 'Birth-cohort trends in rates of major depressive disorder among relatives of patients with affective disorder', *Archives of General Psychiatry* 42 (7): 689–93.

Koslow, S.H., Maas, J.W., Bowden, C.L., Davis, J.M., Hanin, I. and Javaid, J. (1983) 'CSF and urinary biogenic amines and metabolites in depression and mania', *Archives of General Psychiatry* 40: 999–1010.

Kramer, M. (1961) 'Some problems for international research suggested by observations on differences in first admission rates to the mental hospitals of England and Wales and of the United States', *Proceedings of the Third World Congress of Psychiatry* 3: 153–60.

Kramer, M. (1969) 'Cross-national study of diagnosis of the mental disorders: origin of the problem', *American Journal of Psychiatry* 125: supplement I–II.

Leighton, D.C., Harding, J.S., Macklin, D.B., Macmillan, A.M. and Leighton, A.H. (1963) *The Character of Danger*, New York: Basic Books.

Locke, B.Z. and Gardner, E. (1969) 'Psychiatric disorders among the patients of general practitioners and internists', *Public Health Reports* 84: 167–73.

May, P.R.A. (1968) *Treatment of Schizophrenia: A Comparative Study of Five Treatment Methods*, New York: Science house, Inc.

Medical Research Council Drug Trials Subcommittee (1981) 'Continuation therapy with lithium and amitriptyline in unipolar depressive illness: a controlled trial', *Psychological Medicine* 11: 409–16.

Meinert, C.L. (1986) *Clinical Trials: Design, Conduct, and Analysis, Volume 8*, New York: Oxford University Press.

Morris, J.N. (1964) *Uses of Epidemiology*, Baltimore: Williams & Wilkins.

Myers, J.K., Weissman, M.M., Tischler, G.L., Holzer, C.E., Leaf, P.J., Orvaschel, H., Anthony, J.C., Boyd, J.H., Burke, J.D., Kramer, M. and Stoltzman, R. (1984) 'Six-month prevalence of psychiatric disorders in three communities', *Archives of General Psychiatry* 41 (10): 959–67.

National Institute of Mental Health (1981) *NIMH Diagnostic Interview Schedule: Version III*, Rockville, MD: NIMH mimeo.

Prien, R.F., Klett, C.J. and Caffey, E.M. (1973) 'Lithium carbonate and imipramine in prevention of affective episodes', *Archives of General Psychiatry* 29: 420–25.

The President's Commission on Mental health (1978) *Report to the President from the President's Commission on Mental Health* (Stock No. 040-000-00390-8, Volume 1), Washington, DC.

The President's Commission on Mental Health (1978) *Report to the President from the President's Commission on Mental Health*, (Stock No. 040-000-00390-8, Volume 2), Washington, DC.

Redick, R.W., Manderscheid, R.W., Witkin, M.J. and Rosenstein, M.H. (1983), National Institute of Mental health *A History of the US National Reporting Program for Mental Health Statistics, 1840–1983* (DHHS Pub. No. (ADM) 83–1296), Washington, DC: Superintendent of Documents, US Government Printing Office.

Radloff, L.S. and Locke, B.Z. (1986) 'The Community Mental Health Assessment Survey and the CES-D Scale', In M.M. Weissman *et al.* (eds) *Community Surveys of Psychiatric Disorders*, New Jersey: Rutgers University Press.

Regier, D.A., Goldberg, I.D. and Taube, C.A. (1978) 'The de facto US mental health services system', *Archives of General Psychiatry* 35: 685–93.

Regier, D.A. and Rosenfeld, A.H. (1979) *The Report of the ADAMHA Workgroup on Epidemiology, Health Systems Research, and Statistics/Data Systems*, KHHS/ADAMHA, mimeo.

Regier, D.A., Goldberg, I.D., Burns, B.J., Hankin, J.R., Hoeper, E.W. and Nycz, G.R. (1982) 'Specialist/generalist medical care services by persons with mental disorders', *Archives of General Psychiatry* 39: 219–24.

Regier, D.A. and Burke, J.D. (1984) 'Epidemiology', in H.I. Kaplan and B.J. Sadock (eds) *Comprehensive Textbook of Psychiatry*, fourth edition, Baltimore: Williams & Wilkins.

Regier, D.A., Myers, J.K., Kramer, M., Robins, L.N., Blazer, D.G., Hough, R.L., Eaton, W.W. and Locke, B.Z. (1984) 'The NIMH Epidemiological Catchment Area (ECA) program: historical context, major objectives, and study population characteristics', *Archives of General Psychiatry* 41: 934–41.

Regier, D.A., Burke, J.D., Manderscheid, R.W. and Burns, B.J. (1985) 'The chronically mentally ill in primary care', *Psychological Medicine* 15: 265–73.

Regier, D.A. (1987) 'Nosologic principles and diagnostic criteria (introduction and overview)', in G.L. Tischler (ed.) *Diagnosis and Classification in Psychiatry: A Critical Appraisal of DSM-III*, New York: Cambridge University Press.

Regier, D.L., Boyd, J.H., Burke, J.D., Rae, D.S., Myers, J.K., Kramer, M., Robins, L.N., George, L.K., Karno, M. and Locke, B.Z. (1988) 'One-month prevalence of mental disorders in the U.S. – based on five epidemiological catchment area sites', *Archives of General Psychiatry*, in press.

Robins, L.N., Helzer, J.E., Croughan, J. and Ratcliff, K.S. (1981) 'National Institute of Mental Health Diagnostic Interview Schedule: its history, characteristics, and validity', *Archives of General Psychiatry* 38: 381–9.

Robins, L.N., Helzer, J.E., Weissman, M.M., Orvaschel, H., Gruenberg, E., Burke, J.D. and Regier, D.A. (1984) 'Lifetime prevalence of specific psychiatric disorders in three sites', *Archives of General Psychiatry* 41 (10): 949–58.

Rosen, B.M., Locke, B.Z., Goldberg, I.D. and Babigian, H.M. (1972) 'Identification of emotional disturbance in patients seen in general medical clinics', *Hospital Community Psychiatry* 23: 364–70.

Sartorius, N., Jablensky, A., Korten, A., Ernberg, G., Anker, M., Cooper, J.E. and Day, R. (1986) 'Early manifestations and first-contact incidence of schizophrenia in different cultures: a preliminary report on the initial evaluation phase of the WHO Collaborative Study of Determinants of Outcome of Severe Mental Disorders', *Psychological Medicine* 16: 909–28.

Sartorius, N., Shapiro, R. and Jablensky, A. (1974) 'The international pilot study of schizophrenia', *Schizophrenia Bulletin* 1 (experimental issue no. 11) : 21–34.

Shapiro, S., German, P.S., Skinner, E.A., Von Korff, M., Turner, R.W., Klein, L.E., Teitelbaum, M.L., Kramer, M., Burke, J.D. and Burns, B.J. (1987) 'An experiment to change detection and management of mental morbidity in primary care', *Medical Care* 25 (4): 327–39.

Shapiro, S., Skinner, E.A., Kessler, L.G., von Korff, M., German, P.S., Tischler, G.L., Leaf, P.J., Benham, L., Cottler, L. and Regier, D.A. (1984) 'Utilization of health and mental health services', *Archives of General Psychiatry* 41 (10): 971–8.

Shepherd, M. (1978) 'Epidemiology and clinical psychiatry', *Journal of Psychiatry* 133: 289–98.

Shepherd, M., Cooper, B., Brown, A.C. and Kalton, G.W. (1966) *Psychiatric Illness in General Practice*, London: Oxford University Press.

Sokoloff, L., Reivich, M., Kennedy, C., Des Rosiers, M.H., Patlak, C.S., Pettigrew, K.D., Sakurada, O. and Shinohara, M. (1977) 'The [14C]Deoxyglucose method for the measurement of local cerebral glucose utilization: theory, procedure, and normal values in the conscious and anesthetized albino rat[1]', *Journal of neurochemistry* 28: 897–916.

Spitzer, R.L., Endicott, J. and Robins, E. (1978) 'Research diagnostic criteria: rationale and reliability', *Archives of General Psychiatry* 35: 773–83.

Srole, L. (1962) *Mental Health in the Metropolis: The Midtown Manhattan Study*, New York: McGraw-Hill.

Taube, C.A., Thompson, J.W., Burns, B.J., Widem, P. and Prevost, C. (1985) 'Prospective payment and psychiatric discharges from general hospitals with and without psychiatric units', *Hospital and Community Psychiatry* 36 (7): 754–60.

Weissman, M. and Myers, J.K. (1978) 'Affective disorders in a U.S. urban community: the use of research diagnostic criteria in an epidemiological survey', *Archives of General Psychiatry* 35: 1304–11.

The White House (1977) 'Executive Order No. 11973 – President's Commission of Mental Health', Office of the White House Press Secretary.

Wing, J.H., Cooper, J.E. and Sartorius, N. (1974) *The Description and Classification of Psychiatric Symptoms: An Instruction Manual for the PSE and CATEGO system*, London: Cambridge University Press.

WHO/ADAMHA (1985) *Mental Disorders, Alcohol – Drug-Related Problems*, New York: Elsevier.

World Health Organization (1973) *The International Pilot Study of Schizophrenia, Volume I*, Geneva: WHO.

31

Case Definition and Case Identification in Cross-cultural Perspective

Jair Mari, Biswajit Sen, and Tai-Ann Cheng

While psychopathology may imply that there is an inner core of suffering shared by human beings, unanswered questions remain about whether concepts and definitions of psychiatric disturbance developed in western societies can equally be applied to other cultures or whether there are culturally specific psychiatric entities which do not fit into a global classification.

The concept of culture itself can be used in different senses. Operationally, culture can be equated with a nation. This involves two basic assumptions: first, that each nation contains distinctive cultural features and, second, that the possible ethnic differences within a nation are less prominent than those between two nations under scrutiny. Culture can also be used in the traditional anthropological tribal sense and as an ethnic concept in reference to the pluralistic multi-cultural groups within a nation (Murphy 1982).

A variety of standardized psychiatric interviews have been developed in the last two decades, and a number of such instruments have been applied in several nations and to different ethnic groups (the assumptions which have been made about the development of such instruments were described by Wing *et al.* 1981). This article will focus on the methodology adopted in the development of such instruments by highlighting the limitations and achievements of their use in Brazil, India, and Taiwan.

CULTURAL BACKGROUND

Brazil

Brazil has a population of approximately 140 million inhabitants, the spoken language throughout the country is Portuguese (except for some tribal groups accounting for less than 0.5 per cent of the population), and illiteracy is around 30 per cent. Although the 'official' religion of the majority of the population is Roman Catholic, the folk religions 'Umbanda' and 'Kardecismo' are widespread and have a strong influence. These two religions have places of worship, *centros espiritas*, where ill people can be advised and where 'bad spirits' can be expelled; as these *centros* are very accessible (no bureaucracy, queueing, or appointments), families with psychiatrically disturbed members resort to them. There is approximately one of these *centros* per 20,000 inhabitants (Mari 1983).

Neither religion makes a distinction between body and mind. The ceremonies of Umbanda are related to the worship of black ancestors, Indian ancestors, and Catholic saints. In the last century, the slaves used to mask their *Orishas* (literally master of the head; god or goddess) with Catholic saints because they were not free to celebrate their original African rituals. The Umbanda religion is regarded as 'low spiritism' and is deeply rooted in the community. 'Disease' (*Encosto*) is said to be caused by 'spirits without light' (Exus and Qiumbas) wandering around and possessing people. Treatment of such 'disease' consists in exorcising the 'spirit without light'.

Kardecismo is a philosophico-religious system based on the Hindu idea of Karma. There is a belief in the idea of reincarnation and in communication between the dead and the living. It is regarded as 'high spiritism', probably due to the strong influence of the white middle class in this religion. Disease (Karmica disease) is thought to be caused because the spirit has committed faults in a previous life, and is seen as a kind of test which the patient must face. The treatment is based on the development of the spirit.

Although there is no 'official' integration between the 'formal' and 'informal' care systems in Brazil, it is well known that psychiatrists rarely discourage patients from participating in spiritist cults and, in many cases, psychiatrists make referrals and co-operate with them. For instance, Brody gives an interesting account of the way doctors and spiritists work together in 'The Hospital Espirita Pedro de Alcantara' in Rio de Janeiro (Brody 1973: 429–31). This hospital combines spiritist sessions and traditional psychiatric treatments, and patients referred to these sessions are required to be functioning reasonably well by the spiritual leader (*chefe do terreiro*) before attendance. For instance, treatment is not given to those who are hypertensive, receiving insulin, agitated, or very depressed.

Brody randomly selected twenty first admissions from a psychiatric hospital in Rio de Janeiro to investigate how many sought a *centro espirita* and the reasons for doing so: fourteen patients turned out to have attended religious ceremonies at least once, largely because either the patient or a relative believed that spirits were causing the psychiatric condition. Richeport (1984) interviewed 220 families living in a *favela*, in the outskirts of Natal, to compare the pattern of use of 'formal' and 'informal' systems of care in this population. The majority of people had consulted both health professionals and 'spiritists' for problems such as physical symptoms, depression, difficulties arising from unemployment, marital tensions, dealing with retarded children, and alcoholism.

India

India has a population of about 800 million, speaking more than a score of languages and several hundred dialects. The rate of illiteracy is 65 per cent. Approximately 80 per cent of the population are Hindu, believing in the concept of rebirth and explaining human suffering in terms of expiation of accumulated sins in the former and present incarnations (the doctrine of Karma). Between 12 per cent and 14 per cent of the population are Muslim, the rest being Christians, Sikhs, Jains, Buddhists, Parsees, and 'animists', i.e., tribes like Santals, Mundas, etc. While cultural differences undoubtedly exist between these groups, it is believed that 'idioms of distress' are broadly similar across them, varying more with the extent of formal education and degree of westernization than religious affiliation per se. No significant differences in the prevalence of mental illness have been found between important religious groups. However, the prevalence of mental illness among the tribes is known to be fairly low (Nandi *et al.* 1980).

Belief in the evil influences of the spirit world controlled by people with supernatural powers and malefic intent is deeply rooted in India, including, for example, many of the urban elite. There is a corresponding belief in faith healers (*ojhas* or *mantarwadis*) who are believed to possess powers to counteract these evil influences, which may give rise to, among other manifestations, mental illness. Even a decade ago it would have been rare for a psychiatrist in the rural areas to see a patient who had not previously visited a faith healer. This picture is now slowly changing, but it is expected that the influence of faith healers will continue to remain substantial.

Taiwan

Taiwan (R.O.C.) has a population of about nineteen million distributed between villages, towns, and cities, each with approximately one-third of the total inhabitants. The main ethnic group is the Chinese who migrated to Taiwan from mainland China and constitute over 98 per cent of the total population. The rest are Malayo-Polynesian aborigines. Eighty per cent of the Chinese are early immigrants whose mother tongues were the southern Fukien and the Hakka dialects. The 20 per cent late immigrants speak a variety of dialects. Mandarin is the official common language which can be well understood by most people under 50 years of age. The proportion of illiteracy was around 8 per cent in 1986 (Ministry of the Interior 1987). The majority of people in Taiwan believe in Chinese folk religion (65 per cent), and the rest have various religious beliefs including Buddhism (15 per cent), Taoism (7 per cent), and Christianity (5 per cent).

Rapid modernization over the past two to three decades has made Taiwan into a newly industrialized country with a commodity-export-oriented economic policy. Although considerable difference in family size has been found across urban-rural communities in recent years, the strong traditional parent-child kinship, emphasizing filial piety (Hsu 1971), still dominates the

491

family relationship in Taiwan. The divorce rate is rather low, being 5.5 per 1,000 currently married population in 1986 (Ministry of the Interior 1987).

The traditional Chinese medical concept mainly emphasizes both a correspondence between macrocosm and microcosm, as well as a harmony between 'yin' and 'yang' of body and environment. 'Yang' signifies not only the apparent, active, excited, external, upward, forward, aggressive, volatile, hard, bright, hot, but also the abstract and functional. In contrast, 'yin' signifies not only the passive, inhibited, unclear, inward, downward, retrogressive, cold, dark, soft, submissive, but also the material and concrete (Lin 1981). Disharmony would bring about either an excessive or an insufficiency of the *jin-Chi* (vital energy) and thus cause illness.

Although this medical concept explicitly includes only physical illness, it implicitly uses physical terms to describe somatic manifestations arising from emotional distress (Tseng 1975; Kleinman 1982). Hence, while psychotics often seek help first from a folk therapist, people with minor psychiatric morbidity largely look for help from both Chinese and western medicine in Taiwan. There, they always report, their somatic discomfort and their psychosocial distress is often neglected. Very few of them would consult mental health professionals and the general practitioner seldom refers them to the psychiatrists.

DEVELOPING INSTRUMENTS FOR CROSS-CULTURAL STUDIES

There are five major aims of cross-cultural research: a) to compare rates of psychiatric morbidity; b) to develop culturally sensitive instruments; c) to investigate the aetiology of psychopathology; d) to study changes in the pattern of psychopathology over time; and e) to investigate the relationship between psychiatric disturbance and cultural determinants. The contrasting perspective between the two leading aims is one of the main problems of developing psychiatric research instruments for cross-cultural comparison: these should be able to identify symptoms and syndromes which represent the same phenomena in different cultural settings and simultaneously be sensitive to cultural variations.

Flaherty (1987) has pointed to five major mutually exclusive dimensions of equivalence to be considered when developing a psychiatric research instrument for cross-cultural application: *Content Equivalence* – each item of the measuring instrument should have a content relevant to each culture under study; *Semantic Equivalence* – each item of the measuring instrument should have the same meaning for each language; *Technical Equivalence* – the act of measuring should be unaffected by the cultural differences; *Criterion Equivalence* – the interpretation of the results of a measure should remain the same when compared against a norm in each culture; and *Conceptual Equivalence* – responses to the measuring instrument should indicate the measurement of the same theoretical construct across cultures. The first three items are mainly related to the structure of the language being used while the last two refer to the psychiatric taxonomy.

There are basically three methods of case identification using standardized research instruments: clinical evaluation by means of a psychiatric interview, the use of screening questionnaires, and the combination of both in a two-way design. The definition of a case will, of course, depend on the purpose of the study, i.e., a case for what (Copeland 1981)? A number of these instruments have now been applied in Brazil, India, and Taiwan.

Brazil

The Present State Examination (PSE) (Wing *et al*. 1974) has been translated into Portuguese by Caetano and Gentil Filho (1983), and Gentil Filho *et al*. (1986) have raised the problems they have had in the translation of the PSE and its use in some training sessions at the psychiatric unit of the University of Sao Paulo. From a semantic point of view, some original English or German words in the glossary would not have the same meaning in Portuguese vocabulary. It was difficult to translate terms such as 'thought broadcast', '*mitgehen*', and idiomatic expressions such as 'knight's move'. From a conceptual point of view, the definition of '*deliroide*' largely applied by Brazilian psychiatrists had no equivalence in the PSE original version. Moreover, they raised difficulties in detecting specific syndromes such as alcoholism, organic brain disorders, endogenous panic anxiety, affective atypical disorders, mental handicap, and atypical non-paranoid states, though the reasons have not been clearly specified.

Caetano (1986) applied the PSE to an in-patient sample in Cambridge (n = 152), from which he selected forty-one cases presenting either a panic disorder or a generalized anxiety disorder according to DSM-III, to carry out a comparison of symptom profiles with an out-patient clinic Brazilian sample. According to the original version, depersonalization can only be rated if lasting for some hours. However, he noticed that patients in both samples would frequently manifest this state over shorter periods of time. Thus, in the Brazilian version, depersonalization has been rated, even when transient, providing there is an important clinical degree of intensity and/or high frequency.

These two studies provide a list of a number of questions which have been misunderstood by Brazilian patients, probably because of the number of those with few years of schooling and/or illiteracy. The validity of the Portuguese version was not checked by back-translation but appears to be good and both authors have emphasized the feasibility of using the PSE in Brazil provided a proper training period is undertaken to acquaint users with the instrument.

The aim of the study conducted by Mari (1987) was to assess the prevalence of psychiatric morbidity in three primary medical care clinics in the city of Sao Paulo and to develop research instruments to be applied in

493

this setting. A time-sample of consecutive attenders were asked to complete two screening questionnaires, the Self Report Questionnaire (SRQ) (Harding *et al.* 1980), and the General Health Questionnaire (GHQ) (Goldberg 1972), and a subsample of the attenders were selected for a psychiatric interview, the Clinical Interview Schedule (CIS) (Goldberg *et al.* 1970).

For the pilot study, the GHQ-30 was translated into Portuguese, back-translated by workers unfamiliar with the original version, and the back-translation checked by a British psychiatrist. Minor adjustments were made to the original translation, so as to keep the original meaning while trying to conform as closely as possible with Brazilian concepts and idioms. However, the GHQ-30 presented several difficulties in the pilot study: the questionnaire was too long and it became apparent that some of the questions were being misunderstood by the subjects. For example, 'concentration' was occasionally understood to mean preparation to contact 'holy spirits' and this was probably due to the strong influence of the folk religions in Brazil (Mari and Williams 1984). So, for the main study it was decided to use a shorter version of the GHQ, the GHQ-12, while rephrasing some of the questions which were poorly understood by the respondents in the pilot study.

A Portuguese version of the SRQ was made available in a previous WHO collaborative study carried out by Harding *et al.* (1980, 1983), and the two screening questionnaires (GHQ-12 and SRQ-20) were found to be equally valid for the detection of minor psychiatric morbidity in the primary medical care setting in the city of Sao Paulo (Mari and Williams 1985, 1986).

The Clinical Interview Schedule is a semi-structured interview developed to study psychiatric morbidity in general practice and community settings. The translation and back-translation of the CIS into Portuguese has been carried out in the same manner as described for the GHQ without major problems (the glossary was, however, used in the original language). A reliability study of the Portuguese version of the CIS was conducted with two other psychiatrists (Mari *et al.* 1986) and there was only one out of twenty-two items where there was no agreement between the investigators: euphoria (ICC via ANOVA $= 0.02$, n.s.). The item 'histrionic' showed the lowest agreement (weighted Kappa $= + 0.48$) in the study conducted by Goldberg *et al.* (1970) and similar findings were reported in the Brazilian assessment and in the pilot study conducted by Campillo-Serrano *et al.* (1981) in Mexico with fifteen interviews. The low agreement found in euphoria was, however, specific to the Brazilian study.

It is plausible to suppose that constant cross-cultural low agreements would point to problems in the way symptoms are defined or interpreted while specific low reliability agreements might indicate transcultural differences in the use of the instrument (or simply be related to observer bias: examples in the literature can be found in Shepherd *et al.* 1968 and Leff 1974).

A few culture-specific screening instruments of psychiatric disorders have been developed and tested in Brazil, without direct reference to foreign scales. Almeida-Filho (1981) developed a 35-item screening questionnaire to identify psychiatric disturbance in children, the Infant Psychiatric Morbidity Questionnaire (QMPI), and Santana (1978) designed a 44-item questionnaire for the detection of psychiatric disorders in adult populations, the Adult Psychiatric Morbidity Questionnaire (QMPA). Both instruments combined questions from well-known screening questionnaires with those derived from the socio-cultural Brazilian context and they showed good validity when tested by means of unstructured psychiatric interviews.

India

The GHQ, SRQ, PSE, and CIS have also been used in India (Harding *et al.* 1983; Bagadia *et al.* 1985; Sen 1987). For the PSE, translation into Hindi and back-translation was carried out, checking the 'semantic equivalence of the items'. Some concepts (e.g. anxiety) proved difficult to translate 'when significant cultural variations in the perception and intrapsychic phenomena existed' (Harding *et al.* 1983). However, in general, the PSE has been found to be acceptable for use in different regions of India with high inter-rater reliability (Verghese *et al.* 1985). The GHQ-60 and GHQ-12 have also been translated into several Indian languages without difficulty and with satisfactory validity indices. Translation and back-translation of the CIS in Bengali have also been carried out without major problems, with more attention being paid to conceptual than semantic equivalence (Sen *et al.* 1987). The use of these instruments in India and Brazilian cultural contexts has also been discussed in Sen and Mari (1986).

Kapur *et al.* (1974a, 1974b) developed the Indian Psychiatric Interview Schedule (IPIS) and the Indian Psychiatric Survey Schedule (IPSS) as a culture-specific (or emic) instrument for detecting mental illness in India because they felt that phenomena like those of spirit possession, preoccupation with symptoms of sexual inadequacy, and the frequency of vague somatic symptoms of psychological origin are not paid sufficient attention in the standardized interview schedules developed in the west (Carstairs and Kapur 1976). The IPSS 'is an instrument designed to investigate the presence or absence of 125 psychiatric symptoms, with special emphasis on those commonly encountered in a Indian setting . . . [it] enquires about symptoms only; no attempt has been made to combine the symptoms into psychiatric syndromes!' The IPSS and the IPIS have been used both in community and primary care settings in India (Carstairs and Kapur 1976, Gautam *et al.* 1980, Mehta *et al.* 1985, Shamasunder *et al.* 1986), but there is no evidence that the cases detected by the instruments differ either qualitatively or quantitatively (i.e., in terms of prevalence) from those detected by other standardized instruments e.g. PSE and CIS.

Taiwan

Over the past two decades, a few psychiatric interview schedules have been

495

translated into Chinese and used in Taiwan. The Chinese version PSE was used in the IPSS (WHO 1973), and the Chinese version DIS was also applied in an epidemiological study in Taiwan (Hwu *et al*. 1986). Although the inter-rater reliability of the PSE in the IPSS was reported to be acceptable, there has been no report about its cross-cultural comparability. Furthermore, the PSE has been criticized as being primarily constructed for the study of psychotic patients (Dohrenwend *et al*. 1978; Williams *et al*. 1980). In a large-scale epidemiological study, the agreement between diagnoses made by the DIS and psychiatrists was found to be rather unsatisfactory (Folstein *et al*. 1985). The authors concluded that the DIS is better regarded as a screen-ing instrument. If this view is taken, then the over-lengthy DIS is obviously not feasible for community study.

Since there was no valid, reliable, and cross-culturally comparable case-finding instrument for use in community studies of minor psychiatric morbidity in Taiwan, a pilot study was conducted to construct such an instru-ment (Cheng 1985). Based on a presumption that certain symptom expres-sions might be common to many cultures, an experimental screening questionnaire – the Chinese Health Questionnaire (CHQ) – was designed by the inclusion of the translated GHQ-30 items, as well as thirty specially designed, culturally relevant items. The resulting 'hybrid' was then tested in a two-stage survey of a representative community sample (n = 150) in Taiwan. The second-stage psychiatric interview was conducted by one of the authors (Cheng), using a Chinese version of the CIS.

The Chinese CIS was derived from a two-stage translation of the English version. Two inter-rater reliability studies were conducted. The first was between two British and one Chinese senior psychiatrists on an English-speaking community sample in London (Cheng *et al*. 1983), and the second between two Chinese psychiatrists on a community sample in Taiwan (Chong and Cheng 1985). Reliability coefficients derived from these two studies were found to be satisfactory. It is believed that the only way to tackle the problem of cross-cultural comparability of any case-finding instrument is to modify the different language version of an instrument based on extensive field experience obtained from that particular culture. This task was carried out in the pilot study and a main community study of minor psychiatric morbidity in Taiwan (Cheng 1987).

The Chinese CIS was found to be feasible for use in the community study of minor psychiatric morbidity in Taiwan. Its first part, concerning physical health, was found to be especially useful in making a good initial contact and establishing rapport. Thus, the following parts covering psychological phenomena became far less sensitive to the respondents. The semi-structured form of the CIS was found to allow for effective and more free elicitation of the respondent's unpleasant emotions. The wording and sequence of the questions were found to be acceptable to the respondents. Many of the CIS questions were found to be culturally relevant to the Chinese in Taiwan.

496

However, modification was still needed, particularly for items concerning emotional distress, and extra questions were added. Any psycholinguistic equivalent expressed by the Chinese respondents to any of the questions of the CIS was taken to substitute the original. A similar exercise was also performed in the Ugandan survey (Orley and Wing 1979). The operational definition of a few items was also modified in order to fit the characteristic of the Chinese culture. These modifications, which were based on field experience, were believed to have contributed to the resolution of psycho-linguistic problems and the cross-cultural comparability of the CIS.

Since it has been suggested that the optimal method in the development of a screening tool would be to apply a discriminant function technique to find the best set of items with the highest classification power (Hand 1979), this method was used on the CHQ data. A classical linear discriminant analysis with stepwise variable selection method and a prior probability equal to group size was applied to 150 community respondents divided into case (n = 38) and non-case (n = 112) groups. Twelve of the items of the CHQ had an overall classification power of 98 per cent: these became the new CHQ-12, a valid screening tool for use in community studies in Taiwan (Cheng and Williams 1986). It is interesting to note that half the CHQ-12 items came from the GHQ-30 and the remaining six items were newly designed. The former were items about anxiety, depression, and sleep disturbance, while the latter could be grouped into two categories – 'somatic symptoms and somatic concern' and 'family and interpersonal difficulties' which were in accordance with the conceptual construct for the thirty new items.

The validity of the CHQ-12 has been further assessed in the main community study (n = 1023) and the classification power was found to be highly satisfactory (88.6 per cent) (Cheng 1988). Further analyses concerning the misclassification and the factorial structure of the CHQ-12 are being undertaken.

IS THERE A CASE FOR THE CULTURE-BOUND SYNDROME?

In Brazil, the evidence that psychiatric patients often resort to spiritist centres probably led some investigators, mainly in the third and fourth decades of this century, to speculate whether these religious practices are related to the onset of psychiatric disorders and/or whether they might be associated with specific psychiatric conditions reflecting this strong cultural influence. The first attempt to link religious experience and a psychiatric disorder was conducted by Roxo (1918) who described a syndrome named *Delirio Espirita Episodico* (Spiritist Episodic Delusion). This syndrome was said to appear in 'an atypical form of psychopathic personality', with repeated short-term hallucinatory states following the emotional shock experienced in spiritist sessions, and Roxo compared this psychotic phenomenon with that of the

French *boufee delirante*. This might be a transmitted state (contagious) being more frequent among black people due to the influence of African religion heritages and their suggestibility. The idea that ceremonies could trigger acute psychiatric states in people who are not mentally ill before attending the rituals was also raised by Ribeiro and Campos (1931), though they emphasized the role of predisposition.

Stainbrook (1952) studied 200 patients admitted to psychiatric hospitals in Salvador, Bahia, with an already existing diagnosis of schizophrenia and reported that female low-class patients were acting out being possessed by an African god or goddess. However, Brody (1973) studied 254 first admissions to three psychiatric hospitals in the city of Rio de Janeiro by means of two questionnaires, one socio-cultural and the other designed to describe psychopathology. The latter, entitled the Initial Interview Inventory, was derived from the Mental Status Schedule (Spitzer and Endicott 1966) by including 'primitive and folkloric references couched in general terms'. He noted that patients would frequently mention magical, spiritual or cult beliefs during the interview but there was no difference between those who attended African spiritist sessions (they comprised 22 per cent of his sample) and the others. Indeed, the Afro-spiritist attenders did not differ from other patients regarding psychotic phenomena: the majority of lower-class men and both lower- and middle-class women did not make reference to religious beliefs in their deluded thinking. According to Brody, 'in only rare instances were the spiritist or cult-related experiences woven into a delusional system. They were most typically offered by patients in order to explain their depression, weakness, confusion or anxiety' (Brody 1973).

During the last three decades, a number of cultural-specific phenomena have been described in Indian literature. Wig (1960) first used the term *'Dhat* syndrome' which typically occurs in a young adult male who presents with a primary complaint of loss of semen either by 'frequent nocturnal emissions' or by 'semen passing in urine'. Singh (1985) studied fifty consecutive patients with male potency disorders attending the psychiatric out-patient department of a teaching hospital and found a primary complaint of *'Dhat'* in thirty one of them. The majority of these patients, Singh states, were suffering from depressive states. However, almost a third of them could not be given a psychiatric diagnosis. Similar clinical manifestations were reported as Bangladeshi syndrome in Bangladesh (Clyne 1964), Prameha disease in Sri Lanka (Obeyesekere 1976), and *'shen-kuei'* syndrome in Taiwan (Wen and Wang 1981). Wen and Wang found that patients consulting a urologist with this as the chief complaint (n = 23) have psychiatric symptoms similar to neurotic out-patients and can be fitted into contemporary psychiatric diagnostic nosology as anxiety neurosis, depression, and hypochondriacal neurosis.

Teja *et al.* (1970) analysed fifteen cases of 'spirit possession' and reclassified all of them in three categories, viz. hysteria (7), schizophrenia (6), and mania (2).

Dutta *et al.* (1982) reported a Koro epidemic – formerly thought to occur exclusively among people from Malaysia, the southern part of China (Rin 1965, Yap 1965) – in the state of Assam in the north-eastern part of India. Nandi *et al.* (1983) reported a similar epidemic from the district of Murshidabad in the state of West Bengal adjoining Assam. Nandi chose to describe the syndrome as an acute anxiety reaction centred around a culturally elaborated fear of the loss of a valued organ, i.e. penis or breast. Nandi *et al.* (1987) described another culturally-specific epidemic, colloquially known in West Bengal as *Jhin-Jhini* (literally meaning 'the tingling disease') which also was thought by him to be a variant of an acute anxiety reaction or panic attack in which tingling and numbness beginning in the legs and spreading throughout the body, along with an overwhelming fear of death, were the main features.

Somatization has repeatedly been described by some researchers as a culture-specific manifestation of neurosis among certain ethnic groups (Dube 1970; Tseng 1975; Lin 1982). However, the rates of somatic symptoms reported by these researchers were no higher than those found in a number of western surveys among depressive patients (Woodruff *et al.* 1967; Mathew *et al.* 1981). The rates of somatic symptoms and somatic concern found in community surveys carried out in London (Jenkins 1985) and Taiwan, using similar case-finding instruments, were very similar. It is argued that this notion of somatization might better be explained by psycholinguistic expression and illness behaviour of the Chinese (Cheng 1988).

The answer to the question of whether there is a case for culture-bound syndromes in non-western countries can be obtained from the fact that epidemiological studies in some of these countries, whether hospital or community, have not found it necessary to postulate the existence of culture-specific entities to classify psychiatric disorder. For instance, the majority of clinicians in India are now of the opinion that the so-called culture-bound syndromes can almost always be re-classified under internationally accepted diagnostic categories and, among Brazilian psychiatrists, such a need seems to have never been mentioned, at least in the clinical realm. Although Lin (1982) emphasized the existence of certain culture-specific neurotic syndromes (such as somatization and *shin-jin-shui-jo*) in the Chinese, Cheng (1987) has argued that they are laymen's terms referring to a mixture of neurotic symptoms in minor psychiatric morbidity.

As Varma (1986) has pointed out, the attention of psychiatric research workers has now shifted from culture-bound syndromes to 'universal' illness, e.g. schizophrenia, depression, and neuroses. According to him, transcultural differences in psychiatric phenomena should now 'be considered with regard to incidence, types, manifestations, natural history, course, outcome and treatment of mental illness' instead of culture-specific diagnostic entities.

CONCLUSIONS AND RECOMMENDATIONS

Cross-cultural research can be divided into two main streams: the *universalist*, which would be more inclined in emphasize the similarities, and the *specificist*, which would tend to show possible differences among the groups compared. As an example of such debate, Singer (1975), when reviewing the literature on depression, concluded that it was not clear whether depressive illness in primitive and other non-western cultures presented outstanding features. This was previously predicted by Yap (1965) who stated that some specific disorders reported in the literature could be regarded as pathoplastic variants of disorders commonly recognized by western psychiatrists. German (1972) further argued that socio-cultural influences on psychopathology are likely to be less prominent as development progresses in non-western cultures. On the other hand, researchers like Kleinman (1987) have heavily criticized this view. Taking the case of depression he pointed out that, if a narrow concept of depression is applied, cross-cultural studies would find solely what is 'universal', missing out aspects which would be striking examples of the influence of culture on depression. The cultural influence on depression, as he has repeatedly mentioned, determines help-seeking, course, and treatment response of the 'disease'.

It is now widely accepted that an integration of culture-general (etic) and culture-specific (emic) approaches are essential for cross-cultural comparisons. For instance, Beiser and Fleming (1986) compared the pattern of psychiatric disorders among south-east Asian refugees with those of Vancouver residents stratified by sex, age and marital status. The authors applied a questionnaire combining questions derived from well-known instruments such as the DIS and the SRQ-24 with emic items extracted from the Vietnamese Depression Scale. The statistical analysis was performed with a principal component factor technique followed by varimax rotation on the mental health items from each of the two survey samples. The factor analysis produced four mental health dimensions (panic, depression, somatization, and well-being) and they found a high correlation across each pair of similar appearing factors. These results suggest that Asians and Caucasians experience depressive symptoms and express them in similar ways though doubt remains on the possible selective migration bias.

The development of the CHQ-12 is another example of attempting to integrate both etic and emic approaches. The production of a 'hybrid' screening instrument might well imply a difference between 'disease phenomenon' and 'illness expression'. Since there was no difference on symptom manifestations between the British and Chinese neurotics on the CIS interview, the 'emic' items in the CHQ-12 would better be regarded as culture-specific expressions of 'etic' symptoms. Here two questions would then be raised:

(a) Will the validity of a screening tool be lowered without the inclusion of emic items?

(b) Will the study of psychopathology be hampered when the case-finding instrument consists only of a self-administered questionnaire?

It is too early to give an affirmative answer to the first question and further investigations are still needed. Although the answer to the second question might be positive, it can reasonably be neglected when a two-stage case-finding strategy is applied.

Cross-cultural psychopharmacology is a promising field for research in cross-cultural psychiatry. The number of cross-ethnic studies is still limited but there is some evidence that Hispanics, for instance, would respond differently to anti-depressant medication (they may need lower doses and display more side-effects with the same dose of medication when compared with other ethnic groups). A research design comparing treatment responses between homogeneous ethnic groups might elucidate whether possible ethnic differences are variants of the same underlying disorder, i.e., a pathoplastic manifestation, or whether they are related to culturally-bound distinct entities.

According to Beiser et al. (1976), 'comparative studies using standardized instruments are going to continue despite their recognized faults, but it is unlikely to satisfy the anthropologist.' In addition, Murphy (1982) stated that 'comparative psychiatry must lean to the etic rather than to the emic position, since with the emic no comparisons are usually possible.' None the less, it might be more appropriate to establish a practical way to combine anthropological and epidemiological methods in the planning and design of new cross-cultural research strategies. For instance, further cross-cultural comparative studies with the integration of both emic and etic approaches by applying the state of the art of these apparent contrasting techniques might be pursued.

Acknowledgements: We are grateful to Mr Jonathan Gabe from the General Practice Research Unit and Dr Naomar Almeida Filho from the Federal University of Bahia for commenting on earlier versions of this paper. J.J. Mari was funded by the Brazilian Research Council (Conselho Nacional de Pesquisa CNPq, II-C) in the Department of Psychiatry of Escola Paulista de Medicina. His contribution to this chapter was written during leave funded by the British Council and the State of Sao Paulo Research Council (Fundacao de Amparo a Pesquisa do Estado de Sao Paulo – FAPESP). Biswajit Sen was supported by a grant from the Strømme Foundation, Norway, while the work by T.A. Cheng was funded by the National Science Council, Taiwan (ROC) (NSC 72–74–0301–H114–01).

501

REFERENCES

Almeida-Filho, N. (1981) 'Development and assessment of the QMPI: a Brazilian children's behaviour questionnaire for completion by parents, *Social Psychiatry* 16: 205–11.

Bagadia, V. N., Ayyar, K.S., Lakdawala, P.D., Susainathan, U., and Pradhan, P.V. (1985) 'Value of the General Health Questionnaire in detecting psychiatric morbidity in a general hospital out-patient population, *Indian Journal of Psychiatry* 27 (4): 293–6.

Beiser, M., Benfari, R.C., Collomb, H., and Ravel, J.C. (1976) 'Measuring psychoneurotic behaviour in cross-cultural surveys', *The Journal of Nervous and Mental Disease* 163: 10–23

Beiser, M. and Fleming, J.A.E. (1986) 'Measuring psychiatric disorder among Southeast Asian refugees', *Psychological Medicine* 16: 627–39.

Brody, E. (1973) *The Lost Ones: Social Forces and Mental Illness in Rio de Janeiro*, New York: International University Press.

Caetano, D. (1986) 'Experiencia com o Present State Examination (PSE) em pacientes ingleses e brasileiros', *Revista da Associacao Brasileira de Psiquiatria*, supplement, 8: 34–43.

Caetano, R. and Gentil-Filho, V. (1983) *P.S.E. – Exame do Estado Psiquico*, Sao Paulo.

Campillo-Serrano, C., Caraveo-Anduaga, J., Mora, M.E.M., and Lanz, P.M. (1981) 'Confiabilidad entre clinicos utilisando la "Entrevista Estandarizada" de Goldberg en una version mexicana', *Acta Psiquiatrica Psicologica de America Latina* 27: 44–53.

Carstairs, G.M. and Kapur, R.L. (1976) *The Great Universe of Kota*, London: Hogarth Press.

Cheng, T.A. (1985) 'A pilot study of mental disorders in Taiwan', *Psychological Medicine* 15: 195–203.

Cheng, T.A. (1987) *A Community Study of Minor Mental Disorders in Taiwan*, unpublished PhD thesis: University of London.

Cheng, T.A. (1988) 'A community study of minor psychiatric morbidity in Taiwan', in preparation.

Cheng, T.A. (1988) 'Symptomatology of minor psychiatric morbidity: a crosscultural comparison between British and Chinese community cases', in preparation.

Cheng, T.A. and Williams, P. (1986) 'The design and development of a screening questionnaire (CHQ) for use in community studies of mental disorders in Taiwan', *Psychological Medicine* 16: 415–22.

Cheng, T.A., Williams, P., and Clare, A.W. (1983) 'Reliability study of the Clinical Interview Schedule (CIS) between the British and Chinese psychiatrists', *Bulletin of the Chinese Society of Neurology and Psychiatry* 9: 54–5.

Chong, M.Y. and Cheng, T.A. (1985) 'Reliability study of the Clinical Interview Schedule (CIS): the use of community sample', *Bulletin of the Chinese Society of Neurology and Psychiatry* 11: 27–34.

Clyne, M.B. (1964) 'Indian patients', *Practitioner* 193: 195–9.

Copeland, J. (1981) 'What is a case? A case for what?', in J.K. Wing, P. Bebbington, and L.N. Robins (eds) *What is a Case? The Problem of Definition in Psychiatric Community Surveys*, London: Grant McIntyre.

Dohrenwend, B.P., Yager, T.J., Egri, F. and Mendelson, F.S. (1978) 'The Psychiatric Status Schedule as a measure of dimensions of psychopathology in the general population', *Archives of General Psychiatry* 35: 731–7.

Dube, K.C. (1970) 'A study of prevalence and biosocial variables in mental illness in rural and urban community in Uttar Pradesh, India', *Acta Psychiatrica Scandinavica* 46, 327–59.

Dutta, D., Phookan, H.R., and DAS, P.O. (1982) 'The Koro epidemic in lower Assam', *Indian Journal of Psychiatry* 24: 370–5.

Flaherty, J.A. (1987) 'Appropriate and inappropriate methodologies for Hispanic mental health', in M. Gaviria and J.D. Arana (eds) *Health and Behaviour: Research Agenda for Hispanics – Research Monograph 1* Chicago: The University of Illinois.

Folstein, M., Romanoski, A.J., Nestadt, G., Chahal, R., Merchant, A., Shapiro, S., Kramer, M., Anthony, J., Gruenberg, E.M., and McHugh, P.R. (1985) 'Brief report on the clinical reappraisal of the Diagnostic Interview Schedule carried out at the Johns Hopkins site of the Epidemiological Catchment Area Program of the NIMH', *Psychological Medicine* 15: 809–14.

Gautam, S., Kapur, R.L., and Shamasundar, C. (1980) 'Psychiatric morbidity and referral in general practice – a survey of general practitioners in Bangalore city', *Indian Journal of Psychiatry* 22: 295–7.

Gentil-Filho, V., Guerra-Andrade, L.H.S., and Lotufo-Neto, F. (1986) 'PSE: traducao, treinamento e limitacoes ao seu uso no Brasil', *Revista da Associacao Brasileira de Psiquiatria* supplement 8, 30–33.

German, G.A. (1972) 'Aspects of clinical psychiatry in Sub-Saharan Africa', *British Journal of Psychiatry* 121: 461–79.

Goldberg, D.P. (1972) *The Detection of Psychiatric Illness by Questionnaire* (Maudsley Monograph no. 21), London: Oxford University Press.

Goldberg, D.P., Cooper, B., Eastwood, M.R., Kedward, H.B., and Shepherd, M. (1970) 'A standardized psychiatric interview for use in community surveys', *British Journal of Preventive and Social Medicine* 24: 18–23.

Hand, D.J. (1979) *Improving questionnaires for detecting psychiatric morbidity*, unpublished paper, Institute of Psychiatry.

Harding, T.W., Arango, M.V., Baltazar, J., Climent, C.E., Ibrahim, H.H.A., Ignacio, L.L., Murthy, R.S., and Wig, N.N. (1980) 'Mental disorders in primary health care: a study of their frequency and diagnosis in four developing countries', *Psychological Medicine* 10: 231–41.

Harding, T.W., Climent, C.E., Diop, M., Giel, R., Ibrahim, H.H.A., Murthy, R.S., Suleiman, M.A., and Wig, N.N. (1983) 'The WHO collaborative study on strategies for extending mental health care: II: the development of new research methods', *American Journal of Psychiatry* 140: 1474–80.

Hsu, F.L.K. (1971) 'Psychosocial homeostasis and Jen: concepts for advancing psychological anthropology', *American Anthropologist* 73: 23–44.

Hwu, H.G., Yeh, E.K., and Chang, L.Y. (1986) 'Chinese diagnostic interview schedule: I: agreement with psychiatrist's diagnosis', *Acta Psychiatrica Scandinavica* 73: 225–33.

Jenkins, R. (1985) *Sex Differences in Minor Psychiatric Morbidity: Psychological Medicine* (Monograph Supplement 7), Cambridge: Cambridge University Press.

Kapur, R.L., Kapur, M., and Carstairs, G.M. (1974a) 'Indian Psychiatric Survey Schedule: IPSS', *Social Psychiatry* 9: 71–9.

Kapur, R.L., Kapur, M., and Carstairs, G.M. (1974b) 'Indian Psychiatric Survey Schedule: IPSS', *Social Psychiatry* 9: 61–70.

Kleinman, A.M. (1977) 'Depression, somatization and the "New cross-cultural psychiatry"', *Social Science & Medicine* 11: 3–10.

Kleinman, A. (1982) 'Neurasthenia and depression: a study of somatisation and culture in China', *Culture, Medicine, and Psychiatry* 6: 117–89.

Kleinman, A. (1987) 'Anthropology and psychiatry: the role of culture in cross-cultural research on illness', *British Journal of Psychiatry* 151: 447–54.

Leff, J. (1974) 'Transcultural influences on psychiatrists' rating of verbally expressed emotion', *British Journal of Psychiatry* 125: 336–40.

Lin, K.M. (1981) 'Traditional Chinese medical beliefs and their relevance for mental illness and psychiatry', in A. Kleinman and T.Y. Lin (eds) *Normal and Abnormal Behaviour in Chinese Culture*, Dordrecht, Boston, London: Reidel, pp. 95–111.

Lin, T.Y. (1982) 'Culture and psychiatry: a Chinese perspective', *Australian and New Zealand Journal of Psychiatry* 16: 235–45.

Mari, J.J. (1983) 'Psychiatric care in Brazil', in S. Brown (ed.) *Psychiatry in Developing Countries*, London: Gaskell Books.

Mari, J.J. (1987) 'Minor psychiatric morbidity in three primary medical care clinics in the city of Sao Paulo: issues on the mental health of the urban poor', *Social Psychiatry*, 22: 129–138.

Mari, J.J. and Williams, P. (1984) 'Minor psychiatric disorder in primary care in Brazil: a pilot study', *Psychological Medicine* 14: 223–7.

Mari, J.J. and Williams, P. (1985) 'A comparison of the validity of two psychiatric screening questionnaires (GHQ-12 and SRQ-20) in Brazil, using Relative Operating Characteristics (ROC) analysis', *Psychological Medicine* 15: 651–9.

Mari, J.J. and Williams, P. (1986) 'A validity of a psychiatric screening questionnaire (SRQ-20) in primary care in the city of Sao Paulo', *British Journal of Psychiatry* 148: 23–6.

Mari, J.J., Blay, S.L., and Iacoponi, E. (1986) 'Um estudo de confiabilidade da versao brasileira da Clinical Interview Schedule', *Boletim de la Oficina Sanitaria Panamericana* 100 (1): 77–83.

Matthew, R.J., Weinman, M.L., and Mirabi, M. (1981) 'Physical symptoms of depression', *British Journal of Psychiatry* 139: 293–6.

Mehta, P., Joseph, A., and Verghese, A. (1985) 'An epidemiologic study of psychiatric disorders in a rural community in Tamilnadu', *Indian Journal of Psychiatry* 27 (2): 153–8.

Ministry of the Interior (1987) *Taiwan-Fukien Demographic Fact Book*, Taipei.

Murphy, H.B.M. (1982) *Comparative Psychiatry: The International and Intercultural Distribution of Mental Illness*, Berlin: Springer-Verlag.

Nandi, D.N., Mukherjee, S.P., Boral, G.C., Banerjee, G., Ghosh, A., Sarkar, S., and Ajmany, S. (1980) 'Socio-economic status and mental morbidity in certain tribes and castes in India: a cross-cultural study', *British Journal of Psychiatry* 136: 73–85.

Nandi, D.N., Banerjee, G., Saha, H., and Boral, G.C. (1983) 'Epidemic Koro in West Bengal, India', *The International Journal of Social Psychiatry* 83: 265–8.

Nandi, D.N., Saha, H., Banerjee, G., Mukherjee, A., Sarkar, S., Bhattacharya, A., Boral, G.C. (1987) 'An epidemic of "Jhin-Jhini" – a strange contagious disorder – in a village in West Bengal', paper read at the third annual conference of the *Indian Association for Social Psychiatry* in Hyderabad in March 1987.

Obeyesekere, G. (1976) 'The impact of Ayurvedic ideas on the culture and the individual in Sri Lanka', in C. Leslie (ed.) *Asian Medical Systems: A Comparative Study*, Berkeley: University of California Press, 201–26.

Orley, J. and Wing, J.K. (1979) 'Psychiatric disorder in two African villages', *Archives of General Psychiatry* 36: 513–20.

Ribeiro, L. and Campos, M. (1931) *O Espiritismo no Brasil*, Sao Paulo: Companhia Editora Nacional.

Richeport, M. (1984) 'Strategies and outcomes of introducing a mental health plan in Brazil', *Social Science and Medicine* 19: 261–71.

Rin, H. (1965) 'A study of the aetiology of koro in respect of the Chinese concept of illness', *International Journal of Social Psychiatry* 11: 7–13.

Roxo, H.B.B. (1918) 'Delirio Espirita Episodico', in L. Guanabara (ed.) (1946) *Manual de Psiquiatria*, Rio de Janeiro: Livraria Guanabara.

Santana, V. (1978) *Estudo Epidemiologico das Doencas Mentais em um Bairro de Salvador*, M.Sc. thesis, Federal University of Bahia, Salvador.

Sen, B. (1987) 'Psychiatric phenomena in primary health care: their extent and nature', *Indian Journal of Psychiatry* 29 (1): 33–40.

Sen, B. and Mari, J.J. (1986) 'Psychiatric research instruments in the transcultural setting: experiences in India and Brazil', *Social Science & Medicine* 23 (3): 277–81.

Sen, B., Wilkinson, G., and Mari, J.J. (1987) 'Psychiatric morbidity in primary health care: a two-stage screening procedure for developing countries – choice of instruments and cost-effectiveness', *British Journal of Psychiatry* 151: 33–8.

Shamasundar, C., Murthy, K., Prakash, O., Prabhakar, N., and Subba, K.D.K. (1986) 'Psychiatric morbidity in a general practice in an Indian city', *British Medical Journal* 292: 1713–15.

Shepherd, M., Brooke, E.M., and Cooper, J.E. (1968) 'An experimental approach to psychiatric diagnosis', *Acta Psychiatrica Scandinavica*, supplementum 201: 13–26.

Singer, K. (1975) 'Depressive disorders from a transcultural perspective', *Social Science & Medicine* 9: 289–301.

Singh, G. (1985) 'Dhat syndrome revisited', *Indian Journal of Psychiatry* 27 (2): 119–22.

Spitzer, R.L. and Endicott, J. (1966) *Mental Status Schedule*, New York: Department of Psychiatry, Columbia University.

Stainbrook, E. (1952) 'Some characteristics of the schizophrenic behavior in Bahian society', *American Journal of Psychiatry* 109: 330–5.

Teja, J.S., Khanna, S., and Subramanyam, J.B. (1970) '"Possession states" in Indian patients', *Indian Journal of Psychiatry* 12: 71–87.

Tseng, W.S. (1975) 'The nature of somatic complaints among psychiatric patients: the Chinese case', *Comprehensive Psychiatry* 16: 237–45.

Varma, V.K. (1986) 'Cultural psychodynamics and mental illness', *Indian Journal of Psychiatry* 28 (10): 13–34.

Verghese, A., Dube, K.C., Menon, J.J., Menon, M.S., Rajkumar, S., Richard, S., Richard, J., Sethi, B.B., Trivedi, J.K., and Wig, N.N. (1985) 'Factors associated with the course and outcome of schizophrenia: a multi-centred follow up study; Part I: objectives and methodology', *Indian Journal of Psychiatry* 27 (3): 201–6.

Wen, J.K. and Wang, C.L. (1981) 'Shen-K'uei Syndrome: a culture-specific sexual neurosis in Taiwan', in A. Kleinman and T.Y. Lin (eds) *Normal and Abnormal Behaviour in Chinese Culture*, Dordrecht, Boston, London: Reidel, pp. 357–69.

Wig, N.N. (1960) 'Problems of mental health in India', *Journal of Clinical Society*, Medical College, Lucknow, 17: 48–56.

Williams, P., Tarnopolsky, A., and Hand, D.J. (1980) 'Case-definition and case-identification in psychiatric epidemiology: review and reassessment', *Psychological Medicine* 10: 101–14.

Wing, J.K., Cooper, J.E., and Sartorius, N. (1974) *The Measurement and Classification of Psychiatric Symptoms*, Cambridge: Cambridge University Press.

Wing, J.K., Bebbington, R., and Robin, L.N. (1981) (eds) *What is a Case? The Problem of Definition in Psychiatric Community Surveys*, London: Grant McIntyre.

Woodruff, R.A., Murphy, G.E., and Herjanic, M. (1967) 'The natural history of affective disorders; 1: symptoms of 72 patients at the time of index hospital admission', *Journal of Psychiatric Research* 5: 255–63.

World Health Organization (1973) *Report of the International Pilot Study of Schizophrenia, volume 1*, Geneva: WHO.

Yap, P.M. (1965) 'Koro – a culture-bound depersonalisation syndrome', *British Journal of Psychiatry* 111: 43–50.

Yap, P.M. (1965) 'Phenomenology of affective disorder in Chinese and other cultures', in A. Rueck and R. Porter (eds) *Transcultural Psychiatry*, Boston: Little, Brown, & Co.

Section Five

The Scientific Approach to Epidemiological and Social Psychiatry: The Contribution of Michael Shepherd

32

The Contribution of Michael Shepherd

Kenneth Rawnsley

In 1943 John Ryle vacated the Regius Chair of Physic at Cambridge to become the first Professor of Social Medicine in the University of Oxford. Many of his colleagues reacted much as one imagines did those of John Elliotson who, in the early nineteenth century, resigned his position as Professor of Medicine in the University of London to take up Mesmerism. Ryle's standing, however, as a teacher and clinician of the highest calibre, compelled attention to this 'new' subject and focused interest especially on the epidemiology of non-infective disorders. Among those sensitized was Michael Shepherd, then a young medical student in Oxford.

Writing some 35 years later about the training of psychiatrists for research, Shepherd used Ryle's perspective to point the way ahead. After commenting on the agonizing reappraisal within medicine of the pre-eminence of biotechnology and the increasing awareness even among the arch representatives of that approach of the importance of social factors, he says:

> At the core of Ryle's position was his defence of the clinician as an observer, a naturalist with an essentially holistic view of man in disease, for whom scrupulous clinical inquiry is as much a scientific procedure as any other measure of research. Here may be found a key to the dilemma of clinical research in psychiatry. A determined attack on the lacunae in knowledge relating to the clinical epidemiology of mental disorders would help bridge the gap between clinical and basic research casting clinicians in a more substantial role than that of medically qualified entrepreneurs or laboratory ancillaries.　　　　　　　　　　　　(Shepherd 1981a)

In the early 1950s, during his apprenticeship to psychiatry at the Maudsley Hospital, Shepherd's interest in the social aspects of mental illness was stimulated and nurtured by the commanding presence of Professor Aubrey Lewis, his illustrious mentor. Lewis combined a rare clinical expertise with a profound interest in many of the sciences cognate to psychiatry, not least those in the social and epidemiological sphere (Shepherd 1980).

Psychiatry in Britain during the first half of the 1950s was beginning to tingle. The new psychotropic drugs had not yet entered the arena but a few pioneers were setting in train the 'open door' policies in mental hospitals which would revolutionize practice. Others were exploring new ways of helping patients with disordered characters and were raising the curtain on the 'therapeutic community' movement. Psychotherapy was breaking new ground, for example in the use of 'group' approaches. Lysergic acid diethylamide was to be the key to the understanding of the chemistry of endogenous psychoses.

Lewis filled the Maudsley with a rich and varied assortment of senior psychiatrists representing the many facets of this diverse and rapidly growing branch of medicine. The young post-graduate doctors were often hard put to it to find their bearings in this bewildering broth and many responded to the siren call from some dogmatic safe haven, be it psychoanalytic or organic in timbre.

In the midst of this clamour, Shepherd was quietly getting on with some epidemiological spade-work in a study of the pattern of major psychoses hospitalized in the county of Buckinghamshire during two periods 1931–3 and 1945–7. This material was to form the basis of his DM thesis and was published as a Maudsley Monograph (Shepherd 1957). Basically, it was an exercise in counting declared cases from a defined catchment area. The use of the results to illuminate the impact of changing styles of patient management and of specific treatments will be mentioned later in this paper.

At about the same time he was collecting material of a very different stamp, culled from his own clinical practice and from that of colleagues, which was to form the basis of an important contribution to the literature on morbid jealousy (Shepherd 1961). The subtitle of the paper is significant, 'Some clinical and social aspects of a psychiatric symptom'. His analysis of the complex interweaving of these two inseparable elements in the disorder provide a pointer to the development of his theoretical thinking in clinical epidemiology.

Not that he distanced himself or retired from the intellectual market-place of the Maudsley. His approach was that of the acutely interested sceptic, possessed of a zealous, burning curiosity, endlessly questing, requiring evidence of validity beyond mere assertion, scraping down to the bedrock of truth through the detritus of speculation.

Studies of the frequency of mental disorders based on counting cases entering psychiatric hospitals had been pursued for over a century but the limitations of these materials weighed increasingly with epidemiologists. The undeclared, submerged part of the clinical iceberg became an object of study in a number of large-scale population surveys in many parts of the world, though the theoretical and practical problems of defining boundaries between the ice and the surrounding water were manifold.

Moving beyond his studies of mental hospital populations, Shepherd very

510

shrewdly chose a middle ground which, to a degree, avoided the formidable problems of method attending case definition in straight general population sample surveys. In Britain, most people are registered with a general practitioner in the National Health Service and the majority of the population actually consult their doctors at least once in the course of a year. Here, then, was a laboratory in which psychiatric morbidity could be studied from a variety of angles and with a very practical flavour to the findings. The small beginnings of this work were given a fine boost in 1958 through a grant from the Nuffield Foundation, allowing the establishment of a research unit which still exists, though funded from other sources. The work of the first few years was collated and published in book form in 1966. In his foreword to the volume Aubrey Lewis neatly summarizes the intention and the product:

> The study has been conducted with a close regard to the many problems of method involved. It was exploratory in design, as the nature of the problem required; a survey of this kind helps to provide the baseline from which future controlled studies may be carried out and hypotheses tested. It is not surprising that the present findings pose as many questions as they answer. The authors do not pretend otherwise; they are content to have been employed, in Locke's words, 'in clearing the ground a little, and removing some of the rubbish that lies in the way of knowledge'.
>
> (Shepherd *et al.* 1966)

This characteristically low-key summing up of achievement by Lewis should not deflect attention from the substantive results of this large-scale work. The pooled inception rate for a period of one year was fifty-two per 1,000 which placed psychiatric illness among the commoner causes of consultation in general practice. The distribution by diagnosis was sharply different from that found in hospital patients, neuroses and psychophysiological disorders predominating.

One finding of great interest was that, during the survey year, of the identified psychiatric cases only one in twenty had been under specialist care. It was noted that the treatment of minor psychiatric disorders in general practice is often haphazard and inadequate. Despite this, practitioners regarded the management of these conditions as an integral part of their work but wished for better training to deal more effectively with them. An important conclusion follows:

> Administrative and medical logic alike therefore suggest that the . . . cardinal requirement for improvement of the mental health services . . . in this country is not a large expansion and proliferation of . . . psychiatric agencies, but rather a strengthening of the family . . . doctor in his therapeutic role. (Shepherd *et al.* 1966)

511

From the small beginnings of this epidemiological work in the field of primary care an enduring framework of operations had been rapidly created. A base was firmly established at the Institute of Psychiatry of the University of London situated at the Maudsley Hospital. Very fundamental questions were being asked about psychiatric morbidity and ways in which answers might be obtained were being carefully explored. Resources were building up, and among these the most important of all was the recruitment of a cadre of investigators which, over the years, was to include individuals of the highest calibre, many of whom went on to occupy senior academic posts in Britain and abroad.

A *tour d'horizon* was provided in 1979 by two of these collaborators in a book entitled *Psychosocial Disorders in General Practice* (Williams and Clare 1979). Many of the papers brought together in that volume had been written by members of the Shepherd Unit and provide some notion of the wide field of endeavour which had been cultivated during the previous two decades. The evolution of standard reproducible measures of psychiatric morbidity and of social adjustment are a basic feature of the whole undertaking and certain of the instruments devised are now used throughout the world.

In the primary care laboratory, grounded upon the trust and good will developing between participating GPs and researchers, together with sound and acceptable methodology, new and important questions were now addressed. What is the link between onset of neurotic illness and life events? How frequently are psychotropic drugs prescribed in general practice and what are the consequences of this? What is the optimum division of labour between the GP and the psychiatrist? What is the most effective and appropriate pattern of working relationship between doctors and para-medical workers in the extramural setting?

Population surveys in many parts of the world, using representative samples, had revealed a large pool of psychiatric morbidity of which only a fraction was ever brought to medical attention. Workers from the General Practice Unit were able to throw some light on the factors which influenced decisions to consult a general practitioner, through secondary analysis of data originally assembled by Unit colleagues to study the possible effects of aircraft noise on mental health. This West London material was drawn from the largest general population psychiatric survey mounted to date in Britain. It revealed that about one-fifth of GP consultations could be attributed to minor psychiatric morbidity and that the presence of such morbidity doubles the probability of consulting. Health-related factors appeared to exert more influence on decisions to consult than did socio-demographic variables (Williams *et al.* 1986).

Introducing a recent conference on 'Mental Illness in Primary Care Settings' held at the Institute of Psychiatry, the Chief Medical Officer for England and Wales made the comment,

Within the structure of the National Health Service, the medical responsibility for the care of these [psychiatric] patients falls principally on the general practitioner. Much of what we know about the nature and extent of their disorders derives from the work of Michael Shepherd and his colleagues in the distinguished General Practice Research Unit.

(Acheson 1986)

In 1964 a World Health Organization Scientific Group on Mental Health Research called for (a) development of a Classification of Mental Disorders internationally acceptable and capable of uniform application and (b) development of standardized procedures for case-finding and for the assessment of severity of illness.

This was followed in 1965 by a WHO seminar held in London on 'Standardization of Psychiatric Diagnosis, Classification and Mental Health Statistics' in which Shepherd played a leading role. An experimental approach to the problem of observer variation in diagnosis was applied by the use of written case vignettes and also by the exhibition of video recordings of samples of psychiatric interviews. The fact that the expert doctors present differed in their diagnoses is perhaps not surprising to anyone familiar with the cut and thrust of psychiatric case conferences but a dissection of the basis of these differences, succinctly presented in the conclusions to the Report, pointed to future hopes of refinement.

The factors which lead to disagreements and difficulties of . . . communication can be regarded as deriving from three principal . . . sources. These comprise, first, variations at the level of observation and perception by the clinician; secondly, variations . . . in the inferences drawn from such observation; and, thirdly, variation in the nosological schemata employed by the individual clinicians. These sources of variation are open to investigation. (Shepherd *et al.* 1968)

The WHO chariot of fire thus launched was set to roll for a decade ahead pursuing four linked programmes of enquiry. It was hoped that these programmes would, first, illuminate the ninth revision of ICD due in 1975; second, test the applicability of definition and criteria agreed for a particular disease in different countries of contrasting cultures and differing schools of psychiatry: the International Pilot Study of Schizophrenia (WHO 1979) was the vehicle for this endeavour. The other two programmes were to result in comprehensive epidemiological study of geographically defined populations and also in the education of research scientists to embark on work of this nature through training courses and workshops, to which Shepherd made a particular contribution (Shepherd 1982a).

The products of all this labour were indeed fed into the revision process which culminated in Section 5 of ICD-9. They also contributed to the

513

updating of the remarkable glossary of diagnostic terms published in 1974 which owed much in its original form to Sir Aubrey Lewis. This set of definition/descriptions of the categories in Section 5 was a major landmark in the attempt to bring some measure of uniformity to the usage of diagnostic categories, vital for comparative epidemiology.

Paradoxically, the evolution of a successful and reliable classification applicable to the variety of psychiatric problems common in Shepherd's field of primary care has proved elusive to date (Shepherd 1987). The ICD itself has serious limitations in this arena and this led in 1979 to the development of the special International Classification of Health Problems in Primary Care (ICHPPC) (Froom 1976; WONCA 1979). An experimental examination of the reliability of this system by Shepherd and colleagues (Jenkins *et al.* 1985) revealed a high level of observer variation – a disappointing lacuna which awaits further research.

One of the uses of epidemiology is in deepening knowledge of the clinical progress and outcome of particular categories of illness and the work of Shepherd's General Practice Unit in the field of neurosis has already been mentioned. Working with other colleagues, he turned his attention in 1980 to a follow-up study of a group of schizophrenics studied earlier by him for another purpose (Watt *et al.* 1983). They comprised a cohort of patients from the county of Buckinghamshire, being all the individuals from that area fulfilling strict clinical criteria admitted to the local psychiatric hospital over a twenty-month period in 1973–4. A very careful follow-up investigation after five years revealed a good outcome in about half the patients. Females fared significantly better than did males.

The hallmarks of this study were the rigorous clinical definition of the cohort; its representative character within the defined catchment population; the thoroughness of the follow-up and the conclusion that in the evaluation of treatment, knowledge of the expected outcome from a representative sample of cases must form an important backdrop.

These patients had originally been investigated in a comparative controlled drug trial of pimozide versus fluphenazine decanoate (Falloon *et al.* 1978a, 1978b). Shepherd always emphasized the epidemiological nature of drug trials.

> the comparative trial is essentially an epidemiological procedure and reflects the outlook of the statistician, who inevitably tends to think less as a physician and more as a metaphysician, specializing therefore in the description of the types of proof which are appropriate to various types of statement. (Shepherd 1959)

He regarded such trials as of fundamental importance in the evaluation and refinement of treatment, provided they were intelligently constructed and properly applied (Shepherd 1970).

In the field of childhood psychiatric disorders Shepherd used an epidemiological approach to address certain questions: how is deviant behaviour in childhood to be conceptualized, identified, and measured? What is the relationship between deviant behaviour and morbidity? What are the influences which determine whether particular 'cases' come within the ambit of services? What are the benefits, if any, of referral to the specialist? (Shepherd *et al.* 1971).

Epidemiological studies of many common ailments in medicine have shown that for every case attending medical services there are many more untreated in the community. The findings of the child study in Buckinghamshire, based upon a random sample of over 6,000 children aged 5–15, were no exception to this rule. Attempts made to discover factors leading to specialist referral pointed the finger at characteristics of parents rather than at the children themselves:

> Thus, the mothers of children attending child-guidance tended to . . . be more anxious, depressed and . . . easily upset by stress. Still more significantly, they were less able to manage their children's . . . disturbances of behaviour and accept them as temporary . . . difficulties; at the same time they were more liable to discuss their problems with and seek advice from other people. (Shepherd 1971)

This conclusion was based on a critical comparison of fifty children attending child-guidance clinics in the county and fifty children with similar levels of disturbance not so attending.

Naturally enough, the question arose as to how these two groups of children fared over time; in effect an evaluation of the therapeutic influence of clinic contact. Two years after the initial appraisal there was found to be no significant difference in the progress of the two groups. In both about two-thirds of the children manifested evidence of improvement.

The importance of this essay into the realm of childhood disorders lies, first, in the clear exposition of the criteria employed for measuring 'deviance' and in the explicit correlation of deviance with functional disturbance; second, in the scrutiny of factors which appear to bring a particular child to the specialist service; third, in the assessment of the results of specialist intervention in terms of outcome after two years. The study follows good epidemiologic precepts in the unambiguous definition of numerators and denominators and in the utilization of findings to illuminate questions concerning the effectiveness and efficiency of services.

A further contribution to child psychiatry was the publication, following a pioneering exercise, of the first tri-axial system of classification of mental disorders of childhood by the World Health Organization (Rutter *et al.* 1975).

In the scientific study of drugs, clinical and experimental approaches spring to mind as the traditional methods. In compiling what was, in fact, the first textbook of clinical psychopharmacology Shepherd and his colleagues also inserted the epidemiological approach as a third methodology (Shepherd *et al.* 1968). The social angle on psychotropic drug use was discussed in more detail in a later monograph (Shepherd 1981b).

Reference is made in that book to a retrospective study which Shepherd mounted drawing on material from the survey of mental hospital patients in Buckinghamshire already mentioned (Shepherd 1957) when the movement of patients over a four-year period from 1954–57 was scrutinized. 1954 was the year prior to the introduction of the new psychotropic drugs and by 1957 they were in common use:

> The results of a study of this type, depend on detailed . . . statistical analysis and they showed that very little change . . . had occurred during this period. The major movement of the hospital population, defined in terms of a higher discharge . . . rate and shorter hospital stay, had in fact taken place ten . . . years earlier and was attributable partly to the somatic treatments of the day but much more to the setting up of an . . . unusually progressive mental health service in the area.   (Shepherd 1981c)

Similar findings were reported from Norway by Ødegaard who commented:

> in hospitals with a favourable situation the psychotropic . . . drugs brought little or no improvement or even a decrease in . . . the rate of discharges. In hospitals with a low pre-drug discharge rate, on the other hand, the improvement was considerable.   (Ødegaard 1964)

In his Maudsley Bequest lecture (1978) Shepherd set out very clearly the wide-ranging importance of epidemiology, not only as a discipline in its own right but as the fundamental basis of clinical psychiatry. The transmission of mental disorder in populations and indeed in families by the process of psychic contagion affecting vulnerable individuals exemplifies the lay concept of 'epidemic'. However, the epidemiologist may contribute to a deeper understanding of the phenomena of illness:

> We now know from epidemiological inquiries that psychiatric illness in the community is composed largely of minor affective disorders. From a clinical standpoint it is apparent that this large pool of affective illnesses not only extends the spectrum of the concept of such disorders but also bears pointedly on the aetiology of these illnesses and on the sterility of much work on their classification based on hospital cases.
>
> (Shepherd 1978)

Shepherd had many dealings with the British Medical Research Council and in the course of these was able occasionally to bring psychiatry into play

516

as a facilitator of research in other medical fields. An example arises in the large-scale MRC trial in the screening and prophylaxis of mild to moderate hypertension. Concern had been expressed about the possible adverse effects of discovering hypertension in subjects and in 'labelling' them. Shepherd was consulted and promoted a trial carried out by Dr A.H. Mann which showed not only that the labelling was innocuous but that it led to an improvement in the emotional state of certain subjects (Mann 1984).

Michael Shepherd is known as an outstanding clinician, a man to whom colleagues will confidently refer difficult and problematic cases for second opinion. As a practising doctor, he brings to bear not only his profound knowledge of psychiatric theory but also those vaguer skills and propensities which inform the clinical art. His attitude, however, to the future of psychiatry is crystal clear: that, for survival, it must rest ever more firmly upon scientific foundations. This view is manifest insistently in his personal teaching, in his professional writings, and in his discussions both public and private.

It has found trenchant expression many a time in a merciless commentary on all unsubstantiated vapourings, whether these spring from psychoanalysis or from the purveyors of psychotropic drugs. He has, on occasion, an arrestingly mordant style of delivery, whether spoken or written, honed to perfection over the years, which is a scourge to the woolly-minded or the pretentious. Like Sherlock Holmes, a character whose name he recently linked in terms of styles of thought with that of Sigmund Freud (Shepherd 1985), he has a disconcerting ability to materialize from the shadows and to deliver a decisive body-blow, but one springing from a sounder basis than the strange inductions of the legendary detective.

It led him to establish in 1969 what has become a prestigious international journal *Psychological Medicine*, subtitled 'A journal for research in psychiatry and the allied sciences' and which he continues to edit. Describing the setting up of this publication in the course of his Presidential address to the Section of Psychiatry of the Royal Society of Medicine, he remarks:

> Our initial task was to tackle three questions – namely the . . . colour of the dust-jacket, an agreement on objectives, and a . . . title. The first was easily resolved: since nothing in psychiatry is black or white, grey was evidently the colour . . . of choice. With regard to objectives, we had thought . . . originally of aiming at the education of professors in psychiatry but their halo of omniscience appeared to be . . . impenetrable, so we settled for the goal of indispensability . . . by determining to concentrate on original, high-quality work across the wide spectrum of both psychiatry and its allied disciplines. In so doing we were virtually compelled to resurrect Winslow's title [Forbes Winslow's *Journal of Psychological Medicine and Mental Pathology*, the first British journal to be concerned exclusively with mental illness, which had appeared in 1848]. (Shepherd 1986b)

The arrangement of the five volumes of his monumental *Handbook of Psychiatry* is significant (Shepherd 1982b). The middle three volumes, devoted to the clinical manifestations of psychiatric illness, are sandwiched between volume 1 on 'General Psychopathology' and volume 5 on 'The Scientific Foundations of Psychiatry'. Furthermore, Shepherd reveals his catholic approach to the proper limits of science in relation to psychiatry; in the introduction of volume 1, he implicitly supports Karl Jaspers:

> Inveighing against the futility of 'endlessness', the attempt to establish absolute knowledge through the application of any one scientific discipline, he [Jaspers] urges the psychiatrist to 'acquire some of the view-points and methods that belong to the world of the Humanities and Social Studies . . . since the methods of almost all the Arts and Sciences converge on psychopathology' (Jaspers 1963). With this ambiguous phrase Jaspers indicates the complex nature of a discipline which, in his view, extended the notion of scientific enquiry as it is usually understood.
>
> (Shepherd 1982b)

This chapter has concerned itself principally with Shepherd's epidemiological and social psychiatric interests and it is for his contributions in this domain that he is best known. It has led to high professional recognition in the presentation of the Donald Reid Medal for Epidemiology in 1982 and the Lapousse Award of the American Public Health Association in 1983. He has laboured steadily in a number of other psychiatric vineyards producing intellectual wine of superb vintage but amazing in its diversity.

What is perhaps less well recognized, however, is that he has also made indirect contributions to other scientific disciplines. One example is statistics. Three of the statisticians appointed to Shepherd's General Practice Research Unit when they were young became, in time, full professors of statistics and leaders in their own fields. While indicating Shepherd's skill in selecting able people, it also underlines his recognition of the growing importance of quantitative methods in psychiatric research and of the need for close collaborative work. Further instances may be cited in his co-directorship of a psychopharmacological research group with Professor Heinz Schild of University College, London; also in his involvement with, and influence upon, professional historians manifest in the volumes, *Anatomy of Madness, Essays in the History of Psychiatry* (Bynum *et al.* 1985).

Shepherd described the career, contributions, and legacies of Sir Aubrey, his great mentor, in the Adolf Meyer Lecture and in the ninth Aubrey Lewis Lecture, later combining these papers within a single cover (Shepherd 1986a). He quotes Lewis on Edward Mapother, the first Professor of Psychiatry at the Maudsley, and observes that Lewis might have been writing a self-description. To carry the argument on to the third generation and adding a few more sentences from Lewis's encomium (Lewis 1969) the pen portrait would supply a fine likeness for the subject of this Festschrift:

> He was intensely distrustful of anything that seemed to him humbug, and he disliked sentimentality almost as much. Anything that savoured of professional commercialism was likewise anathema. His own integrity was beyond question in small matters as well as large ones. He insisted on strict, at times austere, standards of clinical probity. His intellect was sharp and shrewd, with a touch of legal inquisition, and at its best when examining a complex issue or – in a very different way – making the case for some Maudsley need. His wit served as an astringent partner to his zest for controversy. . . . Fundamentally the temper of his mind was partisan, in the good sense; he was not serene and detached, but eager, pertinacious, argumentative, scathing in criticism and powerful in reasoned support. With all his enjoyment of swordplay and iconoclasm, he remained hopeful and positive, by no means a cynic.

Michael Shepherd will, hopefully, remain with us for years to come, continuing to persuade, cajole, nay demand, that while practising our art we base it increasingly and relentlessly on scientific research findings, thereby ensuring the future viability of our subject and the better care of our patients.

REFERENCES

Acheson, E.D. (1986) 'Introduction', in M. Shepherd, G. Wilkinson and P. Williams (eds) *Mental Illness in Primary Care Settings*, London: Tavistock.

Bynum, W.F., Porter, R., and Shepherd, M. (eds) (1985) *The Anatomy of Madness, Essays in the History of Psychiatry*, two volumes, London: Tavistock.

Falloon, I., Watt, D.C., and Shepherd, M. (1978a) 'A comparative controlled trial of pimozide and fluphenazine decanoate in the continuation therapy of schizophrenia', *Psychological Medicine* 8: 59–70.

Falloon, I., Watt, D.C., and Shepherd, M. (1978b) 'The social outcome of patients in a trial of long-term continuation therapy in schizophrenia: pimozide vs fluphenazine', *Psychological Medicine* 8: 265–74.

Froom, J. (1976) 'The international classification of health problems in primary care', *Medical Care* 14: 450–4.

Jaspers, K. (1963) *General Psychopathology*, seventh edition, translated by J. Hoenig and M. Hamilton, Manchester: Manchester University Press.

Jenkins, R., Smeeton, N., Marinker, M., and Shepherd, M. (1985) 'A study of the classification of mental ill-health in general practice', *Psychological Medicine* 15: 403–9.

Lewis, A. (1969) 'Edward Mapother and the making of the Maudsley Hospital', *British Journal of Psychiatry*, 115: 1349–66.

Mann, A.H. (1984) *Hypertension: Psychological Aspects and Diagnostic Impact in a Clinical Trial* (Psychological Medicine Monograph Supplement No. 5) Cambridge: Cambridge University Press.

Ødegaard, Ø. (1964) 'Pattern of discharge from Norwegian psychiatric hospitals before and after the introduction of the psychotropic drugs', *American Journal of Psychiatry* 120: 772–8.

Rutter, M., Shaffer, D., and Shepherd, M. (1975) *A Multi-axial Classification of Child Psychiatric Disorders*, Geneva: WHO.

Shepherd, M. (1957) *A Study of the Major Psychoses in an English County* (Maudsley Monograph Series No. 3) London: Chapman and Hall.

Shepherd, M. (1959) 'Evaluation of drugs in the treatment of depression', *Canadian Psychiatric Association Journal* Supplement 4: S120.

Shepherd, M. (1961) 'Morbid jealousy: some clinical and social aspects of a psychiatric symptom', *Journal of Mental Science* 107: 687–753.

Shepherd, M. (1970) 'A critical review of clinical drug trials', *Excerpta Medica International Congress Series No. 239 Depression in the 1970s. Proceedings of a Symposium.* New York.

Shepherd, M. (1971) 'Childhood behaviour, mental health and medical services', in G. McLachlan (ed.) *Problems and Progress in Medical Care*, Oxford: Nuffield Provincial Hospitals Trust, Oxford University Press.

Shepherd, M. (1978) 'Epidemiology and clinical psychiatry', *British Journal of Psychiatry* 133: 289–98.

Shepherd, M. (1980) 'From social medicine to social psychiatry: the achievement of Sir Aubrey Lewis', *Psychological Medicine* 10: 211–18.

Shepherd, M. (1981a) 'Psychiatric research in medical perspective', *British Medical Journal* 282: 961–3.

Shepherd, M. (1981b) *Psychotropic Drugs in Psychiatry*, New York: Jason Aronson.

Shepherd, M. (1981c) 'The epidemiological impact of psychotropic medication', in G. Tognoni, C. Bellantuono, and M. Lader (eds) *Epidemiological Impact of Psychotropic Drugs*, Elsevier/North-Holland Biomedical Press.

Shepherd, M. (1982a) 'The application of the epidemiological method in psychiatry', in T.A. Baasher, J.E. Cooper, H. Davidian, A. Jablensky, N. Sartorius, and E. Strömgren (eds) *Acta Psychiatrica Scandinavica*, Supplement 296, volume 65, Copenhagen: Munksgaard.

Shepherd, M. (1982b) *Handbook of Psychiatry Volume 1: General Psychopathology*, Cambridge: Cambridge University Press

Shepherd, M. (1983) *The Psychosocial Matrix of Psychiatry: Collected Papers*, London: Tavistock.

Shepherd, M. (1985) *Sherlock Holmes and the Case of Dr Freud*, London: Tavistock.

Shepherd, M. (1986a) *A Representative Psychiatrist: the Career, Contributions and Legacies of Sir Aubrey Lewis* (Psychological Medicine Monograph Supplement 10) Cambridge: Cambridge University Press.

Shepherd, M. (1986b) 'Psychological medicine redivivus: concept and communication', *Journal of the Royal Society of Medicine* 79: 639–45.

Shepherd, M. (1987) 'Classification of mental disorders', *Practitioner* 231: 985.

Shepherd, M., Brooke, E.M., Cooper, J.E., and Lin, T. (1968) *An Experimental Approach to Psychiatric Diagnosis*, Acta Psychiatrica Scandinavica Supplement 201, Copenhagen: Munksgaard.

Shepherd, M., Cooper, B., Brown, A.C., and Kalton, G.W. (1966) *Psychiatric Illness in General Practice*, (1981) Second edition (additional material jointly with A.W. Clare), London: Oxford University Press.

Shepherd, M., Lader, M.H., and Rodnight, R. (1968) *Clinical Psychopharmacology*, London: English Universities Press.

Shepherd, M., Oppenheim, A.N., and Mitchell, S. (1971) *Childhood Behaviour and Mental Health*, London: University Press.

Watt, D.C., Katz, K., and Shepherd, M. (1983) 'The natural history of schizophrenia: a 5-year prospective follow-up of a representative sample of schizophrenics by means of a standardised clinical and social assessment', *Psychological Medicine* 13: 663–70.

Williams, P. and Clare, A. (1979) *Psychosocial Disorders in General Practice*, London: Academic Press.

Williams, P. Tarnopolsky, A., Hand, D., and Shepherd, M. (1986) *Minor Psychiatric Morbidity and General Practice Consultations: the West London Survey* (Psychological Medicine Monograph Supplement 9), Cambridge: Cambridge University Press.

WONCA (World Organization of National Colleges, Academies and Academic Associations of General Practitioners/Family Physicians) *International Classification of Health Problems in Primary Care* (1979 Revision) (ICHPPC-2), Oxford: Oxford University Press.

World Health Organization (1979) *Schizophrenia: An International Follow-up Study*, Chichester: Wiley.

Name Index

Abrams, Philip, 38
Acheson, E.D., 388, 513
Adelstein, A.M., 174, 267
Akesson, H.O., 267
Akinsola, H.A., 229
Albee, G., 231
Alexander, J., 199–202
Allgulander, C., 281
Allport, G.W., 199
Almeida-Filho, N., 495
Alvear, J., 252–3
Amaducci, L.A., 270–1, 273–5
Ananth, J., 288
Anderson, J.R., 198, 206
Anderson, Olive, 29–30
Anderson, R., 66
Andrews, G., 214
Angst, J., 189, 191
Anthony, J., 105, 111
Appleby, L.A., 201
Asberg, M., 350
Ashford, J.R., 168–9
Ashton, H., 330
Asperger, H., 231
Asscher, A.W., 314
Aubrée, J.C., 316
Ausland, O.G., 109
Avorn, J., 326
Axelrod, Julius, 472
Ayd, F.J., 313

Baastrup, P.C., 480
Babb, L., 152
Bachrach, L.L., 387
Bacon, Francis, 436
Baert, A.E., 160
Bagadia, V.N., 495
Baillargeon, J.G., 111
Baines, M.J., 252
Bakwin, H., 245
Balestrieri, M., 394, 397, 415
Balint, E., 413
Balint, Michael, 413
Ball, M.J., 275
Ballinger, B.R., 204
Ballinger, C.B., 294–5, 410
Baltimore, David, 436
Bamborough, J.B., 154
Bandura, A., 198
Barker, D.J.P., 56
Barre-Sinoussi, F., 437
Bartholomaeus Anglicus, 149–50
Bash, K.W. and Bash-Liechti, J., 291

Bayle, Pierre, 20
Bebbington, P., 55, 291
Beck, A.T., 200, 347, 350
Beiser, M., 500–1
Bellantuono, C., 123, 332
Belloc, N.B., 333
Beloff, J., 53
Bergen, S., 250
Bergin, A.E., 345
Bergmann, K., 267, 270, 279
Berkey, C.S., 250
Bernstein, B.B., 60
Berridge, V., 328
Berrueta-Clement, J.R., 443
Besson, J., 282
Best, D.L., 297
Bharucha, N.E., 270
Bickel, H., 267, 269, 276–9
Bielicki, T., 242, 244
Birley, J.L.T., 232, 343, 355
Bishop, Y.M.M., 129
Black, A.E., 251
Blackburn, I.M., 425
Blacker, C.V.R., 214, 412, 425
Blackwell, B., 168, 213, 313, 331, 404,
    406, 480
Blazer, D., 478
Bleuler, Eugen, 26, 461
Bleuler, Manfred, 161, 233
Block, J., 299
Blomfield, J.M., 247
Boardman, A.P., 408
Bodmer, Sir Walter, 439
Bøjholm, S., 164
Boldsen, J.L., 244
Booth, A., 298
Booth, W., 441
Bowen, B.A., 414
Bower, E., 231
Bowlby, J., 55
Boyd, J.H., 190–1, 229
Brenner, B., 82–3
Bridges, K.W., 110, 121, 123, 213, 404
Briscoe, Monica E., xiii, 11, 53–60, 299,
    414
Brody, E., 490, 498
Brook, A., 415
Brooke, E.M., 87
Broverman, L., 299
Brown, G.W., 45, 55, 207, 232–2, 298,
    343, 355, 362, 381, 383–4, 409
Brown, R., 59
Brown, R.M.A., 426, 429

522

527

Subject Index